Navy

Hospital Corpsman

NAVEDTRA 14295
Following the Model for Military Education

Navy
Hospital Corpsman

NAVEDTRA 14295
Following the Model for Military Education

Navy Hospital Corpsman: NAVEDTRA 14295 Following the Model for Military Education

Copyright © 2004 by Integrated Development, LLC, Copyright © 2010 by PharmaLogika, Inc.

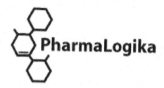

PharmaLogika, Inc.
PO Box 461
Willow Springs, NC 27592

www.pharmalogika.com

Author / Editor: Mindy J. Allport-Settle

Published by PharmaLogika, Inc.

Printed in the United States of America. First Printing.

ISBN-13 978-0-9821476-9-6

Contents

Advancement Handbook for Hospital Corpsman
HM3, HM2, HM1, HMC...591

Overview and Orientation

About this Book

The United States Navy Hospital Corpsman training program has long been the standard used as the pinnacle of training achievement for medical professionals. The program builds a broad foundation that enables hospital corpsman to act independently in the field to preserve the health and safety of the public and their crew mates. This manual has been continuously tested and updated to successfully educate every hospital corpsman of the United States Navy since its inception. The needs of the instructor, the student, the patient, and the Navy are perfectly balanced. This is the model all educators should follow when developing training programs.

This book provides an example of how training materials should be designed for any adult education training program, but especially for any industry that is subject to government regulation. In addition to the Hospital Corpsman manual, the Hospital Corpsman Advancement Handbook has also been included as an example of a properly designed long-term training curriculum.

Included Documents and Features

Hospital Corpsman (NAVEDTRA 14295)

United States Navy Hospital Corpsman

A Hospital Corpsman (HM) is frequently the only medical care-giver available in many fleet or Marine units on extended deployment. Hospital Corpsmen serve as enlisted medical specialists for the United States Navy and the United States Marine Corps. The Hospital Corpsman works in a wide variety of capacities and locations, including shore establishments such as naval hospitals and clinics, aboard ships, as the primary medical caregivers for sailors while underway. Hospital Corpsman perform duties as assistants in the prevention and treatment of disease and injury and assist health care professionals in providing medical care to Navy people and their families. They may function as clinical or specialty technicians, medical administrative personnel and health care providers at medical treatment facilities. They also serve as battlefield corpsmen with the Marine Corps, rendering emergency medical treatment to include initial treatment in a combat environment. Qualified hospital corpsmen may be assigned the responsibility of independent duty aboard ships and submarines; Fleet Marine Force, Special Forces and Seabee units, and at isolated duty stations where no medical officer is available.

The colloquial form of address for a Hospital Corpsman is "Doc." In the U.S. Marine Corps, this term is generally used as a sign of respect.

Organization

Because of the need for Hospital Corpsmen in a vast array of foreign, domestic, and shipboard duty stations, as well as with United States Marine Corps units, the Hospital Corps is the largest rating in the United States Navy.

The basic training for Hospital Corpsmen is Naval Hospital Corps School, located in Great Lakes, IL, one of the Navy's "A" schools (primary rating training). Upon graduation, the Hospital Corpsman is given the Navy Enlisted Classification (NEC) code of HM-0000, or "quad-zero" in common usage. NECs are analogous to MOS in the United States Army and Marine Corps, or AFSC in the Air Force. There are primary NECs, and secondary NECs. For example, a Hospital Corpsman who completes Field Medical Training Battalion (FMTB) and earns the NEC HM-8404, moves that NEC to primary and has a secondary NEC of HM-0000. If that Hospital Corpsman attends a "C" School, then the NEC earned at the "C" School becomes their primary and HM-8404 becomes the secondary. Some Hospital Corpsmen go on to receive more specialized training in roles such as Medical Laboratory Technician, Radiology Technician, Aviation/Aerospace Medicine Specialist, Pharmacy Technician, Operating Room Technician, etcetera. This advanced education is done through "C" schools, which confer additional NECs. Additionally, Hospital Corpsmen E-5 and above may attend Surface Force Independent Duty training, qualifying for independent duty in surface ships and submarines, with diving teams, and Fleet Marine Force Recon teams, as well as at remote shore installations. In addition to advanced medical training, these Hospital Corpsmen receive qualification in sanitation and public health.

Hospital Corpsmen who have received the warfare designator of Enlisted Fleet Marine Force Warfare Specialist are highly trained members of the Hospital Corps who specialize in all aspects of working with the United States Marine Corps operating forces. Attainment of this designation is highly prized among all Corpsmen. The Enlisted Fleet Marine Force Warfare designation for Hospital Corpsmen is the only US Navy warfare device awarded solely by a US Marine Corps General Officer. This awarding authority cannot be delegated to US Navy Officers. However, obtaining the title of "FMF" is a rigorous procedure and not every Hospital Corpsman who has been with a Marine Corps unit will wear the FMF warfare device. U.S. Navy officers in the medical community(Medical Corps (Doctor), Nurse Corps, Dental Corps) can earn and wear the officer equivalent to this insignia. Additionally any sailor attached to a Marine unit can earn and wear an FMF warfare device. (Example, administrative rates such as Logistic Specialists).

The first Physician Assistants were selected from Navy Corpsmen who had combat experience in Vietnam. The Navy trained its own Physician Assistants drawing from the ranks of qualified Independent Duty Hospital Corpsmen at the Naval School of Health Sciences in Portmouth, VA until 1985, then at San Diego, CA. Navy Hospital

Corpsmen are also represented in many medical disciplines, as Physicians, Nurses, Medical Administrators and other walks of life.

Be they assigned to hospital ships, reservist installations, recruiter offices, or Marine Corps combat units, the rating of Hospital Corpsman is the most decorated in the United States Navy with 22 Medals of Honor, 174 Navy Crosses, 31 Distinguished Service Medals, 946 Silver Stars, and 1,582 Bronze Stars.[1] There have been 20 naval ships that have been named after hospital corpsmen.

Hospital Corpsman Pledge

"I solemnly pledge myself before God and these witnesses to practice faithfully all of my duties as a member of the Hospital Corps. I hold the care of the sick and injured to be a privilege and a sacred trust and will assist the Medical Officer with loyalty and honesty. I will not knowingly permit harm to come to any patient. I will not partake of nor administer any unauthorized medication. I will hold all personal matters pertaining to the private lives of patients in strict confidence. I dedicate my heart, mind and strength to the work before me. I shall do all within my power to show in myself an example of all that is honorable and good throughout my naval career."

Rate / Rating Structure

- HR -Hospitalman Recruit (E-1)
- HA -Hospitalman Apprentice (E-2)
- HN -Hospitalman (E-3) (See USN Apprenticeships)
- HM3 -Hospital Corpsman Third Class (E-4)
- HM2 -Hospital Corpsman Second Class (E-5)
- HM1 -Hospital Corpsman First Class (E-6)
- HMC -Chief Hospital Corpsman (E-7)
- HMCS-Senior Chief Hospital Corpsman (E-8)
- HMCM-Master Chief Hospital Corpsman (E-9)

The Role of Education in the Military

Military education and training is a process which intends to establish and improve the capabilities of military personnel in their respective roles.

Military education can be voluntary or compulsory duty. Before any person gets authorization to operate technical equipment or be on the battle field, they must take a medical and often a physical test. If passed, they may begin primary training. The primary training is recruit training. Recruit training attempts to teach the basic information and training in techniques necessary to be an effective service

---

[1] BMC Mayport (2003-06-19). "Happy 105th Birthday To The Hospital Corps"

member. To achieve this, service members are drilled physically, technically and psychologically. The drill instructor has the task of making the service members fit for military use.

After finishing basic training, many service members undergo advanced training more in line with their chosen or assigned specialties. This range from navy training to studies of explosives. In advanced training, military technology and equipment is often taught.

Many large countries have several military academies, one for each branch of the service, that offer college degrees in a variety of subjects, similar to other colleges. However, academy graduates usually rank as officers, and as such have many options besides civilian work in their major subject. Higher ranking officers also have further educational opportunities.

Personnel Resocialization

While regulated industry does not seek to create soldiers and certainly does not want to employ all of the standard military training techniques, it does need to make certain personnel are trained to follow directions precisely and respect the authority of the regulatory agencies as well as their internal command chain (supervisors, managers, and executives).

Resocialization is an important aspect of inducting a civilian into a military team. Resocialization is a sociological concept dealing with the process of mentally and emotionally "re-training" a person so they can operate in an environment other than what they are accustomed to. Successful resocialization into a total institution involves changes to an individual's personality.

Key examples include the process of resocializing new recruits into the military so that they can operate as soldiers – or, in other words, as members of a cohesive unit. Another example is the reverse process, in which those who have become accustomed to such roles return to society after military discharge.

Resocialization from the life of a combat soldier to a civilian member of society is often difficult because of what that soldier saw and did in his military experience. In the transition from civilian to soldier, the individual is trained to solely follow the command of his superiors. In some cases commands would go against certain natural aversions (such as killing) of the individual based on one's moral and ethical principles.

A leading expert in military training methods, Grossman(2001) gives four types of training techniques used; brutalization, classical conditioning, operant conditioning and role modeling.[2] According to Grossman (2001), these techniques were meant to break down barriers to embrace a new set of norms and way of life (brutalization), condition them to pair killing with something more enjoyable and pleasurable (Classical Conditioning), repeat the stimulus-response reaction to

---

[2] Grossman, D. (2001) Trained to Kill. *Professorenforum-Journal*,2(2).

develop a reflex (Operant Conditioning), and finally the use of a role model of a superior to provide action by example.

While leaders effectively train their soldiers to accomplish the goal of battle preparedness, these techniques increase psychological trauma experienced in veterans post-combat.[3] It is because of the evident psychological problems in post-combat situations (i.e. Post Traumatic Stress Disorder) that pose a threat to public safety because of the conditioning of the individual who might be made unstable because of his actions. Resocialization following such intense training and conditioning should be further researched and developed to better aide those discharged from the military service.

---

[3] Kilner, P. (2002, March). Military Leaders' Obligation to Justify Killing in War. *Military Review*, 32(2).

Hospital Corpsman

NAVEDTRA 14295

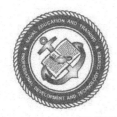

NONRESIDENT TRAINING COURSE

August 2000

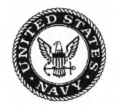

Hospital Corpsman

NAVEDTRA 14295

DISTRIBUTION STATEMENT A: Approved for public release; distribution is unlimited.

Although the words "he," "him," and "his" are used sparingly in this course to enhance communication, they are not intended to be gender driven or to affront or discriminate against anyone.

PREFACE

By enrolling in this self-study course, you have demonstrated a desire to improve yourself and the Navy. Remember, however, this self-study course is only one part of the total Navy training program. Practical experience, schools, selected reading, and your desire to succeed are also necessary to successfully round out a fully meaningful training program.

THE COURSE: This self-study course is organized into subject matter areas, each containing learning objectives to help you determine what you should learn along with text and illustrations to help you understand the information. The subject matter reflects day-to-day requirements and experiences of personnel in the rating or skill area. It also reflects guidance provided by Enlisted Community Managers (ECMs) and other senior personnel, technical references, instructions, etc., and either the occupational or naval standards, which are listed in the *Manual of Navy Enlisted Manpower Personnel Classifications and Occupational Standards*, NAVPERS 18068.

THE QUESTIONS: The questions that appear in this course are designed to help you understand the material in the text.

VALUE: In completing this course, you will improve your military and professional knowledge. Importantly, it can also help you study for the Navy-wide advancement in rate examination. If you are studying and discover a reference in the text to another publication for further information, look it up.

THANKS: A special note of thanks is given to the following activities and their staffs for providing valuable information during the preparation of this course: Bureau of Medicine and Surgery, Washington, DC; Navy Environmental Health Center, Norfolk, Virginia; and Naval Hospital, Pensacola, Florida.

2000 Edition Prepared by
HMCM(SW) Steve Kilroy, USN
HMCM(SW) Lawrence A. Yates, USN
HMCS(AW) Charla Bethune, USN (Ret.)

Published by
NAVAL EDUCATION AND TRAINING
PROFESSIONAL DEVELOPMENT
AND TECHNOLOGY CENTER

NAVSUP Logistics Tracking Number
0504-LP-022-4740

Sailor's Creed

"I am a United States Sailor.

I will support and defend the Constitution of the United States of America and I will obey the orders of those appointed over me.

I represent the fighting spirit of the Navy and those who have gone before me to defend freedom and democracy around the world.

I proudly serve my country's Navy combat team with honor, courage and commitment.

I am committed to excellence and the fair treatment of all."

TABLE OF CONTENTS

INSTRUCTIONS FOR TAKING THE COURSE

ASSIGNMENTS

The text pages that you are to study are listed at the beginning of each assignment. Study these pages carefully before attempting to answer the questions. Pay close attention to tables and illustrations and read the learning objectives. The learning objectives state what you should be able to do after studying the material. Answering the questions correctly helps you accomplish the objectives.

SELECTING YOUR ANSWERS

Read each question carefully, then select the BEST answer. You may refer freely to the text. The answers must be the result of your own work and decisions. You are prohibited from referring to or copying the answers of others and from giving answers to anyone else taking the course.

SUBMITTING YOUR ASSIGNMENTS

To have your assignments graded, you must be enrolled in the course with the Nonresident Training Course Administration Branch at the Naval Education and Training Professional Development and Technology Center (NETPDTC). Following enrollment, there are two ways of having your assignments graded: (1) use the Internet to submit your assignments as you complete them, or (2) send all the assignments at one time by mail to NETPDTC.

Grading on the Internet: Advantages to Internet grading are:

- you may submit your answers as soon as you complete an assignment, and
- you get your results faster; usually by the next working day (approximately 24 hours).

In addition to receiving grade results for each assignment, you will receive course completion confirmation once you have completed all the assignments. To submit your assignment answers via the Internet, go to:

http://courses.cnet.navy.mil

Grading by Mail: When you submit answer sheets by mail, send all of your assignments at one time. Do NOT submit individual answer sheets for grading. Mail all of your assignments in an envelope, which you either provide yourself or obtain from your nearest Educational Services Officer (ESO). Submit answer sheets to:

> COMMANDING OFFICER
> NETPDTC N331
> 6490 SAUFLEY FIELD ROAD
> PENSACOLA FL 32559-5000

Answer Sheets: All courses include one "scannable" answer sheet for each assignment. These answer sheets are preprinted with your SSN, name, assignment number, and course number. Explanations for completing the answer sheets are on the answer sheet.

Do not use answer sheet reproductions: Use only the original answer sheets that we provide—reproductions will not work with our scanning equipment and cannot be processed.

Follow the instructions for marking your answers on the answer sheet. Be sure that blocks 1, 2, and 3 are filled in correctly. This information is necessary for your course to be properly processed and for you to receive credit for your work.

COMPLETION TIME

Courses must be completed within 12 months from the date of enrollment. This includes time required to resubmit failed assignments.

PASS/FAIL ASSIGNMENT PROCEDURES

If your overall course score is 3.2 or higher, you will pass the course and will not be required to resubmit assignments. Once your assignments have been graded you will receive course completion confirmation.

If you receive less than a 3.2 on any assignment and your overall course score is below 3.2, you will be given the opportunity to resubmit failed assignments. **You may resubmit failed** assignments only once. Internet students will receive notification when they have failed an assignment--they may then resubmit failed assignments on the web site. Internet students may view and print results for failed assignments from the web site. Students who submit by mail will receive a failing result letter and a new answer sheet for resubmission of each failed assignment.

COMPLETION CONFIRMATION

After successfully completing this course, you will receive a letter of completion.

ERRATA

Errata are used to correct minor errors or delete obsolete information in a course. Errata may also be used to provide instructions to the student. If a course has an errata, it will be included as the first page(s) after the front cover. Errata for all courses can be accessed and viewed/downloaded at:

http://www.cnet.navy.mil/netpdtc/nac/neas.htm

STUDENT FEEDBACK QUESTIONS

We value your suggestions, questions, and criticisms on our courses. If you would like to communicate with us regarding this course, we encourage you, if possible, to use e-mail. If you write or fax, please use a copy of the Student Comment form that follows this page.

For subject matter questions:

E-mail: n313.products@cnet.navy.mil
Phone: Comm: (850) 452-1001, Ext. 2167
            DSN: 922-1001, Ext. 2167
            FAX: (850) 452-1370
            (Do not fax answer sheets.)
Address: COMMANDING OFFICER
            NETPDTC (CODE N313)
            6490 SAUFLEY FIELD ROAD
            PENSACOLA FL 32509-5000

For enrollment, shipping, grading, or completion letter questions

E-mail: fleetservices@cnet.navy.mil
Phone: Toll Free: 877-264-8583
            Comm: (850) 452-1511/1181/1859
            DSN: 922-1511/1181/1859
            FAX: (850) 452-1370
            (Do not fax answer sheets.)
Address: COMMANDING OFFICER
            NETPDTC (CODE N331)
            6490 SAUFLEY FIELD ROAD
            PENSACOLA FL 32559-5000

NAVAL RESERVE RETIREMENT CREDIT

If you are a member of the Naval Reserve, you will receive retirement points if you are authorized to receive them under current directives governing retirement of Naval Reserve personnel. For Naval Reserve retirement, this course is evaluated at 14 points: 12 points upon satisfactory completion of unit 1, assignments 1-8; and 2 points upon satisfactory completion of unit 2, assignment 9. (Refer to *Administrative Procedures for Naval Reservists on Inactive Duty,* BUPERSINST 1001.39, for more information about retirement points.)

COURSE OBJECTIVES

In completing this nonresident training course, you will demonstrate a knowledge of the subject matter by correctly answering questions on the following subjects: anatomy and physiology; fundamentals of patient care; first aid equipment, supplies, rescue, and transportation; emergency medical care procedures; poisoning, drug abuse, and hazardous material exposure; pharmacy and toxicology; clinical laboratory; medical aspects of chemical, biological, and radiological warfare; diet and nutrition; emergency dental care; preventive medicine; physical examinations; health records; supply; administration; healthcare administration; and decedent affairs.

Student Comments

Course Title: *Hospital Corpsman* _____

NAVEDTRA: 14295 _____ **Date:** _____

We need some information about you:

Rate/Rank and Name: _____ SSN: _____ Command/Unit _____

Street Address: _____ City: _____ State/FPO: _____ Zip _____

Your comments, suggestions, etc.:

NETPDTC 1550/41 (Rev 4-00)

CHAPTER 1

ANATOMY AND PHYSIOLOGY

Knowledge of how the human body is constructed and how it works is an important part of the training of everyone concerned with healing the sick or managing conditions following injury. This chapter will provide you with a general knowledge of the structures and functions of the body.

The human body is a combination of organ systems, with a supporting framework of muscles and bones and an external covering of skin. The study of the body is divided into three sciences:

Anatomy—the study of body structures and the relation of one part to another.

Physiology—the study of the processes and functions of the body tissue and organs. Physiology is the study of how the body works and how the various parts function individually and in relation to each other.

Embryology—the study of the development of the body from a fertilized egg, or ovum.

TERMS OF POSITION AND DIRECTION

LEARNING OBJECTIVE: *Identify anatomical terms of position and direction.*

The planes of the body are imaginary lines dividing it into sections. These planes are used as reference points in locating anatomical structures. As shown in figure 1-1, the **median**, or **midsagittal, plane** divides the body into right and left halves on its vertical axis. This plane passes through the sagittal suture of the cranium; therefore, any plane parallel to it is called a **sagittal plane**. **Frontal planes** are drawn perpendicular to the sagittal lines and divide the body into anterior (front) and posterior (rear) sections. Since this line passes through the coronal suture of the cranium, frontal planes are also called **coronal planes**. The **horizontal**, or **transverse, plane**, which is drawn at right angles to both sagittal and frontal planes, divides the body into superior (upper) and inferior (lower) sections.

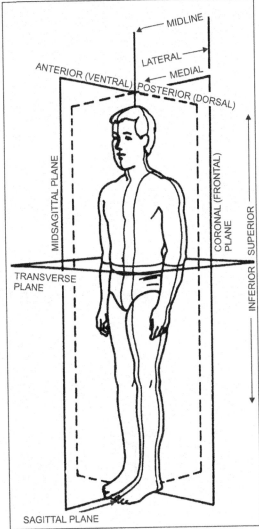

HM3F0101

Figure 1-1.—Planes of the body.

To aid in understanding the location of anatomical structures, you should use a standard body position called the **anatomical position** as a point of reference. This anatomical position is assumed when the body stands erect with the arms hanging at the sides and the palms of the hands turned forward (fig. 1-2).

Other commonly used anatomical terms include the following:

Anterior or ventral—toward the front, or ventral (pertaining to the belly; abdomen), side of the body.

Posterior or dorsal—toward the back, or rear, side of the body.

Medial—near or toward the midline of the body.

Lateral—farther away from the midline of the body.

Internal—inside.

External—outside.

Proximal—nearer the point of origin or closer to the body.

Distal—away from the point of origin or away from the body.

Superior—higher than or above.

Cranial—toward the head.

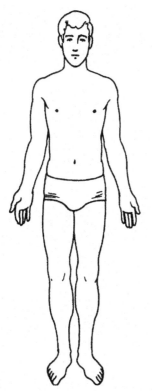

Figure 1-2.—Anatomical position.

Caudal—toward the lower end of the body.

Inferior—lower than or below.

Erect—normal standing position of the body.

Supine—lying position of the body, face up.

Prone—lying position of the body, face down.

Lateral recumbent—lying position of the body on either side.

Peripheral—the outward part or surface of a structure.

CHARACTERISTICS OF LIVING MATTER

LEARNING OBJECTIVE: *Identify the characteristics of living matter.*

All living things, animals and plants, are organisms that undergo chemical processes by which they sustain life and regenerate cells. The difference between animals and plants is that animals have sensations and the power of voluntary movement, and they require oxygen and organic food. On the other hand, plants require only carbon dioxide and inorganic matter for food and have neither voluntary movement nor special sensory organs.

In man, some of the characteristic functions necessary for survival include **digestion**, **metabolism**, and **homeostasis**. Digestion involves the physical and chemical breakdown of the food we eat into its simplest forms. Metabolism is the process of absorption, storage, and use of these foods for body growth, maintenance, and repair. Homeostasis is the body's self-regulated control of its internal environment. It allows the organism to maintain a state of constancy or equilibrium, in spite of vast changes in the external environment.

THE CELL

LEARNING OBJECTIVE: *Identify the parts of the cell and their functions.*

The cell, the smallest unit of life, is the basic structural unit of all living things and a functional unit all by itself. Cells are composed of a viscid, jellylike substance, called **protoplasm**, upon which depend all the vital functions of nutrition, secretion, growth, circulation, reproduction, excitability, and movement. Protoplasm, thus, has often been called "the secret of life."

A typical cell is made up of the plasma membrane, the nucleus, and the cytoplasm.

The **plasma membrane** is a selectively permeable membrane surrounding the cell. In addition to holding the cell together, the membrane selectively controls the exchange of materials between the cell and its environment by physical and chemical means. Gases (such as oxygen) and solids (such as proteins, carbohydrates, and mineral salts) pass through the plasma membrane by a process known as **diffusion**.

The **nucleus** is a small, dense, usually spherical body that controls the chemical reactions occurring in the cell. The substance contained in the nucleus is called **nucleoplasm**. The nucleus is also important in the cell's reproduction, since genetic information for the cell is stored there. Every human cell contains 46 chromosomes, and each chromosome has thousands of genes that determine the cell's function.

The **cytoplasm** is a gelatinous substance surrounding the nucleus and is contained by the plasma membrane. The cytoplasm is composed of all of the cell protoplasm except the nucleus.

The simplest living organism consists of a single cell. The amoeba is a unicellular animal. The single cell of such a one-celled organism must be able to carry on all processes necessary for life. This cell is called a **simple** or **undifferentiated cell**, one that has not acquired distinguishing characteristics.

In multicellular organisms, cells vary in size, shape, and number of nuclei. When stained, the various cell structures can be more readily recognized under a microscope. Other differences such as the number and type of cells can be seen with the aid of a microscope. Many cells are highly specialized. **Specialized cells** perform special functions (e.g., muscle cells, which contract, and epithelial cells, which protect the skin).

TISSUES

LEARNING OBJECTIVES: *Identify the types of tissues in the human body and their functions.*

Tissues are groups of specialized cells similar in structure and function. They are classified into four main groups: epithelial, connective, muscular, and nervous.

EPITHELIAL TISSUE

The lining tissue of the body is called **epithelium**. It forms the outer covering of the body known as the free surface of the skin. It also forms the lining of the digestive, respiratory, and urinary tracts; blood and lymph vessels; serous cavities (cavities which have no communication with the outside of the body, and whose lining membrane secretes a serous fluid), such as the peritoneum or pericardium; and tubules (small tubes which convey fluids) of certain secretory glands, such as the liver and kidneys. Epithelial tissues are classified according to their shape, arrangement, and the function of their cells. For example, epithelial tissues that are composed of single layers of cells are called "simple," while cells with many layers are said to be "stratified." In the following paragraphs we will discuss the three categories of epithelial tissue: columnar, squamous, and cuboidal.

Columnar Epithelial Tissue

Epithelial cells of this type are elongated, longer than they are wide. Columnar tissue is composed of a single layer of cells whose nuclei are located at about the same level as the nuclei in their neighboring cells (fig. 1-3). These cells can be located in the linings of the uterus, in various organs of the digestive system, and in the passages of the respiratory system. In the digestive system, the chief function of columnar tissue is the secretion of digestive fluids and the absorption of nutrients from digested foods. In certain areas (such as the nostrils, bronchial tubes, and trachea), this tissue has a crown of microscopic hairlike processes known as **cilia**. These cilia provide motion to move secretions

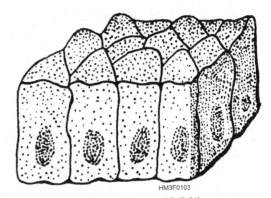

HM3F0103

Figure 1-3.—Columnar epithelial tissue.

and other matter along the surfaces from which they extend. They also act as a barrier, preventing foreign matter from entering these cavities.

Squamous Epithelial Tissue

Squamous epithelial tissue is composed of thin platelike or scalelike cells forming a mosaic pattern (fig. 1-4). This tissue is found in the tympanic membrane (eardrum) as a single layer of cells, or in the free skin surface in multiple layers. Squamous tissue is the main protective tissue of the body.

Cuboidal Epithelial Tissue

The cells of cuboidal tissue are cubical in shape (fig. 1-5) and are found in the more highly specialized organs of the body, such as the ovary and the kidney. In the kidneys, cuboidal tissue functions in the secretion and absorption of fluids.

CONNECTIVE TISSUE

This is the supporting tissue of the various structures of the body. It has many variations and is the most widespread tissue of the body. Connective tissue is highly vascular, surrounds other cells, encases internal organs, sheathes muscles, wraps bones, encloses joints, and provides the supporting framework of the body. Structures of connective tissue differ widely, ranging from delicate tissue-paper membranes to rigid bones. Connective tissue is composed of cells and **extracellular materials** (materials found outside the cells). Extracellular materials include fibers and the **ground substance**. The ground substance contains proteins, water, salts, and other diffusible substances. These extracellular materials give connective tissue varying amounts of elasticity and strength, depending on the type of tissue and location. In the following paragraphs we will discuss the three predominant types of connective tissue: areolar, adipose, and osseous.

Areolar Connective Tissue

Areolar tissue consists of a meshwork of thin fibers that interlace in all directions, giving the tissue both elasticity and tensile strength (fig. 1-6). This type of connective tissue is extensively distributed throughout the body, and its chief function is to bind parts of the body together. Areolar tissue allows a considerable amount of movement to take place because of its elasticity. It is found between muscles and as an outside covering for blood vessels and nerves. The areolar tissue layer connects the blood vessels and nerves to the surrounding structures.

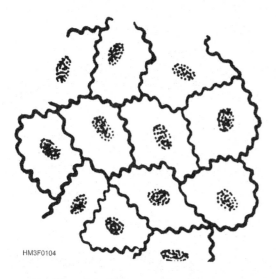

HM3F0104

Figure 1-4.—Squamous epithelial tissue.

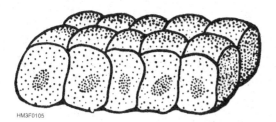

HM3F0105

Figure 1-5.—Cuboidal epithelial tissue.

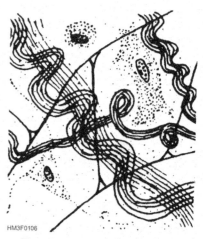

HM3F0106

Figure 1-6.—Areolar connective tissue.

Adipose Connective Tissue

Adipose tissue is "fatty tissue." The adipose cell at first appears star-shaped. When the cell begins to store fat in its cytoplasm, it enlarges, losing its star shape as the nucleus is pushed to one side (fig. 1-7). When this process occurs to many cells, the other cell types are crowded out and adipose tissue is formed. Adipose tissue is found beneath skin, between muscles, and around joints and various organs of the body. Adipose tissue acts as a reservoir for energy-producing foods; helps to reduce body heat loss (because of its poor heat conductivity); and serves as support for various organs and fragile structures, such as the kidneys, blood vessels, and nerves.

Osseous Connective Tissue

This type of tissue, known as "bone tissue," is a dense fibrous connective tissue that forms tendons, ligaments, cartilage, and bones (fig. 1-8). These tissues form the supporting framework of the body.

MUSCULAR TISSUE

Muscular tissue provides for all body movement. Contracting muscles cause body parts to move. The three types of muscle tissue are skeletal, smooth, and cardiac.

Skeletal Muscle Tissue

Skeletal (voluntary) muscle fiber is striated, or striped, and is under the control of the individual's will (fig. 1-9). For this reason, it is often called "voluntary" muscle tissue. Skeletal muscle tissues are usually attached to bones. When muscle fibers are stimulated by an action of a nerve fiber, the fibers contract and relax. This interaction between muscle and nervous fibers produces movement.

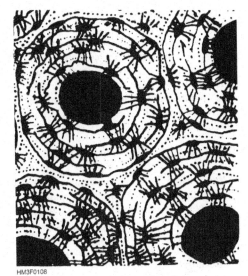

HM3F0108

Figure 1-8.—Osseous (bone) connective tissue.

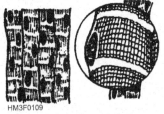

HM3F0109

Figure 1-9.—Skeletal muscle tissue.

Smooth Muscle Tissue

These muscle fibers are smooth, or nonstriated, and are not under the control of the individual's will (fig. 1-10). For this reason, this type of muscle tissue is called "involuntary." Smooth muscle tissue is found in the walls of hollow organs, such as the stomach, intestines, blood vessels, and urinary bladder. Smooth muscle tissues are responsible for the movement of food through the digestive system, constricting blood vessels, and emptying the bladder.

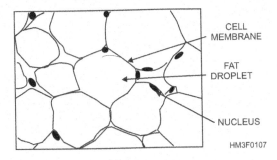

CELL MEMBRANE

FAT DROPLET

NUCLEUS

HM3F0107

Figure 1-7.—Adipose connective tissue.

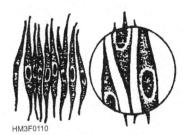

HM3F0110

Figure 1-10.—Smooth muscle tissue.

Cardiac Muscle Tissue

The cardiac muscle cells are striated and are joined end to end, resulting in a complex network of interlocking cells (fig. 1-11). Cardiac muscles are involuntary muscles and are located only in the heart. These tissues are responsible for pumping blood through the heart chambers and into certain blood vessels.

NERVE TISSUE

Nerve tissue is the most complex tissue in the body. It is the substance of the brain, spinal cord, and nerves. Nerve tissue requires more oxygen and nutrients than any other body tissue. The basic cell of the nerve tissue is the **neuron** (fig. 1-12). This highly specialized cell receives stimuli from, and conducts impulses to, all parts of the body.

ORGANS

LEARNING OBJECTIVE: *Recall how organs and body systems are composed of two or more kinds of tissue that perform specialized functions within the body.*

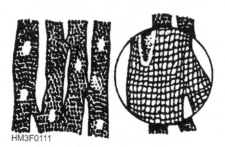

HM3F0111

Figure 1-11.—Cardiac muscle tissue.

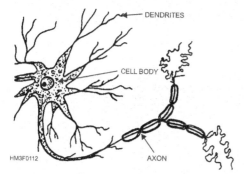

— DENDRITES

CELL BODY

HM3F0112   AXON

Figure 1-12.—Neuron.

As a group of similar cells forms tissues, two or more kinds of tissues grouped together and performing specialized functions constitute an organ. Organs are grouped together to form systems (such as the urinary system, composed of the kidneys, ureters, bladder, and urethra).

THE SKELETAL SYSTEM

LEARNING OBJECTIVE: *Identify the parts of bone and their functions.*

The skeleton, the bony framework of the body, is composed of 206 bones (fig. 1-13). It supports and gives shape to the body; protects vital organs; and provides sites of attachment for tendons, muscles, and ligaments. The skeletal bones are joined members that make muscle movement possible.

ANATOMY OF BONES

Osteology is the study of the structure of bone. Bone is made up of inorganic mineral salts (calcium and phosphorus being the most prevalent) and an organic substance called **ossein**. If human bones were soaked in dilute acid until all inorganic mineral salts were washed out, all that would remain would be a flexible piece of tissue that could be easily bent and twisted. Inorganic mineral salts give bone its strength and hardness.

Bone consists of a hard outer shell, called **compact bone**, and an inner spongy, porous portion, called **cancellous tissue** (fig. 1-14). In the center of the bone is the **medullary canal**, which contains **marrow**. There are two types of marrow, red and yellow. Yellow marrow is ordinary bone marrow in which fat cells predominate. It is found in the medullary canals and cancellous tissue of long bones. Red marrow is one of the manufacturing centers of red blood cells and is found in the articular ends of long bones and in cancellous tissue.

At the ends of the long bones is a smooth, glossy tissue that forms the joint surfaces. This tissue is called **articular cartilage** because it articulates (or joins) with, fits into, or moves in contact with similar surfaces of other bones. The thin outer membrane surrounding the bone is called the **periosteum**. An important function of the periosteum is to supply nourishment to the bone. Capillaries and blood vessels run through the periosteum and dip into the bone surface, supplying it with blood and nutrients. The

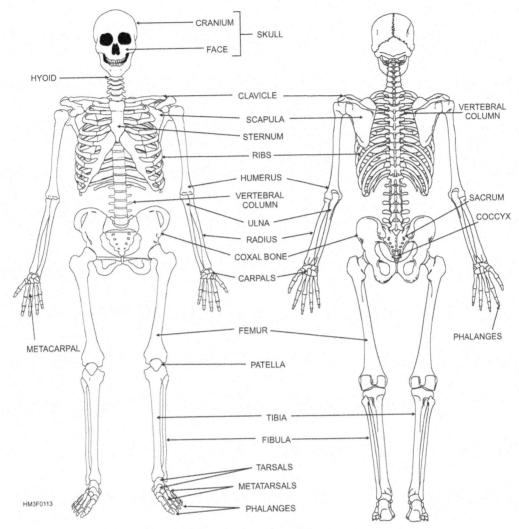

Figure 1-13.—Human skeleton.

periosteum is the pain center of the bone. When a bone fractures, the pain that is felt comes from the periosteum, not the bone proper. Periosteum also forms new bone. The **diaphysis** is the elongated, cylindrical portion (or "shaft") of the bone that is between the **epiphyses** (*sing.* epiphysis) or ends of the bone.

BONE CLASSIFICATIONS

Bones are classified according to their shape. The four bone classifications and examples of each are as follows:

- **Long bones**—femur and humerus

- **Short bones**—wrist and ankle bones

- **Flat bones**—skull, sternum, and scapula

- **Irregular bones**—vertebrae, mandible, and pelvic bones

DIVISIONS OF SKELETON

The human skeleton is divided into two main divisions, the axial skeleton and the appendicular skeleton.

Axial Skeleton

The axial skeleton consists of the skull, the vertebral column, and the thorax.

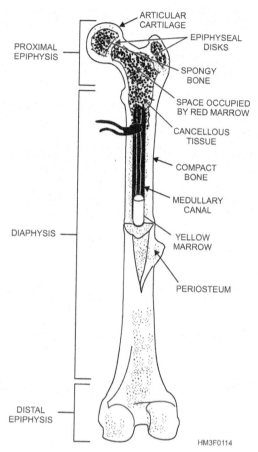

Figure 1-14.—Anatomy of a long bone.

SKULL.—The skull consists of 28 bones (figs. 1-15 and 1-16), 22 of which form the framework of the head and provide protection for the brain, eyes, and ears; six are ear bones. With the exception of the lower jaw bone and the ear bones, all skull bones are joined together and fixed in one position. The seams where they join are known as **sutures**. The bones of the skull are classified as either cranial or facial bones.

Cranial Bones.—The cranium is formed by eight major bones, most of which are in pairs (fig. 1-15). The **frontal bone** forms the forehead and the roof of each orbit (or eye socket) and the nasal cavity. The **parietal bones** form the roof of the skull. The **temporal bones** help form the sides and base of the skull and also house the auditory and hearing organs. The **occipital bone** forms part of the base and back of the skull, and contains a large hole called the foramen magnum. This opening permits passage of the spinal cord from the cranium into the spinal column. The **sphenoid bones** are wedged between several other bones in the anterior portion of the skull. These bones help form the base of the cranium, the sides of the skull, and the floors and sides of the orbits. The **ethmoid bones** are located in front of the sphenoid bone. They form sections of the nasal cavity roof, the cranial floor, and the orbital wall.

Facial Bones.—The facial bones of the skull consists of 14 bones: 13 immovable bones and a movable lower jawbone (fig. 1-16). The facial bones give the face its basic shape and provide attachment sites for various muscles that move the jaw and control facial expressions.

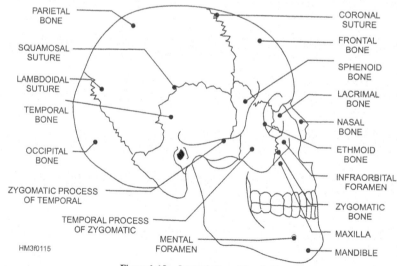

Figure 1-15.—Lateral view of the skull.

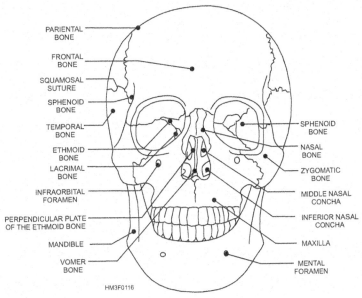

PARIENTAL BONE
FRONTAL BONE
SQUAMOSAL SUTURE
SPHENOID BONE
TEMPORAL BONE
ETHMOID BONE
LACRIMAL BONE
INFRAORBITAL FORAMEN
PERPENDICULAR PLATE OF THE ETHMOID BONE
MANDIBLE
VOMER BONE

SPHENOID BONE
NASAL BONE
ZYGOMATIC BONE
MIDDLE NASAL CONCHA
INFERIOR NASAL CONCHA
MAXILLA
MENTAL FORAMEN

HM3F0116

Figure 1-16.—Facial bones.

The **maxillary bones** form the upper jaw, the anterior roof of the mouth, the floors of the orbits, and the sides and floor of the nasal cavity. The small holes on each side of the nasal opening are called the **infraorbital foramina** (*sing.* foramen). The maxillary bones contain large cavities called **maxillary sinuses**.

The palatine bones are L-shaped bones located behind the maxillary bones. They form the posterior section of the hard palate and the floor of the nasal cavity.

The **zygomatic bones** are responsible for the prominence of the cheeks. The zygomatic bones serve as part of the posterior section of the hard palate and the floor of the nasal cavity.

The **lacrimal bones** provide a pathway for a tube that carries tears from the eye to the nasal cavity. The lacrimal bone is a thin, scalelike structure located in the medial wall of each orbit.

The **nasal bones** have cartilaginous tissues attached to them. These tissues contribute significantly to the shape of the nose. The nasal bones are long, thin, and nearly rectangular in shape. They lie side by side and are fused together to form the bridge of the nose.

The **vomer bone** is connected to the ethmoid bone, and together they form the nasal septum (the wall separating the two nasal cavities).

The **middle and inferior nasal conchae** are fragile, scroll-shaped bones that are attached to the lateral wall of the nasal cavity. The inferior nasal concha provides support for mucous membranes within the nasal cavity.

The lower jawbone is called the **mandible**. The mandible is horseshoe-shaped with flat, bony projections on each end. The two small holes on the jawbone are called the **mental foramina.** The mandible's main function is mastication (chewing food).

VERTEBRAL (SPINAL) COLUMN.—The vertebral column consists of 24 movable or true vertebrae; the sacrum; and the coccyx, or tail bone (fig. 1-17). The vertebrae protect the spinal cord and the nerves that branch out from the spinal cord. Each vertebra has an anterior portion, called the body, which is the large solid segment of the bone (fig. 1-18). This vertebral body supports not only the spinal cord but other structures of the body as well. At the bottom of the spinal column is the **sacrum** and the **coccyx.** Many of the main muscles are attached to the vertebrae.

The **vertebral foramen** is a hole directly behind the body of the vertebrae that forms the passage for the spinal cord. The vertebral projections are for the attachments of muscles and ligaments and for facilitating movement of one vertebra over another. The spinal column is divided into five regions in the following order: cervical (neck), thoracic (chest),

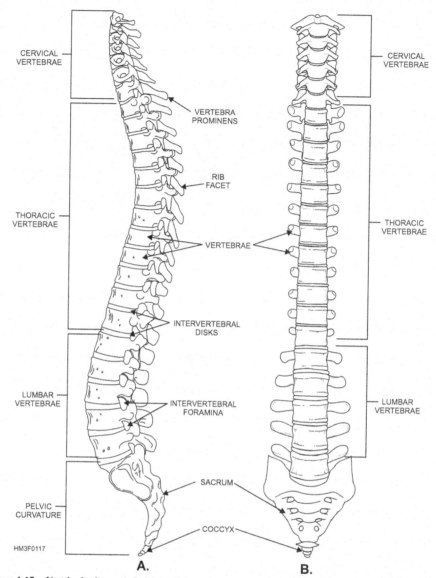

CERVICAL VERTEBRAE

VERTEBRA PROMINENS

RIB FACET

THORACIC VERTEBRAE

VERTEBRAE

INTERVERTEBRAL DISKS

LUMBAR VERTEBRAE

INTERVERTEBRAL FORAMINA

SACRUM

PELVIC CURVATURE

COCCYX

HM3F0117

CERVICAL VERTEBRAE

THORACIC VERTEBRAE

LUMBAR VERTEBRAE

A.   B.

Figure 1-17.—Vertebral column: A. Left lateral view of vertebral column; B. Posterior view of vertebral column.

lumbar (lower back), and sacral and coccygeal (pelvis).

Cervical.—There are seven cervical vertebrae in the neck. The first is called the **atlas** and resembles a bony ring. It supports the head. The second is the highly specialized **axis**. It has a bony prominence that fits into the ring of the atlas, thus permitting the head to rotate from side to side. The atlas and the axis are the only named vertebrae; all others are numbered. See figure 1-19. Each cervical vertebra has a transverse (or

intervertebral) foramen (fig. 1-19) to allow passage of nerves, the vertebral artery, and a vein. The seventh cervical vertebra has a prominent projection that can easily be felt at the nape of the neck. This landmark makes it possible for physicians to count and identify the vertebrae above and below it.

Thoracic.—There are 12 vertebrae in the thoracic region. The thoracic vertebrae articulate with the posterior portion of the 12 ribs to form the posterior wall of the thoracic, or chest, cage.

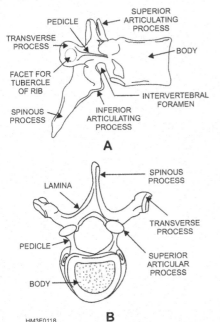

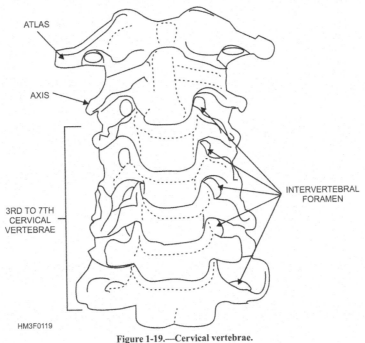

Figure 1-18.—Typical vertebra: A. Lateral view of a typical vertebra; B. Superior view of a typical thoracic vertebra.

Lumbar.—There are five lumbar vertebrae. Located in the small of the back, these vertebrae are the larger and stronger segments of the vertebral column.

Sacrum.—The sacrum is the triangular bone immediately below the lumbar vertebrae. It is composed of five separate vertebrae that gradually fuse together between 18 and 30 years of age. The sacrum is connected on each side with the hip bone and with the **coccyx** to form the posterior wall of the **pelvis**.

THORAX.—This cone-shaped bony cage is about as wide as it is deep (fig. 1-20). The thorax is formed by 12 ribs on each side and articulates posteriorly with the thoracic vertebrae. The first set of ribs are attached to the **manubrium,** a flat irregular bone atop the sternum. The first seven pairs of ribs are called **true ribs**. The remaining five pairs are called **false ribs**. They are called false ribs because their cartilages do not reach the sternum directly. The eighth, ninth, and tenth ribs are united by their cartilages and joined to the rib above. The last two rib pairs, also known as **floating ribs**, have no cartilaginous attachments to the **sternum**. The sternum is an elongated flat bone, forming the middle portion of the upper half of the chest wall in front. The **xiphoid process**, located at the inferior aspect of the sternum, serves as a landmark in the administration of cardiopulmonary resuscitation.

Figure 1-19.—Cervical vertebrae.

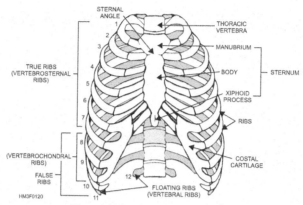

Figure 1-20.—Anterior view of thorax,

Appendicular Skeleton

The appendicular skeleton consists of the bones of the upper and lower extremities.

UPPER EXTREMITY.—The upper extremity consists of the bones of the shoulder, the arm, the forearm, the wrist, and the hand (figs. 1-21 and 1-22). The bones that form the framework for the upper extremities are listed in table 1-1.

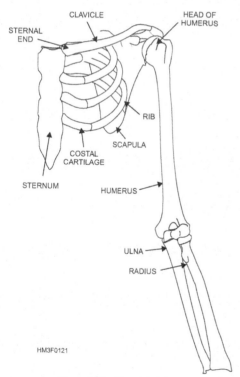

Figure 1-21.—Pectoral girdle.

Table 1-1.—Bones of the Upper Extremities

BONE	COMMON NAME	TOTAL NUMBER IN BODY
clavicle	collar bone	2
scapula	shoulder blade	2
humerus	arm bone	2
radius and ulna	forearm bones	4
carpals	wrist bones	16
metacarpals	bones of the palm	10
phalanges	finger bones	28

Clavicle.—The clavicle (commonly called the collar bone) lies nearly horizontally above the first rib and is shaped like a flat letter S. The clavicle is a thin brace bone that fractures easily. Its inner end is round and attached to the sternum; its outer end is flattened and fixed to the scapula. The clavicle forms the anterior portion of the pectoral girdle (fig. 1-21). The pectoral girdle is composed of the two clavicles and two scapulae (shoulder blades). It functions as a support for the arms and serves as an attachment for several muscles.

Scapula.—The scapula is a triangular bone that lies in the upper part of the back on both sides, between the second and seventh ribs, forming the posterior portion of the pectoral girdle. Its lateral corner forms part of the shoulder joint, articulating with the humerus.

Humerus.—The humerus is the longest bone of the upper extremity and is often called the arm bone (fig. 1-22). It articulates with the pectoral girdle to form the shoulder joint, and with the bones of the

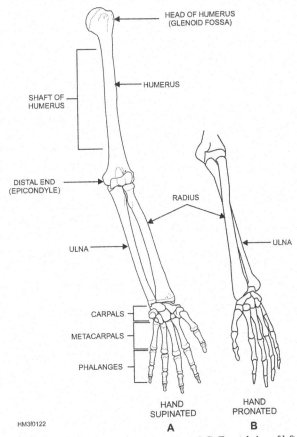

Figure 1-22.—Left arm: A. Frontal view of left arm with hand supinated; B. Frontal view of left arm with hand pronated.

forearm to form the elbow. Its anatomical portions include a head (a rounded portion that fits into a recess of the scapula) called the **glenoid fossa**; the **shaft**, which is the main part of the humerus; and the **distal end**, which includes the prominence (called an **epicondyle**) and the surfaces that articulate with the bones of the forearm.

Radius and Ulna.—When the arm is in the anatomical position with the palm turned forward, the **radius** is on the lateral (thumb) side and the **ulna** is on the medial (little finger) side of the forearm (fig. 1-22). When the hand is pronated (with the palm turned downward), the bones rotate on each other and cross in the middle. This pronation makes it possible to turn the wrist and hand (as when opening doors). The ulna and the radius articulate at their proximal ends with the humerus, at their distal ends with some of the carpal bones, and with each other at both ends.

Carpal.—There are eight carpal bones, arranged in two rows, forming the wrist.

Metacarpal.—The metacarpal bones are numbered one to five, corresponding with the five fingers, or digits, with which they articulate. The fingers are named as follows: 1st—thumb; 2nd—index; 3rd—middle; 4th—ring; and 5th—little.

Phalanges.—The small bones of the fingers are called phalanges, and each one of these bones is called a **phalanx**. Each finger has three phalanges, except the thumb (which has two). The phalanges are named for their anatomical position: The proximal phalanx is the bone closest to the hand; the distal phalanx is the bone at the end of the finger; and the middle phalanx is the bone located between the proximal and distal phalanges.

LOWER EXTREMITY.—The lower extremity includes the bones of the hip, thigh, leg, ankle, and foot. The bones that form the framework of the lower extremities are listed in table 1-2.

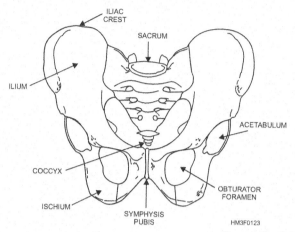

Figure 1-23.—Pelvic girdle.

Table 1-2.—Bones of the Lower Extremities

BONE	COMMON NAME	TOTAL NUMBER IN BODY
innominate	hip bone	2
femur	thigh bone	2
patella	knee cap	2
tibia	leg bone	2
fibula	leg bone	2
tarsals	ankle bones	14
metatarsals	foot bones	10
phalanges	toe bones	28

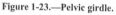
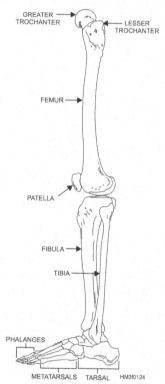

Figure 1-24.—Anterior view of the right leg.

Innominate.—The innominate bone, commonly known as the hip, is a large, irregularly shaped bone composed of three parts: the ilium, ischium, and pubis (fig. 1-23). In children these three parts are separate bones, but in adults they are firmly united to form a cuplike structure, called the **acetabulum**, into which the head of the femur fits. The **ilium** forms the outer prominence of the hip bone (the crest of the ilium, referred to as the **iliac crest**, provides an anatomical landmark above the ilium); the **ischium** forms the hard lower part; and the **pubis** forms the front part of the pelvis.

Symphysis Pubis.—The area where the two pubic bones meet is called the symphysis pubis and is often used in anatomical measurements. The largest foramen, or opening, is located in the hip bone, between the ischium and the pubis, and is called the **obturator foramen** (fig. 1-23). The crest of the ilium

is used in making anatomical and surgical measurements (e.g., location of the appendix, which is approximately halfway between the crest of the ilium and the umbilicus).

Femur.—The femur, or thigh bone, is the longest bone in the body (fig. 1-24). The proximal end is rounded and has a head supported by a constricted neck that fits into the acetabulum. Two processes called the **greater** and **lesser trochanters** are at the proximal end for the attachment of muscles. The neck of the femur, located between the head and the trochanters, is the site on the femur most frequently fractured. At the distal end are two bony prominences, called the **lateral** and **medial condyles**, which articulate with the tibia and the patella.

Patella.—The patella is a small oval-shaped bone overlying the knee joint. It is enclosed within the tendon of the quadriceps muscle of the thigh. Bones like the patella that develop within a tendon are known as **sesamoid** bones.

Tibia.—The tibia, or shin bone, is the larger of the two leg bones and lies at the medial side. The proximal end articulates with the femur and the fibula. Its distal end articulates with the talus (one of the foot bones) and the fibula (fig. 1-25). A prominence easily felt on the inner aspect of the ankle is called the **medial malleolus**.

Fibula.—The fibula, the smaller of the two leg bones, is located on the lateral side of the leg, parallel to the tibia. The prominence at the distal end forms the outer ankle and is known as the **lateral malleolus**.

Tarsus.—The tarsus, or ankle, is formed by seven tarsal bones: **medial cuneiform, intermediate cuneiform, lateral cuneiform, cuboid, navicular, talus,** and **calcaneus**. The strongest of these is the heel bone, or **calcaneus**.

Metatarsus.—The sole and instep of the foot is called the metatarsus and is made up of five metatarsal bones (fig. 1-25). They are similar in arrangement to the metacarpals of the hand.

Phalanges.—The phalanges are the bones of the toes and are similar in number, structure, and arrangement to the bones of the fingers.

JOINTS

LEARNING OBJECTIVE: *Recognize joint classifications and identify joint movements for the key joints in the body.*

Wherever two or more bones meet, a joint is formed. A joint binds various parts of the skeletal system together and enables body parts to move in response to skeletal muscle contractions.

JOINT CLASSIFICATIONS

Joints are classified according to the amount of movement they permit (fig. 1-26). Joint classifications are as follows:

• **Immovable**. Bones of the skull are an example of an immovable joint. Immovable joints are characterized by the bones being in close contact with each other and little or no movement occurring between the bones.

• **Slightly movable**. In slightly movable joints, the bones are held together by broad flattened disks of cartilage and ligaments (e.g., vertebrae and symphysis pubis).

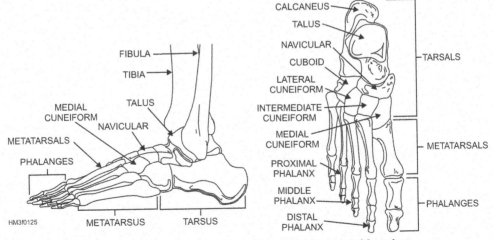

Figure 1-25.—The foot: A. Lateral view of foot; B. Right foot viewed from above.

• **Freely movable**. Most joints in the body are freely movable joints. The joint consists of the **joint capsule, articular cartilage, synovial membrane, and synovial (joint) cavity** (fig. 1-26). There are six classifications of freely movable joints: **ball-in-socket, condyloid, gliding, hinge, pivot**, and **saddle joints** (fig. 1-27). These joints have much more complex structures than the immovable and slightly movable joints. The ends of the bones in this type of joint are covered with a smooth layer of cartilage. The whole joint is enclosed in a watertight sac or membrane containing a small amount of lubricating fluid. This lubrication enables the joint to work with little friction. **Ligaments** (cords or sheets of connective tissue) reach across the joints from one bone to another and keep the bone stable. When ligaments are torn, we call the injury a sprain; when bones are out of place, we refer to this as a dislocation; and when bones are chipped or broken, the injury is called a fracture.

TYPES OF JOINT MOVEMENTS

Joint movements are generally divided into four types: gliding, angular, rotation, and circumduction.

Gliding

Gliding is the simplest type of motion. It is one surface moving over another without any rotary or angular motion. This motion exists between two adjacent surfaces.

Angular

Angular motion decreases or increases the angle between two adjoining bones. The more common types of angular motion are as follows:

• **Flexion**—bending the arm or leg.

• **Extension**—straightening or unbending, as in straightening the forearm, leg, or fingers.

• **Abduction**—moving an extremity away from the body.

• **Adduction**—bringing an extremity toward the body.

Rotation

Rotation is a movement in which the bone moves around a central point without being displaced, such as turning the head from side to side.

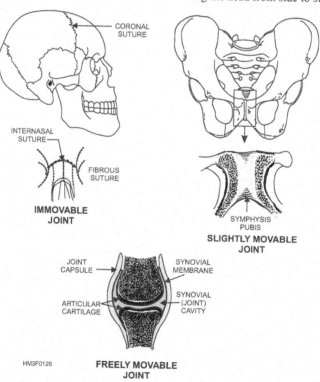

Figure 1-26.—Example of immovable, slightly movable, and freely movable joints.

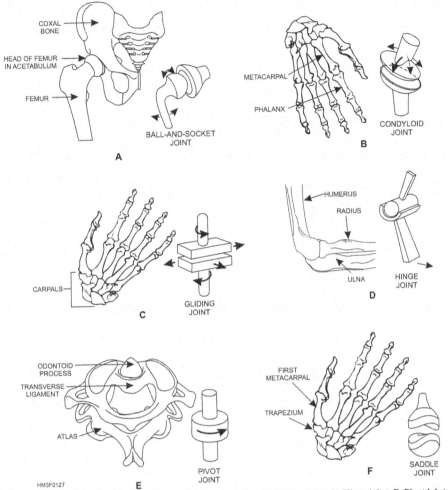

Figure 1-27.—Types of joints: A. Ball-in-socket joint; B. Condyloid joint; C. Gliding joint; D. Hinge joint; E. Pivot joint; F. Saddle joint.

Circumduction

Circumduction is the movement of the hips and shoulders.

Other Types of Movement

Other types of movement generally used to indicate specific anatomical positions include the following:

- **Supination**—turning upward, as in placing the palm of the hand up.

- **Pronation**—turning downward, as in placing the palm of the hand down.

- **Eversion**—turning outward, as in turning the sole of the foot to the outside.

- **Inversion**—turning inward, as in turning the sole of the foot inward.

MUSCLES

LEARNING OBJECTIVE: *Identify primary muscle functions, muscle characteristics, types of muscle tissue, and important functional muscles.*

Muscles are responsible for many different types of body movements. The action of the muscle is determined mainly by the kind of joint it is associated with and the way the muscle is attached to the joint. At one end of some muscles are long white **tendons** that attach the muscles to bone. The point of fixed attachment of a muscle to bone is called the **origin**. The more flexible attachments, especially attachments to a movable bone, are termed **insertions**.

Muscles seldom act alone; they usually work in groups held together by sheets of a white fibrous tissue called **fascia**. Muscles make up about one-half of the total body weight. Their main functions are threefold:

• **Providing movement**—including internal functions such as peristalsis (rhythmic waves of muscular contraction within the intestines).

• **Maintaining body posture**—through muscle tone, as in the muscles of the head, neck and shoulders, which keep the head up.

• **Providing heat**—through chemical changes that take place during muscle activity, such as exercise that warms the body.

In addition, muscles are involved in such essential bodily functions as respiration, blood circulation, digestion, and other functions such as speaking and seeing.

MUSCLE CONTRACTION

Muscle tissue has a highly developed ability to contract. **Contractibility** enables a muscle to become shorter or thicker, and this ability, along with interaction with other muscles, produces movement of internal and external body parts. Muscle contraction in a tissue or organ produces motion and provides power and speed for body activity. A contracting muscle is referred to as a **prime mover**. A muscle that is relaxing while a prime mover is contracting is called the **antagonist**.

STIMULUS FOR CONTRACTION

All muscles respond to stimulus. This property is called **excitability** or **irritability**. The mechanical muscular action of shortening or thickening (also called contraction) is activated by a stimulus sent through a motor nerve. All muscles are linked to nerve fibers that carry messages from the central nervous system.

CONTRACTION AND RECOVERY

The chemical action of muscle fibers consists of two stages, **contraction** and **recovery**. In the contraction stage, two protein substances (actin and myosin) react to provide energy through the breakdown of glycogen into lactic acid. In the recovery stage, oxygen reacts with lactic acid to release carbon dioxide and water.

MUSCLE FATIGUE

When a muscle contracts, it produces chemical waste products (carbon dioxide, lactic acid, and acid phosphate) which make the muscle more irritable. If contraction is continued, the muscle will cramp and refuse to move. This condition is known as **fatigue**. If it is carried too far, the muscle cells will not recover and permanent damage will result. Muscles, therefore, need rest to allow the blood to carry away the waste materials and bring in fresh glucose, oxygen, and protein to restore the muscle protoplasm and the energy that was used.

TONICITY

Tonicity, or muscular tone, is a continual state of partial contraction that gives muscles a certain firmness. **Isometric** muscle contraction occurs when the muscle is stimulated and shortens, but no movement occurs, as when a person tenses his or her muscles against an immovable object. **Isotonic** muscle contraction occurs when the muscle is stimulated. The muscle shortens and movement occurs. An example would be lifting an object.

EXTENSIBILITY AND ELASTICITY

Muscles are also capable of stretching when force is applied (**extensibility**) and regaining their original form when that force is removed (**elasticity**).

MAINTENANCE OF MUSCLE TISSUE

During exercise, massage, or ordinary activities, the blood supply of muscles is increased. This additional blood brings in fresh nutritional material, carries away waste products more rapidly, and enables the muscles to build up and restore their efficiency and tone.

The importance of exercise for normal muscle activity is clear, but excessive muscle strain is damaging. For example, if a gasoline motor stands idle, it eventually becomes rusty and useless. Similarly, a muscle cell that does not work atrophies, becoming weak and decreasing in size. On the other hand, a motor that is never allowed to stop and is forced to run too fast or to do too much heavy work soon wears out so that it cannot be repaired. In the same way, a muscle cell that is forced to work too hard without proper rest will be damaged beyond repair.

When a muscle dies, it becomes solid and rigid and no longer reacts. This stiffening, which occurs from 10 minutes to several hours after death, is called **rigor mortis**.

MUSCLE TISSUES

There are three types of muscle tissue: skeletal, smooth, and cardiac. Each is designed to perform a specific function.

Skeletal

Skeletal, or striated, muscle tissues are attached to the bones and give shape to the body. They are responsible for allowing body movement. This type of muscle is sometimes referred to as **striated** because of the striped appearance of the muscle fibers under a microscope (fig. 1-9). They are also called **voluntary** muscles because they are under the control of our conscious will. These muscles can develop great power.

Smooth

Smooth, or nonstriated, muscle tissues are found in the walls of the stomach, intestines, urinary bladder, and blood vessels, as well as in the duct glands and in the skin. Under a microscope, the smooth muscle fiber lacks the striped appearance of other muscle tissue (fig. 1-10). This tissue is also called **involuntary** muscle because it is not under conscious control.

Cardiac

The cardiac muscle tissue forms the bulk of the walls and septa (or partitions) of the heart, as well as the origins of the large blood vessels. The fibers of the cardiac muscle differ from those of the skeletal and smooth muscles in that they are shorter and branch into a complicated network (fig. 1-11). The cardiac muscle has the most abundant blood supply of any muscle in the body, receiving twice the blood flow of the highly vascular skeletal muscles and far more than the smooth muscles. Cardiac muscles contract to pump blood out of the heart and through the cardiovascular system. Interference with the blood supply to the heart can result in a heart attack.

MAJOR SKELETAL MUSCLES

In the following section, the location, actions, origins, and insertions of some of the major skeletal muscles are covered. In figures 1-28 and 1-29 the superficial skeletal muscles are illustrated. Also note, the names of some of the muscles give you clues to their location, shape, and number of attachments.

Temporalis

The temporalis muscle is a fan-shaped muscle located on the side of the skull, above and in front of the ear. This muscle's fibers assist in raising the jaw and pass downward beneath the zygomatic arch to the mandible (fig. 1-29). The temporalis muscle's origin is the temporal bone. It is inserted in the coronoid process (a prominence of bone) of the mandible.

Masseter

The masseter muscle raises the mandible, or lower jaw, to close the mouth (fig. 1-28). It is the chewing muscle in the mastication of food. It originates in the zygomatic process and adjacent parts of the maxilla and is inserted in the mandible.

Sternocleidomastoid

The sternocleidomastoid muscles are located on both sides of the neck. Acting individually, these muscles rotate the head left or right (figs. 1-28 and 1-29). Acting together, they bend the head forward toward the chest. The sternocleidomastoid muscle originates in the sternum and clavicle and is inserted in the mastoid process of the temporal bone. When this muscle becomes damaged, the result is a common condition known as a "stiff neck."

Trapezius

The trapezius muscles are a broad, trapezium-shaped pair of muscles on the upper back, which raise or lower the shoulders (figs. 1-28 and 1-29). They cover approximately one-third of the back. They originate in a large area which includes the 12 thoracic vertebrae, the seventh cervical vertebra, and the occipital bone. They have their insertion in the clavicle and scapula.

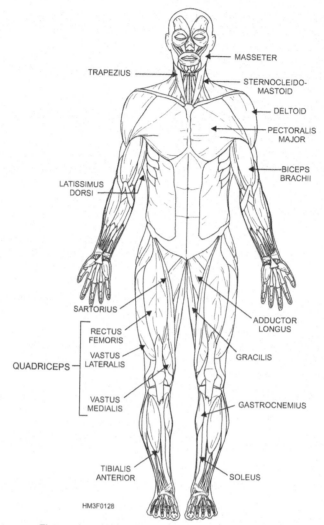

MASSETER

TRAPEZIUS

STERNOCLEIDO-MASTOID

DELTOID

PECTORALIS MAJOR

BICEPS BRACHII

LATISSIMUS DORSI

SARTORIUS

RECTUS FEMORIS

VASTUS LATERALIS

QUADRICEPS

VASTUS MEDIALIS

ADDUCTOR LONGUS

GRACILIS

GASTROCNEMIUS

TIBIALIS ANTERIOR

SOLEUS

HM3F0128

Figure 1-28.—Anterior view of superficial skeletal muscles.

Pectoralis Major

The pectoralis major is the large triangular muscle that forms the prominent chest muscle (fig. 1-28). It rotates the arm inward, pulls a raised arm down toward the chest, and draws the arm across the chest. It originates in the clavicle, sternum, and cartilages of the true ribs, and the external oblique muscle. Its insertion is in the greater tubercle of the humerus.

Deltoid

The deltoid muscle raises the arm and has its origin in the clavicle and the spine of the scapula (figs. 1-28 and 1-29). Its insertion is on the lateral side of the humerus. It fits like a cap over the shoulder and is a frequent site of intramuscular injections.

Biceps Brachii

The biceps brachii is the prominent muscle on the anterior surface of the upper arm (fig. 1-28). Its origin is in the outer edge of the glenoid cavity, and its insertion is in the tuberosity of the radius. This muscle rotates the forearm outward (supination) and, with the aid of the brachial muscle, flexes the forearm at the elbow.

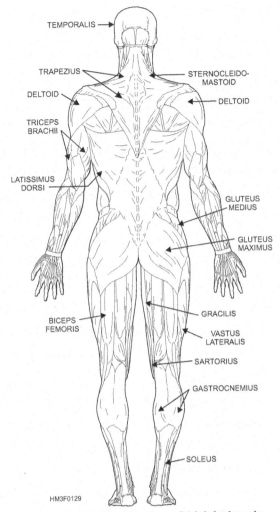

TEMPORALIS

TRAPEZIUS

DELTOID

TRICEPS
BRACHII

LATISSIMUS
DORSI

BICEPS
FEMORIS

STERNOCLEIDO-
MASTOID

DELTOID

GLUTEUS
MEDIUS

GLUTEUS
MAXIMUS

GRACILIS

VASTUS
LATERALIS

SARTORIUS

GASTROCNEMIUS

SOLEUS

HM3F0129

Figure 1-29.—Posterior view of superficial skeletal muscles.

Triceps Brachii

The triceps brachii is the primary extensor of the forearm (the antagonist of the biceps brachii) (fig. 1-29). It originates at two points on the humerus and one on the scapula. These three heads join to form the large muscle on the posterior surface of the upper arm. The point of insertion is the olecranon process of the ulna.

Latissimus Dorsi

The latissimus dorsi is a broad, flat muscle that covers approximately one-third of the back on each side (figs. 1-28 and 1-29). It rotates the arm inward and draws the arm down and back. It originates from the upper thoracic vertebrae to the sacrum and the posterior portion of the crest of the ilium. Its fibers converge to form a flat tendon that has its insertion in the humerus.

Gluteus

The gluteus (**maximus**, **minimus** (not shown), and **medius**) are the large muscles of the buttocks, which extend and laterally rotate the thigh, as well as abduct and medially rotate it (fig. 1-29). They arise from the ilium, the posterior surface of the lower sacrum, and the side of the coccyx. Their points of insertion include the greater trochanter and the gluteal tuberosity of the femur. The gluteus maximus is the site of choice for intramuscular injections.

Quadriceps

The quadriceps is a group of four muscles that make up the anterior portion of the thigh. The four muscles of this group are the **rectus femoris** that originates at the ilium; and the **vastus lateralis, v. medialis, v. intermedius** (not shown), that originate along the femur (fig. 1-28). All four are inserted into the tuberosity of the tibia through a tendon passing over the knee joint. The quadriceps serves as a strong extensor of the leg at the knee and flexes the thigh. Additionally located in the quadriceps area is the **adductor longus** that adducts, rotates, and flexes the thigh.

Biceps Femoris

The biceps femoris (often called the hamstring muscle) originates at the tuberosity of the ischium (the lowest portion of the coxal bone, part of the pelvic girdle) and the middle third of the femur (fig. 1-29). It is inserted on the head of the fibula and the lateral condyle of the tibia. It acts, along with other related muscles, to flex the leg at the knee and to extend the thigh at the hip joint.

Gracilis

The gracilis is a long slender muscle located on the inner aspect of the thigh (figs. 1-28 and 1-29). It adducts the thigh, and flexes and medially rotates the leg. Its origin is in the symphysis pubis, and its insertion is in the medial surface of the tibia, below the condyle.

Sartorius

The sartorius is the longest muscle in the body. It extends diagonally across the front of the thigh from its origin at the ilium, down to its insertion near the tuberosity of the tibia (fig. 1-29). Its function is to flex the thigh and rotate it laterally, and to flex the leg and rotate it slightly medially.

Gastrocnemius and Soleus

The gastrocnemius and soleus (together commonly called the calf muscles) extend the foot at the ankle (figs. 1-28 and 1-29). The gastrocnemius originates at two points on the femur; the soleus originates at the head of the fibula and the medial border of the tibia. Both are inserted in a common tendon called the calcaneus, or Achilles tendon.

Tibialis Anterior

The tibialis anterior originates at the upper half of the tibia and inserts at the first metatarsal and cuneiform bones (fig. 1-28). It flexes the foot.

Diaphragm

The diaphragm (not shown) is an internal (as opposed to superficial) muscle that forms the floor of the thoracic cavity and the ceiling of the abdominal cavity. It is the primary muscle of respiration, modifying the size of the thorax and abdomen vertically. It has three openings for the passage of nerves and blood vessels.

THE INTEGUMENTARY SYSTEM

LEARNING OBJECTIVE: *Identify skin, its functions, structure, and appendages.*

Organ systems are comprised of tissues grouped together to form organs, and groups of organs with specialized functions. Since the skin acts with hair follicles, sebaceous glands, and sweat glands, these organs together constitute the integumentary system.

SKIN FUNCTION

The skin covers almost every visible part of the human body. Even the hair and nails are outgrowths from it. It protects the underlying structures from injury and invasion by foreign organisms; it contains the peripheral endings of many sensory nerves; and it has limited excretory and absorbing powers. The skin also plays an important part in regulating body temperature. In addition, the skin is a waterproof covering that prevents excessive water loss, even in very dry climates.

SKIN STRUCTURE

The skin, or integument, consists of two layers, the epidermis and the dermis, and supporting structures and appendages (fig. 1-30).

Epidermis

The epidermis is the outer skin layer (fig. 1-30). It is made up of tough, flat, scalelike epithelial cells. Five sublayers or strata of epidermal cells have been identified, and, listed from superficial to deep, they are

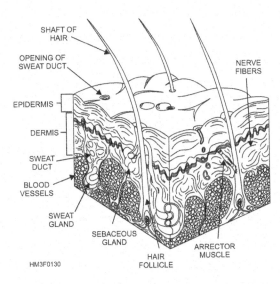

SHAFT OF HAIR

OPENING OF SWEAT DUCT

NERVE FIBERS

EPIDERMIS

DERMIS

SWEAT DUCT

BLOOD VESSELS

SWEAT GLAND

SEBACEOUS GLAND

HAIR FOLLICLE

ARRECTOR MUSCLE

HM3F0130

Figure 1-30.—Cross section of the skin.

the **stratum corneum**, **stratum lucidum** (not always present), **stratum granulosum**, **stratum spinosum**, and **stratum basale**.

Dermis

The dermis, or true skin, lies below the epidermis and gradually blends into the deeper tissues (fig. 1-30). It is a wide area of connective tissue that contains blood vessels, nerve fibers, smooth muscles, and skin appendages.

BLOOD VESSELS.—The blood vessels of the dermis can dilate to contain a significant portion of the body's blood supply (fig. 1-30). This ability, along with the actions of the sweat glands, forms the body's primary temperature-regulating mechanism. The constriction or dilation of these blood vessels also affects blood pressure and the volume of blood available to the internal organs.

NERVE FIBERS.—The skin contains two types of nerve fibers that carry impulses to and from the central nervous system (fig. 1-30). The nerve fibers are distributed to the smooth muscles in the walls of the arteries in the dermis and to the smooth muscles around the sweat glands and hair roots. The first type of nerve fiber carries impulses to the dermal muscles and glands, while the other type carries impulses from sensory receptors (i.e., detecting touch). Both nerve fibers send messages about the external environment to the brain.

SMOOTH MUSCLES.—Smooth involuntary muscles are found in the dermis. They are responsible for controlling the skin surface area. When dilated, these muscles allow for maximum skin surface exposure to aid heat loss. When constricted, the skin surface exposure is decreased, thus impeding heat radiation. Repeated muscle contractions (shivering) are also a rapid means of generating body heat.

Skin Appendages

The appendages of the skin are the nails, hairs, sebaceous glands, sweat glands, and ceruminous glands.

NAILS.—The nails are composed of horny epidermal scales and are found on the dorsal surfaces of the fingers and toes. They protect the many sensitive nerve endings at the ends of these digits. New formation of nail will occur in the epithelium of the nail bed. As a new nail is formed, the whole nail moves forward, becoming longer.

HAIR.—Hair is an epithelial structure found on almost every part of the surface of the body (fig. 1-30). Its color depends on the type of melanin present. The hair has two components: the root below the surface and the shaft projecting above the skin. The root is embedded in a pit-like depression called the hair follicle. Hair grows as a result of the division of the cells of the root. A small muscle, known as the **arrector** (fig. 1-30), fastens to the side of the follicle and is responsible for the gooseflesh appearance of the skin as a reaction to cold or fear. Each hair follicle is associated with two or more sebaceous glands.

SEBACEOUS GLANDS.—Sebaceous glands are found in most parts of the skin except in the soles of the feet and the palms of the hand (fig. 1-30). Their ducts open most frequently into the hair follicles and secrete an oily substance that lubricates the skin and hair, keeping them soft and pliable and preventing bacterial invasion.

SWEAT GLANDS.—Sweat glands are found in almost every part of the skin (fig. 1-30). They are control mechanisms to reduce the body's heat by evaporating water from its surface. The perspiration secreted is a combination of water, salts, amino acids, and urea. Normally, about one liter of this fluid is excreted daily. However, the amount varies with atmospheric temperature and humidity and the amount of exercise taken. When the outside temperature is high, or upon exercise, the glands secrete large amounts to cool the body through evaporation. When evaporation does not remove all the sweat that has been excreted, the sweat collects in beads on the surface of the skin.

CERUMINOUS GLANDS.—Ceruminous glands are modified sweat glands found only in the auditory canal. They secrete a yellow, waxy substance called **cerumen** that protects the eardrum.

THE CIRCULATORY SYSTEM

LEARNING OBJECTIVE: *Identify the parts of the circulatory system, and recognize their major components and functions.*

The circulatory system, also called the **vascular system**, consists of blood, heart, and blood vessels. The circulatory system is close circuited (i.e., there is no opening to external environment of the body). The function of this system is to move blood between the cells and the organs of the integumentary, digestive, respiratory, and urinary system that communicate with the external environment of the body. This function is facilitated by the heart pumping blood through blood vessels. The blood travels throughout the body transporting nutrients and wastes, and permitting the exchange of gases (carbon dioxide and oxygen).

BLOOD

Blood is fluid tissue composed of formed elements (i.e., cells) suspended in plasma. It is pumped by the heart through arteries, capillaries, and veins to all parts of the body. Total blood volume of the average adult is 5 to 6 liters.

Plasma

Plasma is the liquid part of blood (fig. 1-31). Plasma constitutes 55 percent of whole blood (plasma and cells). It is a clear, slightly alkaline, straw-colored liquid consisting of about 92 percent water. The remainder is made up mainly of proteins. One of these proteins, **fibrinogen**, contributes to coagulation.

Blood Cells

The blood cells suspended in the plasma constitute 45 percent of whole blood. Its cells, which are formed mostly in red bone marrow, include red blood cells (RBCs) and white blood cells (WBCs). The blood also contains cellular fragments called blood platelets.

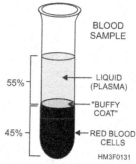

Figure 1-31.—Blood sample illustrating blood components.

When blood components are separated, the WBCs and platelets form a thin layer, called the **buffy coat**, between the layers of plasma and RBCs. These layers are illustrated in figure 1-31.

RED BLOOD CELLS.—Red blood cells, or **erythrocytes**, are small, biconcave, nonnucleated disks, formed in the red bone marrow (fig. 1-32). Blood of the average man contains 5 million red cells per cubic millimeter. Women have fewer red cells, 4.5 million per cubic millimeter. Emotional stress, strenuous exercise, high altitudes, and some diseases may cause an increase in the number of RBCs.

During the development of the red blood cell, a substance called **hemoglobin** is combined with it. Hemoglobin is the key of the red cell's ability to carry oxygen and carbon dioxide. Thus, the main function of erythrocytes is the transportation of respiratory gases. The red cells deliver oxygen to the body tissues, holding some oxygen in reserve for an emergency. Carbon dioxide is picked up by the same cells and discharged via the lungs.

The color of the red blood cell is determined by the hemoglobin content. Bright red (arterial) blood is due to the combination of oxygen and hemoglobin. Dark

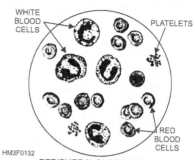

Figure 1-32.—A blood smear showing red blood cells, white blood cells, and platelets.

red (venous) blood is the result of hemoglobin combining with carbon dioxide.

Red blood cells live only about 100 to 120 days in the body. There are several reasons for their short life span. These delicate cells have to withstand constant knocking around as they are pumped into the arteries by the heart. These cells travel through blood vessels at high speed, bumping into other cells, bouncing off the walls of arteries and veins, and squeezing through narrow passages. They must adjust to continual pressure changes. The spleen is the "graveyard" where old, worn out cells are removed from the blood stream. Fragments of red blood cells are found in the spleen and other body tissues.

WHITE BLOOD CELLS.—White blood cells, or leukocytes, are almost colorless, nucleated cells originating in the bone marrow and in certain lymphoid tissues of the body (fig. 1-32). There is only one white cell to every 600 red cells. Normal WBC count is 6,000 to 8,000 per cubic millimeter, although the number of white cells may be 15,000 to 20,000 or higher during infection.

Leukocytes are important for the protection of the body against disease. Leukocytes can squeeze between the cells that form blood cell walls. This movement, called diapedesis, permits them to leave the blood stream through the capillary wall and attack pathogenic bacteria. They can travel anywhere in the body and are often named "the wandering cells." They protect the body tissues by engulfing disease-bearing bacteria and foreign matter, a process called phagocytosis. When white cells are undermanned, more are produced, causing an increase in their number and a condition known as leukocytosis. Another way WBC's protect the body from disease is by producing bacteriolysins that dissolve the foreign bacteria. The secondary function of WBCs is to aid in blood clotting.

BLOOD PLATELETS.—Blood platelets, or thrombocytes, are irregular- or oval-shaped discs in the blood that contain no nucleus, only cytoplasm (fig. 1-32). They are smaller than red blood cells and average about 250,000 per cubic millimeter of blood. Blood platelets play an important role in the process of blood coagulation, clumping together in the presence of jagged, torn tissue.

Blood Coagulation

To protect the body from excessive blood loss, blood has its own power to coagulate, or clot. If blood components and linings of vessels are normal, circulating blood will not clot. Once blood escapes from its vessels, however, a chemical reaction begins that causes it to become solid. Initially a blood clot is a fluid, but soon it becomes thick and then sets into a soft jelly that quickly becomes firm enough to act as a plug. This plug is the result of a swift, sure mechanism that changes one of the soluble blood proteins, fibrinogen, into an insoluble protein, fibrin, whenever injury occurs.

Other necessary elements for blood clotting are calcium salts; a substance called prothrombin, which is formed in the liver; blood platelets; and various factors necessary for the completion of the successive steps in the coagulation process. Once the fibrin plug is formed, it quickly enmeshes red and white blood cells and draws them tightly together. Blood serum, a yellowish clear liquid, is squeezed out of the clot as the mass shrinks. Formation of the clot closes the wound, preventing blood loss. A clot also serves as a network for the growth of new tissues in the process of healing. Normal clotting time is 3 to 5 minutes, but if any of the substances necessary for clotting are absent, severe bleeding will occur.

Hemophilia is an inherited disease characterized by delayed clotting of the blood and consequent difficulty in controlling hemorrhage. Hemophiliacs can bleed to death as a result of minor wounds.

THE HEART

The heart is a hollow, muscular organ, somewhat larger than the closed fist, located anteriorly in the chest and to the left of the midline. It is shaped like a cone, its base directed upward and to the right, the apex down and to the left. Lying obliquely in the chest, much of the base of the heart is immediately posterior to the sternum.

Heart Composition

The heart is enclosed in a membranous sac, the pericardium. The smooth surfaces of the heart and pericardium are lubricated by a serous secretion called pericardial fluid. The inner surface of the heart is lined with a delicate serous membrane, the endocardium, similar to and continuous with that of the inner lining of blood vessels.

The interior of the heart (fig. 1-33) is divided into two parts by a wall called the interventricular septum. In each half is an upper chamber, the atrium, which receives blood from the veins, and a lower chamber, the ventricle, which receives blood from the

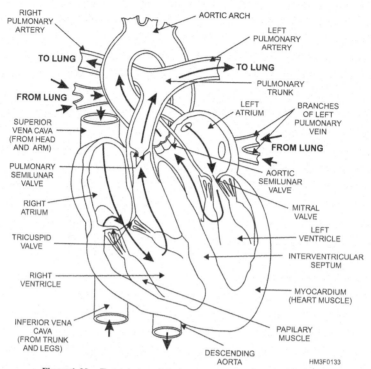

RIGHT PULMONARY ARTERY

AORTIC ARCH

LEFT PULMONARY ARTERY

TO LUNG

TO LUNG

FROM LUNG

PULMONARY TRUNK

LEFT ATRIUM

BRANCHES OF LEFT PULMONARY VEIN

SUPERIOR VENA CAVA (FROM HEAD AND ARM)

FROM LUNG

PULMONARY SEMILUNAR VALVE

AORTIC SEMILUNAR VALVE

RIGHT ATRIUM

MITRAL VALVE

LEFT VENTRICLE

TRICUSPID VALVE

INTERVENTRICULAR SEPTUM

RIGHT VENTRICLE

MYOCARDIUM (HEART MUSCLE)

INFERIOR VENA CAVA (FROM TRUNK AND LEGS)

PAPILARY MUSCLE

DESCENDING AORTA

HM3F0133

Figure 1-33.—Frontal view of the heart—arrows indicate blood flow.

atrium and pumps it out into the arteries. The openings between the chambers on each side of the heart are separated by flaps of tissue that act as valves to prevent backward flow of blood. The valve on the right has three flaps, or cusps, and is called the **tricuspid valve**. The valve on the left has two flaps and is called the **mitral**, or **bicuspid**, **valve**. The outlets of the ventricles are supplied with similar valves. In the right ventricle, the **pulmonary valve** is at the origin of the pulmonary artery. In the left ventricle, the **aortic valve** is at the origin of the aorta. See figure 1-33 for valve locations.

The heart muscle, the **myocardium**, is striated like the skeletal muscles of the body, but involuntary in action, like the smooth muscles. The walls of the atria are thin with relatively little muscle fiber because the blood flows from the atria to the ventricles under low pressure. However, the walls of the ventricles, which comprise the bulk of the heart, are thick and muscular. The wall of the left ventricle is considerably thicker than that of the right, because more force is required to pump the blood into distant or outlying locations of the circulatory system than into the lungs located only a short distance from the heart.

Heart Functions

The heart acts as four interrelated pumps. The right atrium receives deoxygenated blood from the body via the **superior** and **inferior vena cava**. It pumps the deoxygenated blood through the tricuspid valve to the right ventricle. The right ventricle pumps the blood past the pulmonary valve through the **pulmonary artery** to the lungs, where it is oxygenated. The left atrium receives the oxygenated blood from the lungs through four **pulmonary veins** and pumps it to the left ventricle past the mitral valve. The left ventricle pumps the blood to all areas of the body via the aortic valve and the **aorta**.

The heart's constant contracting and relaxing forces blood into the arteries. Each contraction is followed by limited relaxation or dilation. Cardiac muscle never completely relaxes: It always maintains a degree of tone. Contraction of the heart is called **systole** or "the period of work." Relaxation of the heart is called **diastole** or "the period of rest." A complete cardiac cycle is the time from onset of one contraction, or heart beat, to the onset of the next.

Cardiac Cycle

The cardiac cycle is coordinated by specialized tissues that initiate and distribute electrical (cardiac) impulses (fig. 1-34). The contractions of the heart are stimulated and maintained by the **sinoatrial (SA) node**, commonly called the **pacemaker** of the heart. The SA node is an elongated mass of specialized muscle tissue located in the upper part of the right atrium. The SA node sets off cardiac impulses, causing both atria to contract simultaneously. The normal heart rate, or number of contractions, is about 70 to 80 beats per minute.

This same cardiac impulse continues to travel to another group of specialized tissue called the **atrioventricular (AV) node**. The AV node is located in the floor of the right atrium near the septum that separates the atria. The cardiac impulse to the AV node is slowed down by **junctional fibers**. The junctional fibers conduct the cardiac impulse to the AV node; however, these fibers are very small in diameter, causing the impulse to be delayed. This slow arrival of the impulse to the AV node allows time for the atria to empty and the ventricles to fill with blood.

Once the cardiac impulse reaches the far side of the AV node, it quickly passes through a group of large fibers which make up the AV bundle (also called the bundle of His). The AV bundle starts at the upper part of the interventricular septum and divides into right and left branches. About halfway down the interventricular septum, the right and left branches terminate into **Purkinje fibers**. The Purkinje fibers spread from the interventricular septum into the papillary muscles, which project inward from the ventricular walls. As the cardiac impulse passes through the Purkinje fibers, these fibers in turn stimulate the cardiac muscle of the ventricles. This stimulation of the cardiac muscles causes the walls of the ventricles to contract with a twisting motion. This action squeezes the blood out of the ventricular chambers and forces it into the arteries. This is the conclusion of one cardiac cycle.

Blood Pressure

Blood pressure is the pressure the blood exerts on the walls of the arteries. The highest pressure is called **systolic** pressure, because it is caused when the heart is in systole, or contraction. A certain amount of blood pressure is maintained in the arteries even when the heart is relaxed. This pressure is the **diastolic** pressure, because it is present during diastole, or relaxation of the heart. The difference between systolic and diastolic pressure is known as **pulse pressure**.

Normal blood pressure can vary considerably with an individual's age, weight, and general condition. For young adults, the systolic pressure is normally between 120 and 150 mm of mercury, and the diastolic pressure is normally between 70 and 90 mm of mercury. On average, women have lower blood pressure than men.

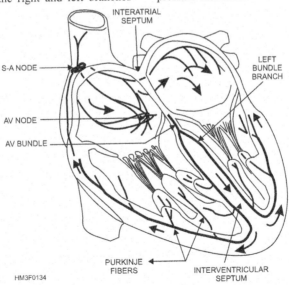

Figure 1-34.—Cardiac cycle.

BLOOD VESSELS

Blood vessels form a closed circuit of tubes that transport blood between the heart and body cells. The several types of blood vessels include arteries, arterioles, capillaries, venules, and veins.

Blood Vessel Classifications

The blood vessels of the body fall into three classifications:

- **Arteries and arterioles**—distributors
- **Capillaries**—exchangers
- **Veins and venules**—collectors

Arteries and Arterioles

Arteries are elastic tubes constructed to withstand high pressure. They carry blood away from the heart to all parts of the body. The smallest branches of the arteries are called **arterioles**. The walls of arteries and arterioles consist of layers of endothelium, smooth muscle, and connective tissue. The smooth muscles of arteries and arterioles constrict and dilate in response to electrical impulses received from the autonomic nervous system.

Capillaries

At the end of the arterioles is a system of minute vessels that vary in structure, but which are spoken of collectively as capillaries. It is from these capillaries that the tissues of the body are fed. There are approximately 60,000 miles of capillaries in the body. As the blood passes through the capillaries, it releases oxygen and nutritive substances to the tissues and takes up various waste products to be carried away by **venules**. Venules continue from capillaries and merge to form veins.

Veins and Venules

Veins and venules form the venous system. The venous system is comprised of vessels that collect blood from the capillaries and carry it back to the heart. Veins begin as tiny venules formed from the capillaries. Joining together as tiny rivulets, veins connect and form a small stream. The force of muscles contracting adjacent to veins aids in the forward propulsion of blood on its return to the heart. Valves, spaced frequently along the larger veins, prevent the backflow of blood. The walls of veins are similar to arteries, but are thinner and contain less muscle and elastic tissue.

Arterial System

Arterial circulation is responsible for taking freshly oxygenated blood from the heart to the cells of the body (fig. 1-35). To take this oxygenated blood from the heart to the entire body, the arterial system begins with the contraction of blood from the left ventricle into the aorta and its branches.

AORTA.—The aorta, largest artery in the body, is a large tube-like structure arising from the left ventricle of the heart. It arches upward over the left lung and then down along the spinal column through the thorax and the abdomen, where it divides and sends arteries down both legs (fig. 1-35).

KEY BRANCHES OF THE AORTA.—Key arterial branches of the aorta are the coronary, innominate (brachiocephalic), left common carotid, and left subclavian. The coronary arteries are branches of what is called the **ascending aorta**. The coronary arteries supply the heart with blood. There are three large arteries that arise from the aorta as it arches over the left lung. First is the **innominate artery**, which divides into the **right subclavian artery** to supply the right arm, and the **right common carotid** to supply the right side of the head. The second branch is the **left common carotid**, which supplies the left side of the head. The third branch is the **left subclavian**, which supplies the left arm.

ARTERIES OF THE HEAD, NECK, AND BRAIN.—The **carotid arteries** divide into internal and external branches, the external supplying the muscle and skin of the face and the internal supplying the brain and the eyes.

ARTERIES OF THE UPPER EXTREM-ITIES.—The **subclavian arteries** are so named because they run underneath the clavicle. They supply the upper extremities, branching off to the back, chest, neck, and brain through the spinal column (fig. 1-35).

The large artery going to the arm is called the **axillary**. The axillary artery becomes the **brachial artery** as it travels down the arm and divides into the **ulnar** and **radial arteries**. The radial artery is the artery at the wrist that you feel when you take the pulse of your patient (fig. 1-35).

ARTERIES OF THE ABDOMEN.—In the abdomen, the aorta gives off branches to the abdominal viscera, including the stomach, liver, spleen, kidneys,

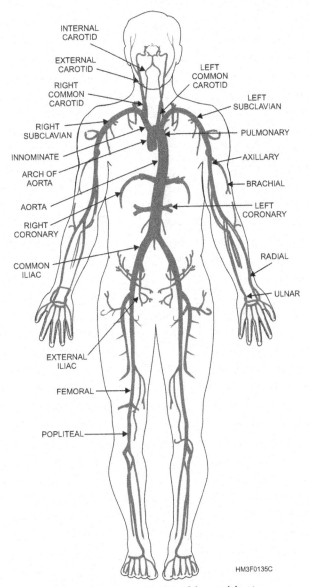

INTERNAL
CAROTID

EXTERNAL
CAROTID

RIGHT
COMMON
CAROTID

LEFT
COMMON
CAROTID

LEFT
SUBCLAVIAN

RIGHT
SUBCLAVIAN

PULMONARY

INNOMINATE

AXILLARY

ARCH OF
AORTA

BRACHIAL

AORTA

LEFT
CORONARY

RIGHT
CORONARY

COMMON
ILIAC

RADIAL

ULNAR

EXTERNAL
ILIAC

FEMORAL

POPLITEAL

HM3F0135C

Figure 1-35.—Principal vessels of the arterial system.

and intestines. The aorta later divides into the **left** and **right common iliacs**, which supply the lower extremities (fig. 1-35).

ARTERIES OF THE LOWER EXTREM- ITIES.—The left and right common iliacs, upon entering the thigh, become the **femoral artery**. At the knee, this same vessel is named the **popliteal artery** (fig. 1-35).

Venous System

Venous circulation is responsible for returning the blood to the heart after exchanges of gases, nutrients, and wastes have occurred between the blood and body cells (fig. 1-36). To return this blood to the heart for reoxygenation, the venous system begins with the merging of capillaries into venules, venules into small veins, and small veins into larger veins. The blood vessel paths of the venous system are difficult to

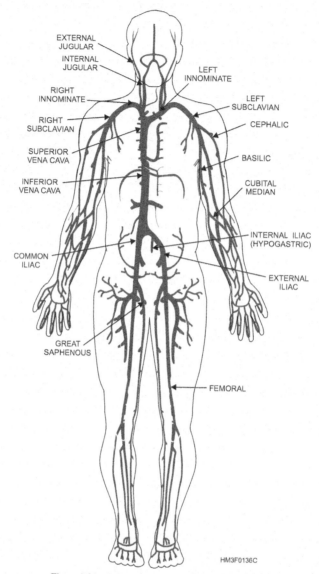

EXTERNAL JUGULAR
INTERNAL JUGULAR
LEFT INNOMINATE
RIGHT INNOMINATE
LEFT SUBCLAVIAN
RIGHT SUBCLAVIAN
CEPHALIC
SUPERIOR VENA CAVA
BASILIC
INFERIOR VENA CAVA
CUBITAL MEDIAN
INTERNAL ILIAC (HYPOGASTRIC)
COMMON ILIAC
EXTERNAL ILIAC
GREAT SAPHENOUS
FEMORAL

HM3F0136C

Figure 1-36.—Principal vessels of the venous system.

follow, unlike the arterial system. However, the larger veins are commonly located parallel to the course taken by their counterpart in the arterial system. For instance, the renal vein parallels the renal artery, the common iliac vein parallels the common iliac artery, and so forth.

THREE PRINCIPAL VENOUS SYSTEMS.—

The three principal venous systems in the body are the **pulmonary, portal**, and **systemic**.

• The **pulmonary system** is composed of four vessels, two from each lung, which empty into the left atrium. These are the only veins in the body that carry freshly oxygenated blood.

• The **portal system** consists of the veins that drain venous blood from the abdominal part of the digestive tract—the spleen, pancreas, and gallbladder, but not the lower rectum—and deliver it to the liver. There, it is distributed by a set of venous capillaries. The blood in the portal system conveys absorbed substances from the intestinal tract to the liver for storage,

1-30

alteration, or detoxification. From the liver the blood flows through the hepatic vein to the inferior vena cava.

• The **systemic system** is divided into the deep and superficial veins. The superficial veins lie immediately under the skin, draining the skin and superficial structures. The deep veins, usually located in the muscle or deeper layers, drain the large muscle masses and various other organs. Deep veins commonly lie close to the large arteries that supply the various organs of the body and typically have the same name as the artery they accompany.

VEINS OF THE HEAD, NECK, AND BRAIN.—The superficial veins of the head unite to form the **external jugular veins**. The external jugular veins drain blood from the scalp, face, and neck, and finally empty into the **subclavian veins**.

The veins draining the brain and internal facial structures are the **internal jugular veins**. These combine with the subclavian veins to form the **innominate veins**, which empty into the **superior vena cava** (fig. 1-36).

VEINS OF THE UPPER EXTREMITIES.—The veins of the upper extremities begin at the hand and extend upward. A vein of great interest to you is the **median cubital**, which crosses the anterior surface of the elbow. It is the vein most commonly used for venipuncture. Also found in this area are the **basilic** and **cephalic veins,** which extend from the midarm to the shoulder.

The deep veins of the upper arm unite to form the **axillary vein**, which unites with the superficial veins to form the subclavian vein. This vein later unites with other veins to form the innominate and eventually, after union with still more veins, the superior vena cava (fig. 1-36).

VEINS OF THE ABDOMEN AND THORACIC REGION.—The veins from the abdominal organs, with the exception of those of the portal system, empty directly or indirectly into the **inferior vena cava**, while those of the thoracic region eventually empty into the superior vena cava (fig. 1-36).

VEINS OF THE LOWER EXTREMTIES.—In the lower extremities (fig. 1-36), a similar system drains the superficial areas. The **great saphenous vein** originates on the inner aspect of the foot and extends up the inside of the leg and thigh to join the **femoral vein** in the upper thigh. The great saphenous vein is used for intravenous injections at the ankle.

The veins from the lower extremities unite to form the femoral vein in the thigh, which becomes the **external iliac vein** in the groin. Higher in this region, external iliac unites the **internal iliac** (hypogastric) **vein** from the lower pelvic region to form the **common iliac veins**. The right and left common iliac veins unite to form the inferior vena cava.

THE LYMPHATIC SYSTEM

LEARNING OBJECTIVE: *Identify the parts of the lymphatic system and their function.*

All tissue cells of the body are continuously bathed in **interstitial fluid**. This fluid is formed by leakage of blood plasma through minute pores of the capillaries. There is a continual interchange of fluids of the blood and tissue spaces with a free interchange of nutrients and other dissolved substances. Most of the tissue fluid returns to the circulatory system by means of capillaries, which feed into larger veins. Large protein molecules that have escaped from the arterial capillaries cannot reenter the circulation through the small pores of the capillaries. However, these large molecules, as well as white blood cells, dead cells, bacterial debris, infected substances, and larger particulate matter, can pass through the larger pores of the lymphatic capillaries and, thus, enter the lymphatic circulatory system with the remainder of the tissue fluid.

The lymphatic system also helps defend the tissues against infections by supporting the activities of the **lymphocytes**, which give immunity, or resistance, to the effects of specific disease-causing agents.

PATHWAYS OF THE LYMPHATIC SYSTEM

The lymphatic pathway begins with lymphatic capillaries. These small tubes merge to form lymphatic vessels, and the lymphatic vessels in turn lead to larger vessels that join with the veins in the thorax.

Lymphatic Capillaries

Lymphatic capillaries are closed-ended tubes of microscopic size (fig. 1-37). They extend into interstitial spaces, forming complex networks that parallel blood capillary networks. The lymphatic capillary wall consists of a single layer of squamous epithelial cells. This thin wall makes it possible for interstitial fluid to enter the lymphatic capillary. Once

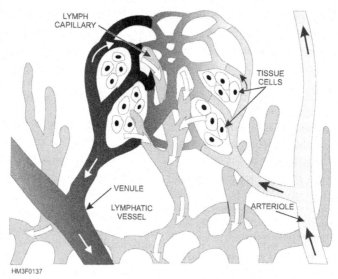

LYMPH
CAPILLARY

TISSUE
CELLS

VENULE

LYMPHATIC
VESSEL

ARTERIOLE

HM3F0137

Figure 1-37.—Lymphatic capillary and vessel.

the interstitial fluid enters the lymphatic capillaries, the fluid is called **lymph**.

Lymphatic Vessels

Lymphatic vessels are formed from the merging of lymphatic capillaries (fig. 1-37). Lymphatic vessels, also known simply as **lymphatics**, are similar to veins in structure. The vessel walls are composed of three layers: an inner layer of endothelial tissue, a middle layer of smooth muscle and elastic fibers, and an outer layer of connective tissue. Like a vein, the lymphatic vessel has valves to prevent backflow of lymph. The larger lymphatic vessels lead to specialized organs called lymph nodes. After leaving these structures, the vessels merge to form still larger lymphatic trunks.

Lymphatic Trunks and Ducts

Lymphatic trunks drain lymph from large regions in the body. The lymphatic trunks are usually named after the region they serve, such as the subclavian trunk that drains the arm. There are many lymphatic trunks through out the body. These lymphatic trunks then join one of two collecting ducts, the **thoracic duct** and the **right lymphatic duct** (fig. 1-38).

Lymphatic trunks from the upper half of the right side of the body converge to form the right lymphatic duct, which empties into the right subclavian vein. Drainage from the remainder of the body is by way of the thoracic duct, which empties into the left subclavian vein.

LYMPH NODES

Lymph nodes, which are frequently called glands but are not true glands, are small bean-shaped bodies of lymphatic tissue found in groups of two to fifteen along the course of the lymph vessels (fig. 1-38). Major locations of lymph nodes are in the following regions: cervical, axillary, inguinal, pelvic cavity, abdominal cavity, and thoracic cavity. Lymph nodes vary in size and act as filters to remove bacteria and particles from the lymph stream. Lymph nodes produce lymphocytes, which help defend the body against harmful foreign particles, such as bacteria, cells, and viruses. Lymph nodes also contain **macrophages**, which engulf and destroy foreign substances, damaged cells, and cellular debris.

THE RESPIRATORY SYSTEM

LEARNING OBJECTIVE: *Identify the location and function of each part of the respiratory system, and recall the process of respiration.*

Respiration is the exchange of oxygen and carbon dioxide between the atmosphere and the cells of the body. There are two phases of respiration:

• **Physical**, or **mechanical**, **respiration** involves the motion of the diaphragm and rib cage. The

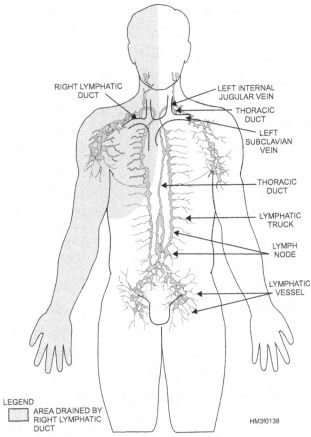

RIGHT LYMPHATIC
DUCT

LEFT INTERNAL
JUGULAR VEIN

THORACIC
DUCT

LEFT
SUBCLAVIAN
VEIN

THORACIC
DUCT

LYMPHATIC
TRUCK

LYMPH
NODE

LYMPHATIC
VESSEL

LEGEND

AREA DRAINED BY
RIGHT LYMPHATIC
DUCT

HM3f0138

Figure 1-38.—Pathway of right lymphatic duct and thoracic duct.

musculoskeletal action, which resembles that of a bellows, causes air to be inhaled or exhaled.

• **Physiological respiration** involves an exchange of gases, oxygen and carbon dioxide, at two points in the body. The first is the transfer that occurs in the lungs between the incoming oxygen and the carbon dioxide present in the capillaries of the lungs (external respiration). The second transfer occurs when oxygen brought into the body replaces carbon dioxide build up in the cellular tissue (internal respiration).

Normally, oxygen and carbon dioxide exchange in equal volumes; however, certain physiological conditions may throw this balance off. For example, heavy smokers will find that the ability of their lungs to exchange gases is impaired, leading to shortness of breath and fatigue during even slight physical exertion. This debilitating situation is the direct result of their inability to draw a sufficient amount of oxygen into the body to replace the carbon dioxide build-up and

sustain further muscular exertion. On the other hand, hyperventilation brings too much oxygen into the body, overloading the system with oxygen, and depleting the carbon dioxide needed for balance.

ANATOMY OF THE RESPIRATORY SYSTEM

Air enters the nasal chambers and the mouth, then passes through the pharynx, larynx, trachea, and bronchi into the bronchioles. Each bronchiole is surrounded by a cluster of alveoli (fig. 1-39).

Nasal Cavity

Air enters the nasal cavity through the nostrils (**nares**). Lining the nasal passages are hairs, which, together with the mucous membrane, entrap and filter out dust and other minute particles that could irritate the lungs. Incoming air is warmed and moistened in the

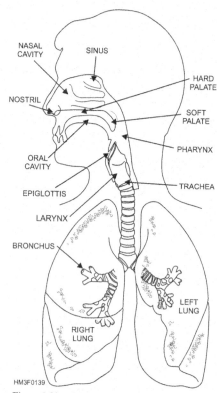

NASAL CAVITY

SINUS

HARD PALATE

NOSTRIL

SOFT PALATE

PHARYNX

ORAL CAVITY

TRACHEA

EPIGLOTTIS

LARYNX

BRONCHUS

LEFT LUNG

RIGHT LUNG

HM3F0139

Figure 1-39.—Organs of the respiratory system.

chambers of the nasal cavity to prevent damage to the lungs. The nasal and oral cavities are separated by the **palate**. The anterior, rigid portion is called the **hard palate**, and the posterior fleshy part is called the **soft palate**. The mouth and nose serve as secondary respiratory structures.

Pharynx

The pharynx, or throat, serves both the respiratory and digestive systems and aids in speech. It has a mucous membrane lining that traps microscopic particles in the air and aids in adjusting temperature and humidifying inspired (inhaled) air. The pharynx connects with the mouth and nasal chambers posteriorly. According to its location, the pharynx is referred to as the **nasopharynx** posterior to the nasal chambers), the **oropharynx** (posterior to the mouth), or the **laryngopharynx** (posterior to the pharynx).

Epiglottis

The epiglottis is a lidlike, cartilaginous structure that covers the entrance to the larynx and separates it from the pharynx. It acts as a trap door to deflect food particles and liquids from the entrance to the larynx and trachea.

Larynx

The larynx, or voice box, is a triangular cartilaginous structure located between the tongue and the trachea. It is protected anteriorly by the thyroid cartilage (commonly called the Adam's apple), which is usually larger and more prominent in men than in women. During the act of swallowing, it is pulled upward and forward toward the base of the tongue. The larynx is responsible for the production of vocal sound (voice). This sound production is accomplished by the passing of air over the vocal cords. The ensuing vibrations can be controlled to produce the sounds of speech or singing. The nose, mouth, throat, bone sinuses, and chest serve as resonating chambers to further refine and individualize the voice.

Trachea

The trachea, or windpipe, begins at the lower end of the larynx and terminates by dividing into the right and left bronchi. It is a long tube composed of 16 to 20 C-shaped cartilaginous rings, embedded in a fibrous membrane, that support its walls, preventing their collapse (fig. 1-39).

The trachea has a ciliated mucous membrane lining that entraps dust and foreign material. It also propels secretions and exudates from the lungs to the pharynx, where they can be expectorated.

Bronchi

The bronchi are the terminal branches of the trachea, which carry air to each lung and further divide into the bronchioles.

Bronchioles

The bronchioles are much smaller than the bronchi and lack supporting rings of cartilage. They terminate at the alveoli (fig. 1-40).

Alveoli

The alveoli are thin, microscopic air sacs within the lungs (fig. 1-40). They are in direct contact with the pulmonary capillaries. It is here that fresh oxygen exchanges with carbon dioxide by means of a diffusion process through the alveolar and capillary cell walls

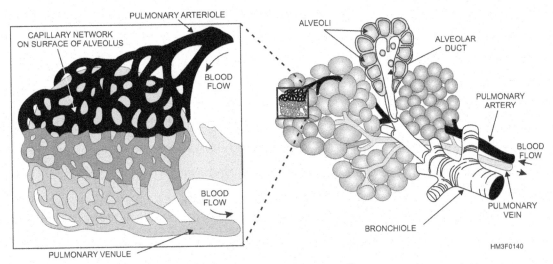

Figure 1-40.—Bronchiole and alveoli.

HM3F0140

(fig. 1-41). The **lungs** are cone-shaped organs that lie in the thoracic cavity. Each lung contains thousands of alveoli with their capillaries. The right lung is larger than the left lung and is divided into superior, middle, and inferior lobes. The left lung has two lobes, the superior and the inferior.

Pleurae

The pleurae are airtight membranes that cover the outer surface of the lungs and line the chest wall. They secrete a serous fluid that prevents friction during movements of respiration.

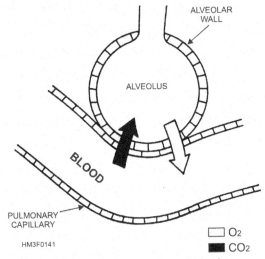

HM3F0141

Figure 1-41.—Pulmonary exchange at alveolus.

Mediastinum

The mediastinum is the tissue and organs of the thoracic cavity that form a septum between the lungs. It extends from the sternum to the thoracic vertebrae and from the fascia of the neck to the diaphragm. The mediastinum contains the heart, the great blood vessels, the esophagus, a portion of the trachea, and the primary bronchi.

Diaphragm

The diaphragm is the primary muscle of respiration. It is a dome-shaped muscle and separates the thoracic and abdominal cavities. Contraction of this muscle flattens the dome and expands the vertical diameter of the chest cavity.

Intercostal Muscles

The intercostal muscles are situated between the ribs. Their contraction pulls the ribs upward and outward, resulting in an increase in the transverse diameter of the chest (chest expansion).

Inhalation is the direct result of the expansion caused by the action of the diaphragm and intercostal muscles. The increase in chest volume creates a negative (lower than atmospheric) pressure in the pleural cavity and lungs. Air rushes into the lungs through the mouth and nose to equalize the pressure. **Exhalation** results when the muscles of respiration relax. Pressure is exerted inwardly as muscles and bones return to their normal position, forcing air from the lungs.

THE PROCESS OF RESPIRATION

The rhythmical movements of breathing are controlled by the respiratory center in the brain. Nerves from the brain pass down through the neck to the chest wall and diaphragm. The nerve that controls the diaphragm is called the **phrenic nerve**; the nerve that controls the larynx is the **vagus nerve**; and the nerves that control the muscles between the ribs are the **intercostal nerves**.

The respiratory center is stimulated by chemical changes in the blood. When too much carbon dioxide accumulates in the blood stream, causing the blood to become acidic, the respiratory center signals the lungs to breathe faster to get rid of the carbon dioxide.

The respiratory center can also be stimulated or depressed by a signal from the brain. For example, changes in one's emotional state can alter respiration through laughter, crying, emotional shock, or panic.

The muscles of respiration normally act automatically, with normal respiration being 14 to 18 cycles per minute. The lungs, when filled to capacity, hold about 6,500 ml of air, but only 500 ml of air is exchanged with each normal respiration. This exchanged air is called **tidal air**. The amount of air left in the lungs after forceful exhalation is about 1,200 ml and is known as **residual air**.

THE NERVOUS SYSTEM

LEARNING OBJECTIVE: *Identify the components and function of a neuron, recall the process of impulse transmission, and identify the components and functions of the central and peripheral nervous systems.*

The activities of the widely diverse cells, tissues, and organs of the body must be monitored, regulated, and coordinated to effectively support human life. The interaction of the nervous and endocrine systems provides the needed control.

The nervous system is specifically adapted to the rapid transmission of impulses from one area of the body to another. On the other hand, the endocrine system, working at a far slower pace, maintains body metabolism at a fairly constant level.

In this section, you will study the **neuron**, the basic functional unit of the nervous system. Also, you will study the components and functions of the different divisions of the nervous system. The nervous system is divided into two major groups, the **central nervous system** (CNS) and the **peripheral nervous system** (PNS). Another division of the nervous system is the **autonomic nervous system** (ANS), which is further subdivided into the **sympathetic** and **parasympathetic nervous systems**.

THE NEURON

The structure and functional unit of the nervous system is the nerve cell, or neuron, which can be classified into three types. The first is the **sensory** neuron, which conveys sensory impulses inward from the receptors. The second is the **motor** neuron, which carries command impulses from a central area to the responding muscles or organs. The third type is the **interneuron**, which links the sensory neurons to the motor neurons.

The neuron is composed of dendrites, a cyton, and an axon (fig. 1-42). The **dendrites** are thin receptive branches, and vary greatly in size, shape, and number with different types of neurons. They serve as receptors, conveying impulses toward the **cyton**. The cyton is the cell body containing the nucleus. The single, thin extension of the cell outward from the cyton is called the **axon**. It conducts impulses away from the cyton to its **terminal branches**, which transmit the impulses to the dendrites of the next neuron.

Large axons of the peripheral nerves are commonly enclosed in a sheath, called **neurilemma**, composed of **Schwann cells** (fig. 1-42). Schwann cells wrap around the axon and act as an electrical insulator.

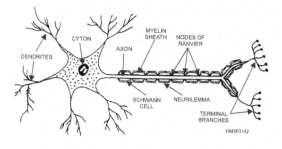

Figure 1-42.—The neuron and its parts.

The membranes of the Schwann cell are composed largely of a lipid-protein called **myelin**, which forms a **myelin sheath** on the outside of an axon. The myelin sheath has gaps between adjacent Schwann cells called **nodes of Ranvier**. Nerve cells without Schwann cells also lack myelin and neurilemma sheaths.

IMPULSE TRANSMISSION

When dendrites receive a sufficiently strong stimulus, a short and rapid change in electrical charge, or polarity, of the neuron is triggered. Sodium ions rush through the plasma membrane into the cell, potassium ions leave, and an electrical impulse is formed, which is conducted toward the cyton. The cyton receives the impulse and transmits it to the terminal filaments of the axon. At this point a chemical transmitter such as acetylcholine is released into the **synapse**, a space between the axon of the activated nerve and the dendrite receptors of another neuron. This chemical transmitter activates the next nerve. In this manner, the impulse is passed from neuron to neuron down the nerve line to a central area at approximately the speed of a bullet.

Almost immediately after being activated, the chemical transmitter in the synapse is neutralized by the enzyme acetylcholinesterase, and the first neuron returns to its normal state by pumping out the sodium ions and drawing potassium ions back in through the plasma membrane. When these actions are completed, the nerve is ready to be triggered again. A particularly strong stimulus will cause the nerve to fire in rapid succession, or will trigger many other neurons, thus giving a feeling of intensity to the perceived sensation.

NERVES

A nerve is a cordlike bundle of nerve fibers held together with connective tissue. Each nerve fiber is an extension of a neuron. Nerves that conduct impulses into the brain or the spinal cord are called **sensory nerves**, and those that carry impulses to muscles and glands are termed **motor nerves**. Most nerves, however, include both sensory and motor fibers, and they are called **mixed nerves**.

CENTRAL NERVOUS SYSTEM

The central nervous system (CNS) consists of the brain and spinal cord. The brain is almost entirely enclosed in the skull, but it is connected with the spinal cord, which lies in the canal formed by the vertebral column.

Brain

The brain has two main divisions, the **cerebrum** and the **cerebellum**. The cerebrum is the largest and most superiorly situated portion of the brain. It occupies most of the cranial cavity. The outer surface is called the **cortex**. This portion of the brain is also called "gray matter" because the nerve fibers are unmyelinated (not covered by a myelin sheath), causing them to appear gray. Beneath this layer is the **medulla**, often called the white matter of the brain because the nerves are myelinated (covered with a myelin sheath), giving them their white appearance.

CEREBRUM.—The cortex of the cerebrum is irregular in shape. It bends on itself in folds called **convolutions**, which are separated from each other by grooves, also known as **fissures**. The deep **sagittal cleft**, a longitudinal fissure, divides the cerebrum into two hemispheres. Other fissures further subdivide the cerebrum into lobes, each of which serves a localized, specific brain function (fig. 1-43). For example, the **frontal lobe** is associated with the higher mental processes such as memory, the **parietal lobe** is concerned primarily with general sensations, the **occipital lobe** is related to the sense of sight, and the **temporal lobe** is concerned with hearing.

CEREBELLUM.—The cerebellum is situated posteriorly to the brain stem (which is made up of the pons, mid-brain, and medulla oblongata) and inferior to the occipital lobe. The cerebellum is concerned chiefly with bringing balance, harmony, and coordination to the motions initiated by the cerebrum.

PONS AND MEDULLA OBLONGATA.— Two smaller divisions of the brain vital to life are the pons and the medulla oblongata. Together, the pons and medulla form the **brain stem** (fig. 1-43). The pons consists chiefly of a mass of white fibers connecting the other three parts of the brain (the cerebrum, cerebellum, and medulla oblongata).

The medulla oblongata is the inferior portion of the brain, the last division before the beginning of the spinal cord. It connects to the spinal cord at the upper level of the first cervical vertebra (C-1). In the medulla oblongata are the centers for the control of heart action, breathing, circulation, and other vital processes such as blood pressure.

MENINGES.—The outer surface of the brain and spinal cord is covered with three layers of membranes called the meninges. The **dura mater** is the strong outer layer; the **arachnoid membrane** is the delicate

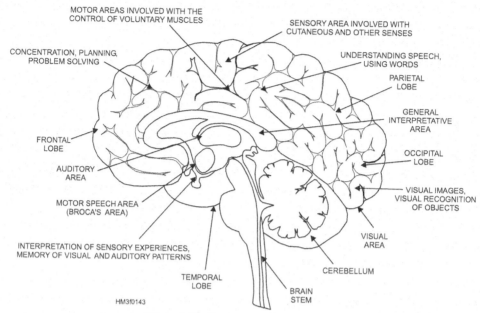

Figure 1-43.—Functional areas of the brain.

middle layer; and the **pia mater** is the vascular inner-most layer that adheres to the surface of the brain and spinal cord. Inflammation of the meninges is called meningitis. The type of meningitis contracted depends upon whether the brain, spinal cord, or both are affected, as well as whether it is caused by viruses, bacteria, protozoa, yeasts, or fungi.

CEREBROSPINAL FLUID.—Cerebrospinal fluid is formed by a plexus, or network, of blood vessels in the central ventricles of the brain. It is a clear, watery solution similar to blood plasma. The total quantity of spinal fluid bathing the spinal cord is about 75 ml. This fluid is constantly being produced and reabsorbed. It circulates over the surface of the brain and spinal cord and serves as a protective cushion as well as a means of exchange for nutrients and waste materials.

Spinal Cord

The spinal cord is continuous with the medulla oblongata and extends from the foramen magnum, through the atlas, to the lower border of the first lumbar vertebra, where it tapers to a point. The spinal cord is surrounded by the bony walls of the vertebral canal (fig. 1-44). Ensheathed in the three protective meninges and surrounded by fatty tissue and blood vessels, the cord does not completely fill the vertebral canal, nor does it extend the full length of it. The nerve roots serving the lumbar and sacral regions must pass some distance down the canal before making their exit. The **sympathetic trunk** contains the **paravertebral ganglia** (*sing.* ganglion), knotlike masses of nerve cell bodies (fig. 1-44).

A cross section of the spinal cord shows white and gray matter (fig. 1-45). The outer white matter is composed of bundles of myelinated nerve fibers arranged in functionally specialized tracts. It establishes motor communication between the brain and the body parts. The inner gray unmyelinated

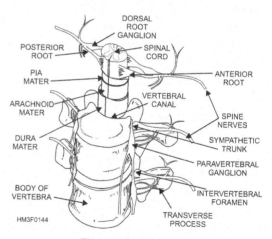

Figure 1-44.—Spinal cord.

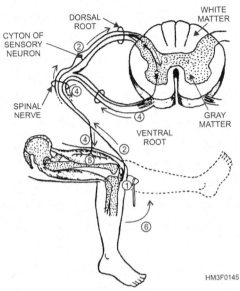

CYTON OF SENSORY NEURON

DORSAL ROOT

WHITE MATTER

SPINAL NERVE

VENTRAL ROOT

GRAY MATTER

HM3F0145

Figure 1-45.—Cross section of the spinal cord and reflex arc—arrows and numbers show impulse pathway.

matter is shaped roughly like the letter H. It establishes sensory communication between the brain and the spinal nerves, conducting sensory impulses from the body parts.

The spinal cord may be thought of as an electric cable containing many wires (nerves) that connect parts of the body with each other and with the brain. Sensations received by a sensory nerve are brought to the spinal cord, and the impulse is transferred either to the brain or to a motor nerve. The majority of impulses go to the brain for action. However, a system exists for quickly handling emergency situations. It is called the **reflex arc**.

If you touch a hot stove, you must remove your hand from the heat source immediately or the skin will burn very quickly. But the passage of a sense impulse to the brain and back again to a motor nerve takes too much time. The reflex arc responds instantaneously to emergency situations like the one just described. The sensation of heat travels to the spinal cord on a sensory nerve. When the sensation reaches the spinal cord, it is picked up by an interneuron in the gray matter. This reception then triggers the appropriate nerve to stimulate a muscle reflex drawing the hand away. An illustrated example of the reflex arc is shown in figure 1-45.

The reflex arc works well in simple situations requiring no action of the brain. Consider, however, what action is involved if the individual touching the stove pulls back and, in so doing, loses balance and has to grab a chair to regain stability. Then the entire spinal cord is involved. Additional impulses must travel to the brain, then down to the muscles of the legs and arms to enable the individual to maintain balance and to hold on to a steadying object. While all this activity is going on, the stimulus is relayed through the sympathetic autonomic nerve fibers to the adrenal glands, causing adrenalin to flow, which stimulates heart action. The stimulus then moves to the brain, making the individual conscious of pain. In this example, the spinal cord has functioned not only as a center for spinal relaxes, but also as a conduction pathway for other areas of the spinal cord to the autonomic nervous system and to the brain.

PERIPHERAL NERVOUS SYSTEM

The peripheral nervous system (PNS) consists of the nerves that branch out from the CNS and connect it to the other parts of the body. The PNS includes 12 pairs of cranial nerves and 31 pairs of spinal nerves. Cranial and spinal nerves carry both voluntary and involuntary impulses.

Cranial Nerves

The 12 pairs of cranial nerves are sensory, motor, or mixed (sensory and motor). Table 1-3 shows the 12 cranial nerves and parts of the body they service.

Spinal Nerves

There are 31 pairs of spinal nerves that originate from the spinal cord. Although spinal nerves are not named individually, they are grouped according to the level from which they arise, and each nerve is numbered in sequence. Thus, there are 8 pairs of **cervical** nerves, 12 pairs of **thoracic** nerves, 5 pairs of **lumbar** nerves, 5 pairs of **sacral** nerves, and 1 pair of **coccygeal** nerves. See figure 1-46.

Spinal nerves (mixed) send fibers to sensory surfaces and muscles of the trunk and extremities. Nerve fibers are also sent to involuntary smooth muscles and glands of the gastrointestinal tract, urogenital system, and cardiovascular system.

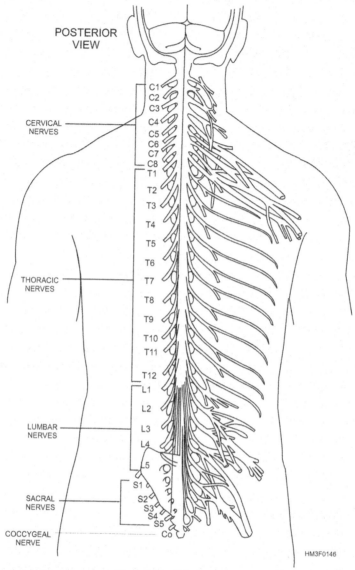

POSTERIOR
VIEW

CERVICAL
NERVES

C1
C2
C3
C4
C5
C6
C7
C8

T1
T2
T3
T4
T5
T6

THORACIC
NERVES

T7
T8
T9
T10
T11
T12

L1
L2

LUMBAR
NERVES

L3
L4
L5

SACRAL
NERVES

S1
S2
S3
S4
S5

COCCYGEAL
NERVE

Co

HM3F0146

Figure 1-46.—Spinal nerves.

AUTONOMIC NERVOUS SYSTEM

The autonomic nervous system (ANS) is the portion of the PNS that functions independently, automatically, and continuously, without conscious effort. It helps to regulate the smooth muscles, cardiac muscle, digestive tube, blood vessels, sweat and digestive glands, and certain endocrine glands. The autonomic nervous system is not directly under the control of the brain but usually works in harmony with the nerves that are under the brain's control. The autonomic nervous system includes two subdivisions (the sympathetic and parasympathetic nervous systems) that act together.

The sympathetic nervous system's primary concern is to prepare the body for energy-expending, stressful, or emergency situations. On the other hand, the parasympathetic nervous system is most active under routine, restful situations. The parasympathetic system also counterbalances the effects of the sympathetic system, and restores the body to a resting

Table 1-3.—Cranial Nerves

CRANIAL NERVE	FUNCTION(S)
Olfactory	Sense of smell.
Optic	Vision.
Oculomotor	Eye movement, size of pupil, and eye focus.
Trochlear	Eye movements.
Trigeminal	Sensations of head and face and chewing movements.
Abducens	Abduction of eye (muscles that turn eye outward).
Facial	Facial expressions, secretion of saliva, and sense of taste.
Acoustic	Sense of hearing and balance or equilibrium sense.
Glossopharyngeal	Taste and other sensations of the tongue, swallowing movements, secretion of saliva.
Vagus	Sensations of movement (e.g., decrease in heart rate, increase in peristalsis, and contracting of muscles for voice production).
Accessory	Shoulder movements, turning movements of the head, and voice production.
Hypoglossal	Tongue movements.

state. For example, during an emergency the body's heart and respiration rate increases. After the emergency, the parasympathetic system will decrease heart and respiration rate to normal. The sympathetic and parasympathetic systems counterbalance each other to preserve a harmonious balance of body functions and activities.

THE ENDOCRINE SYSTEM

LEARNING OBJECTIVE: *Identify endocrine glands and the hormone(s) they produce, and determine the effect each hormone has on the body.*

Homeostasis, the self-balancing of the body's internal environment, is achieved and maintained by the endocrine system and the nervous systems. These systems work alone and together to perform similar functions in the body: communication, integration, and control. Their communication capabilities provide the means for controlling and integrating the many different functions performed by organs, tissues, and cells. The endocrine system, however, performs these functions by different mechanisms than the nervous system.

The endocrine system sends messages by way of chemical messengers called **hormones**. Minute amounts of these hormones are secreted from endocrine gland cells into the blood and distributed by the circulatory system. Endocrine glands secrete hormones directly into the blood, because they have no duct system. The glands of this system are often called **ductless glands**. Cells that are affected by the hormone are referred to as **target organ cells**.

Today, many hormones can be extracted from the glands of animals or produced synthetically. Medical officers may prescribe these naturally derived or synthetic hormones for patients who are deficient in them or who might otherwise benefit from their use. For example, oxytocin (the hormone which stimulates uterine contractions during pregnancy) has been synthesized and is used during the delivery process for women who are deficient in this hormone.

The hormone-producing glands include the hypothalamus, pituitary, thyroid, parathyroids, adrenals, pancreas, and gonads (the testes and ovaries) (fig. 1-47).

HYPOTHALAMUS

The hypothalamus, a structure in the brain, synthesizes chemicals that are secreted to the pituitary

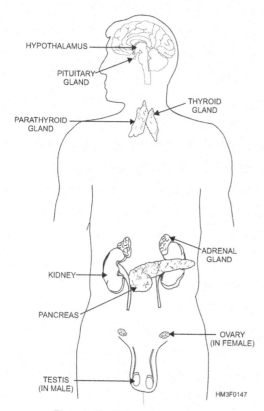

Figure 1-47.—Major endocrine glands.

gland to stimulate the release of its hormones and to help regulate body temperature (fig. 1-47).

PITUITARY GLAND

The pituitary is a small, pea-sized gland located at the base of the brain in the sella turcica, the saddle-shape depression of the sphenoid bone (fig. 1-47). It is often called the master gland of the body because it influences many other endocrine glands. Although the pituitary looks like just one gland, it actually consists of two separate glands, the anterior pituitary gland and the posterior pituitary gland.

Anterior Pituitary Gland

The anterior pituitary gland plays the more important role in influencing body functions. The hormones produced by the anterior pituitary gland have a broad and significant range of effects.

SOMATOTROPIN.—Somatotropin, the growth hormone, influences body growth and development. During the growth years, an overproduction of somatotropin causes giantism, while the lack of it causes dwarfism. An overproduction after the growth years causes **acromegaly**, which is characterized by the development of abnormally large hands, feet, and jaw.

THYROTROPIN.—Thyrotropin, or the thyroid-stimulating hormone (TSH), influences the growth, development, and secreting activities of the thyroid gland.

GONADOTROPIN.—Gonadotropin influences the gonads and is essential for the normal development and functioning of both male and female reproductive systems.

ADRENOCORTICOTROPIN.—The adrenocorticotropin hormone (ACTH) acts primarily on the adrenal cortex (the outer portion of the adrenal glands), stimulating its growth and its secretion of corticosteroids. Corticosteroid hormones affect every cell in the body and are discussed in more detail later in this section.

Posterior Pituitary Gland

The posterior pituitary gland produces two hormones, antidiuretic hormone (ADH) and oxytocin.

ANTIDIURETIC.—The ADH hormone, promotes the conservation of water by the kidney. When ADH is not produced in adequate amounts, the daily urine volume is between 10 and 15 liters instead of the normal 1.5 liters. This condition is known as diabetes insipidus.

OXYTOCIN.—Oxytocin stimulates contraction of the muscles of the uterus, particularly during pregnancy. It also plays an important role in the production of milk in the mammary glands of nursing mothers.

THYROID GLAND

The thyroid gland, shaped like a butterfly, lies in the anterior part of the neck, below the larynx (fig. 1-47). It consists of two lobes, one on each side of the upper trachea, connected by a strip of tissue called the isthmus. The thyroid secretes the iodine containing hormone **thyroxin**, which controls the rate of cell metabolism. Excessive secretion of thyroxin raises the metabolic rate and causes hyperthyroidism. This condition is characterized by a fast pulse rate, dizziness, increased basal metabolism, profuse sweating, tremors, nervousness, and a tremendous appetite coupled with a loss of weight.

Iodine is essential for the formation of thyroxin. **Simple goiter**, a diffuse and painless enlargement of the thyroid gland, was once common in areas of the United States where the iodine content of the soil and water was inadequate. In simple goiter, the gland enlarges to compensate for the lack of iodine. To prevent formation of a simple goiter, iodine-containing foods, such as vegetables, iodized salt, and seafood, should be eaten.

A condition known as **hypothyroidism** is caused by an insufficient secretion of thyroxin. The patient exhibits a decrease in basal metabolism, and sweating is almost absent. There may be a weight gain and constant fatigue. The heart rate may be slow, and a simple goiter may form. There may also be personality changes characterized by slow, lethargic mental functioning. Hypothyroidism during childhood can lead to the development of **cretinism**. Cretinism is a condition characterized by retarded mental and physical development.

PARATHYROID GLANDS

Parathyroid glands are four small round bodies located just posterior to the thyroid gland (fig. 1-47). Their hormone, **parathormone** (PTH), regulates the calcium and phosphorus content of the blood and bones. The amount of calcium is important in certain tissue activities, such as bone formation, coagulation of blood, maintenance of normal muscular excitability, and milk production in the nursing mother. Diminished function or removal of the parathyroid glands results in a low calcium level in the blood. In extreme cases death may occur, preceded by strong contraction of the muscles (tetany) and convulsions.

Hyperparathyroidism, an excess of parathyroid hormone in the blood, causes calcium levels in the blood to become elevated by the withdrawal of calcium from the bones, leaving the skeleton demineralized and subject to spontaneous fractures. The excess calcium may be deposited as stones in the kidneys.

ADRENAL GLANDS

The adrenal glands are located on the superior surface of each kidney, fitting like a cap (fig. 1-47). They consist of an outer portion, the cortex, and an inner portion, the medulla.

Adrenal Cortex

Specialized cells in the outer layer of the adrenal cortex produce three types of steroid hormones that are of vital importance.

MINERALOCORTICOIDS.—Mineralocorticoids are regulators of fluid and electrolyte balance. They are sometimes called salt and water hormones because they regulate the excretion and absorption of sodium, chlorine, potassium, and water.

GLUCOCORTICOIDS.—Glucocorticoids are essential to metabolism. They increase certain liver functions and have an anti-inflammatory effect. Clinically, they are used to suppress inflammatory reactions, to promote healing, and to treat rheumatoid arthritis.

ANDROGENS AND ESTROGENS.—The adrenal cortex also produces sex hormones, some with male characteristics (**androgens**), others with female characteristics (**estrogens**). These hormones appear in different concentrations in both men and women.

Adrenal Medulla

The adrenal medulla secretes **epinephrine** (**adrenalin**) in the presence of emotional crises, hypoglycemia (low blood sugar), or low blood pressure. Epinephrine causes powerful contractions of many arterioles (especially in the skin, mucous membranes, and kidneys), but it dilates other arterioles (such as those of the coronary system, skeletal muscles, and lungs). Heart rate, respiration rate and depth, blood pressure, blood sugar levels, and metabolism are all increased by epinephrine. It also stimulates the production of other adrenal cortical hormones.

Norepinephrine is also produced in the adrenal medulla. It is a chemical precursor to epinephrine. Its effects are similar to those of epinephrine, but its action differs.

Despite these marked influences, the medullary tissue of the adrenal gland is not essential to life, because its various functions can be assumed by other regulatory mechanisms.

PANCREAS

The pancreas contains two types of secretory tissues. The first secretory tissue secretes digestive juice through a duct to the small intestine, while the other tissue releases hormones into body fluids. The endocrine portion of the pancreas consists of cells arranged in groups, called "**islands (islets) of Langerhans**." The islands (islets) of Langerhans contain three types of endocrine cells: alpha, beta, and delta. The **alpha cells** secrete the hormone glucagon. **Glucagon** causes a temporary rise in blood sugar levels. The **beta cells** secrete insulin, which is essential for carbohydrate metabolism. **Insulin** lowers blood sugar levels by increasing tissue utilization of glucose and stimulating the formation and storage of glycogen in the liver. Together, glucagon and insulin act to regulate sugar metabolism in the body. **Delta cells** produce the hormone **somatostatin**. Somatostatin helps regulate carbohydrates by inhibiting the secretion of glucagon.

When the islet cells are destroyed or stop functioning, the sugar absorbed from the intestine remains in the blood and excess sugar is excreted by the kidneys into the urine. This condition is called **diabetes mellitus**, or sugar diabetes. Insulin, a synthetic hormone, is given to patients having this disease as part of their ongoing treatment.

GONADS (TESTES AND OVARIES)

The term **gonads** refers to the primary sex organs of the reproductive system (male and female).

Testes

The male gonad is the testis (*pl.* testes), and the existence of the testes is the primary male sex characteristic (fig. 1-47). The testes produce and secrete the male hormone **testosterone**, which influences the development and maintenance of the male accessory sex organs and the secondary sex characteristics of the male. The male **accessory sex organs** include two groups of organs: the internal sex organs and the external sex organs. See section titled "Male Reproductive System" for more information on the male accessory sex organs.

Male Secondary Sex Characteristics

Male secondary sex characteristics influenced by the hormone testosterone are as follows:

- Increased growth of hair, particularly in the areas of the face, chest, axilla, and pubic region.

- Enlargement of the larynx (Adam's apple) and thickening of the vocal cords, which produces a lower-pitched voice.

- Thickening of the skin.

- Increased muscle growth, broadening of the shoulder and narrowing of the waist.

- Thickening and strengthening of the bones.

Ovaries

The female gonads, the ovaries, produce the hormones **estrogen** and **progesterone** (fig. 1-47). Estrogen influences the development and maintenance of the female accessory sex organs and the secondary sex characteristics, and promotes changes in the mucous lining of the uterus (endometrium) during the menstrual cycle. Progesterone prepares the uterus for the reception and development of the fertilized ovum and maintains the lining during pregnancy.

Today, progesterone and estrogen hormones (naturally derived) are incorporated into oral contraceptives or birth control pills. The combination of hormones released through this monthly series of pills fools the body into not preparing (building-up of uterine lining) for implantation of an embryo. Because the uterus has not prepared for implantation, pregnancy cannot occur.

Female accessory sex organs are also divided into internal and external accessory sex organs. See section titled "Female Reproductive System" for more information on the female accessory sex organs.

Female Secondary Sex Characteristics

Female secondary sex characteristics influenced by the hormone estrogen are listed below.

- Development of the breasts and the ductile system of the mammary glands within the breasts.

- Increased quantities of fatty (or adipose) tissue in the subcutaneous layer, especially in the breasts, thighs, and buttocks.

- Increased vascularization of the skin.

THE SENSORY SYSTEM

LEARNING OBJECTIVE: *Recognize the senses of the body, and identify their physical characteristics.*

The sensory system informs areas of the cerebral cortex of changes that are taking place within the body or in the external environment. The special sensory receptors respond to special individual stimuli such as sound waves, light, taste, smell, pressure, heat, cold, pain, or touch. Positional changes, balance, hunger, and thirst sensations are also detected and passed on to the brain.

SMELL

Odor is perceived upon stimulation of the receptor cells in the **olfactory** membrane of the nose. The olfactory receptors are very sensitive, but they are easily fatigued. This tendency explains why odors that are initially very noticeable are not sensed after a short time. Smell is not as well developed in man as it is in other mammals.

TASTE

The taste buds are located in the tongue. The sensation of taste is limited to **sour, sweet, bitter**, and **salty**. Many foods and drinks tasted are actually smelled, and their taste depends upon their odor. (This interdependence between taste and smell can be demonstrated by pinching the nose shut when eating onions.) Sight can also affect taste. Several drops of green food coloring in a glass of milk will make it all but unpalatable, even though the true taste has not been affected.

SIGHT

The eye, the organ of sight, is a specialized structure for the reception of light. It is assisted in its function by accessory structures, such as the eye brows, eyelashes, eyelids, and **lacrimal apparatus**. The lacrimal apparatus consists of structures that produce tears and drains them from the surface of the eyeball.

Structure of the Eye

Approximately five-sixths of the eyeball lies recessed in the orbit, protected by a bony socket. Only the small anterior surface of the eyeball is exposed.

The eye is not a solid sphere but contains a large interior cavity that is divided into two cavities, anterior and posterior. The anterior cavity is further subdivided into anterior and posterior chambers (fig. 1-48).

The **anterior cavity** of the eye lies in front of the lens. The **anterior chamber** of the anterior cavity is the space anterior to the iris, but posterior to the cornea. The **posterior chamber** of the anterior cavity consists of a small space directly posterior to the iris, but anterior to the lens. Both chambers of the anterior cavity are filled with a clear, watery fluid called **aqueous humor**. Aqueous humor helps to give the cornea its curved shape.

The **posterior cavity** of the eye is larger than the anterior cavity, since it occupies all the space posterior to the lens, suspensory ligaments, and ciliary body. The posterior cavity contains a substance, with the consistency similar to soft gelatin, called **vitreous humor**. Vitreous humor helps maintain sufficient pressure inside the eye to prevent the eyeball from collapsing.

The eyeball is composed of three layers. From the outside in, they are the sclera, choroid, and retina (fig. 1-48).

OUTER LAYER.—The outer layer of the eye is called the **sclera**. The sclera is the tough, fibrous, protective portion of the globe, commonly called the white of the eye. Anteriorly, the outer layer is transparent and is called the **cornea**, or the window of the eye. It permits light to enter the globe. The exposed sclera is covered with a mucous membrane, the conjunctiva, which is a continuation of the inner lining of the eyelids. The **lacrimal gland** produces tears that constantly wash the front part of the eye and the conjunctiva. The tear gland secretions that do not

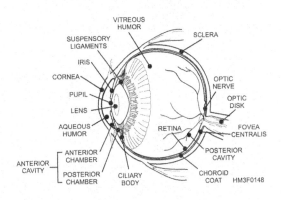

Figure 1-48.—Transverse section of the eye.

evaporate flow toward the inner angle of the eye, where they drain down ducts into the nose.

MIDDLE LAYER.—The middle layer of the eye is called the **choroid**. This layer is a highly vascular, pigmented tissue that provides nourishment to the inner structures. Continuous with the choroid is the **ciliary body**. The ciliary body is formed by a thickening of the choroid and fits like a collar into the area between the retina and iris. Attached to the ciliary the body are the **suspensory ligaments**, which blend with the elastic capsule of the lens and holds it in place.

Iris.—The iris is continuous with the ciliary body. The iris is a circular, pigmented muscular structure that gives color to the eye. The iris separates the anterior cavity into anterior and posterior chambers. The opening in the iris is called the **pupil** (fig. 1-49). The amount of light entering the pupil is regulated through the constriction of radial and circular muscles in the iris. When strong light is flashed into the eye, the circular muscle fibers of the iris contract, reducing the size of the pupil. If the light is dim, the pupil dilates to allow as much of the light in as possible. The size and

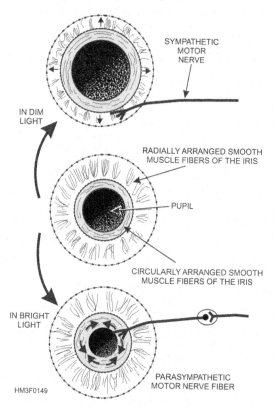

HM3F0149

Figure 1-49.—Anterior view of the eye.

reaction of the pupils of the eyes are an important diagnostic tool.

Lens.—The lens is a transparent, biconvex (having two convex surfaces) structure suspended directly behind the iris. The optic globe posterior to the lens is filled with a jellylike substance called vitreous humor, which helps to maintain the shape of the eyeball by maintaining intraocular pressure. The lens separates the eye into anterior and posterior cavities.

INNER LAYER.—The inner layer of the eye is called the **retina** (fig. 1-48). It contains layers of the nerve cells, **rods**, and **cones** that are the receptors of the sense of vision. The retina is continuous with the **optic nerve**, which enters the back of the globe and carries visual impulses received by the rods and cones to the brain. The area where the optic nerve enters the eyeball contains no rods and cones and is called the **optic disc** (blind spot) (fig. 1-50).

Rods.—Rods respond to low intensities of light and are responsible for night vision. They are located in all areas of the retina, except in the small depression called the **fovea centralis**, where light entering the eye is focused, and which has the clearest vision.

Cones.—Cones require higher light intensities for stimulation and are most densely concentrated in the fovea centralis. The cones are responsible for daytime vision.

Vision Process

The vision process begins with rays of light from an object passing through the cornea. The image is then received by the lens, by way of the iris. Leaving the lens, the image falls on the rods and cones in the retina. The image then is carried to the brain for interpretation by the optic nerve (fig. 1-51). Note the image received by the retina is upside down, but the brain turns it right-side up.

REFRACTION.—Deflection or bending of light rays results when light passes through substances of varying densities in the eye (cornea, aqueous humor, lens, and vitreous humor). The deflection of light in the eye is referred to as **refraction**.

ACCOMMODATION.—Accommodation is the process by which the lens increases or decreases its curvature to refract light rays into focus on the fovea centralis.

CONVERGENCE.—The movement of the globes toward the midline, causes a viewed object to come into focus on corresponding points of the two

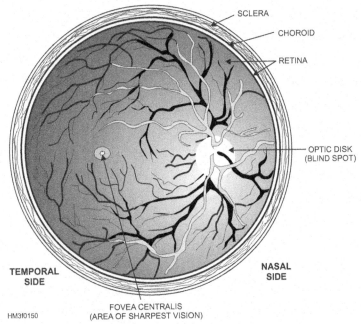

Figure 1-50.—Ophthalmoscope view of the eye.

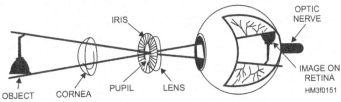

Figure 1-51.—The vision process.

retinas. This process, called **convergence**, produces clear, three-dimensional vision.

HEARING

The ear is the primary organ of hearing. Its major parts are illustrated in figure 1-52. The ear is divided into three parts: the external, middle, and inner ear.

External Ear

The external (outer) ear is composed of two parts, the **auricle** and the **external auditory canal** (fig. 1-52). The auricle, or pinna, is a cartilaginous structure located on each side of the head. The auricle collects sound waves from the environment, which are then conducted by the external auditory canal to the eardrum. The lining of the external auditory canal contains glands that secrete a wax-like substance

called **cerumen**. Cerumen aids in protecting the eardrum against foreign bodies and microorganisms.

The **tympanic membrane**, or eardrum, is an oval sheet of fibrous epithelial tissue that stretches across the inner end of the external auditory canal. The eardrum separates the outer and middle ear. The sound waves cause the eardrum to vibrate, and this vibration transfers the sounds from the external environment to the auditory ossicles.

Middle Ear

The middle ear is a cavity in the temporal bone, lined with epithelium. It contains three **auditory ossicles**—the malleus (hammer), the incus (anvil), and the stapes (stirrup)—which transmit vibrations from the tympanic membrane to the fluid in the inner ear

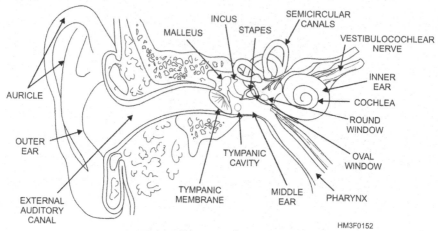

Figure 1-52.—Major parts of the ear.

HM3F0152

(fig. 1-52). The **malleus** is attached to the inner surface of the eardrum and connects with the **incus**, which in turn connects with the **stapes**. The base of the stapes is attached to the **fenestra ovalis** (oval window), the membrane-covered opening of the inner ear. These tiny bones, which span the middle ear, are suspended from bony walls by ligaments. This arrangement provides the mechanical means for transmitting sound vibrations to the inner ear.

The **eustachian tube**, or auditory tube, connects the middle ear with the pharynx. It is lined with a mucous membrane and is about 36 mm long. Its function is to equalize internal and external air pressure. For example, while riding an elevator in a tall building, you may experience a feeling of pressure in the ear. This condition is usually relieved by swallowing, which opens the eustachian tube and allows the pressurized air to escape and equalize with the area of lower pressure. Divers who ascend too fast to allow pressure to adjust may experience rupture of their eardrums. The eustachian tube can also provide a pathway for infection of the middle ear.

Inner Ear

The inner ear is filled with a fluid called **endolymph**. Sound vibrations that cause the stapes to move against the oval window create internal ripples that run through the endolymph. These pressurized ripples move to the **cochlea**, a small snail-shaped structure housing the **organ of Corti**, the hearing organ (fig. 1-52). The cells protruding from the organ of Corti are stimulated by the ripples to convert these mechanical vibrations into nerve impulses, and these

impulses are relayed through the vestibulocochlear (8th cranial) nerve to the auditory area of the cortex in the temporal lobe of the brain. There they are interpreted as the sounds we hear.

Another structure located in the inner ear is composed of the **three semicircular canals**, situated perpendicular to each other. Movement of the endolymph within the canals, caused by general body movements, stimulates nerve endings, which report these changes in body position to the brain, which in turn uses the information to maintain equilibrium.

The **fenestra rotunda** (round window) is another membrane-covered opening of the inner ear. It contracts the middle ear and flexes to accommodate the inner ear ripples caused by the stapes.

TOUCH

Until the beginning of the last century, touch (feeling) was treated as a single sense. Thus, warmth or coldness, pressure, and pain, were thought to be part of a single sense of touch or feeling. It was discovered that different types of nerve ending **receptors** are widely and unevenly distributed in the skin and mucous membranes. For example, the skin of the back possesses relatively few touch and pressure receptors while the fingertips have many. The skin of the face has relatively few cold receptors, and mucous membranes have few heat receptors. The cornea of the eye is sensitive to pain, and when pain sensation is abolished by a local anesthetic, a sensation of touch can be experienced.

Receptors are considered to be sensory organs. They provide the body with the general senses of touch, temperature, and pain. In addition, these receptors initiate reactions or reflexes in the body to maintain homeostasis. For example, receptors in the skin perceive cold, resulting in goosebumps. This reaction is the body's attempt to maintain internal warmth.

Receptors are classified according to location, structure, and types of stimuli activating them. Classified according to location, the three types of receptors are as follows: **superficial receptors** (exteroceptors), **deep receptors** (proprioceptors), and **internal receptors** (visceroceptors). See table 1-4 for receptor locations and the senses resulting from the stimulation of these receptors.

THE DIGESTIVE SYSTEM

LEARNING OBJECTIVE: *Identify the location and function of each part of the digestive system.*

The digestive system includes the organs that digest and absorb food substances, and eliminate the unused residuals. The digestive system consists of the **alimentary canal** and several accessory organs. The accessory organs release secretions into the canal. These secretions assist in preparing food for absorption and use by the tissues of the body. Table 1-5 illustrates principal digestive juices (secretions) produced by alimentary and accessory organs.

Digestion is both mechanical and chemical. Mechanical digestion occurs when food is chewed, swallowed, and propelled by a wave-like motion called **peristalsis**. When peristalsis occurs, a ring of contraction appears in the walls of the alimentary canal. At the same time, the muscular wall just ahead of the ring relaxes. This phenomenon is called **receptive relaxation**. As the wave moves along, it pushes the canal's contents ahead of it. Chemical digestion consists of changing the various food substances, with the aid of digestive enzymes, into solutions and simple compounds. Carbohydrates (starches and sugars) change into simple sugars (glucose); fats change into fatty acids; and proteins change into amino acids. Once the food substances have been broken down into simple compounds, the cells of the body can absorb and use them.

THE ALIMENTARY CANAL

The alimentary canal (tract) is 9 meters in length, tubular, and includes the mouth, pharynx, esophagus, stomach, small intestine, and large intestine (fig. 1-53).

Mouth

The mouth, which is the first portion of the alimentary canal, is adapted to receive food and prepare it for digestion (fig. 1-53). The mouth mechanically reduces the size of solid particles and mixes them with saliva. This process is called **mastication**. Saliva, produced by the **salivary gland**, moistens food making it easier to chew. Saliva also lubricates the food mass to aid swallowing. The tongue assists with both mastication and swallowing.

Pharynx

The pharynx (covered earlier in "The Respiratory System") is the passageway between the mouth and the esophagus and is shared with the respiratory tract (fig. 1-53). The **epiglottis** is a cartilaginous flap that

Table 1-4.—Types of Receptors, Their Location, and Affected Sense

TYPES	LOCATIONS	SENSES
Superficial receptors	At or near surface of body	Touch, pressure, heat, cold, and pain
Deep receptors	In muscles, tendons, and joints	Sense of position and movement
Internal receptors	In the internal organs and blood vessel walls	Usually none (except hunger, nausea, pain from stimuli such as chemicals (e.g., aspirin) and distension (e.g., stomach expansion from gas))

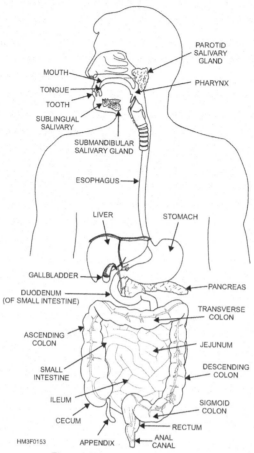

Figure 1-53.—The digestive system.

Table 1-5.—Principal Digestive Juices

Digestive Juice	Source	Substance Acted Upon	Product
Amylase	Salivary glands and pancreas	Starch	Complex sugars (maltose)
Hydrochloric acid	Gastric glands	Pepsinogen (Proteins)	Pepsin (Split proteins)
Bile	Liver	Fats	Emulsified fats
Proteinase	Pancreas	Proteins and split proteins	Peptides and polypeptides
Lipase	Pancreas	Fats (triglycerides)	Fatty acids and glycerol
Carbohydrase	Intestinal glands	Complex sugars (maltose, sucrose, and lactose)	Simple sugars (glucose, fructose, and galactose)
Peptidase	Intestinal glands	Peptides and polypeptides	Amino acids

closes the opening to the larynx when food is being swallowed down the pharynx. Food is deflected away from the trachea to prevent particle aspiration (inhalation).

Esophagus

The esophagus is a muscular tube about 25 cm (10 inches) long (fig. 1-53). It is the passageway between the pharynx and the stomach. By means of peristalsis, food is pushed along this tube to the stomach. When peristalsis is reversed, vomiting occurs.

Stomach

The stomach acts as an initial storehouse for swallowed material and helps in the chemical breakdown of food substances. The stomach is a saccular enlargement of the gastrointestinal tube and lies in the left upper quadrant of the abdomen (fig. 1-53). It connects the lower end of the esophagus with the first portion of the small intestine (the duodenum). The stomach is divided into the **cardiac, fundic, body**, and **pyloric** regions (fig. 1-54). At each end of the stomach, muscular rings (or sphincters) form valves to close off the stomach. The sphincters prevent the stomach's contents from escaping in either direction while food substances are being mixed by peristaltic muscular contractions of the stomach wall. The sphincter at the esophageal end is the **cardiac sphincter**; at the duodenal end it is the **pyloric sphincter**.

The chemical breakdown of food in the stomach is accomplished through the production of digestive juices (**enzymes**) by small (**gastric**) glands in the wall of the stomach. The principal digestive enzymes produced by the gastric glands are **hydrochloric acid** and **pepsinogen**. Hydrochloric acid activates pepsin from pepsinogen, kills bacteria that enter the stomach, inhibits the digestive action of amylase, and helps regulate the opening and closing of the pyloric sphincter. **Pepsin** is a protein-splitting enzyme capable of beginning the digestion of nearly all types of dietary protein.

Most food absorption takes place in the small intestine. In general, food is not absorbed in the stomach. An exception is alcohol, which is absorbed directly through the stomach wall. It is for this reason that intoxication occurs quickly when alcohol is taken on an empty stomach.

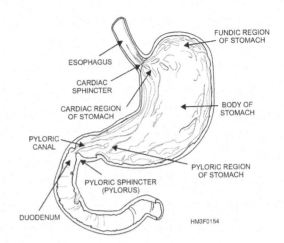

Figure 1-54.—Major regions of the stomach.

Abdominal Cavity

The stomach and intestines are enclosed in the abdominal cavity, the space between the diaphragm and the pelvis. This cavity is lined with serous membrane called the **peritoneum**. The peritoneum covers the intestines and the organs and, by secreting a serous fluid, prevents friction between adjacent organs. The **mesentery** (double folds of peritoneum) extends from the cavity walls to the organs of the abdominal cavity, suspending them in position and carrying blood vessels to the organs.

Small Intestine

The small intestine is a muscular, convoluted, coiled tube, about 7 meters (23 feet) long and attached to the posterior abdominal wall by its mesentery (fig. 1-53).

The small intestine is divided into three contiguous parts: the duodenum, jejunum, and ileum. It receives digestive juices from three accessory organs of digestion: the pancreas, liver, and gallbladder.

DUODENUM.—The duodenum is approximately 25 cm (10 inches) long and forms a C-shaped curve around the head of the pancreas, posterior to the liver. It is lined with a mucous membrane that contains small glands. These glands secrete intestinal juices containing the enzymes carbohydrase, peptidase, and lipase.

JEJUNUM.—The jejunum is the middle part of the small intestine and is approximately 2.5 meters (8.2 feet) long. Its enzymes continue the digestive process.

ILEUM.—The ileum is the last and longest part of the small intestine. It is approximately 3.5 meters (11.5 feet) long. Most of the absorption of food occurs in the ileum, where fingerlike projections (**villi**) provide a large absorption surface. After ingestion, it takes 20 minutes to 2 hours for the first portion of the food to pass through the small intestine to the beginning of the large intestine.

Large Intestine

The large intestine is so called because it is larger in diameter than the small intestine (fig. 1-53). It is considerably shorter, however, being about 1.5 meters (5 feet) long. It is divided into three distinct parts: the cecum, colon, and rectum.

CECUM AND COLON.—The unabsorbed food or waste material passes through the **cecum** into the **ascending colon**, across the **transverse colon**, and down the **descending colon** through the **sigmoid colon** to the rectum. Twelve hours after the meal, the waste material passes slowly through the colon, building in mass and reaching the rectum 24 hours after the food is ingested.

The **appendix**, a long narrow tube with a blind end, is a pouchlike structure of the cecum located near the junction of the ileum and the cecum (fig. 1-53). There is no known function of this structure. Occasionally, the appendix becomes infected, causing inflammation to develop. This inflammation of the appendix is known as **appendicitis**.

RECTUM.—The rectum is approximately 12.5 cm (5 inches) long and follows the contour of the sacrum and coccyx until it curves back into the short (2.5 to 4 cm) anal canal. The **anus** is the external opening at the lower end of the digestive system. Except during bowel movement (defecation), it is kept closed by a strong muscular ring, the **anal sphincter**.

ACCESSORY ORGANS OF DIGESTION

The accessory organs of digestion include the salivary glands, pancreas, liver, and gallbladder. As stated earlier, during the digestive process, the accessory organs produce secretions that assist the organs of the alimentary canal.

Salivary Glands

The salivary glands are located in the mouth (fig. 1-53). Within the salivary glands are two types of secretory cells, serous cells and mucous cells. The serous cells produce a watery fluid that contains a digestive juice called **amylase**. Amylase splits starch and glycerol into complex sugars. The mucous cells secrete a thick, sticky liquid called **mucus**. Mucus binds food particles together and acts to lubricate during swallowing. The fluids produced by the serous and mucous cells combine to form **saliva**. Approximately 1 liter of saliva is secreted daily.

Pancreas

The pancreas is a large, elongated gland lying posteriorly to the stomach (fig. 1-53). As discussed earlier in "The Endocrine System," the pancreas has two functions: It serves both the endocrine system and the digestive system. The digestive portion of the pancreas produces digestive juices (amylase, proteinase, and lipase) that are secreted through the pancreatic duct to the duodenum. These digestive juices break down carbohydrates (amylase), proteins (proteinase), and fats (lipase) into simpler compounds.

Liver

The liver is the largest gland in the body. It is located in the upper abdomen on the right side, just under the diaphragm and superior to the duodenum and pylorus (fig. 1-53).

Of the liver's many functions, the following are important to remember:

- It metabolizes carbohydrates, fats, and proteins preparatory to their use or excretion.

- It forms and excretes bile salts and pigment from bilirubin, a waste product of red blood cell destruction.

- It stores blood; glycogen; vitamins A, D, and B12; and iron.

- It detoxifies the end products of protein digestion and drugs.

- It produces antibodies and essential elements of the blood-clotting mechanism.

Gallbladder

The gallbladder is a pear-shaped sac, usually stained dark green by the bile it contains. It is located in the hollow underside of the liver (fig. 1-53). Its duct, the **cystic duct,** joins the **hepatic duct** from the liver to form the **common bile duct**, which enters the duodenum. The gallbladder receives bile from the liver and then concentrates and stores it. It secretes bile when the small intestine is stimulated by the entrance of fats.

THE URINARY SYSTEM

LEARNING OBJECTIVE: *Recall the parts of the urinary system and their function(s).*

The urinary system is the primary filtering system of the body (fig. 1-55). This system is composed of two main organs, the **kidneys** and **urinary bladder**. The kidneys produce urine, which is drained from the kidneys by two tubes called **ureters**. Urine flows down both ureters to the bladder. The urinary bladder is a large reservoir where the urine is temporarily stored before excretion from the body. A tube called the **urethra** carries the urine from the bladder to the outside of the body. All these parts, except the length of the urethra, are the same in both sexes.

KIDNEYS

The importance of the kidney can be realized only when its structure and functions are understood. The bladder, ureters, and urethra store and pass the products of the kidneys.

The kidneys are two large, bean-shaped organs designed to filter waste materials from the blood (figs. 1-55 and 1-56). They also assist in controlling the rate of red blood cell formation, and in the regulation of blood pressure, the absorption of calcium ions, and the

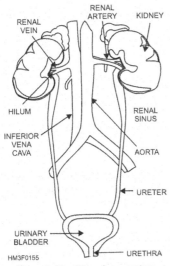

RENAL ARTERY KIDNEY
RENAL VEIN
HILUM
INFERIOR VENA CAVA
RENAL SINUS
AORTA
URETER
URINARY BLADDER
URETHRA
HM3F0155

Figure 1-55.—The urinary system.

volume, composition, and pH of body fluids. The kidneys are located in the upper posterior part of the abdominal cavity, one on each side of the spinal column. The upper end of each kidney reaches above the level of the 12th rib. The suprarenal (adrenal) gland sits like a cap on top of each kidney. The kidneys are protected by a considerable amount of fat and supported by connective tissue and the peritoneum. Attached to the hollow side of each kidney is the dilated upper end of the ureter, forming the **renal pelvis**.

Structure

The lateral surface of the kidneys is convex in shape, and the medial side is deeply concave. The medial side of each kidney possesses a depression that leads to a hollow chamber called the **renal sinus** (fig. 1-55). The entrance of the renal sinus is referred to as the **hilum** (fig. 1-55). Blood vessels, nerves, lymphatic vessels, and the ureters pass through the hilum.

The superior end of the ureter forms a funnel-shaped sac called the **renal pelvis** (fig. 1-56). The renal pelvis is divided into two or three tubes, called **major calyces**. The major calyces (*sing.* calyx) are further subdivided into **minor calyces**.

There are groups of elevated projections in the walls of the renal pelvis. These projections are called **renal papillae**. The renal papillae connect to the minor calyces, through tiny openings in the minor calyces.

The principal portion of the kidney is divided into two distinct regions: an inner medulla and outer cortex (fig. 1-56). The **renal medulla** is composed of pyramid-shaped masses of tubes and tubules called **renal pyramids**. **Renal pyramids** drain the urine to the renal pelvis. The **renal cortex** forms a shell over the renal medulla. Renal cortex tissue dips down, like fingers, between the renal pyramids, and forms what are called **renal columns**. The cortex possesses very small tubes associated with **nephrons**. Nephrons are the functional units of the kidneys.

RENAL BLOOD VESSELS.—The **renal artery** supplies blood to the kidneys (fig. 1-56). The renal artery enters the kidneys through the hilum, and sends off branches to the renal pyramids. These arterial branches are called **interlobar arteries**. At the border between the medulla and cortex, the interlobar arteries branch to form the **arciform arteries**. The arciform arteries branch also and form the **interlobular arteries**.

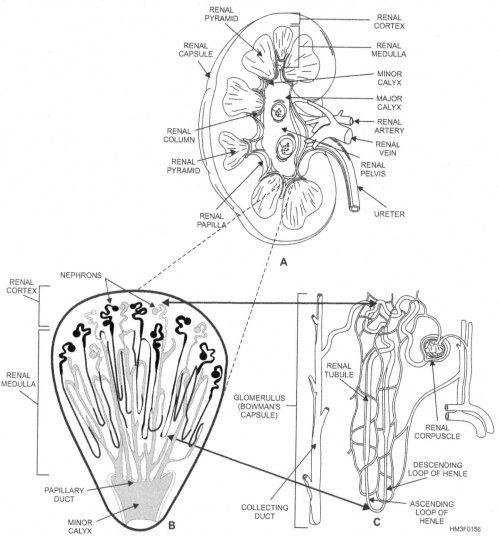

RENAL PYRAMID
RENAL CAPSULE
RENAL COLUMN
RENAL PYRAMID
RENAL PAPILLA
RENAL CORTEX
RENAL MEDULLA
MINOR CALYX
MAJOR CALYX
RENAL ARTERY
RENAL VEIN
RENAL PELVIS
URETER

A

RENAL CORTEX
NEPHRONS
RENAL MEDULLA
PAPILLARY DUCT
MINOR CALYX
B
GLOMERULUS (BOWMAN'S CAPSULE)
COLLECTING DUCT
RENAL TUBULE
RENAL CORPUSCLE
DESCENDING LOOP OF HENLE
ASCENDING LOOP OF HENLE
C
HM3F0156

Figure 1-56.—Principal parts of the kidney: A. Longitudinal section of a kidney; B. A renal pyramid containing nephrons; C. A single nephron.

The venous system of the kidneys generally follow the same paths as the arteries. Venous blood passes through the interlobular, arciform, interlobar, and renal veins (fig. 1-56).

NEPHRONS.—The functional units of the kidneys are called nephrons. There are about 1 million nephrons in each kidney. Each nephron consists of a renal corpuscle and a renal tubule (fig. 1-56, view C).

The **renal corpuscle (Malpighian corpuscle)** is composed of a tangled cluster of blood capillaries called a **glomerulus**. The glomerulus is surrounded by a sac-like structure referred to as the **glomerulus capsule** or **Bowman's capsule** (figs. 1-56, view C, and 1-57).

Leading away from the glomerulus is the renal tubule. The initial portion of the renal tubule is coiled and called the **proximal convoluted** (meaning coiled or twisted) **tubule**. The proximal convoluted tubule dips down to become the **descending loop of Henle**. The tubule then curves upward toward the renal corpuscle and forms the **ascending loop of Henle**.

Once the ascending limb reaches the region of the renal corpuscle, it called the distal convoluted tubule. Several distal convoluted tubules merge in the renal

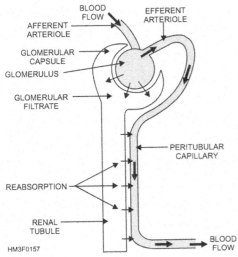

Figure 1-57.—The reabsorption process.

instance, the filtrate entering the renal tubule is high in sugar content, but because of the reabsorption process, urine secreted from the body does not contain sugar.

SECRETION.—Secretion is the process by which the peritubular capillary transports certain substances directly into the fluid of the renal tubule (fig. 1-58). These substances are transported by similar mechanisms as used in the reabsorption process, but done in reverse. For example, certain organic compounds, such as penicillin and histamine, are secreted directly from the proximal convoluted tubule to the renal tubule. Also, large quantities of hydrogen ions are secreted in this same manner. The secretion of hydrogen ions plays an important role in regulating pH of body fluids.

The glomerulus filters gallons of blood each day. It is estimated that 2,500 gallons of blood pass through the kidneys in 24 hours, and about 80 gallons of glomerular filtrate. All the water from this filtrate is reabsorbed in the renal tubules except that containing the concentrated waste products.

cortex to form a **collecting duct**. The collecting duct begins to merge within the renal medulla. The collecting ducts become increasingly larger as they are joined by other collecting ducts. The resulting tube is called the **papillary duct**. The papillary duct empties into the minor calyx through an opening in the renal papilla.

Function

The kidneys are effective blood purifiers and fluid balance regulators. In addition to maintaining a normal pH of the blood (acid-base balance), the kidneys keep the blood slightly alkaline by removing excess substances from the blood. The end product of these functions is the formation of **urine**, which is excreted from the body.

Urine is formed through a series of processes in the nephron. These processes are filtration, reabsorption, and secretion.

FILTRATION.—Urine formation begins when water and various dissolved substances are filtered out of blood plasma from a glomerular capillary into the glomerular capsule. The filtered substance (glomerular filtrate) leaves the glomerular capsule and enters the renal tubule.

REABSORPTION.—As glomerular filtrate passes through the renal tubule, some of the filtrate is reabsorbed into the blood of the **peritubular capillary** (fig. 1-57). The filtrate entering the peritubular capillary will repeat the filtration cycle. This process of reabsorption changes the composition of urine. For

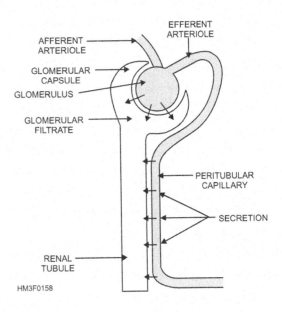

Figure 1-58.—The secretion process.

1-55

The average amount of urine an adult excretes varies from 1,000 to 1,500 ml per day. However, the amount of urine excreted varies greatly with temperature, water intake, and state of health. No matter how much water one drinks, the blood will always remain at a constant concentration, and the excess water will be excreted by the kidneys. A large water intake does not put a strain on the kidneys. Instead it eases the load of concentration placed on the kidneys.

URETERS

The ureters' only function is to carry urine from each kidney to the urinary bladder. The ureters are two membranous tubes 1 mm to 1 cm in diameter and about 25 cm in length. Urine is transported through the ureters by peristaltic waves (produced by the ureter's muscular walls).

URINARY BLADDER

The urinary bladder functions as a temporary reservoir for urine. The bladder possesses features that enable urine to enter, be stored, and later be released for evacuation from the body.

Structure

The bladder is a hollow, expandable, muscular organ located in the pelvic girdle (fig. 1-59). Although the shape of the bladder is spherical, its shape is altered by the pressures of surrounding organs. When it is empty, the inner walls of the bladder form folds. But as the bladder fills with urine, the walls become smoother.

The internal floor of the bladder includes a triangular area called the **trigone** (fig. 1-59). The trigone has three openings at each of its angles. The ureters are attached to the two posterior openings. The anterior opening, at the apex of the trigone, contains a funnel-like continuation called the **neck** of the bladder. The neck leads to the urethra.

The wall of the bladder consists of four bundles of smooth muscle fibers. These muscle fibers, interlaced, form the **detrusor muscle** (which surrounds the bladder neck) and comprise what is called the **internal urethral sphincter**. The internal urethral sphincter prevents urine from escaping the bladder until the pressure inside the bladder reaches a certain level. Parasympathetic nerve fibers in the detrusor muscle function in the micturition (urination) process. The

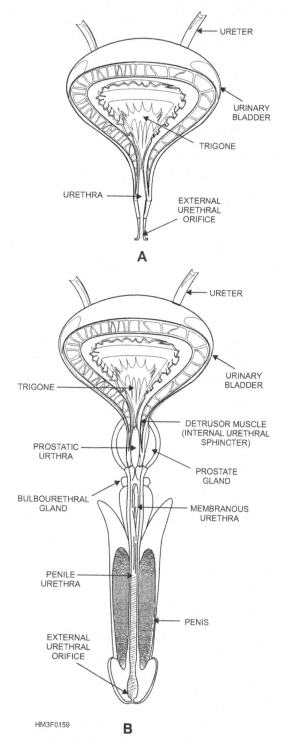

HM3F0159

Figure 1-59.—Urinary bladder and urethra:
A. Frontal section of the female urinary bladder and urethra;
B. Frontal section of the male urinary bladder and urethra.

outer layer (**serous coat**) of the bladder wall consists of two types of tissue, **parietal peritoneum** and **fibrous connective tissue**.

Micturition (Urination)

Micturition is the process by which urine is expelled from the bladder. It involves the contraction of the detrusor muscle, and pressure from surrounding structures. Urination also involves the relaxation of the **external urethral sphincter**. The external urethral sphincter surrounds the urethra about 3 centimeters from the bladder, and is composed of voluntary muscular tissue.

Urination is usually stimulated by the distention of the bladder as it fills with urine. When the walls of the bladder contract, nerve receptors are stimulated, and the urination reflex is triggered. The urination reflex causes the internal urethral sphincter to open and the external urethral sphincter to relax. This relaxation allows the bladder to empty. The bladder can hold up to 600 ml of urine. The desire to urinate may not occur until the bladder contains 250-300 ml.

URETHRA

The urethra is the tube that carries urine from the bladder to the outside of the body (fig. 1-59, views A and B). The **urinary meatus** is the external urethral orifice. In the male, the urethra is common to the urinary and reproductive systems; in the female, it belongs only to the urinary system.

Female Urethra

The female urethra is about 4 cm long, extending from the bladder to the external orifice, (fig. 1-59, view A).

Male Urethra

The male urethra is about 20 cm long and is divided into three parts: the prostatic, membranous, and penile portions. See view B of figure 1-59 for an illustration of the male urethra.

PROSTATIC URETHRA.—The prostatic urethra is surrounded by the prostate gland; it contains the orifices of the prostatic and ejaculatory ducts. This portion of the male urethra is about 2.5 cm long.

MEMBRANOUS URETHRA.—The membranous urethra is about 2 cm in length and is surrounded by the external urethral sphincter.

PENILE URETHRA.—The penile urethra, the longest portion, is about 15 cm long. It lies in the ventral portion of the penis. The urethra terminates with the external orifice at the tip of the penis.

MALE REPRODUCTIVE SYSTEM

LEARNING OBJECTIVE: *Recall the parts of the male reproductive system and their function(s).*

The organs of the male and female reproductive systems are concerned with the process of reproducing offspring, and each organ is adapted to perform specialized tasks. The primary male sex organs of the reproductive system are the testes. The other structures of the male reproductive system are termed accessory reproductive organs. The accessory organs include both internal and external reproductive organs. See figure 1-60 for an illustration of the male reproductive system.

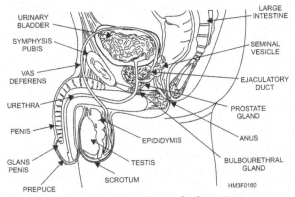

Figure 1-60.—The male reproductive system.

TESTES

The testes, as stated earlier, are the primary male reproductive organs. They produce sperm cells (spermatozoa) and male hormones, both necessary for reproduction.

Structure

The testes are oval glands suspended inside a sac (the scrotum) by a **spermatic cord**. The spermatic cords are formed by the vas deferens, arteries, veins, lymphatics, and nerves, all bound together by connective tissue.

Each testis is encapsulated by a tough, white, fibrous tissue called the tunica albuginea. The interior of the testis is divided into 250 lobules (small lobes). Each lobule contains 1 to 4 highly coiled, convoluted tubules called **seminiferous tubules**. These tubules unite to form a complex network of channels called the **rete testis**. The rete testis give rise to several ducts that join a tube called the **epididymis** (fig. 1-60).

Functions

The testes perform two functions: to produce sperm cells and to secrete male sex hormones. The process by which sperm cells are produced is called **spermatogenesis**. Spermatogenesis occurs in the seminiferous tubules of the testes. Once the sperm cells are formed, they collect in the lumen of each seminiferous tubule. When the sperm cells are ready, they pass through the rete testis to the epididymis, where they remain for a time to mature. The production of sperm cells occurs continually throughout the reproductive life of a male.

The male hormone **testosterone** is produced in the testes. This hormone is initially responsible for the formation of the male reproductive organs. During puberty, testosterone stimulates the enlargement of the testes and various other accessory reproductive organs. It also causes the development of the male secondary sexual characteristics. Refer to the section titled "The Endocrine System" for more detailed discussion on male secondary sexual characteristics.

Other actions of testosterone include increasing the production of red blood cells. As a result, the average number of red blood cells in blood is usually greater in males than in females.

INTERNAL ACCESSORY ORGANS

The internal accessory organs of the male reproductive system include the epididymis, vas deferens, ejaculatory ducts, seminal vesicle, urethra, prostate gland, bulbourethral glands, and semen (fig. 1-60).

Epididymis

Each epididymis is a tightly coiled, thread-like tube that is approximately 6 meters long. This tube is connected to the ducts within the testis. The epididymis covers the top of the testis, runs down the testis' posterior surface, and then courses upward to form the vas deferens.

The epididymis secretes the hormone glycogen, which helps sustain the lives of stored sperm cells and promotes their maturation. When immature sperm cells enter the epididymis, they are not mobile. However, as the sperm cells travel through the epididymis, they mature and become mobile. Once the sperm cells are mature, they leave the epididymis and enter the vas deferens.

Vas Deferens

The vas deferens is a small tube that connects the epididymis and ejaculatory duct. It ascends as part of the spermatic cord through the inguinal canal of the lower abdominal wall into the pelvic cavity, and transmits the sperm to the ejaculatory ducts.

Ejaculatory Ducts

The vas deferens and the seminal vesicles converge, just before the entrance of the prostate gland, to form the ejaculatory ducts (fig. 1-60). The ejaculatory ducts open into the prostatic urethra. Its function is to convey sperm cells to the urethra.

Seminal Vesicles

The seminal vesicles are two pouches that are attached to the vas deferens near the base of the urinary bladder. The lining of the inner walls of the seminal vesicles secrete a slightly alkaline fluid. This fluid is thought to help regulate the pH of the tubular contents as sperm cells are conveyed to the outside. The secretion produced by the seminal vesicles also contains a variety of nutrients, such as fructose (simple sugar), that provides the sperm cells an energy source.

At the time of ejaculation, the contents of the seminal vesicles are emptied into the ejaculatory ducts. This action greatly increases the volume of fluid that is discharged by the vas deferens.

Urethra

The urethra is an important organ of both the urinary and reproductive systems. The role of the urethra, in the reproductive system, is to transport sperm through the penis to outside the body. See "The Urinary System" section for information on the structure of the urethra.

Prostate Gland

The prostate gland, made of smooth muscle and glandular tissue, surrounds the first part of the urethra. It resembles a chestnut in shape and size, and secretes an alkaline fluid to keep the sperm mobile, protecting it from the acid secretions of the female vagina. This substance is discharged into the urethra as part of the ejaculate, or semen, during the sexual act.

Bulbourethral Glands

Bulbourethral glands, also known as **Cowper's glands**, are two pea-sized bodies located below the prostate gland and lateral to the membranous urethra. These glands are enclosed by fibers of the external urethral sphincter. They release a mucous-like fluid in response to sexual stimulation and provide lubrication to the end of the penis in preparation for sexual intercourse.

Semen

Semen is composed of sperm and secretions from the seminal vesicles, prostate, and bulbourethral glands. It is discharged as the ejaculate during sexual intercourse. There are millions of sperm cells in the semen of each ejaculation, but only one is needed to fertilize the ovum. It is generally considered that fertilization of the ovum occurs while it is still in the fallopian tubes. Therefore, it is apparent that sperm cells can move actively in the seminal fluid deposited in the vagina and through the layers of the secretion lining the uterus and fallopian tubes.

EXTERNAL ACCESSORY ORGANS

The external accessory organs of the male reproductive system include the scrotum and penis (fig. 1-60).

Scrotum

The scrotum is a cutaneous pouch containing the testes and part of the spermatic cord. Immediately beneath the skin is a thin layer of muscular fibers (the cremaster), which is controlled by temperature and contracts or relaxes to lower or raise the testes in relation to the body. This muscular activity of the scrotum is necessary to regulate the temperature of the testes, which is important in the maturation of sperm cells.

Penis

The penis is a cylindrical organ that conveys urine and semen through the urethra to the outside. The penis is composed of three columns of spongy cavernous tissue, bound together by connective tissue and loosely covered by a layer of skin. Two of the columns, the **corpora cavernosa**, lie superiorly side by side; the third column, the **corpus spongiosum**, lies below the other two columns. The urethra is located in the corpus spongiosum. The dilated distal end of the corpus spongiosum is known as the **glans penis** (fig. 1-60). The urethra terminates at the glans penis.

The cavernous tissue becomes greatly distended with blood during sexual excitement, causing an erection of the penis. The loose skin of the penis folds back on itself at the distal end (forming the **prepuce**, or foreskin) and covers the glans. The prepuce is sometimes removed by a surgical procedure called a **circumcision.**

FEMALE REPRODUCTIVE SYSTEM

LEARNING OBJECTIVE: *Recall the parts of the female reproductive system and their function(s).*

The organs of the female reproductive system are specialized to produce and maintain the female sex cells, or egg cells; to transport these cells to the site of fertilization; to provide an environment for a developing offspring; to move the offspring outside; and to produce female sex hormones. The primary female reproductive organs are the ovaries. The other structures of the female reproductive system are considered accessory reproductive organs. The

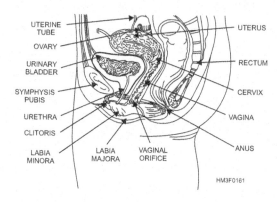

Figure 1-61.—The female reproductive system.

accessory organs include both internal and external reproductive organs (fig. 1-61).

OVARIES

The ovaries, as stated earlier, are the primary female reproductive organs, producing the female sex cells and sex hormones (fig. 1-61).

Structure

The ovaries, or female gonads, are two almond-shaped glands suspended by ligaments in the upper pelvic cavity. There is one ovary on each side of the uterus. The ligaments that suspend the ovaries contain ovarian blood vessels and nerves.

The tissues of an ovary are divided into two regions, an inner **medulla** and an outer **cortex**. The ovarian medulla is largely composed of loose connective tissue, numerous blood vessels, lymph vessels, and nerves. The ovarian cortex is composed of compact tissue containing tiny masses of cells called **ovarian (primordial) follicles**. The follicles contain the female sex cells or **ova**. The external surface of the ovary is covered by a layer of cuboidal epithelium cells. Beneath the epithelium is a layer of dense connective tissue.

Primordial Follicle

In the outer region of the ovarian cortex, microscopic groups of cells are referred to as primordial follicles. The primordial follicles consist of a single large cell, called an **oocyte**, which is surrounded by a layer of flattened epithelial cells called **follicular cells**. The oocyte is an immature egg

cell. Follicular cells surround a developing egg cell and secrete female sex hormones. There are approximately 400,000 primordial follicles at puberty. Of these, probably fewer than 500 will be released from the ovary during the reproductive life of a female.

At puberty, the anterior pituitary gland secretes increased amounts of FSH (follicle-stimulating hormone). In response, the ovaries enlarge and many of the primordial follicles begin to mature. During this maturation process, the oocyte enlarges and the follicle cells multiply until there are 6 to 12 layers. Fluid-filled spaces begin to appear among the follicle cells. These spaces join to form a single cavity called the antrum. Ten to fourteen days after this process begins, the primordial follicle reaches maturity. The mature primordial follicle (preovulatory or graafian follicle) and its fluid-filled cavity bulges outward on the surface of the ovary, like a blister.

Ovulation

Ovulation is the process by which the mature oocyte is released from the primordial follicle (fig. 1-62). Ovulation is stimulated by hormones from the anterior pituitary gland. These hormones cause the mature follicle to swell rapidly and its walls to weaken. Eventually the wall ruptures, permitting the oocyte and 1 or 2 layers of follicle cells to be released from the ovary's surface.

After ovulation, the oocyte is usually propelled to the opening of a nearby fallopian tube. If the oocyte is not fertilized by a sperm cell within a relatively short time, it will degenerate.

This process of ovulation occurs once a month. Each ovary normally releases an ovum every 56 days. The right and left ovary alternately discharge an ovum approximately every 28 days. The menstrual cycle in most women is therefore approximately 28 days.

Female Sex Hormones

Female sex hormones are produced by the ovaries and various other tissues, such as the adrenal glands, pituitary gland, and placenta (during pregnancy). These female sex hormones are **estrogen** and **progesterone**.

The primary source for estrogen is the ovaries. At puberty, estrogen stimulates enlargement of various accessory organs, which include the vagina, uterus, fallopian tubes, and external structures. Estrogen is also responsible for the development and maintenance

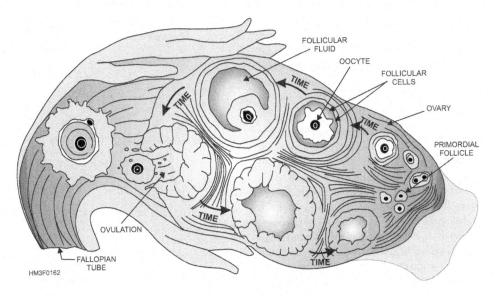

Figure 1-62.—Ovulation process.

of female secondary sexual characteristics. See section titled "Endocrine System" for listing of secondary female sexual characteristics.

The ovaries are also the primary source of progesterone (in a nonpregnant female). This hormone promotes changes that occur in the uterus during the female reproductive cycle. In addition, progesterone stimulates the enlargement of mammary glands and ducts, and increases fat deposits in female breasts during puberty.

INTERNAL ACCESSORY ORGANS

The internal accessory organs of the female reproductive system include a pair of fallopian tubes, the uterus, and the vagina (fig. 1-61).

Fallopian Tubes

The fallopian tubes, also known as uterine tubes, serve as ducts for the ovaries, providing a passageway to the uterus. The fallopian tubes are composed of three tissue layers. These tissue layers include an inner mucosal layer, a middle muscular layer, and an outer serous layer, and they are continuous with the layers of the uterus. The fallopian tubes are in contact with the ovaries but are not continuous with them. Their funnel-shaped openings, called **free openings**, are fringed with fingerlike processes that pick up an ovum and draw it into the fallopian tubes. Once the ovum enters the fallopian tubes, it is transported to the uterus

by peristalsis and gravity. Fertilization of an ovum normally takes place in the fallopian tubes.

Uterus

The function of the uterus is to receive the embryo that results from the fertilization of an egg cell, and to sustain its life during development. The uterus, or womb, is a hollow, pear-shaped organ with thick, muscular walls. The uterus is divided into two main regions, the **body** and **cervix** (fig. 1-61). The body of the uterus consists of the upper two-thirds of the uterus. The cervix is the lower one-third portion of the uterus that projects into the upper part of the vagina. The cervical opening into the vagina is called the **external os.**

The uterine wall is composed of three layers: the endometrium, the myometrium, and the perimetrium. The inner lining consists of specialized epithelium, called **endometrium**, which undergoes partial destruction approximately every 28 days in the nonpregnant female. The middle layer, the **myometrium**, consists of bundles of interlaced muscular fibers. The muscular layer produces powerful rhythmic contractions that are important in the expulsion of the fetus at birth. The **perimetrium** consists of an outer serosal layer that covers the body of the uterus and part of the cervix. The uterus also has three openings: superiorly and laterally, two openings connect the fallopian tubes to the uterus, and inferiorly, an opening leading to the vagina.

Vagina

The vagina is the organ that receives the male sperm during intercourse. It also forms the lower portion of the birth canal, stretching widely during delivery. In addition, it serves as an excretory duct for uterine secretions and menstrual flow.

The vagina is a fibromuscular tube capable of great distention. The canal is approximately 9 cm long and extends from the uterus to the outside. The vaginal orifice is partially closed by a thin membrane of tissue called the **hymen**. The wall of the vagina consists of three layers. The inner **mucosal layer** does not have mucous glands; the mucous found in the vagina comes from the glands of the cervix. The middle **muscular layer** consists mainly of smooth muscles fibers. At the lower end of the vagina is a thin band of smooth muscle that helps close the vaginal opening. The outer **fibrous layer** consists of dense fibrous connective tissue interlaced with elastic fibers. These fibers attach the vagina to the surrounding organs.

EXTERNAL ACCESSORY ORGANS

Many of the external accessory organs of the female reproductive system are referred to collectively as the **vulva**. The vulva includes the labia majora, the labia minora, the clitoris, and the vestibular glands (fig. 1-63). The mammary glands are also considered an accessory organ of the female reproductive system.

Labia Majora

The function of the labia majora is to enclose and protect the other external reproductive organs. The labia majora are composed of two round folds of fat tissue and a thin layer of smooth muscle, covered by skin. On the outer portion of the labia majora, the skin has numerous hairs, sweat glands, and sebaceous glands. The inner portion of skin is thin and hairless. The labia majora extend from the mons pubis anteriorly to the perineum (the region between the vaginal orifice and the anus). The **mons pubis** is the pad of fatty tissue beneath the skin, which overlies the symphysis pubis.

Labia Minora

Within the labia majora folds are two smaller folds, called the labia minora. The labia minora extend from the clitoris to either side of the vaginal orifice.

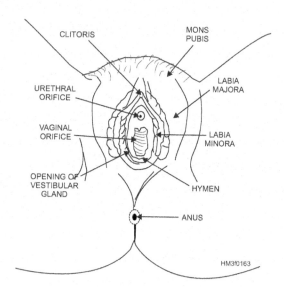

Figure 1-63.—External reproductive organs.

Clitoris

The clitoris is a small projectile at the anterior end of the vulva between the labia minora. It is richly endowed with sensory nerves that are associated with the feeling of pleasure during sexual stimulation.

Vestibule

The vestibule is the area enclosed by the labia minora that includes that vaginal and urethral openings. The vestibule contains a pair of vestibular glands, more commonly known as the **Bartholin's glands**. The Bartholin's glands lay on each side of the vaginal opening. The ducts of these glands secrete fluid that moistens and lubricates the vestibule.

Mammary Glands

The mammary glands, or breasts, are accessory organs of the female reproductive system. They develop during puberty under the influence of the hormones estrogen and progesterone. The breasts are responsible for the secretion of milk (**lactation**) for the nourishment of newborn infants.

Structurally, the breasts resemble sweat glands. At the center is a nipple containing 15 to 20 depressions into which ducts from the lobes of the gland empty. During pregnancy, placental estrogen and progesterone stimulate further development of the mammary glands in preparation for lactation. After childbirth, hormones secreted by the anterior lobe of the pituitary gland stimulate production for 6 to 9 months.

FEMALE REPRODUCTIVE CYCLE

Females around age 11 begin to experience the female reproductive cycle and continue into middle age, after which it ceases. The female reproductive cycle, or menstrual cycle, is characterized by regular, recurring changes in the uterine lining, resulting in menstrual bleeding (**menses**). The first phase of the recurring reproductive cycle is menstrual bleeding. Menstrual bleeding begins when the endometrial lining starts to slough off from the walls of the uterus, and it is characterized by bleeding from the vagina. This is day 1 of the cycle, and this phase usually lasts through day 5. The time between the last day of the menses and ovulation is known as the postmenstrual phase. It lasts from day 6 through day 13 or 14 and is characterized by proliferation of endometrial cells in the uterus, which develop under the influence of the hormone estrogen. Ovulation, as discussed earlier in this section, is the rupture of a primordial follicle with the release of a mature ovum into the fallopian tubes. It usually occurs on day 14 or 15 of the cycle. The postovulatory (premenstrual) phase is the time between ovulation and the onset of the menstrual bleeding and normally lasts 14 days. During this phase the ovum travels through the fallopian tubes to the uterus. If the ovum becomes fertilized during this passage, it will become implanted in and nurtured by the newly developed endometrial lining. However, if fertilization does not take place, the lining deteriorates and eventually sloughs off, marking day 1 of the next cycle.

SUMMARY

In this chapter, you have learned about the basic structures of the cell to the many complex systems of the human body. In addition, you have acquired the understanding of how each body system functions and how each system is interdependent upon each other. You will use this knowledge of human anatomy and physiology throughout your career in the medical services. For example, the anatomical terminology will be used in describing location of injuries or conditions. Also, when you perform patient assessments, a clear and thorough understanding of anatomy and physiology is essential. Patient assessment and documentation procedures will be discussed in the next chapter, entitled "Fundamentals of Patient Care."

CHAPTER 2

FUNDAMENTALS OF PATIENT CARE

Twentieth century advances in the medical and technological sciences have made a significant impact on the methods of marketing healthcare services. The numbers and kinds of healthcare providers have expanded greatly. Patients have become more informed about both their healthcare needs and expectations. Additionally, patients have become more vocal, seeking answers for the "what's" and "why's" of the entire spectrum of healthcare services.

The goal of this chapter is to give the Hospital Corpsman basic theory concerning the multidisciplinary aspects of patient care. This chapter is an introduction to some of the critical basic concepts for providing care to individuals seeking healthcare services.

HEALTH AND ILLNESS

LEARNING OBJECTIVE: *Recognize the concepts of health and illness.*

To intelligently and skillfully discharge your duties as a member of the Navy Medical Department healthcare team, you must first understand the concepts of health and illness.

The concept of health includes the physical, mental, and emotional condition of human beings that provide for the normal and proper performance of one's vital functions. Not only is health the absence of disease or disability; health is also a state of soundness of the body, mind, and spirit. Conversely, the concept of illness includes conditions often accompanied by pain or discomfort that inhibit a human being's ability to physically, mentally, or emotionally perform in a normal and proper manner.

In most cultures, when people need assistance in maintaining their health, dealing with illness, or coping with problems related to health and illness, they seek assistance from personnel specialized in the fields of healthcare.

Physicians, nurses, and Hospital Corpsmen are frequently referred to as the core team. All health personnel comprise the total healthcare team. Obviously, individual members of the team use their skills differently, depending upon their personal, professional, and technical preparation and experience. Nevertheless—and despite the differences in clinical expertise—they all share one common objective: to respond to the patient's health needs. The overall goal of this response is to assist the patient to maintain, sustain, and restore or rehabilitate a physical or psychological function.

THE PATIENT

LEARNING OBJECTIVE: *Recognize the Patients' Bill of Rights and Responsibilities.*

No discussion about healthcare or the healthcare team would be complete without including the patient, often referred to as the consumer. A patient is a human being under the care of one or more healthcare providers. The patient may or may not be hospitalized. However, regardless of healthcare needs or environmental disposition, the patient is the most important part of the healthcare team. Without a patient, the healthcare team has little, if any, reason for existence.

As a Hospital Corpsman, you are tasked to provide every patient committed to your charge with the best care possible. This care must reflect your belief in the value and dignity of every person as an individual. Additionally, you must understand the patient's rights and responsibilities as they apply to providing and receiving healthcare services.

The Joint Commission on Accreditation of Healthcare Organizations (JCAHO) has developed standards that address the rights and responsibilities of patients. Because the goal of JCAHO is to promote excellence in providing healthcare services, this goal is compatible with that of the Navy Medical Department. The next two sections review the rights and responsibilities of patients when they enter a relationship with a healthcare service facility. Students seeking additional detailed information should refer to the *Patients' Bill of Rights and Responsibilities* (an enclosure to BUMEDINST 6300.10) and the *Accreditation Manual for Hospitals* published by the JCAHO.

PATIENT'S RIGHTS

The following are the patient's rights:

- **Medical Care and Dental Care**—A patient has the right to quality care and treatment consistent with available resources and generally accepted standards. The patient has the right to refuse treatment to the extent permitted by law and government regulations. However, the patient should be informed of the consequences of refusal.

- **Respectful Treatment**—A patient has the right to considerate and respectful care, with recognition of his personal dignity.

- **Privacy and Confidentiality**—A patient, within law and military regulations, is entitled to privacy and confidentiality concerning medical care.

- **Identity**—A patient has the right to know, at all times, the identity, professional status, and professional credentials of healthcare personnel, as well as the name of the healthcare provider primarily responsible for his care.

- **Explanation of Care**—A patient has the right to an explanation concerning his diagnosis, treatment, procedures, and prognosis of illness in terms the patient can understand.

- **Informed Consent**—A patient has the right to be advised in nonclinical terms of information needed to make knowledgeable decisions on consent or refusal of treatments. Such information should include significant complications, risks, benefits, and alternative treatments available.

- **Research Projects**—A patient has the right to be advised if the facility proposes to engage in or perform research associated with his care or treatment. The patient has the right to refuse to participate in any research projects.

- **Safe Environment**—A patient has the right to care and treatment in a safe environment.

- **Medical Treatment Facility (MTF) or Dental Treatment Facility (DTF) Rules and Regulations**—A patient has the right to be informed of the facility's rules and regulations that relate to patient or visitor conduct. The patient is entitled to information for the initiation, review, and resolution of patient complaints.

PATIENT'S RESPONSIBILITIES

The following are the patient's responsibilities:

- **Providing Information**—A patient has the responsibility to provide, to the best of his knowledge, accurate and complete information about complaints, past illnesses, hospitalizations, medications, and other matters relating to his personal health.

- **Respect and Consideration**—A patient has the responsibility to be considerate of the rights of other patients and MTF or DTF healthcare personnel, and to assist in the control of noise, smoking, and the number of visitors. The patient is responsible for being respectful of the property of other persons and of the facility.

- **Compliance with Medical Care**—A patient is responsible for complying with the medical and nursing treatment plan, including followup care recommended by healthcare providers.

- **Medical Records**—A patient is responsible for ensuring that medical records are promptly returned to the medical facility for appropriate filing and maintenance when those records are transported by the patient for the purpose of medical appointments or consultation, etc.

- **MTF and DTF Rules and Regulations**—A patient is responsible for following the MTF or DTF rules and regulations affecting patient care.

- **Reporting of Patient Complaints**—A patient is responsible for helping the MTF or DTF commander provide the best possible care to all beneficiaries. The patient's recommendations, questions, or complaints should be reported to the patient contact representative.

PROFESSIONAL PRACTICE

LEARNING OBJECTIVE: *Recognize the key elements of professional practice.*

Each member of the healthcare team has specific responsibilities and limitations that define his area of practice. To fulfill your role as a member of the Hospital Corps within the context of the total mission of the Navy Medical Department, it is imperative that your practice be based on a sound body of knowledge and the development of well-defined technical skills. The rate training manual (TRAMAN) contributes to the development of your body of knowledge. The HM occupational standards (NAVPERS 18068F, chapter 40) define minimal technical skills required of a Hospital Corpsman. As a member of the healthcare team, the mechanism of on-the-job training, in-service classes, and continuing education programs contribute significantly to your continued growth in both healthcare knowledge and skills.

PROFESSIONAL LIMITATIONS

In conjunction with their professional responsibilities, all healthcare providers should realize that they are subject to certain limitations in providing healthcare services. These standards of practice are based on the amount and kind of education, training, experience, local regulations, and guidelines possessed by the healthcare provider. The mature, responsible individual will recognize, accept, and demand that these limitations be respected. In clinical settings, Hospital Corpsmen are tasked with administering medication, performing treatments, and providing individual patient care in compliance with the orders of the senior healthcare provider. In the hospital and some clinical environments, a Nurse Corps officer divides and delegates portions of the patient's care to other members of the team based on the skills and experiences of each member. In situations where a Nurse Corps officer is not a member of the team, such delegation of duties will generally be made by an experienced chief petty officer or a senior petty officer of the Hospital Corps.

ACCOUNTABILITY

Regardless of rank, rate, or corps membership, all members of the healthcare team are held accountable for their performance. Being accountable means being held responsible for your actions. As a healthcare provider, you should continue to acquire new knowledge and skills and to strive for clinical competency. Equally important is your ability to apply new knowledge and acquired skills as a competent professional in providing total healthcare.

Accountability becomes a critical issue when determining issues of malpractice. Malpractice occurs when an individual delivers improper care because of negligence or practicing outside of his area of expertise. Because the areas of expertise and responsibility in medicine frequently overlap, legal limits of practice are defined by each state. The assignments and responsibilities of Hospital Corpsmen frequently include areas of practice usually provided by physicians and nurses in the civilian sector. **These responsibilities are only legal when Hospital Corpsmen are performing such duties while under the authority of the United States Government**. Because of this requirement, it is vital that you thoroughly understand your legal rights and limitations when providing patient care services both in government and civilian sectors.

PATIENT ADVICE

Another area that has potential medical and legal implications regarding your role as a healthcare provider is that of giving advice or opinions. As a result of your frequent and close contact with patients, you will often be asked your opinion of the care or the proposed care a patient is undergoing. Often, these questions are extremely difficult to respond to, regardless of who the healthcare provider is. No one is ever totally prepared or has so much wisdom that he can respond spontaneously in such situations. In such cases, it is best to refer the question to the nurse or physician responsible for the patient's care.

You must always be conscious that you are seen as a representative of Navy medicine by the recipients of your care. As such, you will be accorded the respect that goes with having a specialized body of knowledge and an inventory of unique skills. A caduceus on the sleeve of the Hospital Corpsman marks that person as a member of a prestigious corps worthy of respect.

PATIENT BEHAVIOR

Remember, you have been charged to provide care to a total, feeling, human person. The person seeking healthcare service has the same needs for security, safety, love, respect, and self-fulfillment as everyone else. When something threatens the soundness of the body, mind, or spirit, an individual may behave inappropriately. Occasionally, there are temper outbursts, episodes of pouting, sarcastic remarks, unreasonable demands, or other inappropriate responses, often to the point of disruptive behavior. The healthcare provider is challenged to look beyond the behavior being displayed to identify the underlying stress and to attempt to relieve the immediate and obvious source of anxiety. This may be as simple as communicating, through your care and understanding of the patient as an individual, that Navy medicine is pleased to provide a caring service.

PROFESSIONAL ETHICS

LEARNING OBJECTIVE: *Recognize the concept of professional ethics.*

The word **ethics** is derived from the Greek "ethos," meaning custom or practice, a characteristic manner of acting, or a more-or-less constant style of behavior in the deliberate actions of people. When we speak of ethics, we refer to a set of rules or a body of principles. Every social, religious, and professional group has a body of principles or standards of conduct that provides ethical guidance to its members.

During your indoctrination into the military, you were introduced to the Code of the U.S. Fighting Forces. This code of conduct is an ethical guide that charges you with certain high standards of general behavior as a member of the Armed Forces.

All professional interactions must be directly related to codes of behavior that support the principles of justice, equality of human beings as persons, and respect for the dignity of human beings. Upholding medical ethics is the responsibility of all Hospital Corpsmen. Upon completion of basic Hospital Corps School, you took the following pledge:

I solemnly pledge myself before God and these witnesses to practice faithfully all of my duties as a member of the Hospital Corps. I hold the care of the sick and injured to be a privilege and a sacred trust and will assist the Medical Officer with loyalty and honesty. I will hold all personal matters pertaining to the private lives of patients in strict confidence. I dedicate my heart, mind, and strength to the work before me. I shall do all within my power

to show in myself an example of all that is honorable and good throughout my naval career.

This pledge morally binds you to certain responsibilities and rules that are included in the science of medical ethics. Ethics, whether they be classified general or special (e.g., legal or medical), teach us how to judge accurately the moral rightness and wrongness of our actions. The one element that makes healthcare ethics different from general ethics is the inclusion of the moral rule, "Do your duty." This statement is a moral rule because it involves expectations (e.g., of confidentiality). It involves what others have every reason to believe will be forthcoming. Failure to fulfill these expectations is to do harm to your clients (i.e., your patients) and/or your colleagues. Through the Hospital Corpsman Pledge, you committed yourself to fulfilling certain duties, not only to those entrusted to your care, but also to all members of the healthcare team. It is this commitment to service and to mankind that has traditionally distinguished the United States Navy Hospital Corps wherever its members have served.

PERSONAL TRAITS

LEARNING OBJECTIVE: *Recognize important personality traits of a healthcare professional.*

A Hospital Corpsman must develop many personal traits that apply to all petty officers. You can get a general understanding of them by referring to *Military Requirements for Petty Officer Third Class* (NAVEDTRA 12024).

The following traits, however, apply especially to your Hospital Corps duties and are essential for good performance.

INTEGRITY

Nowhere in the Navy is the need for personal integrity so great as in the Hospital Corps, where we deal continually with people, their illnesses, and their personal problems. The information that we have access to falls into the category of "privileged communication." We, as Hospital Corpsmen, have no right whatsoever to divulge any medical information, however trivial, to any unauthorized individuals.

Medical information is prime gossip material. The prohibition on the release of medical information is sometimes difficult to remember, but it is essential to the maintenance of professional integrity.

One important commitment that all Corps personnel have is the obligation never to abuse the controlled substances that we have access to—or to tolerate abuse by others. These substances are on the ward or in the mount-out block for use, under a medical officer's supervision, for the care of patients. Any other use must not be tolerated.

PERSONAL APPEARANCE

Excellent personal hygiene habits, including cleanliness, neat hair styles, and spotless, correct uniforms are essential for the Hospital Corps. Our appearance can positively or negatively influence the opinion the public has of the medical community. Both a professional appearance and attitude enhance the overall reputation of the Navy Medical Department and reinforce our role as competent healthcare providers.

LEADERSHIP

Naval leadership is based on personal example, good management, and moral responsibility. All of the personal traits previously discussed are also considered leadership traits. You will learn that many examples of effective leadership are those that are set by officers, chief petty officers, and senior petty officers. The success of the Medical Department rests heavily on the petty officer. Good petty officers are the backbone of the Medical Department, whether they are supervising military personnel or conducting specialist duties.

INTERPERSONAL RELATIONS

LEARNING OBJECTIVE: *Recognize how an understanding of a patient's culture, race, religion, sex, and age can affect interpersonal relations.*

As a healthcare provider, you must be able to identify, understand, and use various kinds of information. In addition, it is important that you develop good "interpersonal relations" skills. In providing total patient care, it is important that you see the individual not only as a biological being, but also as a thinking, feeling person. Your commitment to understanding this concept is the key to your developing good interpersonal relationships.

Simply stated, your interpersonal relationships are the result of how you regard and respond to people. Many elements influence the development of that regard and those responses. In the following discussion, some of these elements will be discussed as they apply to your involvement in the military service and to your relationships with other healthcare providers and the patient.

CULTURE

Because of the multi- and cross-cultural nature and military mission of the Navy Medical Department, you will frequently encounter members of various cultures. **Culture** is defined as a group of socially learned, shared standards (norms) and behavior patterns. Concepts such as perceptions, values, beliefs, and goals are examples of shared norms. In addition, apparel, eating habits, and personal hygiene reflect common behavior patterns of specific groups of people. An understanding of common norms and behavior patterns enhances the quality—and often the quantity—of service a provider is able to make available. An individual's cultural background has an effect on every area of healthcare service, ranging from a simple technical procedure to the content and effectiveness of health education activities. Becoming familiar with the beliefs and practices of different cultural and subcultural groups (the military community, for example) is not only enriching to the healthcare provider, but also promotes an understanding and acceptance of the various peoples in the world community.

RACE

The term **race** is a classification assigned to a group of people who share inherited physical characteristics. This term becomes a socially significant reality since people tend to attach great importance to assuming or designating a racial identity. Information identifying racial affiliation can be an asset to the healthcare provider in assessing the patient's needs, carrying out direct-care activities, and planning and implementing patient education programs. Racial identification has the potential to create a negative environment in the healthcare setting when factors such as skin color differences motivate prejudicial and segregational behaviors. When this is permitted to occur, an environment that feeds a multitude of social illnesses and destructive behaviors develops. In the Navy Medical Department, no expressions or actions based on prejudicial attitudes will be tolerated.

It is both the moral and legal responsibility of the healthcare provider to render services with respect for the life and human dignity of the individual without regard to race, creed, gender, political views, or social status.

RELIGION

A large majority of people have some form of belief system that guides many of their life decisions and to which they turn to in times of distress. A person's religious beliefs frequently help give meaning to suffering and illness; those beliefs may also be helpful in the acceptance of future incapacities or death.

As a healthcare professional, you must accept in a nonjudgmental way the religious or nonreligious beliefs of others as valid for them, even if you personally disagree with such beliefs. Although you may offer religious support when asked and should always provide chaplain referrals when requested or indicated, it is not ethical for you to abuse your patients by forcing your beliefs (or nonbeliefs) upon them. You must respect their freedom of choice, offering your support for whatever their needs or desires may be.

GENDER

In today's Navy, you will encounter many situations where you are responsible for the care and treatment of service members of the opposite sex. When you treat service members of the opposite sex, you must always conduct yourself in a professional manner.

To ensure the professional conduct of a healthcare provider is not called into question, the Navy Medical Department provides specific guidelines in BUMEDINST 6320.83, *Provisions of Standbys During Medical Examinations*. Some of these guidelines are as follows:

- A standby should be present when you are examining or treating a member of the opposite sex. Whether this standby is a member of the

same sex as the patient may be dictated by the availability of personnel.

- Common sense dictates that when you are caring for a patient, sensitivity to both verbal and nonverbal communication is paramount. A grin, a frown, or an expression of surprise may all be misinterpreted by the patient.

- Explanations and reassurances will go far in preventing misunderstandings of actions or intentions.

Knowledge, empathy, and mature judgment should guide the care provided to any patient. This is especially crucial when the care involves touching. As a member of the healthcare team, you are responsible for providing complete, quality care to those who need and seek your service. This care must also be provided in a manner compatible with your technical capabilities.

AGE

The age of the patient must be considered in performance of patient care. As a Hospital Corpsman, you will be responsible for the care of infants, children, adults, and the elderly. Communication techniques and patient handling may need to be modified because of the age of the patient.

Infants and Children

Infants can communicate their feelings in a variety of positive and negative ways, and they exhibit their needs by crying, kicking, or grabbing at the affected area of pain. An infant, however, usually responds positively to cuddling, rocking, touching, and soothing sounds.

Children need emotional support and display the same feelings an adult would when ill: fear, anger, worry, and so on. When ill, children may display behavior typical for an earlier age. For example, when hospitalized, a child who has been toilet trained may soil himself. This is not unusual, and parents should be informed that this behavior change is temporary. While the child is under your care in the hospital, you are a parent substitute and must gain the child's confidence and trust. Offer explanations of what you are going to do in ways the child will understand.

Elderly

In taking care of the elderly patient, a healthcare professional must be alert to the patient's mental and physical capabilities (i.e., physical coordination, mental orientation, reduced eyesight). Medical management should be modified to accommodate the individual patient. Show genuine respect and warmth with the elderly. Avoid using terms like "gramps" or "granny." You should always show the elderly respect by treating them as the adults they are.

Give older patients the opportunity to control as many aspects of their self-care as possible. Allowing patients to self-pace their own care may take more time, but it will result in reducing their feelings of frustration, anger, and resentment. Listen to patients and allow them to reminisce if they wish to. The conversation can be used as a vehicle to bring today's events into focus for the patient. Remember to involve family members, as needed, into the patient education process. Some of your elderly patients will require assistance from family members for their medical needs once they are back home.

COMMUNICATION SKILLS

LEARNING OBJECTIVE: *Recognize communication techniques used in a healthcare setting.*

Communication is a highly complicated interpersonal process of people relating to each other through conversation, writing, gestures, appearance, behavior, and, at times, even silence. Such communications not only occur among healthcare providers and patients, but also among healthcare providers and support personnel. Support personnel may include housekeeping, maintenance, security, supply, and food service staff. Another critical communication interaction occurs among healthcare providers and visitors. Because of the critical nature of communication in healthcare delivery, it is important that you understand the communication process and the techniques used to promote open, honest, and effective interactions. It is only through effective communication that you are able to identify the goals of the individual and the Navy healthcare system.

THE COMMUNICATION PROCESS

The human communication process consists of four basic parts: the sender of the message, the message, the receiver of the message, and feedback.

The sender of the message starts the process. The message is the body of information the sender wishes to transmit to the receiver. The receiver is the individual intended to receive the message. Feedback is the response given by the receiver to the message. Feedback, at times, is used to validate whether effective communication has taken place.

Verbal and Nonverbal Communication

The two basic modes of communication are verbal and nonverbal. Verbal communication is either spoken or written. Verbal communication involves the use of words. Nonverbal communication, on the other hand, does not involve the use of words. Dress, gestures, touching, body language, face and eye behavior, and even silence are forms of nonverbal communication. Remember that even though there are two forms of communication, both the verbal and the nonverbal are inseparable in the total communication process. Conscious awareness of this fact is extremely important because your professional effectiveness is highly dependent upon successful communication.

Barriers to Effective Communication

Ineffective communication occurs when obstacles or barriers are present. These barriers are classified as physiological, physical, or psychosocial. **Physiological barriers** result from some kind of sensory dysfunction on the part of either the sender or the receiver. Such things as hearing impairments, speech defects, and even vision problems influence the effectiveness of communication. **Physical barriers** consist of elements in the environment (such as noise) that contribute to the development of physiological barriers (such as the inability to hear). **Psychosocial barriers** are usually the result of one's inaccurate perception of self or others; the presence of some defense mechanism employed to cope with some form of threatening anxiety; or the existence of factors such as age, education, culture, language, nationality, or a multitude of other socioeconomic factors. Psychological barriers are the most difficult to identify and the most common cause of communication failure or breakdown. A person's true feelings are often communicated more accurately through nonverbal communication than through verbal communication.

Listening

Listening, a critical element of the communication process, becomes the primary activity for the healthcare provider, who must use communication as a tool for collecting or giving information. When one is engaged in listening, it is important to direct attention to both the verbal and nonverbal cues provided by the other person. Like many other skills necessary for providing a healthcare service, listening requires conscious effort and constant practice. Your listening skills can be improved and enhanced by developing the following attitudes and skills:

- Hear the speaker out.

- Focus on ideas.

- Remove or adjust distractions.

- Maintain objectivity.

- Concentrate on the immediate interaction.

As a healthcare provider, you will be using the communication process to service a patient's needs, both short and long-term. To simplify this discussion, short-term needs will be discussed under the heading of "patient contact point." Long-term needs will be discussed under the heading of "therapeutic communications."

PATIENT CONTACT POINT

To give you a frame of reference for the following discussion, the following definitions will clarify and standardize some critical terms:

- **Initial contact point**—The physical location where patients experience their first communication encounter with a person representing, in some role, the healthcare facility.

- **Contact point**—The place or event where the contact point person and the patient meet. The contact point meeting can occur anywhere in a facility and also includes telephone events.

- **Contact point person**—The healthcare provider in any healthcare experience who is tasked by role and responsibility to provide a service to the patient.

The contact point person has certain criteria to meet in establishing a good relationship with the patient. Helping the patient through trying experiences is partially the responsibility of all contact point personnel. Such healthcare providers must not only have skills related to their professional assignment, but they must also have the ability to interact in a positive, meaningful way to communicate concern and the desire to provide a service.

Consumers of healthcare services expect to be treated promptly, courteously, and correctly. They expect their care to be personalized and communicated to them in terms they understand. The Navy healthcare system is a service system, and it is the responsibility of every healthcare provider to give professional, quality customer service.

The significance of the contact point and the responsibility of the personnel staffing this area are important to emphasize. The following message from a former Surgeon General of the Navy reflects the philosophy of the Navy Medical Department regarding contact point interactions.

Some of the most frequent complaints received by the Commander, Bureau of Medicine and Surgery, are those pertaining to the lack of courtesy, tact, and sympathetic regard for patients and their families exhibited by Medical Department personnel and initial points of contact within Navy Medical facilities. These points of initial patient contact, which include central appointment desks, telephones, patient affairs offices, emergency rooms, pharmacies, laboratories, record offices, information desks, walk-in and specialty clinics, and gate guards, are critical in conveying to the entering patient the sense that Navy Medicine is there to help them. The personnel, both military and civilian, who man these critical areas are responsible for ensuring that the assistance that they provide is truly reflective of the spirit of "caring" for which the Navy Medical Department must stand.

No matter how excellent and expert the care in the facility may be, an early impression of nonchalance, disregard, rudeness, or neglect of the needs of patients reflects poorly on its efforts and achievements. Our personnel must be constantly on their guard to refrain from off-hand remarks or jokes in the presence of patients or their families. We must insist that our personnel in all patient areas are professional in their attitudes. What may be commonplace to us may be to a patient frightening or subject to misinterpretation.

By example and precept, we must insist that, in dealing with our beneficiaries, no complaint is ever too trivial not to deserve the best response of which we are capable. . . .

THERAPEUTIC COMMUNICATION

A distinguishing aspect of therapeutic communication is its application to long-term communication interactions. Therapeutic communication is defined as the face-to-face process of interacting that focuses on advancing the physical and emotional well-being of a patient. This kind of communication has three general purposes: collecting information to determine illness, assessing and modifying behavior, and providing health education. By using therapeutic communication, we attempt to learn as much as we can about the patient in relation to his illness. To accomplish this learning, both the sender and the receiver must be consciously aware of the confidentiality of the information disclosed and received during the communication process. You must always have a therapeutic reason for invading a patient's privacy.

When used to collect information, therapeutic communication requires a great deal of sensitivity as well as expertise in using interviewing skills. To ensure the identification and clarification of the patient's thoughts and feelings, you, as the interviewer, must observe his behavior. Listen to the patient and watch how he listens to you. Observe how he gives and receives both verbal and nonverbal responses. Finally, interpret and record the data you have observed.

As mentioned earlier, listening is one of the most difficult skills to master. It requires you to maintain an open mind, eliminate both internal and external noise and distractions, and channel attention to all verbal and nonverbal messages. Listening involves the ability to recognize pitch and tone of voice, evaluate vocabulary and choice of words, and recognize hesitancy or intensity of speech as part of the total communication attempt. The patient crying aloud for help after a fall is communicating a need for assistance. This cry for help sounds very different from the call for assistance you might make when requesting help in transcribing a physician's order.

The ability to recognize and interpret nonverbal responses depends upon consistent development of observation skills. As you continue to mature in your role and responsibilities as a member of the healthcare team, both your clinical knowledge and understanding of human behavior will also grow. Your growth in both knowledge and understanding will contribute to your ability to recognize and interpret many kinds of nonverbal communication. Your sensitivity in

listening with your eyes will become as refined as—if not better than—listening with your ears.

The effectiveness of an interview is influenced by both the amount of information and the degree of motivation possessed by the patient (interviewee). Factors that enhance the quality of an interview consist of the participant's knowledge of the subject under consideration; his patience, temperament, and listening skills; and your attention to both verbal and nonverbal cues. Courtesy, understanding, and nonjudgmental attitudes must be mutual goals of both the interviewee and the interviewer.

Finally, to function effectively in the therapeutic communication process, you must be an informed and skilled practitioner. Your development of the required knowledge and skills is dependent upon your commitment to seeking out and participating in continuing education learning experiences across the entire spectrum of healthcare services.

PATIENT EDUCATION

LEARNING OBJECTIVE: *Recognize the importance of patient education.*

Patient (health) education is an essential part of the healthcare delivery system. In the Navy Medical Department, patient education is defined as "the process that informs, motivates, and helps people adapt and maintain healthful practices and life styles." Specifically, the goals of this process are to

- assist individuals acquire knowledge and skills that will promote their ability to care for themselves more adequately;

- influence individual attitudinal changes from an orientation that emphasizes disease to an orientation that emphasizes health; and

- support behavioral changes to the extent that individuals are willing and able to maintain their health.

All healthcare providers, whether they recognize it or not, are teaching almost constantly. Teaching is a unique skill that is developed through the application of principles of learning. Patient teaching begins with an assessment of the patient's knowledge. Through this assessment, learning needs are identified. For example, a diabetic patient may have a need to learn how to self-administer an injection. After the learner's needs have been established, goals and objectives are developed. Objectives inform the learner of what kind of (learned) behavior is expected. Objectives also assist the healthcare provider in determining how effective the teaching has been. These basic principles of teaching/learning are applicable to all patient-education activities, from the simple procedure of teaching a patient how to measure and record fluid intake/output to the more complex programs of behavior modification in situations of substance abuse (i.e., drug or alcohol) or weight control.

As a member of the healthcare team, you share a responsibility with all other members of the team to be alert to patient education needs, to undertake patient teaching within the limitation of your own knowledge and skills, and to communicate to other team members the need for patient education in areas you are not personally qualified to undertake.

REPORTING AND ASSESSMENT PROCEDURES

LEARNING OBJECTIVE: *Recall proper patient care reporting and assessment procedures.*

Although physicians determine the overall medical management of a person requiring healthcare services, they depend upon the assistance of other members of the healthcare team when implementing and evaluating that patient's ongoing treatment. Nurses and Hospital Corpsmen spend more time with hospitalized patients than all other providers. This situation places them in a key position as data-collecting and -reporting resource persons.

The systematic gathering of information is called **data collection** and is an essential aspect in assessing an individual's health status, identifying existing problems, and developing a combined plan of action to assist the patient in his health needs. The initial assessment is usually accomplished by establishing a health history. Included in this history are elements such as previous and current health problems; patterns of daily living activities, medication, and dietary requirements; and other relevant occupational, social, and psychological data. Additionally, both subjective and objective observations are included in the initial

assessment gathering interview and throughout the course of hospitalization.

REPORTING

Accurate and intelligent assessments are the basis of good patient care and are essential elements for providing a total healthcare service. You must know what to watch for and what to expect. It is important to be able to recognize even the slightest change in a patient's condition, since such changes indicate a definite improvement or deterioration. You must be able to recognize the desired effects of medication and treatments, as well as any undesirable reactions to them. Both of these factors may influence the physician's decision to continue, modify, or discontinue parts or all of the treatment plan.

Oral and Written Reporting

Equally as important as assessments is the reporting of data and observations to the appropriate team members. Reporting consists of both oral and written communications and, to be effective, must be done accurately, completely, and in a timely manner. Written reporting, commonly called **recording**, is documented in a patient's clinical record. Maintaining an accurate, descriptive clinical record serves a dual purpose: It provides a written report of the information gathered about the patient, and it serves as a means of communication to everyone involved in the patient's care. The clinical record also serves as a valuable source of information for developing a variety of care-planning activities. Additionally, the clinical record is a legal document and is admissible as evidence in a court of law in claims of negligence and malpractice. Finally, these records serve as an important source of material that can be used for educating and training healthcare personnel and for conducting research and compiling statistical data.

Basic Guidelines for Written Entries

It is imperative that you follow some basic guidelines when you make written entries in the clinical record. All entries must be recorded accurately and truthfully. Omitting an entry is as harmful as making an incorrect recording. Each entry should be concise and brief; therefore, avoid extra words and vague notations. Recordings must be legible. If an error is made, it must be deleted following the standard Navy policy for correcting erroneous written notations. Finally, your entries in the clinical record must include the time and date, your signature, and your rate or rank.

SOAP Note Format

SOAP stands for SUBJECTIVE, OBJECTIVE, ASSESSMENT, and PLAN. Medical documentation of patient complaint(s) and treatment must be consistent, concise, and comprehensive. The Navy Medical Department uses the SOAP note format to standardize medical evaluation entries made in clinical records. The four parts of a SOAP note are discussed below. For more detailed instructions, refer to chapter 16 of the MANMED.

SUBJECTIVE.—The initial portion of the SOAP note format consists of subjective observations. These are symptoms verbally given to you by the patient or by a significant other (family or friend). These subjective observations include the patient's descriptions of pain or discomfort, the presence of nausea or dizziness, and a multitude of other descriptions of dysfunction, discomfort, or illness.

OBJECTIVE.—The next part of the format is the objective observation. These objective observations include symptoms that you can actually see, hear, touch, feel, or smell. Included in objective observations are measurements such as temperature, pulse, respiration, skin color, swelling, and the results of tests.

ASSESSMENT.—Assessment follows the objective observations. Assessment is the diagnosis of the patient's condition. In some cases the diagnosis may be clear, such as a contusion. However, an assessment may not be clear and could include several diagnosis possibilities.

PLAN.—The last part of the SOAP note is the plan. The plan may include laboratory and/or radiologic tests ordered for the patient, medications ordered, treatments performed (e.g., minor surgery procedure), patient referrals (sending patient to a specialist), patient disposition (e.g., binnacle list, Sick-in-Quarters (SIQ), admission to hospital), patient directions, and follow-up directions for the patient.

SELF-QUESTIONING TECHNIQUES FOR PATIENT ASSESSMENT AND REPORTING

Table 2-1 outlines the self-questioning techniques for patient assessment and reporting is a good guide to assist you in developing proficiency in assessing and reporting patient conditions.

INPATIENT CARE

A patient will often require inpatient care, whether due to injury or illness. Frequently, the inpatient will need specialized treatments, perhaps even surgery. In this part of the chapter, we will discuss the procedures for assisting both the medical inpatient and the surgical inpatient.

THE MEDICAL PATIENT

LEARNING OBJECTIVE: *Evaluate the needs of a medical patient.*

For purposes of this discussion, the term **medical patient** applies to any person who is receiving diagnostic, therapeutic, and/or supportive care for a condition that is not managed by surgical-, orthopedic-, psychiatric-, or maternity-related therapy. This is not to infer that patients in these other categories are not treated for medical problems. Many surgical, orthopedic, psychiatric, and maternity patients do have secondary medical problems that are treated while they are undergoing management for their primary condition. Although many medical problems can be treated on an outpatient basis, this discussion will address the hospitalized medical patient. It should be noted that the basic principles of management are essentially the same for both the inpatient and outpatient.

The medical management of the patient generally consists of laboratory and diagnostic tests and procedures, medication, food and fluid therapy, and patient teaching. Additionally, for many medical patients, particularly during the initial treatment phase, rest is a part of the prescribed treatment.

Laboratory Tests And Diagnostic Procedures

A variety of laboratory and diagnostic tests and procedures are commonly ordered for the medical patient. Frequently, the Hospital Corpsman is assigned to prepare the patient for the procedure, collect the specimens, or assist with both the procedure and specimen collection. Whether a specimen is to be collected or a procedure is to be performed, the patient needs a clear and simple explanation about what is to

Table 2–1.—Self-Questioning Techniques for Patient Assessment and Reporting

Area of Concern	Assessment Criteria
General Appearance	Is the patient • of average build, short, tall, thin, or obese? • well-groomed? • apparently in pain? • walking with a limp, wearing a cast, walking on crutches, or wearing a prosthetic extremity?
Behavior	Does the patient • appear worried, nervous, excited, depressed, angry, disoriented, confused, or unconscious? • refuse to talk? • communicate thoughts in a logical order or erratically? • lisp, stutter, or have slurred speech? • appear sullen, bored, aggressive, friendly, or cooperative? • sleep well or arouse early? • sleep poorly, moan, talk, or cry out when sleeping? • join ward activities? • react well toward other patients, staff, and visitors?
Position	Does the patient • remain in one position in bed? • have difficulty breathing while in any position? • use just one pillow or require more pillows to sleep well? • move about in bed without difficulty?
Skin	Is the patient's skin • flushed, pale, cyanotic (bluish hue), hot, moist, clammy, cool, or dry? • bruised, scarred, lacerated, scratched, or showing a rash, lumps, or ulcerations? • showing signs of pressure, redness, mottling, edema, or pitting edema? • appearing shiny or stretched? • perspiring profusely? • infested with lice?
Eyes	Are the patient's • eyelids swollen, bruised, discolored, or dropping? • sclera (whites of eyes) clear, dull, yellow, or bloodshot? • pupils constricted or dilated, equal in size, react equally to light? • eyes tearing or showing signs of inflammation or discharge? • complaints about pain; burning; itching; sensitivity to light; or blurred, double, or lack of vision?
Ears	Does the patient • hear well bilaterally? • hold or pull on his ears? • complain of a buzzing or ringing sound? • have a discharge or wax accumulation? • complain of pain?
Nose	Is the patient's • nose bruised, bleeding, or difficult to breathe through? • nose excessively dry or dripping? Are the patient's nares (nasal openings) equal in size? Is the patient sniffling excessively?
Mouth	Does the patient's • mouth appear excessively dry? • breath smell sweet, sour, or of alcohol? • tongue appear dry, moist, clean, coated, cracked, red, or swollen? • gums appear inflamed, ulcerated, swollen, or discolored? • teeth appear white, discolored, broken, or absent? Does the patient • wear dentures, braces, or partial plates? • complain of mouth pain or ulcerations? • complain of an unpleasant taste?

Area of Concern	Assessment Criteria

Chest	Does the patient
	• have shortness of breath, wheezing, gasping, or noisy respirations? cough?
	• have a dry, moist, hacking, productive, deep, or persistent cough?
	• have white, yellow, rusty, or bloody sputum?
	   – Is it thin and watery or thick and purulent (containing pus)?
	   – How much is produced?
	   – Does it have an odor?
	• complain of chest pain?
	   – Where is the pain?
	   – Is the pain a dull ache, sharp, crushing, or radiating?
	   – Is the pain relieved by resting?
	   – Is the patient using medication to control the pain (i.e., nitroglycerin)?

Abdomen	Does the patient
	• have an abdomen that looks or feels distended, boardlike, or soft?
	• have a distended abdomen, and, if so, is the abdomen distended above or below the umbilicus or over the entire abdomen?
	• belch excessively?
	• feel nauseated, or has he vomited?
	   – If so, how often, and when?
	   – What is the volume, consistency, and odor of the vomitus?
	   – Is it coffee ground, bilious (containing bile), or bloody in appearance?
	   – Is patient vomiting with projectile force?

Bladder & Bowel	Does the patient have
	• bladder and bowel control?
	• normal urination volume and frequency?
	   – Does the urine have an odor?
	   – Is the urine dark amber or bloody?
	   – Is the urine cloudy; does it have sediment in it?
	   – Is there pain, burning, or difficulty when voiding?
	• diarrhea, soft stools, or constipation?
	   – What is the color of the stool?
	   – Does the stool contain blood, pus, fat, or worms?
	   – Does the patient have hemorrhoids, fistulas, or rectal pain?

Vagina or Penis	Does the patient have
	• ulcerations or irritations?
	• a discharge or foul odor?
	   – If there is a discharge present, is it bloody, purulent, mucoid (containing mucous), or watery?
	   – What is the amount?
	• associated pain?
	   – If pain is present, where is it located?
	   – Is it constant or intermittent?
	   – Is it tingling, dull, aching, burning, gnawing, cramping, or crushing?

Food & Fluid Intake	Does the patient • have a good, fair, or poor appetite? • get thirsty often? • have any kind of food intolerance?
Medications	Does the patient • take any medications? (If so: what, why, and when last taken?) • have medications with him? • have any history of medication reactions or allergies?

be done and what the patient can do to assist with the activity. Often the success of the test or procedure is dependent upon the patient's informed cooperation. When collecting specimens, the Hospital Corpsman must complete the following procedures:

- Collect the correct kind and amount of specimen at the right time.

- Place the specimen in the correct container.

- Label the container completely and accurately. This often differs somewhat for each facility, and local policies should be consulted.

- Complete the laboratory request form accurately.

- Record on the patient's record or other forms, as appropriate; the date, time, kind of specimen collected; the disposition of the specimen; and anything unusual about the appearance of the specimen or the patient during the collection.

When assisting with a diagnostic procedure, the Hospital Corpsman must understand the sequence of steps of the procedure and exactly how the assistance can best be provided. Since many procedures terminate in the collection of a specimen, the above principles of specimen collecting must be followed.

Following the completion of a procedure or specimen collection, it is the responsibility of the assisting Hospital Corpsman to ensure that the patient's safety and comfort are attended to, the physician's orders accurately followed, and any supplies or equipment used appropriately discarded.

Medications

A major form of therapy for the treatment of illness is the use of drugs. It is not uncommon for the medical patient to be treated with several drugs. As members of the healthcare team, Hospital Corpsmen assigned to preparing and administering medications are given a serious responsibility demanding constant vigilance, integrity, and special knowledge and skills. The preparation and administration of medications were addressed in great detail in the Hospital Corps School curriculum. References and the continued in-service training devoted to medication administration at all medical facilities support the importance of accurate preparation and administration of drugs.

An error—which also includes omissions—can seriously affect a patient, even to the point of causing death. Each Hospital Corpsman is responsible for his own actions, and this responsibility cannot be transferred to another. No one individual is expected to know all there is to know about all patients and medications. However, in every healthcare environment, the Hospital Corpsman can access other healthcare providers who can assist in clarifying orders; explaining the purposes, actions, and effects of drugs; and, in general, answering any questions that may arise concerning a particular patient and that patient's medications. There should be basic drug references available to all personnel handling medications, including the *Physicians' Desk Reference* and a hospital formulary. As a Hospital Corpsman, it is your responsibility to consult these members of the team and these references for assistance in any area in which you are not knowledgeable or whenever you have questions or doubts. You are also responsible for knowing and following local policies and procedures regarding the administration of medications.

Food and Fluid Therapy

The following brief discussion covers food and fluid and how it relates specifically to the medical patient. Loss of appetite, food intolerance, digestive disturbances, lack of exercise, and even excessive weight gain influence a medical patient's intake requirements. Regardless of their medical problems, patients have basic nutritional needs that frequently differ from those of the healthy person. As a part of the patient's therapeutic regimen, food is usually prescribed in the form of a special diet. Regardless of the kind of diet prescribed, the patient must understand why certain foods are ordered or eliminated, and how compliance with the regimen will assist in his total care. It is the responsibility of the Corpsman to assist the patient in understanding the importance of the prescribed diet and to ensure that accurate recording of the patient's dietary intake is made on the clinical record.

In many disease conditions, the patient is unable to tolerate food or fluids or may lose these through vomiting, diarrhea, or both. In these cases, replacement fluids as well as nutrients are an important part of the patient's medical management. On the other hand, there are several disease conditions in which fluid restrictions are important aspects of the patient's therapy. In both of these instances, accurate measurement and recording of fluid intake and output must be carefully performed. Very frequently this becomes a major task of the staff Hospital Corpsman.

Patient Teaching

Earlier in this chapter, under "Patient Education," the goals and principles of patient teaching were addressed. When taken in the context of the medical patient, there are some general areas of patient teaching needs that must be considered, particularly as the patient approaches discharge from an inpatient status. Those areas include the following:

- Follow-up appointments

- Modification in daily living activities and habits

- Modification in diet, including fluid intake

- Medications and treatment to be continued after discharge

- Measures to be taken to promote health and prevent illness

Rest

The primary reason for prescribing rest as a therapeutic measure for the medical patient is to prevent further damage to the body or a part of the body when the normal demand of use exceeds the ability to respond. However, prolonged or indiscriminate use of rest—particularly bed rest—is potentially hazardous. Some of the common complications occurring as a result of prolonged bed rest are

- circulatory problems (such as development of thrombi and emboli) and subsequent skin problems (such as decubiti);

- respiratory problems (such as atelectasis and pneumonia);

- gastrointestinal problems (such as anorexia, constipation, and fecal impactions);

- urinary tract problems (such as retention, infection, or the formation of calculi);

- musculoskeletal problems (such as weakness, atrophy, and the development of contractures); and

- psychological problems (such as apathy, depression, and temporary personality changes).

The prevention of complications is the key concept in therapeutic management for the patient on prolonged bed rest. Awareness of the potential hazards is the first step in prevention. Alert observations are essential: Skin condition, respirations, food and fluid intake, urinary and bowel habits, evidence of discomfort, range of motion, and mood are all critical elements that provide indications of impending problems. When this data is properly reported, the healthcare team has time to employ measures that will arrest the development of preventable complications.

THE SURGICAL PATIENT

LEARNING OBJECTIVE: *Evaluate the needs of a surgical patient during the preoperative, operative, recovery, and postoperative phases of his treatment.*

Surgical procedures are classified into two major categories: emergency and elective. Emergency surgery is that required immediately to save a life or maintain a necessary function. Elective surgery is that which, in most cases, needs to be done but can be scheduled at a time beneficial to both the patient and the provider. Regardless of the type of surgery, every surgical patient requires specialized care at each of four phases. These phases are classified as **preoperative**, **operative**, **recovery**, and **postoperative**. The following discussion will address the basic concepts of care in each phase.

Preoperative Phase

Before undergoing a surgical procedure, the patient must be in the best possible psychological, spiritual, and physical condition. Psychological preparation begins the moment the patient learns of the necessity of the operation. The physician is responsible for explaining the surgical procedure to the patient, including the events that can be expected after the procedure. Since other staff personnel reinforce the physician's explanation, all members of the team must know what the physician has told the patient. In this manner, they are better able to answer the patient's questions. All patients approaching surgery are fearful and anxious. The staff can assist in reducing this fear by instilling confidence in the patient regarding the competence of those providing care. The patient should be given the opportunity and freedom to express any feelings or fears concerning the proposed procedure. Even in an emergency, it is possible to give a patient and the family psychological support. Often this is accomplished simply by the confident and skillful manner in which the administrative and physical preoperative preparation is performed.

The fears of presurgical patients derive from their insecurities in the areas of anesthesia, body disfigurement, pain, and even death. Frequently, religious faith is a source of strength and courage for these patients. If a patient expresses a desire to see a clergyman, every attempt should be made to arrange a visit.

ADMINISTRATIVE PREPARATION.— Except in emergencies, the administrative preparation usually begins before surgery. A step-by-step procedure is outlined in *Fundamental Skills and Concepts in Patient Care,* "Caring for the Patient Undergoing Surgery." Only the Request for Administration of Anesthesia and for Performance of Operations and Other Procedures (SF 522) will be addressed here. The SF 522 identifies the operation or procedure to be performed; has a statement written for the patient indicating in lay terms a description of the procedure; and includes the signatures of the physician, patient, and a staff member who serves as a witness. An SF 522 must be completed before any preoperative medications are administered. If the patient is not capable of signing the document, a parent, legal guardian, or spouse may sign it. It is customary to require the signature of a parent or legal guardian if the patient is under 21 years of age, unless the patient is married or a member of the Armed Forces. In these latter two cases, the patient may sign his own permit, regardless of age.

Normally, the physical preparation of the patient begins in the late afternoon or early evening the day before surgery. As with the administrative preparation, each step is clearly outlined in *Fundamental Skills and Concepts in Patient Care,* "Caring for the Patient Undergoing Surgery."

PREOPERATIVE INSTRUCTIONS.— Preoperative instructions are an important part of the total preparation. The exact time that preoperative teaching should be initiated greatly depends upon the individual patient and the type of surgical procedure. Most experts recommend that preoperative instructions be given as close as possible to the time of surgery. Appropriate preoperative instructions given in sufficient detail and at the proper time greatly reduce operative and postoperative complications.

Operative Phase

The operative (or intra-operative) phase begins the moment the patient is taken into the operating room.

Two of the major factors to consider at this phase are positioning and anesthesia.

POSITIONING.—The specific surgical procedure will dictate the general position of the patient. For example, the **lithotomy** position is used for a vaginal hysterectomy, while the **dorsal recumbent** position is used for a herniorrhaphy. Regardless of the specific position the patient is placed in, there are some general patient safety guidelines that must be observed. When positioning a patient on the operating table, remember the following:

- Whether the patient is awake or asleep, place the patient in as comfortable a position as possible.

- Strap the patient to the table in a manner that allows for adequate exposure of the operative site and is secure enough to prevent the patient from falling, but that does not cut off circulation or contribute to nerve damage.

- Secure all the patient's extremities in a manner that will prevent them from dangling over the side of the table.

- Pad all bony prominences to prevent the development of pressure areas or nerve damage.

- Make sure the patient is adequately grounded to avoid burns or electrical shock to either the patient or the surgical team.

ANESTHESIA.—One of the greatest contributions to medical science was the introduction of anesthesia. It relieves unnecessary pain and increases the potential and scope of many kinds of surgical procedures. Therefore, healthcare providers must understand the nature of anesthetic agents and their effect on the human body.

Anesthesia may be defined as a loss of sensation that makes a person insensible to pain, with or without loss of consciousness. Some specific anesthetic agents are discussed in the "Pharmacy" chapter of this manual. Healthcare providers must understand the basics of anesthesiology as well as a specific drug's usage.

The two major classifications of anesthesia are regional and general.

Regional Anesthesia.—Regional anesthetics reduce all painful sensations in a particular area of the body without causing unconsciousness. The following is a listing of the various methods and a brief description of each.

- **Topical** anesthesia is administered topically to desensitize a small area of the body for a very short period.

- **Local blocks** consist of the subcutaneous infiltration of a small area of the body with a desensitizing agent. Local anesthesia generally lasts a little longer than topical.

- **Nerve blocks** consist of injecting the agent into the region of a nerve trunk or other large nerve branches. This form of anesthesia blocks all impulses to and from the injected nerves.

- **Spinal** anesthesia consists of injecting the agent into the subarachnoid space of the spinal canal between the third and fourth lumbar space or between the fifth lumbar and first sacral space of the spinal column. This form of anesthesia blocks all impulses to and from the entire area below the point of insertion, provided the patient's position is not changed following injection of the agent. If the patient's position is changed, for example, from dorsal recumbent to Trendelenburg's, the anesthetic agent will move up the spinal column and the level of the anesthesia will also move up. Because of this reaction, care must be exercised in positioning the patient's head and chest above the level of insertion to prevent paralysis (by anesthesia) of the respiratory muscles. In general, spinal anesthesia is considered the safest for most routine major surgery.

- **Epidural blocks** consist of injecting the agent into the epidural space of the spinal canal at any level of the spinal column. The area of anesthesia obtained is similar to that of the subarachnoid spinal method. The epidural method is frequently used when continuous anesthesia is desired for a prolonged period. In these cases, a catheter is inserted into the epidural space through a spinal needle. The needle is removed, but the catheter is left in place. This provides for continuous access to the epidural space.

- **Saddle blocks** consist of injecting the agent into the dural sac at the third and fourth lumbar space. This form of anesthesia blocks all impulses to and from the perineal area of the body.

- **Caudal blocks** consist of injecting the agent into the sacral canal. With this method, anesthesia is obtained from the umbilicus to the toes.

General Anesthesia.—General anesthetics cause total loss of sensation and complete loss of consciousness in the patient. They are administered by inhalation of certain gases or vaporized liquids, intravenous infusion, or rectal induction. The induction of inhalation anesthesia is divided into four stages. These stages and the body's main physiological reaction in each phase are explained below and depicted in figure 2–1.

- **Stage 1** is called the stage of analgesia or induction. During this period, the patient experiences dizziness, a sense of unreality, and a lessening sensitivity to touch and pain. At this stage, the patient's sense of hearing is increased, and responses to noises are intensified (fig. 2-1).

- **Stage 2** is the stage of excitement. During this period, there is a variety of reactions involving muscular activity and delirium. At this stage, the vital signs show evidence of physiological stimulation. It is important to remember that during this stage the patient may respond violently to very little stimulation (fig. 2–1).

- **Stage 3** is called the surgical or operative stage. There are four levels of consciousness (also called planes) to this stage. It is the responsibility of the anesthetist or anesthesiologist to determine which plane is optimal for the procedure. The determination is made according to specific tissue sensitivity of

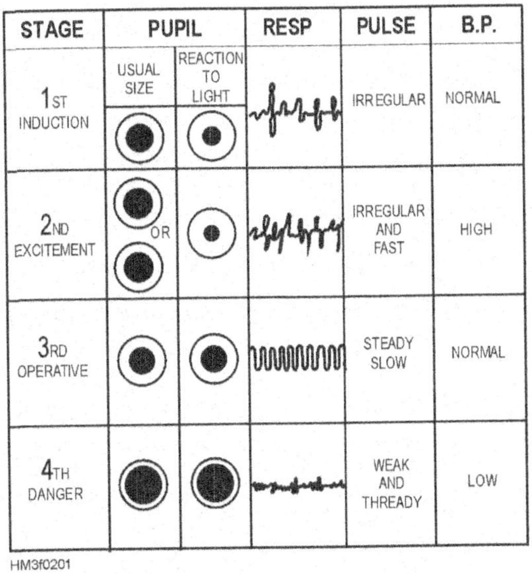

STAGE	PUPIL		RESP	PULSE	B.P.
1ST INDUCTION	USUAL SIZE	REACTION TO LIGHT		IRREGULAR	NORMAL
2ND EXCITEMENT	OR			IRREGULAR AND FAST	HIGH
3RD OPERATIVE				STEADY SLOW	NORMAL
4TH DANGER				WEAK AND THREADY	LOW

HM3f0201

Figure 2–1.—Stages of anesthesia.

the individual and the surgical site. Each successive plane is achieved by increasing the concentration of the anesthetic agent in the tissue (fig. 2–1).

- **Stage 4** is called the toxic or danger stage. Obviously, this is never a desired stage of anesthesia. At this point, cardiopulmonary failure and death can occur. Once surgical anesthesia has been obtained, the healthcare provider must exercise care to control the level of anesthesia. The fourth level of consciousness of stage 3 is demonstrated by cardiovascular impairment that results from diaphragmatic paralysis. If this plane is not corrected immediately, stage 4 quickly ensues (fig. 2–1).

Recovery Stage

For purposes of this discussion, the recovery phase consists of the period that begins at the completion of the operation and extends until the patient has recovered from anesthesia. The recovery phase generally takes place in a specialized area called the recovery room. This unit is usually located near the operating room and has access to the following:

- Surgeons and anesthesiologists or anesthetists

- Nurses and Hospital Corps personnel who are specially prepared to care for immediate postoperative patients

- Special equipment, supplies, medication, and replacement fluids

From the time of admission to patient discharge, routine care in the recovery room consists of the following:

- Measuring temperature and vital signs (taken immediately upon admission and as ordered by the physician thereafter)

- Maintaining airway patency

  —Patients having an artificial airway in place will automatically expel it as they regain consciousness.

  —Have a mechanical suction apparatus available to remove excess excretions from the patient's airway.

- Ensuring the integrity of dressings, tubes, catheters and casts

  —Locate the presence of any of the above.

  —Make notations regarding all drainage, including color, type, and amount.

  —Immediately report the presence of copious amounts of drainage to a nurse or physician.

- Monitoring intravenous therapy (including blood and blood components)

  —Make notations including type of infusion, rate of flow, and condition of the infusion site.

  —Observe patients receiving blood or blood components closely for untoward reactions.

- Monitoring skin color changes

  —Check dressings and casts frequently to ensure they are not interfering with normal blood circulation to the area.

  —Notify a physician or nurse of general skin color changes that may indicate airway obstruction, hemorrhage, or shock.

- Assessing level of responsiveness

  —For general anesthetics, check for orientation to the environment each time vital signs are taken.

  —For regular anesthetics, check for return of sensory perception and voluntary movement each time vital signs are taken.

- Observing for side effects of the anesthetic agent

  —Each agent has the potential for causing specific side effects. Some common major side effects that may occur following the administration of both spinal and general anesthesia consist of the following:

    - Hypotension/shock

    - Respiratory paralysis

    - Neurological complications

    - Headache

    - Cardiac arrest

    - Respiratory depression

    - Bronchospasm/laryngospasm

    - Diminished circulation

    - Vomiting/aspiration

Postoperative Phase

After the patient's condition has been stabilized in the recovery room, a physician will order the patient's transfer to another area of the facility. Generally, this transfer is to the unit that the patient was assigned to preoperatively. Since both surgery and anesthesia have unavoidable temporary ill effects on normal physiological functions, every effort must be made to prevent postoperative complications.

POSTOPERATIVE GOALS.—From the time the patient is admitted to the recovery room to the time recovery from the operation is complete, there are definite goals of care that guide the entire postoperative course. These goals are as follows:

- Promoting respiratory function
- Promoting cardiovascular function
- Promoting renal function
- Promoting nutrition and elimination
- Promoting fluid and electrolyte balance
- Promoting wound healing
- Encouraging rest and comfort
- Encouraging movement and ambulation
- Preventing postoperative complications

The physician will write orders for postoperative care that are directed at accomplishing the above goals. Although the orders will be based on each individual patient's needs, there will be some common orders that apply to all patients. These orders will center around the promotion of certain physiological functions and areas addressed in the following paragraphs.

Respiratory function is promoted by encouraging frequent coughing and deep breathing. Early movement and ambulation also help improve respiratory function. For some patients, oxygen therapy may also be ordered to assist respiratory function. **Cardiovascular function** is assisted by frequent position changes, early movement and ambulation, and, in some cases, intravenous therapy. **Renal function** is promoted by adequate fluid intake and early movement and ambulation. **Nutritional status** is promoted by ensuring adequate oral and correct intravenous intake and by maintaining accurate intake and output records. **Elimination functions** are promoted by adequate diet and fluid intake. Postoperative patients should be advanced to a normal dietary regimen as soon as possible, since this, too,

promotes elimination functions. Early movement and ambulation also help to restore normal elimination activities.

In addition to various medications and dressing change procedures ordered by the physician, **wound healing** is promoted by good nutritional intake and by early movement and ambulation. **Rest and comfort** are supported by properly positioning the patient, providing a restful environment, encouraging good basic hygiene measures, ensuring optimal bladder and bowel output, and promptly administering pain-relieving medications. Early **movement and ambulation** are assisted by ensuring maximum comfort for the patient and providing the encouragement and support for ambulating the patient, particularly in the early postoperative period. As indicated in the above discussion, the value of early movement and ambulation, when permissible, cannot be overemphasized.

POSTOPERATIVE COMPLICATIONS.— During the early postoperative phase, the major complications to be guarded against are respiratory obstruction, shock, and hemorrhage. As the patient progresses in the postoperative period, other complications to avoid are the development of pneumonia, phlebitis and subsequent thrombophlebitis, gastrointestinal problems ranging from abdominal distention to intestinal obstruction, and, finally, wound infections. Accurate implementation of the physician's orders and careful observation, reporting, and recording of the patient's condition will contribute markedly to an optimal and timely postoperative recovery course for the patient.

THE ORTHOPEDIC PATIENT

LEARNING OBJECTIVE: *Evaluate the needs of the orthopedic patient.*

Patients receiving orthopedic services are those who require treatment for fractures, deformities, and diseases or injuries of some part of the musculoskeletal system. Some patients will require surgery, immobilization, or both to correct their condition.

General Care

The basic principles and concepts of care for the surgical patient will apply to orthopedic patients. The majority of patients not requiring surgical intervention will be managed by bed rest, immobilization, and rehabilitation. Many of the basic concepts of care of the medical patient are applicable for orthopedic patient care. In the military, the usual orthopedic patient is fairly young and in good general physical condition. For these patients, bed rest is prescribed only because other kinds of activity are limited by their condition on admission.

Immobilization

Rehabilitation is the ultimate goal when planning the orthopedic patient's total management. Whether the patient requires surgical or conservative treatment, immobilization is often a part of the overall therapy. Immobilization may consist of applying casts or traction, or using equipment (such as orthopedic frames). During the immobilization phase, simple basic patient care is extremely important. Such things as skin care, active-passive exercises, position changes in bed (as permitted), good nutrition, adequate fluid intake, regularity in elimination, and basic hygiene contribute to both the patient's physical and psychological well-being.

Lengthy periods of immobilization are emotionally stressful for patients, particularly those who are essentially healthy except for the limitations imposed by their condition. Prolonged inactivity contributes to boredom that is frequently manifested by various kinds of acting-out behavior.

Often, the orthopedic patient experiences exaggerated levels of pain. Orthopedic pain is commonly described as sore and aching. Because this condition requires long periods of treatment and hospitalization, the wise management of pain is an important aspect of care. Constant pain, regardless of severity, is energy consuming. You should make every effort to assist the patient in conserving this energy. There are times when the patient's pain can and should be relieved by medications. There are, however, numerous occasions when effective pain relief can be provided by basic patient-care measures such as proper body alignment, change of position, use of heat or cold (if permitted by a physician's orders), back rubs and massages, and even simple conversation with the patient. Meaningful activity also has been found to help relieve pain. Whenever possible, a well-planned physical/occupational therapy regimen should be an integral part of the total rehabilitation plan.

CAST FABRICATION.—As mentioned previously, immobilization is often a part of the overall therapy of the orthopedic patient, and casting is the most common and well-known form of long-term immobilization. In some instances, a Corpsman may be required to assist in applying a cast or be directed to apply or change a cast. In this section, we will discuss the method of applying a short and long arm cast, and a short leg cast.

In applying any cast, the basic materials are the same: webril or cotton bunting, plaster of Paris, a bucket or basin of tepid water, a water source (tap water), protective linen, gloves, a working surface, a cast saw, and seating surfaces for the patient and the Corpsman. Some specific types of casts may require additional material.

SHORT ARM CAST.—A short arm cast extends from the metacarpal-phalangeal joints of the hand to just below the elbow joint. Depending on the location and type of fracture, the physician may order a specific position for the arm to be casted. Generally, the wrist is in a neutral (straight) position, with the fingers slightly flexed in the position of function.

Beginning at the wrist, apply three layers of webril (fig. 2–2A). Then apply webril to the forearm and the hand, making sure that each layer overlaps the other by a third (as shown in figure 2–2B). Check for lumps or wrinkles and correct any by tearing the webril and smoothing it.

Dip the plaster of Paris into the water for approximately 5 seconds. Gently squeeze to remove excess water, but do not wring out. Beginning at the wrist (fig. 2–2C) wrap the plaster in a spiral motion, overlapping each layer by one-third to one-half. Smooth out the layers with a gentle palmar motion. When applying the plaster, make tucks by grasping the excess material and folding it under as if making a pleat. Successive layers cover and smooth over this fold. When the plaster is anchored on the wrist, cover the hand and the palmar surface before continuing up the arm (figs. 2–2D and 2–2E). Repeat this procedure until the cast is thick enough to provide adequate support, generally 4 to 5 layers. The final step is to remove any rough edges and smooth the cast surface (fig. 2–2F). Turn the ends of the cast back and cover with the final layer of plaster, and allow the plaster to set for approximately 15 minutes. Trim with a cast saw, as needed.

LONG ARM CAST.—The procedure for a long arm cast is basically the same as for a short arm cast, except the elbow is maintained in a 90° position, the

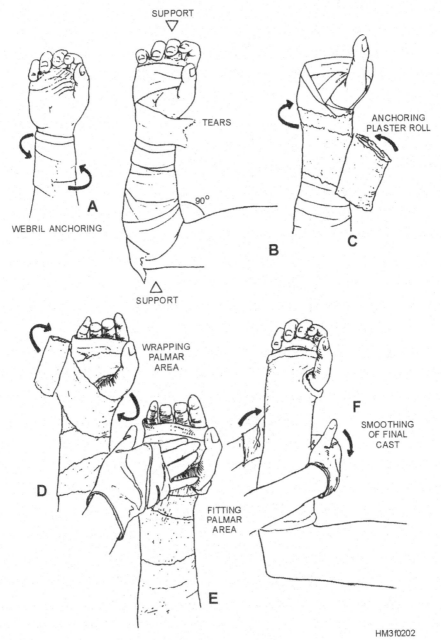

SUPPORT

TEARS

90°

SUPPORT

WEBRIL ANCHORING

ANCHORING
PLASTER ROLL

A

B

C

WRAPPING
PALMAR
AREA

SMOOTHING
OF FINAL
CAST

FITTING
PALMAR
AREA

D

E

F

HM3f0202

Figure 2–2.—Applying a short arm cast.

cast begins at the wrist and ends on the upper arm below the axilla, and the hand is not wrapped.

SHORT LEG CAST.—In applying a short leg cast, seat the patient on a table with both legs over the side, flexed at the knee. Instruct the patient to hold the affected leg, with the ankle in a neutral position (90°). Make sure that the foot is not rotated medially or laterally. Beginning at the toes, apply webril (figs. 2–3A, 2–3B, and 2–3C) in the same manner as for the short arm cast, ensuring that there are no lumps or

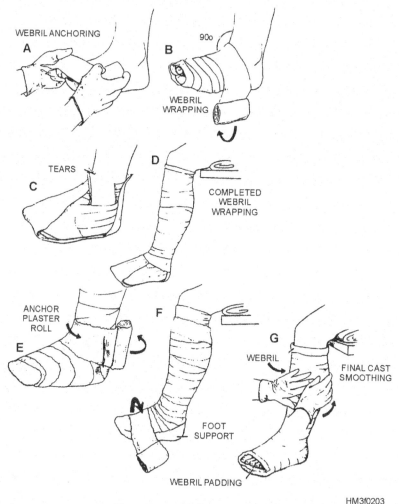

WEBRIL ANCHORING

A

90o

B

WEBRIL WRAPPING

TEARS

C

D

COMPLETED WEBRIL WRAPPING

ANCHOR PLASTER ROLL

E

F

G

WEBRIL

FINAL CAST SMOOTHING

FOOT SUPPORT

WEBRIL PADDING

HM3f0203

Figure 2–3.—Applying a short leg cast.

wrinkles. Apply the plaster beginning at the toes (fig. 2–3E), using the same technique of tucks and folds and smoothing as for the short arm cast. Before applying the last layer, expose the toes and fold back the webril. As the final step, apply a footplate to the plantar surface of the cast, using a generous thickness of plaster splints secured with one or two rolls of plaster (fig. 2–3F). This area provides support to the cast and a weight-bearing surface when used with a walking boot.

Whenever a cast is applied, you must give the patient written and verbal instruction for cast care and circulation checks (i.e., numbness, cyanosis, tingling of extremities). Instruct the patient to return immediately should any of these conditions occur.

When a leg cast is applied, the patient must also receive instructions in the proper use of crutches. The cast will take 24 to 48 hours to completely dry, and it must be treated gently during this time. Since plaster is water-soluble, the cast must be protected with a waterproof covering when bathing or during wet weather. Nothing must be inserted down the cast (e.g., coat hangers) since this action can cause bunching of the padding and result in pressure sores. If swelling occurs, the cast may be split and wrapped with an elastic wrap to alleviate pressure.

Cast Removal

A cast can be removed in two ways: by soaking in warm vinegar-water solution until it dissolves, or by cutting. To remove by cutting, cast cutters, spreaders, and bandage scissors are necessary. Cuts are made laterally and medially along the long axis of the cast, then widened with the use of spreaders. The padding is then cut with the scissors.

THE TERMINALLY ILL PATIENT

LEARNING OBJECTIVE: *Evaluate the needs of the terminally ill patient.*

The terminally ill patient has many needs that are basically the same as those of other patients: spiritual, psychological, cultural, economic, and physical. What differs in these patients may be best expressed as the urgency to resolve the majority of these needs within a limited time frame. Death comes to everyone in different ways and at different times. For some patients, death is sudden following an acute illness. For others, death follows a lengthy illness. Death not only affects the individual patient; it also affects family and friends, staff, and even other patients. Because of this, it is essential that all healthcare providers understand the process of dying and its possible effects on people.

Individual's Perspective on Death

People view death from their individual and cultural value perspectives. Many people find the courage and strength to face death through their religious beliefs. These patients and their families often seek support from representatives of their religious faith. In many cases, patients who previously could not identify with a religious belief or the concept of a Supreme Being may indicate (verbally or nonverbally) a desire to speak with a spiritual representative. There will also be patients who, through the whole dying experience, will neither desire nor need spiritual support and assistance. In all these cases, it is the responsibility of the healthcare provider to be attentive and perceptive to the patient's needs and to provide whatever support personnel the patient may require.

Cultural Influences

An individual's cultural system influences behavior patterns. When we speak of cultural systems, we refer to certain norms, values, and action patterns of specific groups of people to various aspects of life.

Dying is an aspect of life, and it is often referred to as the final crisis of living. In all of our actions, culturally approved roles frequently encourage specific behavior responses. For example, in the Caucasian, Anglo-European culture, a dying patient is expected to show peaceful acceptance of the prognosis; the bereaved is expected to communicate grief. When people behave differently, the healthcare provider frequently has difficulty responding appropriately.

Five Stages of Death

A theory of death and dying has developed that provides highly meaningful knowledge and skills to all persons involved with the experience. In this theory of death and dying (as formulated by Dr. Elizabeth Kubler-Ross in her book *On Death and Dying*), it is suggested that most people (both patients and significant others) go through five stages: **denial, anger, bargaining, depression**, and **acceptance**.

The first stage, **denial**, is one of nonacceptance. "No, it can't be me! There must be a mistake!" It is not only important for the healthcare provider to recognize the denial stage with its behavior responses, but also to realize that some people maintain denial up to the point of impending death. The next stage is **anger**. This is a period of hostility and questioning: "Why me?" The third stage is **bargaining**. At this point, people revert to a culturally reinforced concept that good behavior is rewarded. Patients are often heard stating, "I'd do anything if I could just turn this thing around." Once patients realize that bargaining is futile, they quickly enter into the stage of **depression**. In addition to grieving because of their personal loss, it is at this point that patients become concerned about their family and "putting affairs in order." The final stage comes when the patient finally **accepts** death and is prepared for it. It is usually at this time that the patient's family requires more support than the patient. It is important to remember that one or more stages may be skipped, and that the last stage may never be reached.

Support for the Dying

Despite the fact that we all realize our mortality, there is no easy way to discuss death. To the strong and healthy, death is a frightening thought. The fact that sooner or later everyone dies does not make death easier. There are no procedure books that tell healthcare providers "how to do" death. The "how to" will only come from the individual healthcare provider who understands that patients are people, and that, more than any other time in life, the dying patient needs to be treated as an individual person.

An element of uncertainty and helplessness is almost always present when death occurs. Assessment and respect for the patient's individual and cultural value system are of key importance in planning the care of the dying. As healthcare personnel, we often approach a dying patient with some feelings of uncertainty, helplessness, and anxiety. We feel helpless in being unable to perform tasks that will keep the patient alive, uncertain that we are doing all that we can do to either make the patient as comfortable as possible or to postpone or prevent death altogether. We feel anxious about how to communicate effectively with patients, their family, or even among ourselves. This is a normal response since any discussion about death carries a high emotional risk for the patient as well as the healthcare provider. Nevertheless, communicating can provide both strength and comfort to all if done with sensitivity and dignity, and it is sensitivity and dignity that is the essence of all healthcare services.

PATIENT SAFETY

LEARNING OBJECTIVE: *Identify patient safety concerns in a medical treatment facility.*

The primary goal of the healthcare provider is maintaining, sustaining, restoring, and rehabilitating a physical or psychological function of the patient. To achieve this goal, healthcare facilities and providers are charged with developing policies and implementing mechanisms that ensure safe, efficient, and therapeutically effective care. The theme of this discussion is safety and will address the major aspects of both environmental and personal safety.

ENVIRONMENTAL SAFETY

For purposes of this discussion, the environment is defined as the physical surroundings of the patient and includes such things as lighting, equipment, supplies, chemicals, architectural structure, and the activities of both patient and staff personnel. Maintaining safety becomes even more difficult when working with people who are ill or anxious and who cannot exercise their usual control over their environment. Loss of strength, decreased sensory input, and disability often accompany illness. Because of this, you must be constantly alert and responsive to maintaining a safe environment.

Both JCAHO and the National Safety Council of the American Hospital Association (AHA) have identified four major types of accidents that continually occur to patients. These hazards consist of falls, electrical shocks, physical and chemical burns, and fire and explosions.

Patient Fall Precautions

The most basic of hospital equipment, the patient's bed, is a common cause of falls. Falls occur among oriented patients getting in and out of bed at night in situations where there is inadequate lighting. Falls occur among disoriented or confused bed patients when bedrails are not used or are used improperly. Slippery or cluttered floors contribute to patient, staff, and even visitor falls. Patients with physical limitations or patients being treated with sensory-altering medications fall when attempting to ambulate without proper assistance. Falls result from running in passageways, carelessness when going around blind corners, and collisions between personnel and equipment. Unattended and improperly secured patients fall from gurneys and wheelchairs.

Healthcare personnel can do much to prevent the incidence of falls by following some simple procedures. These preventive measures include properly using side rails on beds, gurneys, and cribs; locking the wheels of gurneys and wheelchairs when transferring patients; and not leaving patients unattended. Safety straps must also be used to secure patients on gurneys or in wheelchairs. Maintaining dry and uncluttered floors markedly reduces the number of accidental falls. Patients with physical or sensory deficiencies should always be assisted during ambulation. Patients using crutches, canes, or walkers must receive adequate instructions in the proper use of these aids before being permitted to ambulate independently. The total care environment must be equipped with adequate night lights to assist orientation and to prevent falls resulting from an inability to see.

Electrical Safety Precautions

The expanded variety, quantity, and complexity of electrical and electronic equipment used for diagnostic and therapeutic care has markedly increased the hazards of burns, shock, explosions, and fire. It is imperative that healthcare providers at all levels be alert to such hazards and maintain an electrically safe environment. Knowledge and adherence to the following guidelines will contribute significantly to providing an electrically safe environment for all personnel, whether they be patients, staff, or visitors.

- Do not use electrical equipment with damaged plugs or cords.

- Do not attempt to repair defective equipment.

- Do not use electrical equipment unless it is properly grounded with a three-wire cord and three-prong plug.

- Do not use extension cords or plug adapters unless approved by the Medical Repair Department or the safety officer.

- Do not create a trip hazard by passing electrical cords across doorways or walkways.

- Do not remove a plug from the receptacle by gripping the cord.

- Do not allow the use of personal electrical appliances without the approval of the safety officer.

- Do not put water on an electrical fire.

- Do not work with electrical equipment with wet hands or feet.

- Have newly purchased electronic medical equipment tested for electrical safety by Medical Repair before putting it into service.

- Operate all electrical and electronic equipment according to manufacturer's instructions.

- Remove from service electrical equipment that sparks, smokes, or gives a slight shock. Tag defective equipment and expedite repair.

- Be aware that patients with intravenous therapy and electronic monitoring equipment are at high risk from electrical shocks.

- Call Medical Repair when equipment is not functioning properly or Public Works if there is difficulty with the power distribution system.

Since accidents resulting in physical and chemical burns have initiated numerous consumer claims of healthcare provider and facility malpractice, all healthcare personnel must be thoroughly indoctrinated in the proper use of equipment, supplies, and chemicals.

Physical and Chemical Burn Precautions

The following discussion will address common causes and precautions to be taken to eliminate the occurrence of burn injuries.

HOT WATER BOTTLES.—A common cause of burns—particularly in the elderly, diabetics, and patients with circulatory impairments—is the hot water bottle. When you are filling the bottle, the water temperature must never exceed 125°F (51°C). Test the bottle for leaks and cover it so that there is a protective layer of cloth between the patient and the bottle itself.

HEATING PADS.—Heating pads present a dual hazard of potential burns and electrical shock. The precautions that should be taken when using heating pads are the same ones that should be used for hot water bottles: temperature control and protective cloth padding. Precautions you should observe to avoid shock include properly maintaining the equipment; conducting preuse inspections; testing the equipment for wiring and plug defects; and ensuring periodic safety inspections are conducted by Medical Repair personnel.

ICE BAGS OR COLD PACKS.—Like hot water bottles, ice bags and cold packs (packaged chemical coolant) can cause skin-contact burns. This kind of burn is commonly referred to as local frostbite. The precautions taken for applying ice bags and cold baths are the same as those for hot water bottles with regard to attention to elderly, diabetic, and patients with circulatory impairments.

HYPOTHERMIA BLANKETS.—Like ice bags, hypothermia blankets can also cause contact burns. When using hypothermia blankets, check the patient's skin frequently for signs of marked discoloration (indicating indirect localized tissue damage). Ensure that the bare blanket does not come in direct contact with the patient's unprotected skin. This precaution is easily accomplished by using sheets or cotton blankets between the patient and the hypothermia blanket itself. When using this form of therapy, follow both the physician's orders and the manufacturer's instructions in managing the temperature control of the equipment.

HEAT (BED) CRADLE.—When using the heat (bed) cradle, protect the patient from burns resulting from overexposure or placement of the equipment too close to the area of the patient being treated. As with heating pads, heat cradles present the dual hazard of potential burns and electrical shock. Another hazard to keep in mind is that of fire. Ensure that the bedding and the heat source do not come in direct contact and cause the bedding to ignite. Occasionally, heat lamps are used to accomplish the same results as a heat cradle. Do not use towels, pillow cases, or linen of any kind to drape over heat lamps. In fact, no lamps of any kind should be draped with any kind of material, regardless of the purpose of the draping.

STEAM VAPORIZERS AND HOT FOODS AND LIQUIDS.—Steam vaporizers and hot foods and liquids are common causes of patient burns. When using steam vaporizers, ensure that the vapor of steam does not flow directly on the patient as a result of the initial positioning of the equipment or by accidental movement or bumping. Patients sensitive to hot foods and liquids are more likely burned. Also, because of lack of coordination, weakness, or medication, patients may be less able to handle hot foods and liquids safely without spilling them.

In the direct patient care units as well as in diagnostic and treatment areas, there is unlimited potential for inflicting burns on patients. When the modern electrical and electronic equipment and the potent chemicals used for diagnosis and treatment are used properly, they contribute to the patient's recovery and rehabilitation. When they are used carelessly or improperly, these same sources may cause patients additional pain and discomfort, serious illness, and, in some cases, death.

Fire and Explosion Precautions

Often when we speak of safety measures, one of our first thoughts is of a fire or an explosion involving the loss of life or injury to a number of people. Good housekeeping, maintenance, and discipline help prevent such mishaps. Remember that buildings constructed of fire-resistant materials may not be fireproof, and they are certainly not explosion proof. Good maintenance includes checking, reporting, and ensuring correct repair of electrical equipment, and routine checking of fire fighting equipment by qualified personnel. The education and training of personnel are the most effective means of preventing fires. Used in the context of fire safety measures, good discipline means developing a fire plan to use as outlined in a fire bill, having periodic fire drills, and enforcing no-smoking regulations.

FIRE EVACUATION PROCEDURES.—Staff members should be familiar with the fire regulations at their duty station and know what to do in case of fire. Staff should know how to report a fire, use a fire extinguisher, and evacuate patients. When a fire occurs, there are certain basic rules to follow: The senior person should take charge and appoint someone to notify the fire department and the officer of the day of the exact location of the fire. Everyone should remain calm. All oxygen equipment and electrical appliances must be turned off unless such equipment is necessary to sustain life. All windows and doors should be closed and all possible exits cleared. When necessary and directed by proper authority, patients should be removed in a calm and orderly fashion and mustered outside.

SMOKING REGULATIONS.—By regulation (BUMEDINST 6200.12, *Tobacco Use in Navy Medical Department Activities*), smoking is no longer permitted in Navy hospitals. To ensure general safety and awareness of this prohibition, inform patients, visitors, and staff of the facility's no-smoking status by prominently displaying "No Smoking" signs throughout the hospital—especially in rooms and areas where oxygen and flammable agents are used and stored.

Safety Precautions in the Operating Room

Since safety practices are important to emphasize, this section will cover some of the situations that are potentially hazardous in the operating room and discuss what might be done to eliminate the hazard.

All personnel should know the location of all emergency medications and equipment in the operating room. This includes drugs, cardiac arrest equipment, and resuscitators. All electrical equipment and plugs must be of the explosion-proof type and bear a label stating such. There should be written schedules of inspections and maintenance of all electrical equipment. Navy regulations prohibit the use of explosive anesthetics in the operating room. These regulations, however, do not mean we can lessen our concern for fire and explosion hazards. The surface of all floors in the operating room must provide a path of electrical conductivity between all persons and equipment making contact with the floor to prevent the accumulation of dangerous electrostatic charges. All furniture and equipment should be constructed of metal or of other electrically conductive material and should be equipped with conductive leg tips, casters, or equivalent devices. Periodic inspections should be made of leg tips, tires, casters, or other conductive devices of furniture and equipment. These inspections will ensure that they are maintained free of wax, lint, or other foreign material that may insulate them and defeat the purpose for which they are used. Excess lubrication of casters should be avoided to prevent accumulation of oil on conductive wheels. Dry graphite and graphite oil are the preferred lubricants.

Rubber accessories for anesthesia machines should be of the conductive type, plainly labeled as such, and routinely tested to ensure that conductivity is maintained. It is essential that all replacement items be of conductive material.

All personnel entering the operating room should be in electrical contact with the conductive floor by wearing conductive footwear or an alternative method of providing a path of conductivity. Conductive footwear and other personnel-to-floor conductive equipment should be tested on a regularly scheduled basis.

All apparel worn in the operating room should be made of a nonstatic-producing material. Fabrics of 100 percent cotton are the most acceptable. Fabrics made of synthetic blends may be used only if they have been treated by the manufacturer for use in the operating room. Wool blankets and apparel made of untreated synthetic fabrics are not permitted in the operating room.

Operating rooms must have adequate air-conditioning equipment to maintain relative humidity and temperature within a constant range. The relative humidity should be kept at 55 to 60 percent. This level will reduce the possibility of electrostatic discharge and possible explosion of combustible gases. The temperature should be chosen on the basis of the well-being of the patient. The recommended temperature is between 65° and 74°F. The control of bacteria carried on dust particles is facilitated when the recommended humidity and temperature are maintained.

All oxygen cylinders in use or in storage will be tagged with DD Form 1191, Warning Tag for Medical Oxygen Equipment, and measures will be taken to ensure compliance with instructions 1 through 7 printed on the form. An additional tag is required on all cylinders to indicate "EMPTY," "IN USE," or "FULL." Safety precautions should be conspicuously posted in all areas in which oxygen cylinders are stored and in which oxygen therapy is being administered. This posting should be made so it will immediately make all personnel aware of the precautionary measures required in the area.

All electrical service equipment, switchboards, or panelboards should be installed in a nonhazardous location. Devices or apparatus that tend to create an arc, sparks, or high temperatures must not be installed in hazardous locations unless these devices are in compliance with the National Electrical Code. Lamps in a fixed position will be enclosed and will be properly protected by substantial metal guards or other means where exposed to breakage. Cords for portable lamps or portable electrical appliances must be continuous and without switches from the appliance to the attachment plug. Such cords must contain an insulated conductor to form a grounding connection between the electrical outlet and the appliance.

GENERAL SAFETY

In addition to the specifics presented earlier, some other basic principles are relevant to patient safety. They are:

- Ensure your patients are familiar with their environment, thus making it less hazardous to them. This familiarization can be accomplished in many ways, such as by showing your patients the floor plan of the ward they have been admitted to and by indicating key areas (lounge, bathrooms, nursing station, etc.) that may be of interest to them.

- Be aware of patient sensory impairment and incorporate precautionary procedures into their patient-care plan. For example, this principle can be applied to patients who have been given a pain medication, such as morphine or Demerol®. Medications such as these dull body senses. If a patient in this condition wishes to walk around, precautionary actions dictate that you either be close at hand to prevent the patient from accidental falls or that you do not permit the patient to ambulate until the effects of the medication have stopped.

- Understand that all diagnostic and therapeutic measures have the potential to cause a patient harm.

- Ensure that all accidents and incidents are documented and analyzed to identify and correct high-risk safety hazards.

ENVIRONMENTAL HYGIENE

LEARNING OBJECTIVE: *Identify environmental hygiene concerns in a medical treatment facility.*

Today's public is very much aware of the environment and its effect on the health and comfort of human beings. The healthcare setting is a unique environment and has a distinct character of its own. You need to be aware of that character and ensure that the environment will support the optimum in health maintenance, care, and rehabilitation.

In the context of the environment, hygiene may best be described as practices that provide a healthy environment. Basically, environmental hygiene practices include the following three areas of concern: safety (which has already been addressed); environmental comfort and stimuli; and, finally, infection control (which will be discussed briefly here, but in greater detail later in this chapter under "Medical Asepsis"). You have certain responsibilities for helping to control the facility's general environment as well as the patient's immediate surroundings.

CONCURRENT AND TERMINAL CLEANING

Maintaining cleanliness is a major responsibility of all members of the healthcare team, regardless of their position on the team. Cleanliness not only provides for patient comfort and a positive stimulus, it also impacts on infection control. The Hospital Corpsman is often directly responsible for the maintenance of patient care areas. The management of cleanliness in patient care areas is conducted concurrently and terminally. **Concurrent cleaning** is the disinfection and sterilization of patient supplies and equipment during hospitalization. **Terminal cleaning** is the disinfection and sterilization of patient supplies and equipment after the patient is discharged from the unit or hospital. Both concurrent and terminal cleaning are extremely important procedures that not only aid the patient's comfort and psychological outlook, but also contribute to both efficient physical care and control of the complications of illness and injury.

AESTHETICS

Aesthetically, an uncluttered look is far more appealing to the eye than an untidy one. Other environmental factors, such as color and noise, can also enhance or hinder the progress of a person's physical condition. In the past, almost all healthcare facilities used white as a basic color for walls and bedside equipment. However, research has shown that the use of color is calming and restful to the patient, and, as has been previously stated, rest is a very important healing agent in any kind of illness. Noise control is another environmental element that requires your attention. The large number of people and the amount of equipment traffic in a facility serve to create a high noise level that must be monitored. Add to that the noise of multiple radios and televisions, and it is understandable why noise control is necessary if a healing environment is to be created and maintained.

CLIMATE CONTROL

Another important aspect of environmental hygiene is climate control. Many facilities use air conditioning or similar control systems to maintain proper ventilation, humidity, and temperature control. In facilities without air conditioning, windows should be opened from the top and bottom to provide for cross-ventilation. Ensure that patients are not located in a drafty area. Window sill deflectors or patient screens are often used to redirect drafty airflows. Maintain facility temperatures at recommended energy-conservation levels that are also acceptable as health-promoting temperatures. In addition to maintaining a healthy climate, good ventilation is necessary in controlling and eliminating disagreeable odors. In cases where airflow does not control odors, room fresheners should be discretely used. Offensive, odor-producing articles (such as soiled dressings, used bedpans, and urinals) should be removed to appropriate disposal and disinfecting areas as rapidly as possible. Objectionable odors (such as bad breath or perspiration of patients) are best controlled by proper personal hygiene and clean clothing.

LIGHTING

Natural light is important in the care of the sick. Sunlight usually brightens the area and helps to improve the mental well-being of the patient. However, light can be a source of irritation if it shines directly in the patient's eyes or produces a glare from the furniture, linen, or walls. Adjust shades or blinds for the patient's comfort. Artificial light should be strong enough to prevent eyestrain and diffuse enough to prevent glare. Whenever possible, provide a bed lamp for the patient. As discussed earlier under "Safety Aspect," a dim light is valuable as a comfort and safety measure at night. This light should be situated so it will not shine in the patient's eyes and yet provide sufficient light along the floor so that all obstructions can be seen. A night light may help orient elderly patients if they are confused as to their surroundings upon awakening.

In conclusion, it is important that you understand the effects of the environment on patients. People are more sensitive to excessive stimuli in the environment when they are ill, and they often become irritable and unable to cooperate in their care because of these excesses. This is particularly apparent in critical care areas (e.g., in CCUs and ICUs) and isolation, terminal, and geriatric units. You must realize and respond to the vital importance of the environment in the total medical management plan of your patients.

PATHOGENIC ORGANISM CONTROL

LEARNING OBJECTIVE: *Recall medical asepsis principles and recognize medical asepsis practices.*

All health care, regardless of who provides it or where it is provided, must be directed toward maintaining, promoting, and restoring health. Because of this goal, all persons seeking assistance in a healthcare facility must be protected from additional injury, disease, or infection. Adherence to good safety principles and practices protects a patient from personal injury. Additionally, attention to personal and environmental hygiene not only protects against further injury, but also constitutes the first step in controlling the presence, growth, and spread of pathogenic organisms. The discussion that follows addresses infection control, particularly in the context of medical and surgical aseptic practices.

MEDICAL ASEPSIS

Medical asepsis is the term used to describe those practices used to prevent the transfer of pathogenic organisms from person to person, place to place, or person to place. Medical aseptic practices are routinely used in direct patient care areas, as well as in

other service areas in the healthcare environment, to interrupt a chain of events necessary for the continuation of an infectious process. The components of this chain of events consist of the elements defined below.

Infectious Agent

An infectious agent is an organism that is capable of producing an infection or infectious disease.

Reservoir of Infectious Agents

A reservoir of infectious agents is the carrier on which the infectious agent primarily depends for survival. The agent lives, multiplies, and reproduces so that it can be transferred to a susceptible host. Reservoirs of infectious agents could be man, animal, plants, or soil. Man himself is the most frequent reservoir of infectious agents pathogenic to man.

PORTAL OF EXIT.—The portal of exit is the avenue by which the infectious agent leaves its reservoir. When the reservoir is man, these avenues include various body systems (such as respiratory, intestinal, and genitourinary tracts) and open lesions.

MODE OF TRANSMISSION.—The mode of transmission is the mechanism by which the infectious agent is transmitted from its reservoir to a susceptible being (host). Air, water, food, dust, dirt, insects, inanimate objects, and other persons are examples of modes of transmission.

PORTAL OF ENTRY.—The portal of entry is the avenue by which the infectious agent enters the susceptible host. In man, these portals correspond to the exit route avenues, including the respiratory and gastrointestinal tracts, through a break in the skin, or by direct infection of the mucous membrane.

SUSCEPTIBLE HOST.—The susceptible host is man or another living organism that affords an infectious agent nourishment or protection to survive and multiply.

Removal or control of any one component in the above chain of events will control the infectious process.

Two Basic Medical Asepsis Practices

The two basic medical asepsis practices that are absolutely essential in preventing and controlling the spread of infection and transmittable diseases are frequent hand washing and proper linen-handling procedures.

HAND WASHING.—The following are some common instances when provider hand washing is imperative:

- Before and after each patient contact

- Before handling food and medications

- After coughing, sneezing, or blowing your nose

- After using the toilet

LINEN HANDLING.—Improper handling of linen results in the transfer of pathogenic organisms through direct contact with the healthcare provider's clothing and subsequent contact with the patient, patient-care items, or other materials in the care environment. Proper linen handling is such an elementary procedure that, in theory, it seems almost unnecessary to mention. However, it is a procedure so frequently ignored that emphasis is justified.

All linen, whether clean or used, must never be held against one's clothing or placed on the floor. The floors of a healthcare facility are considered to be grossly contaminated, and, thus, any article coming in contact with the floor will also be contaminated. Place all dirty linen in appropriate laundry bags. Linen from patients having infectious or communicable diseases must be handled in a special manner.

Isolation Technique

Isolation technique, a medical aseptic practice, inhibits the spread and transfer of pathogenic organisms by limiting the contacts of the patient and creating some kind of physical barrier between the patient and others. Isolation precautions in hospitals must meet the following objectives. They must

- be epidemiologically sound;

- recognize the importance that body fluids, secretions, and excretions may have in the transmission of nosocomial (hospital originating) pathogens;

- contain adequate precautions for infections transmitted by airborne droplets and other routes of transmission; and

- be as simple and as patient friendly as possible.

In isolation techniques, disinfection procedures are employed to control contaminated items and areas. For purposes of this discussion, disinfection is described as the killing of certain infectious (pathogenic) agents outside the body by a physical or chemical means. Isolation techniques employ two kinds of disinfection practices, concurrent and terminal.

CONCURRENT DISINFECTION.— Concurrent disinfection consists of the daily measures taken to control the spread of pathogenic organisms while the patient is still considered infectious.

TERMINAL DISINFECTION.—Terminal disinfection consists of those measures taken to destroy pathogenic organisms remaining after the patient is discharged from isolation. There are a variety of chemical and physical means used to disinfect supplies, equipment, and environmental areas, and each facility will determine its own protocols based on the recommendation of an Infection Control Committee.

SURGICAL ASEPTIC TECHNIQUE

LEARNING OBJECTIVE: *Recall the principles and guidelines for surgical aseptic technique, and determine the correct sterilization process for different types of materials.*

As used in this discussion, surgical aseptic technique is the term used to describe the sterilization, storage, and handling of articles to keep them free of pathogenic organisms. The following discussion will address the preparation and sterilization of surgical equipment and supplies, and the preparation of the operating room for performing a surgical procedure. It should be noted that specific methods of preparation will vary from place to place, but the basic principles of surgical aseptic technique will remain the same. This discussion will present general guidelines, and individual providers are advised to refer to local instructions regarding the particular routines of a specific facility.

Before an operation, it is necessary to sterilize and keep sterile all instruments, materials, and supplies that come in contact with the surgical site. Every item handled by the surgeon and the surgeon's assistants must be sterile. The patient's skin and the hands of the members of the surgical team must be thoroughly scrubbed, prepared, and kept as aseptic as possible.

During the operation, the surgeon, surgeon's assistants, and the scrub corpsman must wear sterile gowns and gloves and must not touch anything that is not sterile. Maintaining sterile technique is a cooperative responsibility of the entire surgical team. Each member must develop a surgical conscience, a willingness to supervise and be supervised by others regarding the adherence to standards. Without this cooperative and vigilant effort, a break in sterile technique may go unnoticed or not be corrected, and an otherwise successful surgical procedure may result in complete failure.

Basic Guidelines

To assist in maintaining the aseptic technique, all members of the surgical team must adhere to the following principles:

- All personnel assigned to the operating room must practice good personal hygiene. This includes daily bathing and clothing change.

- Those personnel having colds, sore throats, open sores, and/or other infections should not be permitted in the operating room.

- Operating room attire (which includes scrub suits, gowns, head coverings, and face masks) should not be worn outside the operating room suite. If such occurs, change all attire before re-entering the clean area. (The operating room and adjacent supporting areas are classified as "clean areas.")

- All members of the surgical team having direct contact with the surgical site must perform the surgical hand scrub before the operation.

- All materials and instruments used in contact with the site must be sterile.

- The gowns worn by surgeons and scrub corpsmen are considered sterile from shoulder to waist (in the front only), including the gown sleeves.

- If sterile surgical gloves are torn, punctured, or have touched an unsterile surface or item, they are considered contaminated.

- The safest, most practical method of sterilization for most articles is steam under pressure.

- Label all prepared, packaged, and sterilized items with an expiration date.

- Use articles packaged and sterilized in cotton muslin wrappers within 28 calendar days.

- Use articles sterilized in cotton muslin wrappers and sealed in plastic within 180 calendar days.

- Unsterile articles must not come in contact with sterile articles.

- Make sure the patient's skin is as clean as possible before a surgical procedure.

- Take every precaution to prevent contamination of sterile areas or supplies by airborne organisms.

Methods of Sterilization

Sterilization refers to the complete destruction of all living organisms, including bacterial spores and viruses. The word "sterile" means free from or the absence of all living organisms. Any item to be sterilized must be thoroughly cleaned mechanically or by hand, using soap or detergent and water. When cleaning by hand, apply friction to the item using a brush. After cleaning, thoroughly rinse the item with clean, running water before sterilization. The appropriate sterilization method is determined according to how the item will be used, the material from which the item is made, and the sterilization methods available. The physical methods of sterilization are moist heat and dry heat. Chemical methods include gas and liquid solutions.

PHYSICAL METHODS.—Steam under pressure (autoclave) is the most dependable and economical method of sterilization. It is the method of choice for metalware, glassware, most rubber goods, and dry goods. All articles must be correctly wrapped or packaged so that the steam will come in contact with all surfaces of the article. Similar items should be sterilized together, especially those requiring the same time and temperature exposure. Articles that will collect water must be placed so that the water will drain out of the article during the sterilization cycle. A sterilizer should be loaded in a manner that will allow the free flow of steam in and around all articles. Each item sterilized must be dated with the expiration of sterility. Sterilization indicators must be used in each load that is put through the sterilization process. This verifies proper steam and temperature penetration.

The operating procedures for a steam sterilizer will vary according to the type and manufacturer. There are a number of manufacturers, but there are only two types of steam-under-pressure sterilizers. They are the downward displacement and the prevacuum, high-temperature autoclaves.

Downward Displacement Autoclave.—In the downward (gravity) displacement autoclave, air in the chamber is forced downward from the top of the chamber. The temperature in the sterilizer gradually increases as the steam heats the chamber and its contents. The actual timing does not begin until the temperature is above 245°F (118°C).

Prevacuum, High-temperature Autoclave.— The prevacuum, high-temperature autoclave is the most modern and economical to operate and requires the least time to sterilize a single load. By use of a vacuum pump, air is extracted from the chamber before admitting steam. This prevacuum process permits instant steam penetration to all articles and through all cotton or linen dry goods. The sterilization time is reduced to 4 minutes. The temperature of the chamber is rapidly raised and held at 274°F (134°C). The cycle is timed automatically.

Sterilizing Times.—If the temperature is increased, the sterilization time may be decreased. The following are some practical sterilization time periods.

- 3 minutes at 270°F (132°C)

- 8 minutes at 257°F (125°C)

- 18 minutes at 245°F (118°C)

All operating rooms are equipped with high-speed (flash) sterilizers. Wrapped, covered, opened instruments placed in perforated trays are "flash" sterilized for 3 minutes at 270°F (132°C). Sterilization timing begins when the above temperature is reached, not before.

Dry-Heat Sterilization.—The use of dry heat as a sterilizing agent has limitations. It should be restricted to items that are unsuitable for exposure to moist heat. High temperatures and extended time periods are required when using dry heat. In most instances, this method often proves impractical. The temperature must be 320°F (160°C), and the time period must be at least 2 hours.

CHEMICAL STERILIZATION.—Only one liquid chemical, if properly used, is capable of rendering an item sterile. That chemical is **glutaraldehyde**. The item to be sterilized must be totally submerged in the glutaraldehyde solution for 10 hours. Before immersion, the item must be thoroughly cleansed and rinsed with sterile water or sterile normal saline. It should be noted that this chemical is extremely caustic to skin, mucous membranes, and other tissues.

The most effective method of gas chemical sterilization presently available is the use of **ethylene oxide (ETO) gas**. ETO gas sterilization should be used only for material and supplies that will not withstand sterilization by steam under pressure. Never gas-sterilize any item that can be steam-sterilized. The concentration of the gas and the temperature and humidity inside the sterilizer are vital factors that affect the gas-sterilization process.

ETO gas-sterilization periods range from 3 to 7 hours. All items gas-sterilized must be allowed an aeration (airing out) period. During this period, the ETO gas is expelled from the surface of the item. It is not practical here to present all exposure times, gas concentrations, and aeration times for various items to be gas-sterilized. When using an ETO gas-sterilizer, you must be extremely cautious and follow the manufacturer's instructions carefully.

Preparation of Supplies for Autoclaving

Comply with the following guidelines in preparing supplies that are to be autoclaved.

- Inspect all articles to be sterilized, making sure they are clean, in good condition, and in working order.

- Wrap instruments and materials in double muslin wrappers or two layers of disposable sterilization wrappers.

- When muslin wrappers are routinely used, launder them after each use, and carefully inspect them for holes and tears before use.

- When articles are placed in glass or metal containers for autoclaving, place the lid of the container so the steam will penetrate the entire inside of the container.

- Arrange the contents of a linen pack in such a way that the articles on top are used first.

- Label every item that is packaged for sterilization to specify the contents and expiration date.

- Do not place surgical knife blades or suture materials inside linen packs or on instrument trays before sterilization.

The following are specific guidelines for sterilizing instruments, glassware, suture materials, and rubber latex materials.

Instruments:

- Wash each instrument after use with an antiseptic detergent solution. When washing by hand, pay particular attention to hinged parts and serrated surfaces. Rinse all instruments, and dry them thoroughly.

- Use an instrument washer/sterilizer, if available, to decontaminate instruments and utensils following each surgical procedure.

- Following cleaning and decontamination, leave hinged instruments unclasped and wrapped singly or placed on trays for resterilization.

Glassware:

- Inspect all reusable glassware for cracks or chips.

- Wash all reusable glassware with soap or detergent and water after use, and rinse it completely.

- When preparing reusable glass syringes

  —match numbers or syringe parts;

  —wrap each plunger and barrel separately in gauze; and

  —wrap each complete syringe in a double muslin wrapper.

- When glassware, tubes, medicine glasses, and beakers are part of a sterile tray, wrap each glass item in gauze before placing it on the tray.

Suture Material: Suture materials are available in two major categories: **absorbable** and **nonabsorbable**. Absorbable suture materials can be digested by the tissues during the healing process. Absorbable sutures are made from collagen (an animal protein derived from healthy animals) or from synthetic polymers. Nonabsorbable suture materials are those that effectively resist the enzymatic digestion process in living tissue. These sutures are made of metal or other inorganic materials. In both types, each strand of specifically sized suture material is uniform in diameter and is predictable in performance.

Modern manufacturing processes make all suture materials available in individual packages, presterilized,

with or without a surgical needle attached. Once opened, **do not resterilize** either the individual package or an individual strand of suture material.

NOTE: The only exception to this rule involves the use of surgical stainless steel. This material is often provided in unsterile packages or tubes. Individual strands or entire packages of surgical stainless steel must be sterilized before use.

Rubber Latex Materials:

- Wash rubber tubing in an antiseptic detergent solution.

  —Pay attention to the inside of the tubing. Rinse all tubing well and place it flat or loosely coiled in a wrapper or container.

  —When packing latex surgical drains for sterilization, place a piece of gauze in the lumen of the tray. **Never resterilize surgical drains.**

  —**Never resterilize rubber catheters bearing a disposable label.**

  —**Never resterilize surgeon's disposable (rubber) gloves.** These gloves are for one-time use only.

Handling Sterile Articles

LEARNING OBJECTIVE: *Recall sterile article handling and surgical hand scrubbing techniques, donning procedure for gowning and gloving, and the steps to clean an operating/treatment room.*

When you are changing a dressing, removing sutures, or preparing the patient for a surgical procedure, it will be necessary to establish a sterile field from which to work. The field should be established on a stable, clean, flat, dry surface. Wrappers from sterile articles may be used as a sterile field as long as the inside of the wrapper remains sterile. If the size of the wrapper does not provide a sufficient working space for the sterile field, use a sterile towel. Once established, only those persons who have donned sterile gloves should touch the sterile field. Additionally, the following basic rules must be adhered to:

- An article is either sterile or unsterile; there is no in-between. If there is doubt about the sterility of an item, consider it unsterile.

- Any time the sterility of a field has been compromised, replace the contaminated field and setup.

- Do not open sterile articles until they are ready for use.

- Do not leave sterile articles unattended once they are opened and placed on a sterile field.

- Do not return sterile articles to a container once they have been removed from the container.

- Never reach over a sterile field.

- When pouring sterile solutions into sterile containers or basins, do not touch the sterile container with the solution bottle. Once opened and first poured, use bottles of liquid entirely. If any liquid is left in the bottle, discard it.

- Never use an outdated article. Unwrap it, inspect it, and, if reusable, rewrap it in a **new** wrapper for sterilization.

Surgical Hand Scrub

The purpose of the surgical hand scrub is to reduce resident and transient skin flora (bacteria) to a minimum. Resident bacteria are often the result of organisms present in the hospital environment. Because these bacteria are firmly attached to the skin, they are difficult to remove. However, their growth is inhibited by the antiseptic action of the scrub detergent used. Transient bacteria are usually acquired by direct contact and are loosely attached to the skin. These are easily removed by the friction created by the scrubbing procedure.

Proper hand scrubbing and the wearing of sterile gloves and a sterile gown provide the patient with the best possible barrier against pathogenic bacteria in the environment and against bacteria from the surgical team. The following steps comprise the generally accepted method for the surgical hand scrub.

1. Before beginning the hand scrub, don a surgical cap or hood that covers all hair, both head and facial, and a disposable mask covering your nose and mouth.

2. Using approximately 6 ml of antiseptic detergent and running water, lather your hands and arms to 2 inches above the elbow. Leave detergent on your arms and do not rinse.

3. Under running water, clean your fingernails and cuticles, using a nail cleaner.

4. Starting with your fingertips, rinse each hand and arm by passing them through the running water. Always keep your hands above the level of your elbows.

5. From a sterile container, take a sterile brush and dispense approximately 6 ml of antiseptic detergent onto the brush and begin scrubbing your hands and arms.

6. Begin with the fingertips. Bring your thumb and fingertips together and, using the brush, scrub across the fingertips using 30 strokes.

7. Now scrub all four surface planes of the thumb and all surfaces of each finger, including the webbed space between the fingers, using 20 strokes for each surface area.

8. Scrub the palm and back of the hand in a circular motion, using 20 strokes each.

9. Visually divide your forearm into two parts, lower and upper. Scrub all surfaces of each division 20 strokes each, beginning at the wrist and progressing to the elbow.

10. Scrub the elbow in a circular motion using 20 strokes.

11. Scrub in a circular motion all surfaces to approximately 2 inches above the elbow.

12. Do not rinse this arm when you have finished scrubbing. Rinse only the brush.

13. Pass the rinsed brush to the scrubbed hand and begin scrubbing your other hand and arm, using the same procedure outlined above.

14. Drop the brush into the sink when you are finished.

15. Rinse both hands and arms, keeping your hands above the level of your elbows, and allow water to drain off the elbows.

16. When rinsing, do not touch anything with your scrubbed hands and arms.

17. The total scrub procedure must include all anatomical surfaces from the fingertips to approximately 2 inches above the elbow.

18. Dry your hands with a sterile towel. Do not allow the towel to touch anything other than your scrubbed hands and arms.

19. Between operations, follow the same hand-scrub procedure.

Gowning and Gloving

If you are the scrub corpsman, you will have opened your sterile gown and glove packages in the operating room before beginning your hand scrub. Having completed the hand scrub, back through the door holding your hands up to avoid touching anything with your hands and arms. Gowning technique is shown in the steps of figure 2–4. Pick up the sterile towel that has been wrapped with your gown (touching only the towel) and proceed as follows:

1. Dry one hand and arm, starting with the hand and ending at the elbow, with one end of the towel. Dry the other hand and arm with the opposite end of the towel. Drop the towel.

2. Pick up the gown in such a manner that hands touch only the inside surface at the neck and shoulder seams.

3. Allow the gown to unfold downward in front of you.

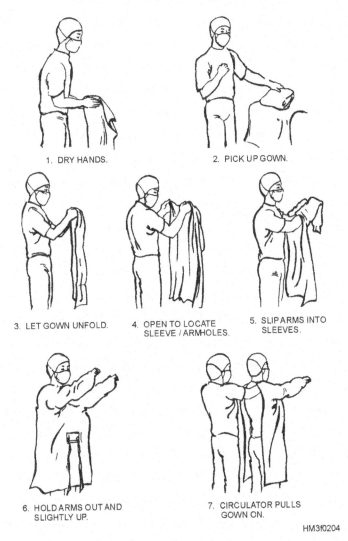

1. DRY HANDS.

2. PICK UP GOWN.

3. LET GOWN UNFOLD.

4. OPEN TO LOCATE SLEEVE / ARMHOLES.

5. SLIP ARMS INTO SLEEVES.

6. HOLD ARMS OUT AND SLIGHTLY UP.

7. CIRCULATOR PULLS GOWN ON.

HM3f0204

Figure 2–4.—Gowning.

4. Locate the arm holes.

5. Place both hands in the sleeves.

6. Hold your arms out and slightly up as you slip your arms into the sleeves.

7. Another person (circulatory) who is not scrubbed will pull your gown onto you as you extend your hands through the gown cuffs.

Continue the process by opening the inner glove packet on the same sterile surface on which you opened the gown. The entire gloving process is shown in the steps of figure 2–5.

1. Pick up one glove by the cuff using your thumb and index finger.

2. Touching only the cuff, pull the glove onto one hand and anchor the cuff over your thumb.

3. Slip your gloved fingers under the cuff of the other glove. Pull the glove over your fingers and hand, using a stretching side-to-side motion.

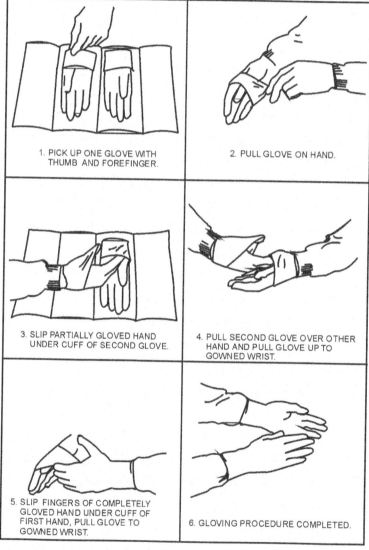

1. PICK UP ONE GLOVE WITH THUMB AND FOREFINGER.

2. PULL GLOVE ON HAND.

3. SLIP PARTIALLY GLOVED HAND UNDER CUFF OF SECOND GLOVE.

4. PULL SECOND GLOVE OVER OTHER HAND AND PULL GLOVE UP TO GOWNED WRIST.

5. SLIP FINGERS OF COMPLETELY GLOVED HAND UNDER CUFF OF FIRST HAND, PULL GLOVE TO GOWNED WRIST.

6. GLOVING PROCEDURE COMPLETED.

HM3f0205

Figure 2–5.—Gloving.

4. Anchor the cuff on your thumb. With your fingers still under the cuff, pull the cuff up and away from your hand and over the knitted cuff of the gown.

5. Repeat the preceding step to glove your other hand.

6. The gloving process is complete.

To gown and glove the surgeon, follow these steps:

1. Pick up a gown from the sterile linen pack. Step back from the sterile field and let the gown unfold in front of you. Hold the gown at the shoulder seams with the gown sleeves facing you.

2. Offer the gown to the surgeon. Once the surgeon's arms are in the sleeves, let go of the gown. Be careful not to touch anything but the sterile gown. The circulator will tie the gown.

3. Pick up the right glove. With the thumb of the glove facing the surgeon, place your fingers and thumbs of both hands in the cuff of the glove and stretch it outward, making a circle of the cuff. Offer the glove to the surgeon. Be careful that the surgeon's bare hand does not touch your gloved hands.

4. Repeat the preceding step for the left glove.

Cleaning the Operating/Treatment Room

Cleanliness in the operating room is an absolute must. Cleaning routines must be clearly understood and carefully followed. The cause of postoperative wound infections have, on occasion, been traced to the operating room. Since no two patients are alike and all patients have their own "resident" bacteria, every surgical case must be considered to be contaminated.

At the beginning of each day, all the fixtures, equipment, and furniture in each operating room will be damp-dusted with an antiseptic germicide solution. During the operation, keep the room clean and orderly at all times. Should sponges be dropped on the floor, or if blood or other body fluids spill, clean the area immediately using a disinfectant germicide solution and a clean cloth. Between operations, clean all used items. The area of the floor occupied by the surgical team must be cleaned using the wet vacuum method. If a wet vacuum is not available, mops may be used, but a clean mop head must be used following each operation. Gowns and gloves must be removed before leaving the room. All linens and surgical drapes must be bagged and removed from the room. All trash and disposable items must be bagged and taken from the room. All instruments must be washed by gloved hands or placed in perforated trays and put through a washer/sterilizer.

At the completion of the day's operations, each operating room should be terminally cleaned using an antiseptic germicide solution and the following tasks accomplished.

- Clean all wall- or ceiling-mounted equipment.

- Clean all spotlights and lights on tracks.

- Thoroughly scrub all furniture used in the room, including the wheels.

- Clean metal buckets and other waste receptacles and, if possible, put them through the washer/sterilizer.

- Clean scrub sinks.

- Machine scrub the entire floor in each room. If a machine is not available, use a large floor brush.

- Suction up the disinfectant germicide solution that is used on the floor, using a wet vacuum. If mops are used, make sure a clean mop head is used for each room.

NOTE: The use of mops in the operating room is the LEAST DESIRABLE method of cleaning.

MANAGEMENT OF INFECTIOUS WASTE

LEARNING OBJECTIVE: *Identify medical waste sorting, packaging, handling, and disposal procedures.*

Concern about potentially adverse effects of infectious waste on public health and the environment has gained widespread media attention. While scientific evidence shows that infectious waste is no greater threat to the environment or public health than residential solid waste, medical facilities are perceived to be a source of pollution. It is, therefore, imperative that a medical facility establish an effective plan for dealing with infectious waste. This plan should include the segregation, packing and handling, storage, transportation, treatment, and disposal of such debris. The management plan should establish recordkeeping systems and personnel training programs, and should incorporate the minimally acceptable management standards for Navy MTFs and DTFs (as contained in BUMEDINST 6280.1, *Management of Infectious Waste*).

INFECTIOUS WASTE

Infectious waste is liquid or solid waste containing pathogens in sufficient numbers and of sufficient virulence to cause infectious disease in susceptible hosts exposed to the waste. Several examples are:

- sharps (needles, scalpel blades),

- microbiology waste (cultures, stocks containing microbes),

- pathological waste (human tissue, body parts),

- liquid waste (blood, cerebrospinal fluid), and

- medical waste from isolation rooms.

TREATMENT AND DISPOSAL METHODS FOR INFECTIOUS WASTE

Several steps should be used in the treatment and disposal of infectious waste. These steps include the identification of waste; segregation, sorting, packaging,

Table 2–2.—Treatment and Disposal Methods for Infectious Waste

Types of Infectious Waste	Methods of Treatment	Methods of Disposal
Microbiological	Steam sterilization [1] Chemical disinfection [2] Incineration [3]	Sanitary landfill
Pathological [5]	Incineration [3 & 4] Cremation	Sanitary landfill Burial [6]
Bulk blood and other potentially infectious liquids	Gelatinization [6]	Sanitary sewer [7] Sanitary landfill [8]
Sharps in sharps containers	Steam sterilization Incineration	Sanitary landfill Sanitary landfill

[1] For effective sterilization, the temperature must be maintained at 121° C (250° F) for at least 90 minutes, at 15 pounds per square inch of gauge pressure. *Bacillus stearothermophilus* spore strips must be used weekly to test the sterilization process.

[2] Chemical disinfection is most appropriate for liquids.

[3] Ash remaining after incineration may go directly to the sanitary landfill, unless state or local regulations require testing the ash for characteristics of hazardous waste.

[4] Disposal of placentas by grinding with subsequent discharge to a sanitary sewer is acceptable unless prohibited by county or local laws/regulations.

[5] Burial or cremation is acceptable.

[6] Must be further treated by steam sterilization or incineration.

[7] Discharge to a sanitary sewer is acceptable unless prohibited by county or local laws/regulations.

[8] Must be treated by steam sterilization or incineration before landfill disposal.

handling, transporting, and treating of waste; and, finally, disposal of the waste. The treatment and disposal methods shown in table 2–2 are the minimally acceptable standards.

SUMMARY

This chapter has introduced you to many basic patient-care procedures and philosophies, such as patient rights and responsibilities, professional conduct, reporting and assessment procedures, patient education, and patient safety precautions. Additionally, you have learned about inpatient care and the various types of patients you will encounter as a Hospital Corpsman. Finally, you have been introduced to standard rules of hygiene, aseptic techniques, and the management of medical waste. Having a good grasp of these areas of patient care will give you a good base from which you can grow as a Hospital Corpsman.

CHAPTER 3

FIRST AID EQUIPMENT, SUPPLIES, RESCUE, AND TRANSPORTATION

This chapter will discuss first aid equipment and supplies, and the rescue and transportation of the injured patient. As a Hospital Corpsman, you will be expected to recognize the uses and application procedures for dressings and bandages, and to be able to identify the protective equipment needed in specific emergencies, along with where and when to use it.

In this chapter, you will learn the phases of a rescue operation and the stages of extrication. You will also learn the precautionary steps that must be taken in special rescue situations. You will learn to recognize the different patient-moving devices and lifting techniques. Additionally, this chapter will familiarize you with the various forms of emergency transportation, and you will learn to identify essential basic life support supplies on Navy ambulances. Finally, this chapter will give you the preparatory, en route, and turnover procedures for patients being transported to medical treatment facilities.

FIRST AID EQUIPMENT AND SUPPLIES

LEARNING OBJECTIVE: *Identify initial equipment and supply needs.*

In a first aid situation, the Corpsman must always be ready to improvise. In many field emergency situations, standard medical supplies and equipment may not be immediately available, or they may run out. When medical supplies and equipment are available, they will probably be found in an ambulance or in the field medical Unit One Bag.

Navy ambulances are stocked in accordance with BUMEDINST 6700.42, *Ambulance Support.* Table 3-1 lists equipment currently required for EMT-Basic level ambulances. Table 3-2 lists the contents of an emergency bag that a Hospital Corpsman might find in an ambulance.

When assigned to Marine Corps Units, Hospital Corpsmen carry their medical equipment and supplies in a special bag. It is referred to as a "Unit One Bag."

The Unit One Bag is made of nylon, weighs about 9 pounds, has an adjustable carrying strap, and contains four strong compartments. The contents of the Unit One Bag are listed below in table 3-3.

Unique operational requirements or command decisions may modify the make-up of these lists. As a Corpsman, it is up to you to be familiar with the emergency medical equipment at the command, since a call may come at a moment's notice and you may have to use these items to help save or sustain a life.

DRESSINGS AND BANDAGES

LEARNING OBJECTIVE: *Recognize the uses and application procedures for dressings and bandages.*

There are many different types of dressings and bandages. You should be familiar with the various standard dressings and bandages, their respective functions, and their proper application in first-aid and emergency situations.

DEFINITION OF A DRESSING

A dressing is a sterile pad or compress (usually made of gauze or cotton wrapped in gauze) used to cover wounds to control bleeding and/or prevent further contamination. Dressings should be large enough to cover the entire area of the wound and to extend at least 1" in every direction beyond the edges. If the dressing is not large enough, the edges of the wound are almost certain to become contaminated. Figure 3-1 shows several commonly used styles of dressings.

Any part of a dressing that is to come in direct contact with a wound should be absolutely sterile (that is, free from microorganisms). The dressings that you will find in first aid kits have been sterilized. However, if you touch them with your fingers, your clothes, or any other unsterile object, they are no longer sterile. If you drag a dressing across the victim's skin or allow it

Table 3-1.—Essential Equipment for Ambulance ETM-Basic Level

ESSENTIAL EQUIPMENT FOR AMBULANCES EMT-BASIC LEVEL		
General Category of Equipment	**Detailed Breakdown**	**Comments**
Patient transfer litter	• Collapsible-wheeled litter	
Ventilation and airway equipment	• Portable suction apparatus • Portable fixed oxygen equipment • Oxygen administration equipment • Bag-valve mask • Airways • Respirator (optional)	• Wide-bore tubing, rigid pharyngeal curved suction cup • Variable flow regulator, humidifier (on fixed equipment) • Adequate length tubing, masks (adult, child, and infant sizes; transparent, non-rebreathing, venture and valveless nasal prongs) • Hand-operated, self-reexpanding bag (adult and infant sizes, ≥0.85), accumulator (Fi02, 0.9), clear mask (adult, child, and infant sizes), valve (clear, easily cleanable, operable in cold weather) • Nasopharyngeal, oropharyngeal (adult, child, and infant sizes) • Volume-cycled valve, on-off operation, 100% oxygen, 40-50 psi pressure
Immobilization devices (splints)	• Traction (adult and pediatric sizes) • Extremity immobilization devices • • Backboards (long, short, and clamshell)	• Lower extremity, limb-support slings, padded ankle hitch, padded pelvic support, traction strap • Joint above and joint below fracture, rigid support, appropriate material (cardboard, metal, pneumatic, wood, plastic, etc.) • Joint above and point below fracture site. Chin strap (should not use for head immobilization), hand holds for moving patient, short (extrication: head-to-pelvis length), long (transport: head-to-feet length)
Bandages	• Burn sheets • Triangle bandages • Dressings • Roller bandages — Soft — Elastic • Vaseline gauze • Adhesive tape	• Two clean (not sterile) • Eight, three safety pins each • Sterile, large and small • — Sterile, 4" or larger — Nonsterile, 4" or larger • Sterile, 3" × 8" or larger • 2" or larger
Pneumatic Antishock Garment (MAST)	• Compartmentalized (legs and abdomen separate), control valves (closed/open), inflation pump, lower leg to lower rib cage (does not include chest)	
Obstetrical equipment	• Sterile obstetrical kit • Aluminum foil roll	• Towels, 4" × 4" dressing, umbilical tape type, bulb syringe, clamps for cords, sterile gloves, blanket • Enough to cover a newborn
Miscellaneous	• Sphygmomanometer • Stethoscope • Heavy bandage scissors for cutting clothing, belts, boots, etc. • Mouth gags (commercial or tongue blades covered with gauze) • C-collar • Flashlight	
Radio communication	• Two-way communication (EMT to physician) • Portable cellular telephone (optional)	• Radio UHF (ultra-high frequency) or VHF (very-high frequency)

Table 3-2.—Ambulance Emergency Bag Contents

AMBULANCE EMERGENCY BAG CONTENTS		
Regular drip IV tubing	Ambu bag	Syrup of Ipecac
Mini drip IV tubing	Trach adaptor	Ace® wrap
IV extension tubing	Suction tubing	Klings®
19-gauge butterflies	Straight & Y-connector	Arm slings
18-gauge Medicut®	Toomey syringe	Safety pins
16-gauge Medicut®	10cc syringe	Tongue blades
Tourniquet	20-gauge needles	Tape
Adult oxygen mask	Alcohol swabs	Stethoscope
Nasal cannula	Examination gloves	4 x 4's
Oxygen tubing	Sodium Chloride ampules	Lubricant
Airways (various sizes)	Ammonia ampules	Grease pencil

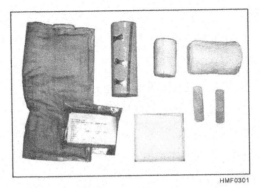
HMF0301

Figure 3–1.—Commonly used styles of dressings.

Table 3–3.—Unit One Bag Contents

UNIT ONE BAG CONTENTS	
One roll wire fabric, 5" x 36"	One tourniquet
Two bottles of aspirin, 324 mg, 100s	One pair scissors, bandage
Three packages of morphine inj., 1/4 g, 5s	Six packages of plastic strip bandages, 6s
One bottle tetracaine hydrochloride ophthalmic sol.	Three bottles povidone-iodine solution, 1/2 fl oz
One airway, plastic, adult/child	One thermometer, oral
Two packages atropine inj., 12s	One card of safety pins, medium, 12s
Two muslin triangular bandages	Two books field medical cards
Two medium battle dressings, 7 1/4" x 8"	One surgical instrument set, minor surgery
Eight small battle dressings 4" x 7"	One pencil, black lead, mechanical
One roll adhesive tape, 3 in x 5 yds	Two packages gauze, rolled, 3 in x 5 yds

to slip after it is in place, the dressing is no longer sterile.

Should an emergency arise when a sterile dressing is not available, the cleanest cloth at hand may be used—a freshly laundered handkerchief, towel, or shirt, for instance. Unfold these materials carefully so that you do not touch the part that goes next to the skin. Always be ready to improvise when necessary, but never put materials directly in contact with wounds if those materials are likely to stick to the wound, leave lint, or be difficult to remove.

DEFINITION OF A BANDAGE

Standard bandages are made of gauze or muslin and are used over a sterile dressing to secure the dressing in place, to close off its edge from dirt and germs, and to create pressure on the wound and control bleeding. A bandage can also support an injured part or secure a splint. The most common types of bandages are the roller and triangular bandages.

Roller Bandage

The roller bandage, shown in figure 3–2, consists of a long strip of material (usually gauze, muslin, or elastic) that is wound into a cylindrical shape. Roller bandages come in various widths and lengths. Most of the roller bandages in the first aid kits have been sterilized, so pieces may be cut off and used as compresses in direct contact with wounds. If you use a piece of roller bandage in this manner, you must be careful not to touch it with your hands or with any other unsterile object.

GENERAL APPLICATION.—In applying a roller bandage, hold the roll in the right hand so that the loose end is on the bottom; the outside surface of the loose or initial end is next applied to and held on the body part by the left hand. The roll is then passed around the body part by the right hand, which controls the tension and application of the bandage. Two or three of the initial turns of a roller bandage should overlie each other to properly secure the bandage (see figure 3–3).

In applying the turns of the bandage, it is often necessary to transfer the roll from one hand to the

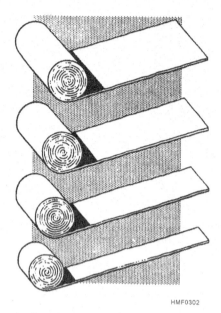

HMF0302

Figure 3-2.—Roller bandages.

other. Bandages should be applied evenly, firmly, but not too tightly. Excessive pressure may cause interference with the circulation and may lead to disastrous consequences. In bandaging an extremity, it is advisable to leave the fingers or toes exposed so the circulation of these parts may be readily observed. It is likewise safer to apply a large number of turns of a bandage, rather than to depend upon a few turns applied too firmly to secure a compress.

In applying a wet bandage, or one that may become wet, you must allow for shrinkage. The turns of a bandage should completely cover the skin, as any uncovered areas of skin may become pinched between the turns, with resulting discomfort. In bandaging any extremity, it is advisable to include the whole member (arm or leg, excepting the fingers or toes) so that uniform pressure may be maintained throughout. It is also desirable in bandaging a limb that the part is placed in the position it will occupy when the dressing is finally completed, as variations in the flexion and extension of the part will cause changes in the pressure of certain parts of the bandage.

The initial turns of a bandage on an extremity (including spica bandages of the hip and shoulder) should be applied securely, and, when possible, around the part of the limb that has the smallest circumference. Thus, in bandaging the arm or hand, the initial turns are usually applied around the wrist, and in bandaging the leg or foot, the initial turns are applied immediately above the ankle.

The final turns of a completed bandage are usually secured in the same manner as the initial turns, by employing two or more overlying circular turns. As both edges of the final circular turns are exposed, they should be folded under to present a neat, cufflike appearance. The terminal end of the completed bandage is turned under and secured to the final turns by either a safety pin or adhesive tape. When these are not available, the end of the bandage may be split lengthwise for several inches, and the two resulting tails may be secured around the part by tying.

ROLLER BANDAGE FOR ELBOW.—A spica or figure-eight type of bandage is used around the elbow joint to retain a compress in the elbow region and to allow a certain amount of movement. Flex the elbow slightly (if you can do so without causing further pain or injury), or anchor a 2- or 3-inch bandage above the elbow and encircle the forearm below the elbow with a circular turn. Continue the bandage upward across the hollow of the elbow to the starting point. Make another circular turn around the upper arm, carry it downward, repeating the figure-eight procedure, and gradually ascend the arm. Overlap each previous turn about two-thirds of the width of the bandage. Secure the bandage with two circular turns above the elbow, and tie. To secure a dressing on the tip of the elbow, reverse the procedure and cross the bandage in the back (fig. 3-4).

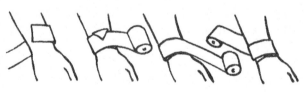

HMF0303

Figure 3-3.—Applying a roller bandage.

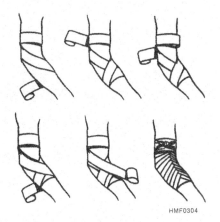

Figure 3-4.—Roller bandage for the elbow.

ROLLER BANDAGE FOR HAND AND WRIST.

—For the hand and wrist, a figure-eight bandage is ideal. Anchor the dressing, whether it is on the hand or wrist, with several turns of a 2- or 3-inch bandage. If on the hand, anchor the dressing with several turns and continue the bandage diagonally upward and around the wrist and back over the palm. Make as many turns as necessary to secure the compress properly (fig. 3-5).

ROLLER BANDAGE FOR ANKLE AND FOOT.

—The figure-eight bandage is also used for dressings of the ankle, as well as for supporting a sprain. While keeping the foot at a right angle, start a 3-inch bandage around the instep for several turns to anchor it. Carry the bandage upward over the instep and around behind the ankle, forward, and again across the instep and down under the arch, thus completing one figure-eight. Continue the figure-eight turns, overlapping one-third to one-half the width of the bandage and with an occasional turn around the ankle, until the compress is secured or until adequate support is obtained (fig. 3-6).

ROLLER BANDAGE FOR HEEL.

—The heel is one of the most difficult parts of the body to bandage. Place the free end of the bandage on the outer part of the ankle and bring the bandage under the foot and up. Then carry the bandage over the instep, around the heel, and back over the instep to the starting point. Overlap the lower border of the first loop around the heel and repeat the turn, overlapping the upper border of the loop around the heel. Continue this procedure until the desired number of turns is obtained, and secure with several turns around the lower leg (fig. 3-7).

ROLLER BANDAGE FOR ARM AND LEG.

—The spiral reverse bandage must be used to cover wounds of the forearms and lower extremities;

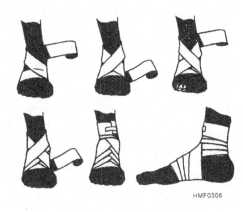

Figure 3-6.—Roller bandage for the ankle and foot.

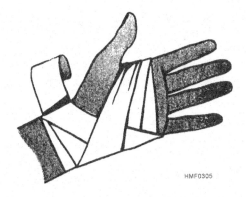

Figure 3-5.—Roller bandage for the hand and wrist.

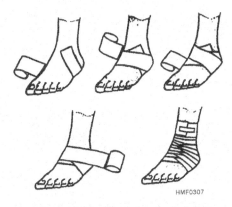

Figure 3-7.—Roller bandage for the heel.

only such bandages can keep the dressing flat and even. Make two or three circular turns around the lower and smaller part of the limb to anchor the bandage and start upward, going around making the reverse laps on each turning, overlapping about one-third to one-half the width of the previous turn. Continue as long as each turn lies flat. Continue the spiral and secure the end when completed (fig. 3–8).

FOUR-TAILED BANDAGE.—A piece of roller bandage may be used to make a four-tailed bandage. The four-tailed bandage is good for bandaging any protruding part of the body because the center portion of the bandage forms a smoothly fitting pocket when the tails are crossed over. This type of bandage is created by splitting the cloth from each end, leaving as large a center area as necessary. Figure 3–9A shows a bandage of this kind. The four-tailed bandage is often used to hold a compress on the chin, as shown in figure 3–9B, or on the nose, as shown in figure 3–9C.

BARTON BANDAGE.—The Barton bandage is frequently used for fractures of the lower jaw and to retain compresses to the chin. As in the progressive steps illustrated in figure 3–10, the initial end of the roller bandage is applied to the head, just behind the right mastoid process. The bandage is then carried under the bony prominence at the back of the head, upward and forward back of the left ear, obliquely across the top of the head. Next bring the bandage downward in front of the right ear. Pass the bandage obliquely across the top of the head, crossing the first turn in the midline of the head, and then backward and downward to the point of origin behind the right mastoid. Now carry the bandage around the back of the

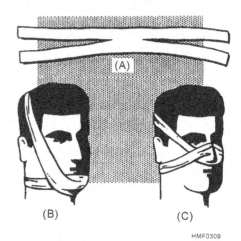

HMF0309

Figure 3–9.—Four-tailed bandages: A. Four-tailed bandage; B. Four-tailed bandage applied to chin; C. Four-tailed bandage applied to nose.

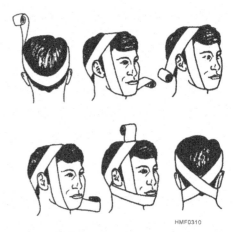

HMF0310

Figure 3–10.—Barton bandage.

head under the left ear, around the front of the chin, and under the right ear to the point of origin. This procedure is repeated several times, each turn exactly overlaying the preceding turn. Secure the bandage with a pin or strip of adhesive tape at the crossing on top of the head.

Triangular Bandage

Triangular bandages are usually made of muslin. They are made by cutting a 36- to 40-inch square of a piece of cloth and then cutting the square diagonally, thus making two triangular bandages (in sterile packs on the Navy's medical stock list). A smaller bandage

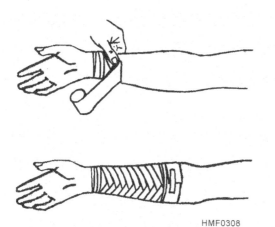

HMF0308

Figure 3–8.—Roller bandage for the arm or leg.

may be made by folding a large handkerchief diagonally. The longest side of the triangular bandage is called the base; the corner directly opposite the middle of the base is called the point; and the other two corners are called ends (fig. 3–11).

The triangular bandage is useful because it can be folded in a variety of ways to fit almost any part of the body. Padding may be added to areas that may become uncomfortable.

TRIANGULAR BANDAGE FOR HEAD.— This bandage is used to retain compresses on the forehead or scalp. Fold back the base about 2 inches to make a hem. Place the middle of the base on the forehead, just above the eyebrows, with the hem on the outside. Let the point fall over the head and down over the back of the head. Bring the ends of the triangle around the back of the head above the ears, cross them over the point, carry them around the forehead, and tie

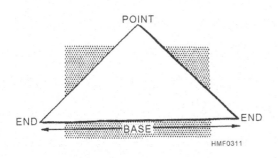

Figure 3–11.—Triangular bandage.

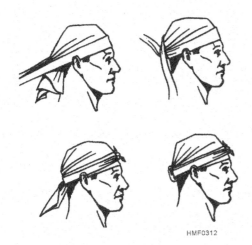

Figure 3–12.—Triangular bandage for the head.

in a SQUARE KNOT. Hold the compress firmly with one hand, and, with the other, gently pull down the point until the compress is snug; then bring the point up and tuck it over and in the bandage where it crosses the back part of the head. Figure 3–12 shows the proper application of a triangular bandage for the head.

TRIANGULAR BANDAGE FOR SHOULDER.— Cut or tear the point, perpendicular to the base, about 10 inches. Tie the two points loosely around the patient's neck, allowing the base to drape down over the compress on the injured side. Fold the base to the desired width, grasp the end, and fold or roll the sides toward the shoulder to store the excess bandage. Wrap the ends snugly around the upper arm, and tie on the outside surface of the arm. Figure 3–13 shows the proper application of a triangular bandage for the shoulder.

TRIANGULAR BANDAGE FOR CHEST.— Cut or tear the point, perpendicular to the base, about 10 inches. Tie the two points loosely around the patient's neck, allowing the bandage to drape down over the chest. Fold the bandage to the desired width, carry the ends around to the back, and secure by tying. Figure 3–14 shows the proper application of a triangular bandage for the chest.

TRIANGULAR BANDAGE FOR HIP OR BUTTOCK.—Cut or tear the point, perpendicular to the base, about 10 inches. Tie the two points around the thigh on the injured side. Lift the base up to the waistline, fold to the desired width, grasp the ends, fold or roll the sides to store the excess bandage, carry the ends around the waist, and tie on the opposite side of the body. Figure 3–15 shows the proper application of a triangular bandage for the hip or buttock.

TRIANGULAR BANDAGE FOR SIDE OF CHEST.—Cut or tear the point, perpendicular to the base, about 10 inches. Place the bandage, points up, under the arm on the injured side. Tie the two points on top of the shoulder. Fold the base to the desired width, carry the ends around the chest, and tie on the opposite side. Figure 3–16 shows the proper application of a triangular bandage for the side of the chest.

TRIANGULAR BANDAGE FOR FOOT OR HAND.—This bandage is used to retain large compresses and dressings on the foot or the hand. **For the foot:** After the compresses are applied, place the foot in the center of a triangular bandage and carry the point over the ends of the toes and over the upper side of the foot to the ankle. Fold in excess bandage at the side of the foot, cross the ends, and tie in a square knot

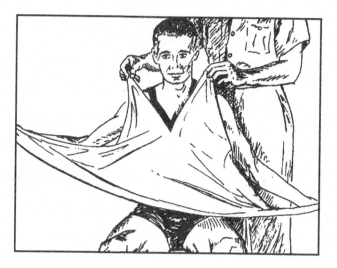

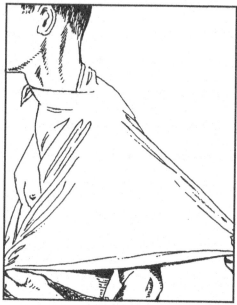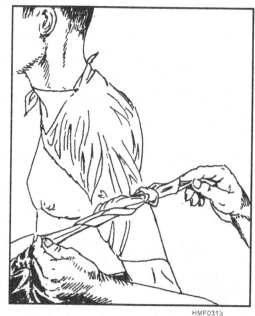

HMF0313

Figure 3–13.—Triangular bandage for the shoulder.

in front. **For the hand:** After the dressings are applied, place the base of the triangle well up in the palmar surface of the wrist. Carry the point over the ends of the fingers and back of the hand well up on the wrist. Fold the excess bandage at the side of the hand, cross the ends around the wrist, and tie a square knot in front. Figure 3–17 shows the proper application of a triangular bandage for either the foot or the hand.

CRAVAT BANDAGE.—A triangular bandage can be folded into a strip for easy application during an emergency. When folded as shown in figure 3–18, the bandage is called a cravat. To make a cravat bandage, bring the point of the triangular bandage to the middle of the base and continue to fold until a 2-inch width is obtained. The cravat may be tied, or it may be secured with safety pins (if the pins are available).

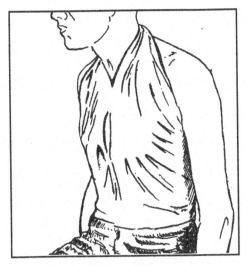

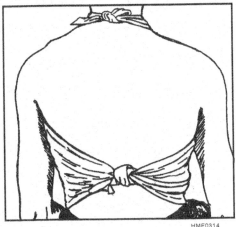

Figure 3–14.—Triangular bandage for the chest.

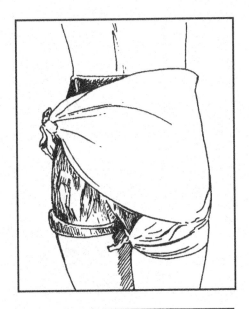

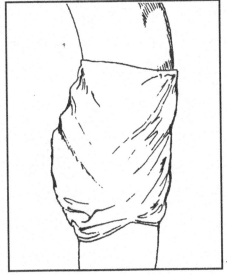

Figure 3–15.—Triangular bandage for the hip or buttock.

When necessary, a cravat can be improvised from common items such as T-shirts, bed linens, trouser legs, scarves, or any other item of pliable and durable material that can be folded, torn, or cut to the desired size.

Cravat Bandage for Head.—This bandage is useful to control bleeding from wounds of the scalp or forehead. After placing a compress over the wound, place the center of the cravat over the compress and carry the ends around to the opposite side; cross them, continue to carry them around to the starting point, and tie in a square knot.

Cravat Bandage for Eye.—After applying a compress to the affected eye, place the center of the cravat over the compress and on a slant so that the lower end is inclined downward. Bring the lower end around under the ear on the opposite side. Cross the ends in back of the head, bring them forward, and tie them over the compress. Figure 3–19 shows the proper application of a cravat bandage for the eye.

3-9

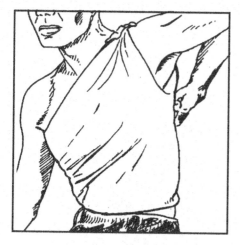

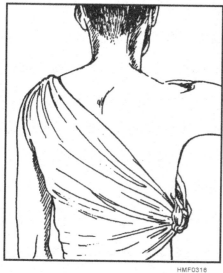

Figure 3–16.—Triangular bandage for the side of the chest.

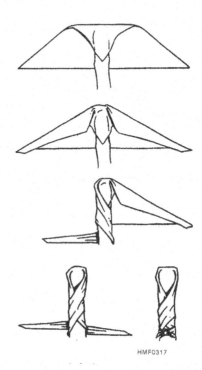

Figure 3–17.—Triangular bandage for the foot or hand.

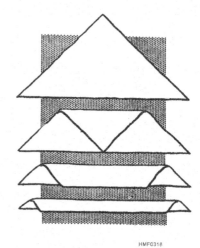

Figure 3–18.—Cravat bandage.

Cravat Bandage for Temple, Cheek, or Ear.—After a compress is applied to the wound, place the center of the cravat over it and hold one end over the top of the head. Carry the other end under the jaw and up the opposite side, over the top of the head, and cross the two ends at right angles over the temple on the injured side. Continue one end around over the forehead and the other around the back of the head to meet over the temple on the uninjured side. Tie the ends in a square knot. (This bandage is also called a Modified Barton.) Figure 3–20 shows the proper

application of a cravat bandage for the temple, cheek, or ear.

Cravat Bandage for Elbow or Knee.—After applying the compress, and if the injury or pain is not too severe, bend the elbow or knee to a right-angle position before applying the bandage. Place the

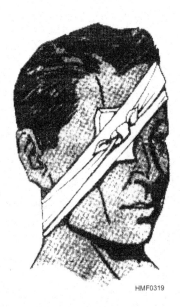

HMF0319

Figure 3–19.—Cravat bandage for the eye.

middle of a rather wide cravat over the point of the elbow or knee, and carry the upper end around the upper part of the elbow or knee, bringing it back to the hollow, and the lower end entirely around the lower part, bringing it back to the hollow. See that the bandage is smooth and fits snugly; then tie in a square knot outside of the hollow. Figure 3–21 shows the proper application of a cravat bandage for the elbow or knee.

Cravat Bandage for Arm or Leg.—The width of the cravat you use will depend upon the extent and area of the injury. For a small area, place a compress over the wound, and center the cravat bandage over the compress. Bring the ends around in back, cross them, and tie over the compress. For a small extremity, it may be necessary to make several turns around to use all the bandage for tying. If the wound covers a larger area, hold one end of the bandage above the compress and wind the other end spirally downward across the compress until it is secure, then upward and around again, and tie a knot where both ends meet. Figure 3–22 shows the proper application of a cravat bandage for the arm, forearm, leg, or thigh.

Cravat Bandage for Axilla (Armpit).—This cravat is used to hold a compress in the axilla. It is similar to the bandage used to control bleeding from the axilla. Place the center of the bandage in the axilla over the compress and carry the ends up over the top of the shoulder and cross them. Continue across the back and chest to the opposite axilla, and tie them. Do not tie

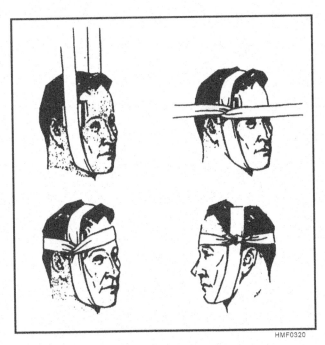

HMF0320

Figure 3–20.—Cravat (Modified Barton) bandage for the temple, cheek, or ear.

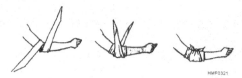

Figure 3–21.—Cravat bandage for the elbow or knee.

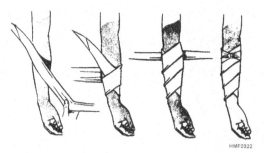

Figure 3–22.—Cravat bandage for the arm, forearm, leg, or thigh.

too tightly or the axillary artery will be compressed, adversely affecting the circulation of the arm. Figure 3–23 shows the proper application of a cravat bandage for the axilla.

BATTLE DRESSING

A battle dressing is a combination compress and bandage in which a sterile gauze pad is fastened to a gauze, muslin, or adhesive bandage (fig. 3–24). Most Navy first aid kits contain both large and small battle dressings of this kind.

RESCUE AND TRANSPORTATION

LEARNING OBJECTIVE: *Identify protective equipment items that are used during patient rescues, and recall how and when each protective equipment item should be used.*

It is a basic principle of first aid that an injured person must be given essential treatment **before** being moved. However, it is impossible to treat an injured person who is in a position of immediate danger. If the victim is drowning, or if his life is endangered by fire, steam, electricity, poisonous or explosive gases, or other hazards, rescue must take place before first aid treatment can be given.

The life of an injured person may well depend upon the manner in which rescue and transportation to a medical treatment facility are accomplished. Rescue operations must be accomplished quickly, but unnecessary haste is both futile and dangerous. After rescue and essential first aid treatment have been given, further transportation must be accomplished in a manner that will not aggravate the injuries. As a Corpsman, it may be your responsibility to direct—and be the primary rescuer in—these operations. The life and safety of the victim and the members of the rescue team may rest on your decisions.

In this section, we will consider the use of common types of protective equipment; rescue procedures; special rescue situations; ways of moving

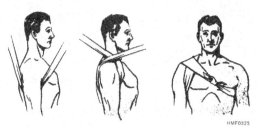

Figure 3–23.—Cravat bandage for the axilla.

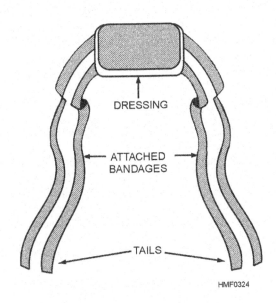

DRESSING

ATTACHED
BANDAGES

TAILS

HMF0324

Figure 3-24.—Battle dressing.

the patient to safety; and procedures for transporting the injured after first aid has been given.

PROTECTIVE EQUIPMENT

The use of appropriate items of protective equipment will increase your ability to effect rescue from life-threatening situations. Protective equipment that is generally available on naval vessels and some shore activities include the oxygen breathing apparatus (OBA); hose (air line) masks; protective (gas) masks; steel-wire lifelines; and devices for detecting oxygen insufficiency, explosive vapors, and some poisonous gases.

Oxygen Breathing Apparatus

An oxygen breathing apparatus (OBA) is provided for emergency use in compartments containing toxic gases. The apparatus is particularly valuable for rescue purposes because it is a self-contained unit. The wearer is not dependent upon outside air or any type of air line within the effective life of the canister.

There are several types of OBAs, but they are all similar in operation. Independence of the outside atmosphere is achieved by having air within the apparatus circulated through a canister. Within the canister, oxygen is continuously generated. The effective life of the canister varies from 20 to 45

minutes, depending on the particular apparatus and the type of work being done. One of the newer types of OBA is designed so that you can change canisters without leaving the toxic atmosphere.

If you are to enter an extremely hazardous area, you should also wear a lifeline. The lifeline should be tended by two persons, one of whom is also wearing a breathing apparatus.

Never allow oil or grease to come in contact with any part of an OBA. Oxygen is violently explosive in the presence of oil or grease. If any part of the apparatus becomes contaminated with oil or grease smudges, clean it before it is stowed. Care should be taken to prevent oil or oily water from entering the canister between the time it is opened and the time of disposal.

Hose (Air Line) Masks

Hose masks are part of the allowance of all ships having repair party lockers. They are smaller than the oxygen breathing outfits and can, therefore, be used by persons who must enter voids or other spaces that have very small access hatches. The hose or air line mask consists essentially of a gas mask facepiece with an adjustable head harness and a length of airhose. Note that the air line mask uses **air** rather than pure oxygen. It must **NEVER** be connected to an oxygen bottle, oxygen cylinder, or other source of oxygen. Even a small amount of oil or grease in the air line could combine rapidly with the oxygen and cause an explosion.

Safety belts are furnished with each air line mask and **MUST BE WORN**. A lifeline must be fastened to the safety belt; and the lifeline should be loosely lashed to the airhose to reduce the possibility of fouling. The airhose and lifeline must be carefully tended at all times so that they do not become fouled or cut. The person wearing the air line mask and the person tending the lines should maintain communication by means of standard divers' signals.

Protective (Gas) Masks

Protective masks provide respiratory protection against chemical, biological, and radiological warfare agents. They do not provide protection from the effects of carbon monoxide, carbon dioxide, and a number of industrial gases. Protection from these gases is discussed in the section, "Rescue from Unventilated Compartments," later in this chapter.

In emergencies, protective masks may be used for passage through a smoke-filled compartment or for entry into such a compartment to perform a job that can be done quickly (such as to close a valve, secure a fan, or de-energize a circuit). However, they provide only limited protection against smoke. The length of time you can remain in a smoke-filled compartment depends on the type of smoke and its concentration.

The most important thing to remember about protective masks is that they do not manufacture or supply oxygen. They merely filter the air as it passes through the canister.

Lifelines

The lifeline is a steel-wire cable, 50 feet long. Each end is equipped with a strong hook that closes with a snap catch. The line is very pliable and will slide freely around obstructions. See figure 3–25.

Lifelines are used as a precautionary measure to aid in the rescue of persons wearing rescue breathing apparatus, hose masks, or similar equipment. Rescue, if necessary should be accomplished by having another person equipped with a breathing apparatus follow the lifeline to the person being rescued, rather than by attempting to drag the person out. Attempts to drag a person from a space may result in fouling the lifeline on some obstruction or in parting the harness, in which case it would still be necessary to send a rescue person into the space.

An important point to remember is that a stricken person must never be hauled by a lifeline attached to the waist. The victim may be dragged along the deck a short distance, but his weight must never be suspended on a line attached to the waist. If not wearing a harness of some kind, pass the line around the chest under the armpits and fasten it in front or in back.

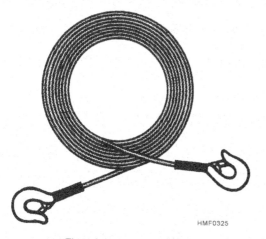

HMF0325

Figure 3–25.—Steel wire lifeline.

When tending a lifeline, you must wear gloves to be able to handle the line properly. Play out the line carefully to keep it from fouling. Try to keep the lifeline in contact with grounded metal; do not allow it to come in contact with any energized electrical equipment.

Detection Devices

The detection devices used to test the atmosphere in closed or poorly ventilated spaces include the **oxygen indicator**, for detecting oxygen deficiency; **combustible-gas indicators**, for determining the concentration of explosive vapors; and **toxic-gas indicators**, such as the **carbon monoxide indicator**, for finding the concentration of certain poisonous gases. The devices are extremely valuable and should be used whenever necessary. However, they **MUST BE USED ONLY AS DIRECTED**. Improper operation of these devices may lead to false assurances of safety or, worse yet, to an increase in the actual danger of the situation. For example, the use of a flame safety lamp in a compartment filled with acetylene or hydrogen could cause a violent explosion.

RESCUE PROCEDURES

LEARNING OBJECTIVE: *Recognize the phases of rescue operations and the stages of extrication.*

If you are faced with the problem of rescuing a person threatened by fire, explosive or poisonous gases, or some other emergency, do not take any action until you have had time to determine the extent of the danger and your ability to cope with it. In a large number of accidents, the rescuer rushes in and becomes the second victim. Do not take unnecessary chances! Do not attempt any rescue that needlessly endangers your own life!

Phases of Rescue Operations

In disasters where there are multiple patients (as in explosions or ship collisions), rescue operations should be performed in phases. These rescue phases apply only to extrication operations.

The first phase is to remove lightly pinned casualties, such as those who can be freed by lifting boxes or removing a small amount of debris.

In the second phase, remove those casualties who are trapped in more difficult circumstances but who can be rescued by use of the equipment at hand and in a minimum amount of time.

In the third phase, remove casualties where extrication is extremely difficult and time consuming. This type of rescue may involve cutting through decks, breaching bulkheads, removing large amounts of debris, or cutting through an expanse of metal. An example would be rescuing a worker from beneath a large, heavy piece of machinery.

The last phase is the removal of dead bodies.

Stages of Extrication

The first stage of extrication within each of the rescue phases outlined above is gaining access to the victim. Much will depend on the location of the accident, damage within the accident site, and the position of the victim. The means of gaining access must also take into account the possibility of causing further injury to the victim since force may be needed. Further injury must be minimized.

The second stage involves giving lifesaving emergency care. If necessary, establish and maintain an open airway, start artificial respiration, and control hemorrhage.

The third stage is disentanglement. The careful removal of debris and other impediments from the victim will prevent further injury to both the victim and the rescuer.

The fourth stage is preparing the victim for removal, with special emphasis on the protection of possible fractures.

The final stage, removing the victim from the trapped area and transporting to an ambulance or sickbay, may be as simple as helping the victim walk out of the area or as difficult as a blanket dragged out of a burning space.

Special Rescue Situations

LEARNING OBJECTIVE: *Recognize the procedural and precautionary steps that must be taken in various rescue situations.*

The procedures you follow in an emergency situation will be determined by the nature of the disaster or emergency you encounter. Some of the more common rescue situations and the appropriate procedures for each are outlined below.

RESCUE FROM FIRE.—If you must go to the aid of a person whose clothing is on fire, try to smother the flames by wrapping the victim in a coat, blanket, or rug. Leave the head **UNCOVERED**. If you have no material with which to smother the fire, roll the victim over—**SLOWLY**—and beat out the flames with your hands. Beat out the flames around the head and shoulders, then work downward toward the feet. If the victim tries to run, throw him down. Remember that the victim **MUST** lie down while you are trying to extinguish the fire. Running will cause the clothing to burn rapidly. Sitting or standing may cause the victim to be killed instantly by inhaling flames or hot air.

CAUTION: Inhaling flames or hot air can kill YOU, too. **Do not get your face directly over the flames. Turn your face away from the flame when you inhale.**

If your own clothing catches fire, roll yourself up in a blanket, coat, or rug. **KEEP YOUR HEAD UNCOVERED.** If material to smother the fire is not available, lie down, roll over slowly, and beat at the flames with your hands.

If you are trying to escape from an upper floor of a burning building, be very cautious about opening doors into hallways or stairways. Always feel a door before you open it. If the door feels hot, do not open it if there is any other possible way out. Remember, also, that opening doors or windows will create a draft and make the fire worse. So do not open any door or window until you are actually ready to get out.

If you are faced with the problem of removing an injured person from an upper story of a burning building, you may be able to improvise a lifeline by tying sheets, blankets, curtains, or other materials together. Use square knots to connect the materials to each other. Secure one end of the line around some heavy object inside the building, and fasten the other end around the casualty under the arms. You can lower the victim to safety and then let yourself down the line. Do not jump from an upper floor of a burning building except as a last resort.

It is often said that the "best" air in a burning room or compartment is near the floor, but this is true only to a limited extent. There is less smoke and flame down low, near the floor, and the air may be cooler. But it is also true that carbon monoxide and other deadly gases are just as likely to be present near the floor as near the ceiling. Therefore, if possible, use an oxygen breathing apparatus or other protective breathing equipment when you go into a burning compartment. If protective equipment is not available, cover your mouth and nose with a wet cloth to reduce the danger of inhaling smoke, flame, or hot air.

CAUTION: A WET CLOTH GIVES YOU NO PROTECTION AGAINST POISONOUS GASES OR LACK OF OXYGEN!

RESCUE FROM STEAM-FILLED SPACES.— It is sometimes possible to rescue a person from a space in which there is a steam leak. Since steam rises, escape upward may not be possible. If the normal exit is blocked by escaping steam, move the casualty to the escape trunk or, if there is none, to the lowest level in the compartment.

RESCUE FROM ELECTRICAL CONTACT.— Rescuing a person who has received an electrical shock is likely to be difficult and dangerous. Extreme caution must be used, or you may be electrocuted yourself.

CAUTION: YOU MUST NOT TOUCH THE VICTIM'S BODY, THE WIRE, OR ANY OTHER OBJECT THAT MAY BE CONDUCTING ELECTRICITY.

First of all, look for the switch. If you find the switch, turn off the current immediately. Do not waste too much time hunting for the switch: Every second is important.

If you cannot find the switch, try to remove the wire from the victim with a **DRY** broom handle, branch, pole, oar, board, or similar **NONCON-DUCTING** object. It may be possible to use a **DRY** rope or **DRY** clothing to pull the wire away from the victim. You can also break the contact by cutting the wire with a **WOODEN-HANDLED** axe, but this is extremely dangerous because the cut ends of the wire are likely to curl and lash back at you before you have time to get out of the way. When you are trying to break an electrical contact, always stand on some nonconducting material such as a **DRY** board, **DRY** newspapers, or **DRY** clothing. See figure 3–26.

RESCUE FROM UNVENTILATED COM-PARTMENTS.—Rescuing a person from a void,

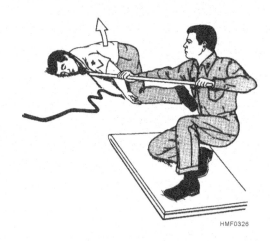

Figure 3–26.—Moving a victim away from an electrical line.

double bottom, gasoline or oil tank, or any closed compartment or unventilated space is generally a very hazardous operation. Aboard naval vessels and at naval shore stations, no person is permitted to enter any such space or compartment until a damage control officer (DCO), or some person designated by the DCO, has indicated that the likelihood of suffocation, poisoning, and fire or explosion has been eliminated as far as possible. The rescue of a person from any closed space should therefore be performed under the supervision of the DCO or in accordance with the DCO's instructions. In general, it is necessary to observe the following precautions when attempting to rescue a person from any closed or poorly ventilated space:

- If possible, test the air for oxygen deficiency, poisonous gases, and explosive vapors.

- Wear a hose (air line) mask or oxygen breathing apparatus. The air line mask is preferred for use in spaces that may contain high concentrations of oil or gasoline vapors. Do not depend upon a protective mask or a wet cloth held over your face to protect you from oxygen deficiency or poisonous gases.

- Before going into a compartment that may contain explosive vapors, be sure that people are stationed nearby with fire-extinguishing equipment.

- When going into any space that may be deficient in oxygen or contain poisonous or explosive vapors, be sure to maintain communication with someone outside. Wear a lifeline, and be sure that it is tended by a competent person.

- Do not use, wear, or carry any object or material that might cause a spark. Matches, cigarette lighters, flashlights, candles or other open flames, and ordinary electrical lights must **NEVER** be taken into a compartment that may contain explosive vapors. The kind of portable light used by cleaning parties in boilers, fuel tanks, and similar places may be taken into a suspect compartment. This is a steam-tight, glove-type light whose exposed metal parts are either made of nonsparking alloy or protected in some way so they will not strike a spark.

An electrical apparatus or tool that might spark must never be taken into a compartment until a DCO has indicated that it is safe to do so. When electrical equipment is used (e.g., an electric blower might be used to vent a compartment of explosive vapors), it must be explosion proof and properly grounded.

If you go into a space that may contain explosive vapors, do not wear clothing that has any exposed spark-producing metal. For example, do not wear boots or shoes that have exposed nailheads or rivets, and do not wear coveralls or other garments that might scrape against metal and cause a spark.

A particular caution must be made concerning the use of the steel-wire lifeline in compartments that may contain explosive vapors. If you use the line, be sure that it is carefully tended and properly grounded at all times. When other considerations permit, you should use a rope line instead of the steel-wire lifeline when entering compartments that may contain explosive vapors.

RESCUE FROM THE WATER.—You should never attempt to swim to the rescue of a drowning person unless you have been trained in lifesaving methods—and then only if there is no better way of reaching the victim. A drowning person may panic and fight against you so violently that you will be unable either to carry out the rescue or to save yourself. Even if you are not a trained lifesaver, however, you can help a drowning person by holding out a pole, oar, branch, or stick for the victim to catch hold of, or by throwing a lifeline or some buoyant object that will support the victim in the water.

Various methods are used aboard ship to pick up survivors from the water. The methods used in any particular instance will depend upon weather conditions, the type of equipment available aboard the rescue vessel, the number of people available for rescue operations, the physical condition of the people requiring rescue, and other factors. In many cases it has been found that the best way to rescue a person from the water is to send out a properly trained and properly equipped swimmer with a lifeline.

It is frequently difficult to get survivors up to the deck of the rescuing vessel, even after they have been brought alongside the vessel. Cargo nets are often used, but many survivors are unable to climb them without assistance. Persons equipped with lifelines (and, if necessary, dressed in anti-exposure suits) can be sent over the side to help survivors up the nets. If survivors are covered with oil, it may take the combined efforts of four or five people to get one survivor up the net.

A seriously injured person should never, except in an extreme emergency, be hauled out of the water by means of a rope or lifeline. Special methods must be devised to provide proper support, both to keep the victim in a horizontal position and to provide protection from any kind of jerking, bending, or twisting motion. The Stokes stretcher (described later in this chapter) can often be used to rescue an injured survivor. People on the deck of the ship can then bring the stretcher up by means of handlines. Life preservers, balsa wood, unicellular material, or other flotation gear can be used, if necessary, to keep the stretcher afloat.

MOVING THE VICTIM TO SAFETY

LEARNING OBJECTIVE: *Recognize the different patient-moving devices and lifting techniques that can be used in patient rescues.*

In an emergency, there are many ways to move a victim to safety, ranging from one-person carries to stretchers and spineboards. The victim's condition and the immediacy of danger will dictate the appropriate method. Remember, however, to give all necessary first aid **BEFORE** moving the victim.

Stretchers

The military uses a number of standard stretchers. The following discussion will familiarize you with the most common types. When using a stretcher, you should consider a few general rules:

- Use standard stretchers when available, but be ready to improvise safe alternatives.

- When possible, bring the stretcher to the casualty.

- Always fasten the victim securely to the stretcher.

- Always move the victim **FEET FIRST** so the rear bearer can watch for signs of breathing difficulty.

STOKES STRETCHER.—The Navy service litter most commonly used for transporting sick or injured persons is called the Stokes stretcher. As shown in figure 3–27, the Stokes stretcher is essentially a wire basket supported by iron rods. Even if the stretcher is tipped or turned, the casualty can be held securely in place, making the Stokes adaptable to a variety of uses. This stretcher is particularly valuable for transferring injured persons to and from boats. As mentioned before, it can also be used with flotation devices to rescue injured survivors from the water. It is also used for direct ship-to-ship transfer of injured persons. Fifteen-foot handling lines are attached to each end for shipboard use in moving the victim.

The Stokes stretcher should be padded with three blankets: two of them should be placed lengthwise (so that one will be under each of the casualty's legs), and the third should be folded in half and placed in the upper part of the stretcher to protect the head and shoulders. The casualty should be lowered gently into the stretcher and made as comfortable as possible. The feet must be fastened to the end of the stretcher so that the casualty will not slide down. Another blanket (or more, if necessary) should be used to cover the casualty. The casualty must be fastened to the stretcher by means of straps that go over the chest, hips, and knees. Note that the straps go **OVER** the blanket or other covering, thus holding it in place.

ARMY LITTER.—The Army litter, shown in figure 3–28, is a collapsible stretcher made of canvas and supported by wooden or aluminum poles. It is very useful for transporting battle casualties in the field. However, it is sometimes difficult to fasten the casualty onto the Army litter, and for this reason its use is somewhat limited aboard ship. The litter legs keep the patient off the ground. The legs fit into the restraining tracks of a jeep or field ambulance to hold the litter in place during transport.

MILLER (FULL BODY) BOARD.—The Miller Board (fig 3-29) is constructed of an outer plastic shell with an injected foam core of polyurethane foam. It is impervious to chemicals and the elements and can be used in virtually every confined-space rescue and vertical extrication. The Miller Board provides for full body immobilization through a harness system, including a hood and two-point contact for the head (forehead and chin) to stabilize the head and cervical spine. The board's narrow design allows passage through hatches and crowded passageways. It fits

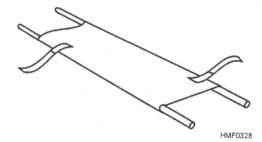

HMF0328

Figure 3–28.—Opening an Army litter.

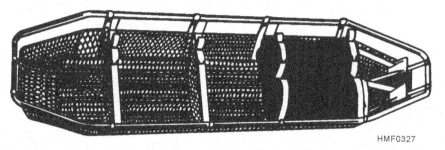

HMF0327

Figure 3–27.—Stokes stretcher.

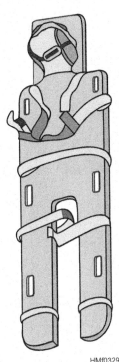

HMf0329

Figure 3–29.—Miller (full body) Board.

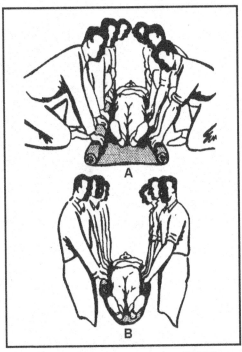

HMF0330

Figure 3–30.—Blanket used as an improvised stretcher.

within a Stokes (basket) stretcher and will float a 250-pound person.

IMPROVISED STRETCHERS.—Standard stretchers should be used whenever possible to transport a seriously injured person. If none are available, it may be necessary for you to improvise. Shutters, doors, boards, and even ladders may be used as stretchers. All stretchers of this kind must be very well padded and great care must be taken to see that the casualty is fastened securely in place.

Sometimes a blanket may be used as a stretcher, as shown in figure 3–30. The casualty is placed in the middle of the blanket in the supine position. Three or four people kneel on each side and roll the edges of the blanket toward the casualty, as shown in figure 3–30A. When the rolled edges are tight and large enough to grasp securely, the casualty should be lifted and carried as shown in figure 3–30B.

Stretchers may also be improvised by using two long poles (about 7 feet long) and strong cloth (such as a rug, a blanket, a sheet, a mattress cover, two or three gunny sacks, or two coats). Figure 3–31 shows an improvised stretcher made from two poles and a blanket.

CAUTION: Many improvised stretchers do not give sufficient support in cases where there are fractures or extensive wounds of the body. They should be used only when the casualty is able to stand some sagging, bending, or twisting without serious consequences. An example of this type of improvised stretcher would be one made of 40 to 50 feet of rope or 1-1/2-inch firehose (fig. 3–32).

Spineboards

Spineboards are essential equipment in the immobilization of suspected or real fractures of the spinal column. Made of fiberglass or exterior plywood, they come in two sizes, short (18" × 32") and long (18" × 72"), and are provided with handholds and straps. Spineboards also have a runner on the bottom to allow clearance to lift (fig. 3–33).

A short spineboard is primarily used in extrication of sitting victims, especially in automobile wrecks (where it would be difficult to maneuver the victim out of position without doing additional damage to the spine). The long board makes a firm litter, protecting the back and neck, and providing a good surface for

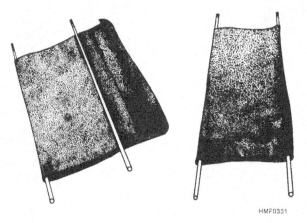

Figure 3–31.—Improvised stretcher using blankets and poles.

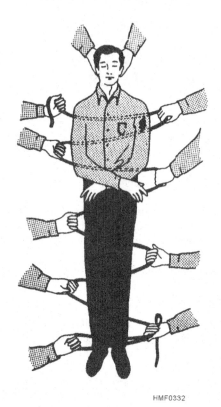

Figure 3–32.—Improvised stretcher using rope or firehose.

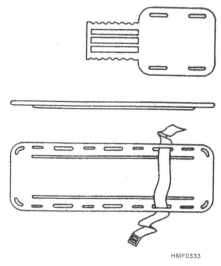

Figure 3–33.—Spineboards.

CPR and a good sliding surface for difficult extractions.

The short and long boards are often used together. For example, at an automobile accident site, the Corpsman's first task is to assess the whole situation and to plan the rescue. If bystanders must be used, it is essential that they be briefed in thorough detail on what you want them to do. After all accessible bleeding has been controlled and the fractures splinted, the short spineboard should be moved into position behind the victim. A neck collar should be applied in all cases and will aid in the immobilization of the head and neck. The head should then be secured to the board with a headband or a 6-inch self-adhering roller bandage. The victim's body should then be secured to the board by use of the supplied straps around the chest and thighs. The victim may then be lifted out. If, however, the victim is too large, or further immobilization of the lower extremities is necessary, the long spineboard may be slid at a right angle behind the short spineboard, and the victim maneuvered onto his side and secured to the longboard.

The possible uses of the spineboard in an emergency situation are limited only by the imagination of the rescuers.

Emergency Rescue Lines

As previously mentioned, the steel-wire lifeline can often be used to haul a person to safety. An emergency rescue line can also be made from any strong fiber line. Both should be used only in extreme emergencies, when an injured person must be moved and no other means is available. Figure 3–34 shows an emergency rescue line that could be used to hoist a person from a void or small compartment. Notice that a running bowline is passed around the body, just below the hips, and a half hitch is placed just under the arms. Notice also that a guideline is tied to the casualty's ankles to prevent banging against bulkheads and hatchways.

Rescue Drag and Carry Techniques

There will be times when you, as a Corpsman, will be required to evacuate a sick or injured person from an

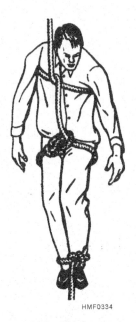

HMF0334

Figure 3–34.—Hoisting a person.

emergency scene to a location of safety. Casualties carried by manual means must be carefully and correctly handled, otherwise their injuries may become more serious or possibly fatal. Situation permitting, evacuation or transport of a casualty should be organized and unhurried. Each movement should be performed as deliberately and gently as possible.

Manual carries are tiring for the bearer(s) and involve the risk of increasing the severity of the casualty's injury. In some instances, however, they are essential to save the casualty's life. Although manual carries are accomplished by one or two bearers, the two-man carries are used whenever possible. They provide more comfort to the casualty, are less likely to aggravate his injuries, and are also less tiring for the bearers, thus enabling them to carry him farther. The distance a casualty can be carried depends on many factors, such as

- strength and endurance of the bearer(s),

- weight of the casualty,

- nature of the casualty's injury, and

- obstacles encountered during transport.

You should choose the evacuation technique that will be the least harmful, both to you and the victim. When necessary and appropriate, use a one-rescuer technique (several of which are described in the following section). Two-rescuer techniques and the circumstances under which those techniques are appropriate are also listed below.

ONE-RESCUER TECHNIQUES.—If a victim can stand or walk, assist him to a safe place. If there are no indications of injury to the spine or an extremity but the casualty is not ambulatory, he can be carried by means of any of the following:

- **Fireman's Carry**: One of the easiest ways to carry an unconscious person is by means of the fireman's carry. Figure 3–35 shows the steps of this procedure.

- **Pack-strap Carry**: With the pack-strap carry, shown in figure 3–36, it is possible to carry a heavy person for some distance. Use the following procedure:

1. Place the casualty in a supine position.

2. Lie down on your side along the casualty's uninjured or less injured side. Your shoulder should be next to the casualty's armpit.

3. Pull the casualty's far leg over your own, holding it there if necessary.

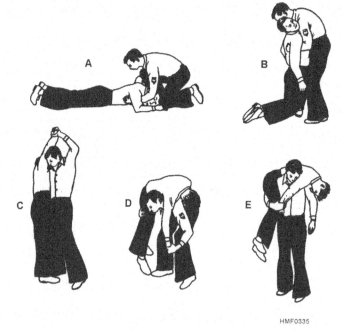

Figure 3–35.—Fireman's carry.

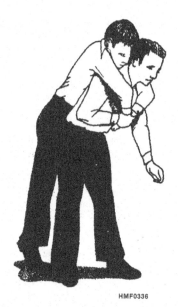

Figure 3–36.—Pack-strap carry.

4. Grasp the casualty's far arm at the wrist and bring it over your upper shoulder as you roll and pull the casualty onto your back.

5. Raise up your knees, holding your free arm for balance and support. Hold both the casualty's wrists close against your chest with your other hand.

6. Lean forward as you rise to your feet, and keep both of your shoulders under the casualty's armpits.

Do not attempt to carry a seriously injured person by means of the pack-strap carry, especially if the arms, spine, neck, or ribs are fractured.

• **Arm Carry**: The technique for a one-person arm carry is shown in figure 3–37. However, you should never try to carry a person who is seriously injured with this method. Unless considerably smaller than you are, you will not be able to carry the casualty very far using this technique.

• **Blanket Drag**: The blanket drag, shown in figure 3–38, can be used to move a person who, due to the severity of the injury, should not be lifted or carried by one person alone. Place the casualty in the supine position on a blanket and pull the blanket along the floor or deck. Always pull the casualty head first, with the head and shoulders slightly raised so that the head will not bump against the deck.

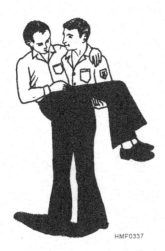

Figure 3-37.—One-person arm carry.

A variant of the blanket drag is the **clothes drag**, where the rescuer drags the victim by the clothing on the victim's upper body.

• **Tied-hands Crawl**: The tied-hands crawl, shown in figure 3-39, may be used to drag an unconscious person for a short distance. It is particularly useful when you must crawl underneath a low structure, but it is the least desirable because the victim's head is not supported.

To be carried by this method, the casualty must be in the supine position. Cross the wrists and tie them together. Kneel astride the casualty and lift the arms over your head so that the wrists are at the back of your neck. When you crawl forward, raise your shoulders high enough so that the casualty's head will not bump against the deck.

TWO-RESCUER TECHNIQUES.—If the casualty is ambulatory, you and your partner should assist him to safety. However, if the victim has either a spinal injury or a fractured extremity, there are a number of two-rescuer techniques that can be used to move him to safety.

• Chair Carry: The chair carry can often be used to move a sick or injured person away from a position of danger. The casualty is seated on a chair, as shown in figure 3-40, and the chair is carried by two rescuers. This is a particularly good method to use when you must carry a person up or down stairs or through narrow, winding passageways. **This carry must NEVER be used to move a person who has an injured neck, back, or pelvis.**

• **Arm Carry**: The two-person arm carry, shown in figures 3-41 and 3-42, can be used in some cases to move an injured person. However, **this carry should not be used to carry a person who has serious wounds or broken bones.**

Another two-person carry that can be used in emergencies is shown in figure 3-43. Two rescuers position themselves beside the casualty, on the same side, one at the level of the chest and the other at the thighs. The rescuers interlock adjacent arms as shown, while they support the victim at the shoulders and knees. In unison, they lift the victim and roll his front toward theirs. **This carry must not be used to move seriously injured persons.**

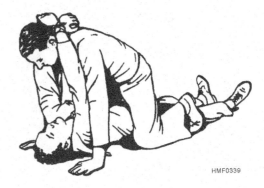

Figure 3-39.—Tied-hands crawl.

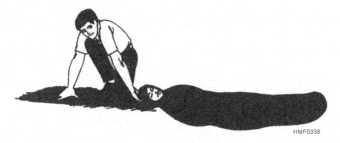

Figure 3-38.—Blanket drag.

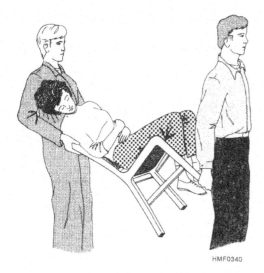

Figure 3–40.—Chair carry.

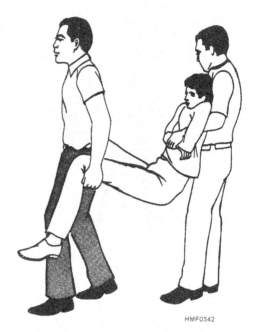

Figure 3–42.—Two-person arm carry (alternate).

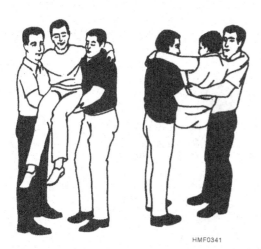

Figure 3–41.—Two-person arm carry.

TRANSPORTATION OF THE INJURED

LEARNING OBJECTIVE: *Recognize the different forms of emergency transportation, and identify essential BLS equipment and supplies on Navy ambulances.*

Thus far we have dealt with emergency methods used to move an injured person out of danger and into a position where first aid can be administered. As we have seen, these emergency rescue procedures often involve substantial risk to the casualty and should be used only when clearly necessary.

Once you have rescued the casualty from the immediate danger, **SLOW DOWN!** Casualties should not be moved before the type and extent of injuries are evaluated and the required emergency medical treatment is given. (The exception to this occurs, of course, when the situation dictates immediate movement for safety purposes. For example, it may be necessary to remove a casualty from a burning vehicle. The situation dictates that the urgency of casualty movement outweighs the need to administer emergency medical treatment.)

From this point on, handle and transport the casualty with every regard for the injuries that have been sustained. In the excitement and confusion that almost always accompany an accident, you are likely to feel rushed, wanting to do everything rapidly. To a certain extent, this is a reasonable feeling. Speed is essential in treating many injuries and in getting the casualty to a medical treatment facility. However, it is not reasonable to let yourself feel so hurried that you

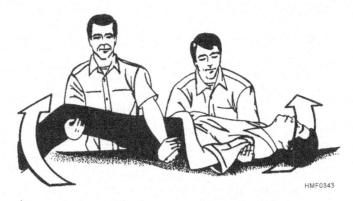

Figure 3–43.—Two-person arm carry (alternate).

become careless and transport the victim in a way that will aggravate the injuries.

Emergency Vehicles

In most peacetime emergency situations, some form of ambulance will be available to transport the victim to a medical treatment facility. Navy ambulances vary in size and shape from the old "gray ghost" to modern van and modular units. Although there are many differences in design and storage capacity, most Navy ambulances are equipped to meet the same basic emergency requirements. They contain equipment and supplies for emergency airway care, artificial ventilation, suction, oxygenation, hemorrhage control, fracture immobilization, shock control, blood pressure monitoring, and poisoning. They will also contain litters, spineboards, and other supplies and equipment as mandated in BUMEDINST 6700.42. (Table 3–1, at the beginning of this chapter, lists the currently required equipment for EMT-Basic level ambulances, and table 3–2 lists the contents of an emergency bag that a Hospital Corpsman might find in that ambulance.)

Deployed units at sea and in the field and certain commands near air stations will also have access to helicopter MEDEVAC support. Helicopters are ideal for use in isolated areas but are of limited practical use at night, in adverse weather, under certain tactical conditions, or in developed areas where building and power lines interfere. In addition to taking these factors into consideration, the Corpsman must decide if the victim's condition is serious enough to justify a call for a helicopter.

Some injuries require very smooth transportation or are affected by pressure changes that occur in flight. The final decision will be made by the unit commander, who is responsible for requesting the helicopter support.

Preparing the Patient for Transport

LEARNING OBJECTIVE: *Recall preparatory, en route, and turnover procedures for patients being transported to medical treatment facilities.*

Once emergency medical care has been completed on-scene, the patient must be transferred to the medical treatment facility. A process known as **packaging** provides the means of properly positioning, covering, and securing the patient to avoid any unnecessary aggravation to the patient's condition. (Covering helps maintain the patient's body temperature, prevents exposure to the elements, and provides privacy.) Do not "package" a badly traumatized patient; it is more important to transport the critical or unstable patient to the medical treatment facility quickly. The most important aspect of each rescue or transfer is to complete it as safely and efficiently as possible.

Care of Patient en Route

The emergency care a Corpsman can offer patients en route is limited only by the availability of supplies, the level of external noise and vibrations, and the degree and ingenuity the Corpsman possesses.

Care at the Medical Treatment Facility

Do not turn the victim over to anyone without giving a complete account of the situation, especially if a tourniquet was used or medications administered. If possible, while en route, write down the circumstances of the accident, the treatment given, and keep a log of vital signs. After turning the patient over to the medical treatment facility, ensure that depleted ambulance supplies are replaced so that the vehicle is in every way ready to handle another emergency.

SUMMARY

This chapter covered first aid equipment and supplies, and rescue and transportation of the injured patient. You should now be able to recognize the various types of dressings and bandages, as well as how and when to apply them. You should be familiar with protective equipment, rescue operations, the stages of extrication, and the precautionary steps that must be taken in special rescue situations. Additionally, you should be acquainted with the different patient-moving devices and lifting techniques. Further, you should be able to identify essential basic life support equipment and supplies on Navy ambulances, and you should be able to recognize different forms of emergency transportation. Finally, you should now be able to recall preparatory, en route, and turnover procedures for patients being transported to medical treatment facilities.

CHAPTER 4

EMERGENCY MEDICAL CARE PROCEDURES

For a Navy Corpsman, the terms "first aid" and "emergency medical procedures" relate to the professional care of the sick and injured before in-depth medical attention can be obtained. Appropriate care procedures may range from providing an encouraging word to performing a dramatic struggle to draw a person back from the brink of death. Always remember, however, that first aid measures are temporary expedients to save life, to prevent further injury, and to preserve resistance and vitality. These measures are not meant to replace proper medical diagnosis and treatment procedures. Hospital Corpsmen will be able to provide the competent care that makes the difference between life or death, temporary or permanent injury, and rapid recovery or long-term disability if they

- understand the relationship between first aid and proper medical diagnosis and treatment,

- know the limits of the professional care Corpsmen can offer, and

- keep abreast of new emergency medical equipment.

GENERAL FIRST AID RULES

LEARNING OBJECTIVE: *Recall general first aid rules.*

There are a few general first aid rules that you should follow in any emergency:

1. Take a moment to get organized. On your way to an accident scene, use a few seconds to remember the basic rules of first aid. Remain calm as you take charge of the situation, and act quickly but efficiently. Decide as soon as possible what has to be done and which one of the patient's injuries needs attention first.

2. Unless contraindicated, make your preliminary examination in the position and place you find the victim. Moving the victim before this check could gravely endanger life, especially if the neck, back, or ribs are broken. Of course, if the situation is such that you or the victim is in danger, you must weigh this threat against the potential damage caused by premature transportation. If you decide to move the victim, do it quickly and gently to a safe location where proper first aid can be administered.

3. In a multivictim situation, limit your preliminary survey to observing for airway patency, breathing, and circulation, the **ABC**s of basic life support. Remember, irreversible brain damage can occur within 4 to 6 minutes if breathing has stopped. Bleeding from a severed artery can lethally drain the body in even less time. If both are present and you are alone, quickly handle the major hemorrhage first, and then work to get oxygen back into the system. Shock may allow the rescuer a few minutes of grace but is no less deadly in the long run.

4. Examine the victim for fractures, especially in the skull, neck, spine, and rib areas. If any are present, prematurely moving the patient can easily lead to increased lung damage, permanent injury, or death. Fractures of the hip bone or extremities, though not as immediately life-threatening, may pierce vital tissue or blood vessels if mishandled.

5. Remove enough clothing to get a clear idea of the extent of the injury. Rip along the seams, if possible, or cut. Removal of clothing in the normal way may aggravate hidden injuries. Respect the victim's modesty as you proceed, and do not allow the victim to become chilled.

6. Keep the victim reassured and comfortable. If possible, do not allow the victim to see the wounds. The victim can endure pain and discomfort better if confident in your abilities. This is important because under normal conditions the Corpsman will not have strong pain relief medications right at hand.

7. Avoid touching open wounds or burns with your fingers or unsterile objects, unless clean compresses and bandages are not available and it is imperative to stop severe bleeding.

8. Unless contraindicated, position the unconscious or semiconscious victim on his side or back, with the head turned to the side to minimize choking or the aspirating of vomitus. Never give an unconscious person any substance by mouth.

9. Always carry a litter patient feet first so that the rear bearer can constantly observe the victim for respiratory or circulatory distress.

TRIAGE

LEARNING OBJECTIVE: *Recognize the protocols for tactical and nontactical triage.*

Triage, a French word meaning "to sort," is the process of quickly assessing patients in a multiple-casualty incident and assigning patient a priority (or classification) for receiving treatment according to the severity of his illness or injuries. In the military, there are two types of triage, tactical and nontactical, and each type uses a different set of prioritizing criteria. The person in charge is responsible for balancing the human lives at stake against the realities of the tactical situation, the level of medical stock on hand, and the realistic capabilities of medical personnel on the scene. Triage is a dynamic process, and a patient's priority is subject to change as the situation progresses.

SORTING FOR TREATMENT (TACTICAL)

The following discussion refers primarily to battalion aid stations (BAS) (where neither helicopter nor rapid land evacuation is readily available) and to shipboard battle-dressing stations.

Immediately upon arrival, sort the casualties into groups in the order listed below.

Class I Patients whose injuries require minor professional treatment that can be done on an outpatient or ambulatory basis. These personnel can be returned to duty in a short period of time.

Class II Patients whose injuries require immediate life-sustaining measures or are of a moderate nature. Initially, they require a minimum amount of time, personnel, and supplies.

Class III Patients for whom definitive treatment can be delayed without jeopardy to life or loss of limb.

Class IV Patients whose wounds or injuries would require extensive treatment beyond the immediate medical capabilities. Treatment of these casualties would be to the detriment of others.

SORTING FOR TREATMENT (NONTACTICAL)

In civilian or nontactical situations, sorting of casualties is not significantly different from combat situations. There are four basic classes (priorities) of injuries, and the order of treatment of each is different.

Priority I Patients with correctable life-threatening illnesses or injuries such as respiratory arrest or obstruction, open chest or abdomen wounds, femur fractures, or critical or complicated burns.

Priority II Patients with serious but non-life-threatening illnesses or injuries such as moderate blood loss, open or multiple fractures (open increases priority), or eye injuries.

Priority III Patients with minor injuries such as soft tissue injuries, simple fractures, or minor to moderate burns.

Priority IV Patients who are dead or fatally injured. Fatal injuries include exposed brain matter, decapitation, and incineration.

As mentioned before, triage is an ongoing process. Depending on the treatment rendered, the amount of time elapsed, and the constitution of the casualty, you may have to reassign priorities. What may appear to be a minor wound on initial evaluation could develop into a case of profound shock. Or a casualty who required initial immediate treatment may be stabilized and downgraded to a delayed status.

SORTING FOR EVACUATION

During the Vietnam war, the techniques for helicopter medical evacuation (MEDEVAC) were so effective that most casualties could be evacuated to a major medical facility within minutes of their injury. This considerably lightened the load of the Hospital Corpsman in the field, since provision for long-term care before the evacuation was not normally required. However, rapid aeromedical response did not relieve the Corpsman of the responsibility for giving the best emergency care within the field limitations to stabilize the victim before the helicopter arrived. Triage was seldom needed since most of the injured could be evacuated quickly.

New developments in warfare, along with changes in the theaters of deployment, indicate that the helicopter evacuation system may no longer be viable in future front-line environments. If this becomes the case, longer ground chains of evacuation to the battalion aid station or division clearing station may be required. This will increase the need for life-stabilizing activities before each step in the chain and in transit. Evacuation triage will normally be used for personnel in the Class II and Class III treatment categories, based on the tactical situation and the nature of the injuries. Class IV casualties may have to receive treatment at the BAS level, and Class I personnel will be treated on the line.

Remember, triage is based on the concept of saving the maximum number of personnel possible. In some cases, a casualty may have the potential to survive, but to ensure that casualty's survival, the treatment necessary may require a great deal of time and supplies. As difficult as it may be, you may have to forsake this patient to preserve the time and supplies necessary to save others who have a greater potential for survival.

PATIENT ASSESSMENT IN THE FIELD

LEARNING OBJECTIVE: *Recognize the assessment sequence for emergency medical care in the field, and identify initial equipment and supply needs.*

Patient assessment is the process of gathering information needed to help determine what is wrong with the patient. Assessments that you conduct in the field (at the emergency scene) or during transport are known as a field assessments.

Field assessments are normally performed in a systematic manner. The formal processes are known as the **primary survey** and the **secondary survey**. The primary survey is a rapid initial assessment to detect and treat life-threatening conditions that require immediate care, followed by a status decision about the patient's stability and priority for immediate transport to a medical facility. The secondary survey is a complete and detailed assessment consisting of a subjective interview and an objective examination, including vital signs and head-to-toe survey. (Both types of surveys will be discussed in more detail later in this chapter.)

BEFORE ARRIVAL AT THE SCENE

Before or during transit to an emergency scene, you may learn about the patient's illness or injury.

Although this information could later prove to be erroneous, you should use this time to consider what equipment you may need and what special procedures you should use immediately upon arrival.

ARRIVAL AT THE SCENE

When you arrive at an emergency scene, you need to start gathering information immediately. First, make sure the scene is safe for yourself, then for the patient or patients. Do not let information you received before your arrival form your complete conclusion concerning the patient's condition. Consider all related factors before you decide what is wrong with the patient and what course of emergency care you will take.

You can quickly gain valuable information as to what may be wrong with the patient. Observe and listen as you proceed to your patient. Do not delay the detection of life-threatening problems. Be alert to clues that are obvious or provided to you by others. Some immediate sources of information may come from the following:

- **The scene**—Is it safe or hazardous? Does the patient have to be moved? Is the weather severe?

- **The patient**—Is the patient conscious, trying to tell you something, or pointing to a part of his body?

- **Bystanders**—Are they trying to tell you something? Listen. They may have witnessed what happened to the patient or have pertinent medical history of the patient (for example, prior heart attacks).

- **Medical identification device**—Is the patient wearing a medical identification device (necklace or bracelet)? Medical identification devices can provide you with crucial information on medical disorders, such as diabetes.

- **Mechanism of injury**—Was there a fire? Did the patient fall or has something fallen on the patient? Is the windshield of vehicle cracked or the steering wheel bent?

- **Deformities or injuries**—Is the patient lying in a strange position? Are there burns, crushed limbs, or other obvious wounds?

- **Signs**—What do you see, hear, or smell? Is there blood around the patient? Has the patient vomited? Is the patient having convulsions? Are the patient's clothes torn?

PRIMARY SURVEY

As stated earlier, the primary survey is a process carried out to detect and treat **life-threatening conditions**. As these conditions are detected, lifesaving measures are taken immediately, and early transport may be initiated. The information acquired before and upon your arrival on the scene provides you with a starting point for the primary survey. The primary survey is a "treat-as-you-go" process. As each major problem is detected, it is treated immediately, before moving on to the next.

During the primary survey, you should be concerned with what are referred to as the **ABCDE**s of emergency care: airway, breathing, circulation, disability, and expose.

A=Airway. An obstructed airway may quickly lead to respiratory arrest and death. Assess responsiveness and, if necessary, open the airway.

B=Breathing. Respiratory arrest will quickly lead to cardiac arrest. Assess breathing, and, if necessary, provide rescue breathing. Look for and treat conditions that may compromise breathing, such as penetrating trauma to the chest.

C=Circulation. If the patient's heart has stopped, blood and oxygen are not being sent to the brain. Irreversible changes will begin to occur in the brain in 4 to 6 minutes; cell death will usually occur within 10 minutes. Assess circulation, and, if necessary, provide cardiopulmonary resuscitation (CPR). Also check for profuse bleeding that can be controlled. Assess and begin treatment for severe shock or the potential for severe shock.

D=Disability. Serious central nervous system injuries can lead to death. Assess the patient's level of consciousness and, if you suspect a head or neck injury, apply a rigid neck collar. Observe the neck before you cover it up. Also do a quick assessment of the patient's ability to move all extremities.

E=Expose. You cannot treat conditions you have not discovered. Remove clothing–especially if the patient is not alert or communicating with you–to see if you missed any life-threatening injuries. Protect the patient's privacy, and keep the patient warm with a blanket if necessary.

As soon as the ABCDE process is completed, you will need to make what is referred to as a **status decision** of the patient's condition. A status decision is a judgment about the severity of the patient's condition and whether the patient requires immediate transport to a medical facility without a secondary survey at the scene. Ideally, the ABCDE steps, status, and transport decision should be completed within 10 minutes of your arrival on the scene.

SECONDARY SURVEY

The object of a secondary survey is to detect medical and injury-related problems that do not pose an immediate threat to survival but that, if left untreated, may do so. Unlike the primary survey, the secondary survey is not a "treat-as-you-go" process. Instead, you should mentally note the injuries and problems as you systematically complete the survey. Then you must formulate priorities and a plan for treatment.

The secondary survey for a patient who presents with medical illness is somewhat different from that of an injured patient. Usually the **trauma assessment** is about 20 percent patient interview and 80 percent physical exam. On the other hand, the **medical assessment** is 80 percent patient interview and 20 percent physical exam. Both the physical exam and patient interview should always be done for all medical and trauma patients.

NOTE: Remember, if the patient's condition deteriorates, it may not be possible to complete the secondary survey before starting to transport the patient.

Subjective Interview

The subjective interview is similar to the interview physicians make before they perform a physical examination. The main objective of the interview is to gather needed information from the patient. Other objectives of the interview are to reduce the patient's fear and promote cooperation. Whenever possible, conduct the subjective interview while you are performing the physical examination.

Relatives and bystanders at the emergency scene may also serve as sources of information, but you should not interrupt interviewing the patient to gather information from a bystander. If the patient is unconscious, you may obtain information from bystanders and medical identification devices while you are conducting the physical examination.

When conducting a patient interview, you should take the following steps:

1. **Place yourself close to the patient.** Position yourself, when practical, so the patient can see your face. If at all possible, position yourself so that the sun or bright lights are not at your back. The glare makes it difficult for the patient to look at you.

2. **Identify yourself and reassure the patient.** Identify yourself and maintain a calm, professional manner. Speak to the patient in your normal voice.

3. **Learn your patient's name.** Once you learn the patient's name, you should use it during the rest of your interview. Children will expect you to use their first name. For military adults, use the appropriate rank. If civilian, use "Mr." or "Ms." unless they introduce themselves by their first name.

4. **Learn your patient's age.** Age information will be needed for reports and communications with the medical facility. You should ask adolescents their age to be certain that you are dealing with a minor. With minors, always ask how you can contact their parent or guardian. Sometimes this question upsets children because it intensifies their fear of being sick or injured. Be prepared to offer comfort and assure children that someone will contact their parents or guardians.

5. **Seek out what is wrong.** During this part of the interview, you are seeking information about the patient's symptoms and what the patient feels or senses (such as pain or nausea). Also, find out what the patient's chief complaint is. Patients may give you several complaints, so ask what is bothering them most. Unless there is a spinal injury that has interrupted nerve pathways, most injured individuals will be able to tell you of painful areas.

6. **Ask the PQRST questions if the patient is experiencing pain or breathing difficulties.**

   P=**Provocation**—What brought this on?

   Q=**Quality**—What does it feel like?

   R=**Region**—Where is it located?

   R=**Referral**—Does it go anywhere (e.g., "into my shoulder")?

   R=**Recurrence**—Has this happened before?

   R=**Relief**—Does anything make it feel better?

   S=**Severity**—How bad is it on a scale of 1 to 10?

   T =**Time**—When did it begin?

7. **Obtain the patient's history by asking the AMPLE questions.**

   A=**Allergies**—Are you allergic to any medication or anything else?

   M=**Medications**—Are you currently taking any medication?

   P=**Previous medical history**—Have you been having any medical problems? Have you been feeling ill? Have you been seen by a physician recently?

   L=**Last meal**—When did you eat or drink last? (Keep in mind, food could cause the symptoms or aggravate a medical problem. Also, if the patient requires surgery, the hospital staff will need to know when the patient has eaten last.)

   E=**Events**—What events led to today's problem (e.g., the patient passed out and then got into a car crash)?

Objective Examination

The objective examination is a comprehensive, hands-on survey of the patient's body. During this examination, check the patient's vital signs and observe the signs and symptoms of injuries or the effects of illness.

When you begin your examination of the patient, you should heed the following rules:

1. Obtain the patient's consent (if the patient is alert).

2. Tell the patient what you are going to do.

3. Always assume trauma patients have a spinal injury, especially unconscious trauma patients, unless you are certain you are dealing with a patient free from spinal injury (e.g., a medical patient with no trauma).

HEAD-TO-TOE SURVEY.—The head-to-toe survey is a systematic approach to performing a physical examination. This survey is designed so nothing important is missed during the examination of the patient. There may be variations in the head-to-toe survey depending on local guidelines. Traditionally, the examination is started with the head. However, most medical authorities now recommend that the neck be examined first in an effort to detect possible spinal injuries and any serious injury to the trachea that may lead to an airway obstruction.

During the head-to-toe survey, you should

- **look** for discolorations, deformities, penetrations, wounds, and any unusual chest movements;

- **feel** for deformities, tenderness, pulsations, abnormal hardness or softness, spasms, and skin temperature;

- **listen** for changes in breathing patterns and unusual breathing sounds; and

- **smell** for any unusual odors coming from the patient's body, breath, or clothing.

The head-to-toe survey may appear to be a long process, but as you practice the procedure you will find that it can be done in just a few minutes. All necessary personal protective equipment, such as exam gloves and eye protection, should be worn during your examination.

Begin the survey by kneeling at the side of the patient's head. Quickly take an overview of the patient's body (i.e., general appearance, demeanor, behavior, skin color and characteristics, etc.), then perform the 26 steps described in the following sections.

Step 1.—**Check the cervical spine for point tenderness and deformity.** To perform this procedure, gently slide your hands, palms up, under both sides of the patient's neck. Move your fingertips toward the cervical midline. Check the back of the neck from the shoulders to the base of the skull. Apply gentle finger pressure. A painful response to this pressure is **point tenderness**.

If there are signs of possible spinal injury, such as midline deformities, point tenderness, or muscle spasms, stop the survey and provide stabilization of the head and neck.

NOTE: If a rigid cervical collar is to be applied, make sure you have examined the posterior, anterior, and sides of the neck before applying the collar.

Step 2.—**Inspect the anterior neck for indications of injury and neck breathing.** This procedure consists of exposing the anterior neck to check for injury and to detect the presence of a surgical opening (stoma) or a metal or plastic tube (tracheostomy). The presence of a stoma or tracheostomy indicates the patient is a neck breather. Also, if you have not already done so in the primary survey, check for a medical identification necklace. A necklace may state the patient has a stoma or tracheostomy.

Look for signs of injury, such as the larynx or trachea deviated from the midline of the neck, bruises, deformities, and penetrating injuries. Also, check for distention of the jugular vein. If the jugular vein is distended, there may be an airway obstruction, a cervical spine injury, damage to the trachea, or a serious chest injury. All of these conditions require immediate medical care.

After the anterior neck is inspected and if a spinal injury is suspected, apply a rigid cervical or extrication collar. If the patient is unconscious, assume the patient has a spinal injury.

Step 3.—**Inspect the scalp for wounds.** Use extreme caution when inspecting the scalp for wounds. Pressure on the scalp from your fingers could drive bone fragments or force dirt into wounds. Also, DO NOT move the patient's head, as this could aggravate possible spinal injuries. To inspect the scalp, start at the top of the head and gently run your gloved fingers through the patient's hair. If you come across an injury site, DO NOT separate strands of the hair. To do this could restart bleeding. When the patient is found lying on his back, check the scalp of the back of the head by placing your fingers behind the patient's head. Then slide your fingers upward toward the top of the head. Check your fingers for blood. If a spinal or neck injury is suspected, delay this procedure until the head and neck have been immobilized. Furthermore, if you suspect a neck injury, DO NOT lift the head off the ground to bandage it.

NOTE: You may find upon inspection that the patient is wearing a hairpiece or wig. Hairpieces and wigs may be held in place by adhesive, tape, or permanent glue, so DO NOT remove them unless you suspect profuse bleeding. Attempting removal may aggravate injury or restart bleeding.

Step 4.—Check the skull and face for deformities and depressions. As you feel the scalp, check for depressions or bony projections. Visually examine facial bones for signs of fractures. Unless there are obvious signs of injury, gently palpate the cheekbones, forehead, and lower jaw.

Step 5.—Examine the patient's eyes. After examining the face and scalp, move back to a side position. Begin your examination of the eyes by looking at the patient's eyelids. Do not open the eyelids of patients with burns, cuts, or other injuries to the eyelid(s). Assume there is damage to the eye and treat accordingly. If eyelids are not injured, have patients open their eyes. To examine the eyes of unconscious patients, gently open their eyes by sliding back the upper eyelids. Keep in mind, pressure applied to the eyelid may cause further injury. When the eye has been opened, visually check the globe of the eye.

Step 6.—Check the pupils for size, equality, and reactivity. Using a penlight or flashlight, examine both eyes. Note pupil size and if both pupils are equal in size. Also, see if the pupils react to the beam of light. Note a slow pupil reaction to the light. Look for eye movement. Both eyes should move as a pair when they observe moving persons or objects.

NOTE: Check unconscious patients for contact lenses. Prompt removal of contact lenses is recommended. If removal of the lens is impractical, close the patient's eyes so the contact lenses stay lubricated.

Table 4-1 lists pupil characteristics you may encounter and the possible causes of abnormalities.

Step 7.—Inspect the inner surfaces of the eyelids. If there is no obvious injury to the eye, gently pull the upper lid up and the lower eyelid down, and check the color of the inner surface. Normally, the inner surfaces of the eyelids are pink. However, with blood loss they become pale; with jaundice, the surface is yellow. The inner surface of the eyelid is an excellent location to detect cyanosis (skin discoloration due to lack of

Table 4-1.—Listing of Pupil Characteristics and the Possible Cause of Abnormality

PUPIL CHARACTERISTICS	POSSIBLE CAUSE OF ABNORMALITY
Dilated and unresponsive	• Cardiac arrest • Influence of drugs (e.g., LSD and amphetamines)
Constricted and unresponsive	• Central Nervous System disease or disorder • Influence of narcotics (e.g., heroin, morphine, or codeine)
Unequal	• Stroke • Head injury
Lackluster (dull) and pupils do not appear to focus	• Shock • Coma

oxygen), especially for patients with dark skin pigmentation. Cyanosis is denoted by a blue color.

Step 8.—Inspect the ears and nose for injury and the presence of blood or clear fluids. Without rotating the patient's head, inspect the ears and nose for cuts, tears, or burns. Use a penlight to look in the ears and nose for blood, clear fluids, or bloody fluids. Blood in the ears and clear fluids (cerebrospinal fluid) in the ears or nose are strong indicators of a skull fracture. Also, check for bruises behind the ears, commonly referred to as **Battle's sign.** Bruises behind the ears are strong indicators of skull fracture and cervical spine injury. Burned or singed nasal hairs indicate possible burns in the airway.

Step 9.—Inspect the mouth. Look inside the mouth for signs of airway obstruction that may not have been observed during the primary survey (e.g., loose or broken teeth, dentures, and blood). When you inspect the mouth, remember not to rotate the patient's head.

Step 10.—Smell for odd breath odors. Place your face close to the patient's mouth and nose and note any unusual odors. A fruity smell indicates diabetic coma or prolonged vomiting and diarrhea; a petroleum odor indicates ingested poisoning; and an alcohol odor indicates possible alcohol intoxication.

Step 11.—Inspect the chest for wounds. Expose the chest. For unconscious and trauma patients, you should completely remove clothing to expose the chest. (Try to provide as much privacy as possible for patients.) Look for obvious chest injuries, such as cuts, bruises, penetrations, objects impaled in the chest, deformities, burns, or rashes. If puncture or bullet wounds are found, check for exit wounds when inspecting the back.

Step 12.—**Examine the chest for possible fracture.** Before you begin examining the chest for fractures, warn the patient that the examination may be painful. Begin your examination by gently feeling the clavicles (collarbones). Next, feel the sternum (breastbone). Then examine the rib cage by placing your hands on both sides of the rib cage and applying gentle pressure. This process is known as **compression**. If the patient has a fracture, compression of the rib cage will cause pain. Finally, slide your hands under the patient's scapulae (shoulder blades) to feel for deformities or tenderness.

Point tenderness, painful reaction to compression, deformity, or grating sounds indicate a fracture. If air is felt (like crunching popcorn) or heard (crackling sounds) under the skin, this indicates that at least one rib is fractured or that there is a pneumothorax (punctured lung). You may also observe air escaping the chest cavity and the wound when the patient has a punctured lung.

Step 13.—**Check for equal expansion of the chest.** Check chest movements and feel for equal expansion by placing your hand on both sides of the chest. Be alert to sections of the chest that seem to be "floating" (flail chest) or moving in a direction opposite to the rest of the chest during respiration.

Step 14.—**Listen for sounds of equal air entry.** Using a stethoscope, listen to both sides of the anterior and lateral chest. The sounds of air entry will usually be clearly present or clearly absent. The absence of air movement indicates an obstruction, injury, or illness to the respiratory system. Bubbling, wheezing, rubbing, or crackling sounds may indicate the patient has a medical problem or a trauma-related injury.

Step 15.—**Inspect the abdomen for wounds.** Look for obvious signs of injury (e.g., abdominal distension, cuts, bruises, penetrations, open wounds with protruding organs (evisceration), or burns) in all four quadrants and sides.

Step 16.—**Palpate the abdomen for tenderness.** Look for attempts by the patient to protect his abdomen (e.g., patient drawing up the legs). Gently palpate the entire abdomen. If the patient complains of pain in an area of the abdomen, palpate that area last. Do not palpate over an obvious injury site or where the patient is having severe pain. While palpating the abdomen, check for any tight (rigid) or swollen (distended) areas. Performing abdominal palpation is important because tender areas do not normally hurt until palpated. Note if pain is localized, general, or diffused.

Step 17.—**Feel the lower back for point tenderness and deformity.** Gently slide your hands under the void created by the curve of the spine. Apply gentle pressure to detect point tenderness or any deformities.

NOTE: This examination of the lower back may be performed later, when the patient's entire back is exposed in preparation to being placed on a backboard or stretcher.

Step 18.—**Examine the pelvis for injuries and possible fractures.** Examine the pelvic area for obvious injuries. Next, gently slide your hand down both sides of the small of the patient's back and apply compression downward and then inward to check the stability of the pelvic girdle. Note any painful responses or deformities. If a grating sound is heard, the injury may involve the hip joint, or the pelvis may be fractured.

Step 19.—Note any obvious injury to the genital region. Look for obvious injuries, such as bleeding wounds, objects impaled in the area, or burns. Also, check for **priapism** in male patients. Priapism is a persistent erection of the penis often brought about by spinal injury or certain medical problems, such as sickle cell crisis.

Step 20.—**Examine the lower extremities.** DO NOT move, lift, or rearrange the patient's lower extremities (legs and feet) before or during the examination as further injury to the patient may occur. Check for signs of injury by inspecting each limb, one at a time, from hip to foot. Rearrange or remove clothing and footwear to observe the entire examination site. Pants should be removed in a manner that does not aggravate injuries. Cutting along the seams to remove pants is the best method. If the injury is not obvious, remove the shoe(s) and palpate any suspected fracture sites for point tenderness. Before palpating the site, warn the patient that this examination may cause pain. Before the patient is moved, all suspected or known fractures should be stabilized (with splints, traction splints, or the like).

Step 21.—Check for a distal pulse and capillary refill. To make sure there are no circulatory problems in the legs or feet, check the distal pulse and capillary refill. The **distal pulse** is a pulse taken at the foot or wrist. It is called distal because the pulse is located at the distal end of the limb. The distal pulse of the foot, also referred to as **pedal pulse**, may be taken at either of two sites: the posterior tibial pulse (located behind the medial ankle) or the dorsalis pedis pulse (located on the anterior surface of the foot, lateral to the large tendon of the great toe).

You should compare the quality of the pulses in each lower limb. Absence of a distal pulse usually indicates that a major artery supplying the limb has been pinched or severed. This condition may be caused by a broken or displaced bone end or a blood clot. An absent or weak distal pulse may also result from splints or bandages being applied too tightly.

Check capillary refill by squeezing a toe (usually, the big toe) with your thumb and forefinger. The skin and nail where pressure is applied should blanch (lighten). When you release the pressure, the color (blood) should return immediately. If it takes more than 2 seconds for the color to return, capillary refill is considered delayed.

NOTE: After splints or bandages are applied, check capillary refill to make sure circulation has not been impaired.

Step 22.—Check for nerve function and possible paralysis of the lower extremities (conscious patient). Check the lower extremities of conscious patients for nerve function or paralysis. First, touch a toe and ask the patient which toe it is. Do this to both feet. If the patient cannot feel your touch or if the sensations in each foot are not the same, assume that nerve damage in the limb or a spinal injury has occurred.

If sensations appear normal and no injuries are present, have the patient wave his feet. Finally, ask the patient to gently press the soles of his feet against your hand. The inability of the patient to perform any of these tasks indicates the possibility of nerve damage. When nerve damage is suspected, assume the patient has a spinal injury.

Step 23.—Examine the upper extremities for injury. Check for signs of injury to the upper extremities (arms and hands) by inspecting each limb, one at a time, from clavicle to fingertips. Rearrange or remove items of clothing to observe the entire examination site. Check for point tenderness, swelling, or bruising. Any of these symptoms may indicate a fracture. Immobilize any limb where a fracture is suspected.

Step 24.—Check for a distal pulse and capillary refill. To make sure the circulation to the upper extremities has not been compromised, confirm distal (radial) pulse. Initial check of radial pulse was performed during the primary survey. Check capillary refill of fingers or palm of hand (see step 21 for procedure). If there is no pulse or if capillary refill is delayed, the patient may be in shock or a major artery supplying the limb has been pinched, severed, or blocked.

Step 25.—Check for nerve function and possible paralysis of the upper extremities (conscious patient). Check the upper extremities of conscious patients for nerve function or paralysis. Have the patient identify the finger you touch, wave his hand, and grasp your hand. Do this to both hands. If the patient cannot feel your touch or the sensations in each hand are not the same, assume nerve damage in the limb or a spinal injury has occurred.

WARNING: Be alert for a rapid onset of difficult breathing or respiratory arrest. These conditions may occur to patients who have sustained a cervical injury.

Step 26.—Inspect the back and buttocks for injury. If there is no indication of injury to the skull, neck, spine, or extremities, and you have no evidence of severe injury to the chest or abdomen, gently roll the conscious patient as a unit toward your knees and inspect the surface of the back for bleeding or obvious injuries. The back surface may be inspected prior to positioning the patient for transport or delayed until the patient is transferred to a spineboard or other immobilization device.

VITAL SIGNS.—Vital signs (which generally are taken after primary, secondary, and head-to-toe surveys have been completed) include taking the patient's pulse, respiration, blood pressure, and temperature. Depending on local protocols, the patient's level of consciousness as well as eye pupil size and reactivity may be recorded with vital signs. Skin characteristics, such as temperature, color, and moistness or dryness, can also be conveniently determined at this time.

Pulse.—When taking a patient's pulse, you should be concerned with two factors: rate and character. For **pulse rate**, you will have to determine the number of beats per minute. Pulse rate is classified as normal, rapid, or slow. A normal pulse rate for adults is between 60 to 80 beats per minute. Any pulse rate above 100 beats per minute is rapid (**tachycardia**), while a rate below 60 beats per minute is slow (**bradycardia**).

NOTE: An athlete may have a normal at-rest pulse rate between 40 and 50 beats per minute. This is a slow pulse rate, but is not an indication of poor health.

Pulse character is the rhythm and force of the pulse. **Pulse rhythm** is evaluated as regular or irregular. When intervals between beats are constant, the pulse is regular, and when intervals are not constant, the pulse is described as irregular. **Pulse force** refers to the pressure of the pulse wave as it expands the artery. Pulse force is determined as full or thready. A full pulse feels as if a strong wave has passed under your fingertips. When the pulse feels weak and thin, the pulse is described as thready.

The pulse rate and character can be determined at a number of points throughout the body. The most common site to determine a patient's pulse is the **radial pulse**. The radial pulse (wrist pulse) is named after the radial artery found in the lateral aspect of the forearm.

Respiration.—Respiration is the act of breathing. A single breath is the complete process of breathing in (**inhalation**) followed by breathing out (**exhalation**). When observing respiration in connection to vital signs, you should be concerned with two factors: rate and character.

Respiration rate is the number of breaths a patient takes in 1 minute. The rate of respiration is classified as normal, rapid, or slow. The normal respiration rate for an adult at rest is 12 to 20 breaths per minute. A rapid respiration rate is more than 28 respirations per minute, and a slow respiration rate is less than 10 breaths per minute. A rapid or slow respiration rate indicates the patient is in need of immediate medical attention and should be transported to a medical treatment facility as soon as possible.

Respiration character includes rhythm, depth, ease of breathing, and sound. **Respiration rhythm** refers to the manner in which a person breathes. Respiration rhythm is classified as regular or irregular. A regular rhythm is when the interval between breaths is constant, and an irregular rhythm is when the interval between breaths varies.

Respiration depth refers to the amount of air moved between each breath. Respiration depth is classified as normal, deep, or shallow.

Ease of breathing can be judged while you are judging depth. Ease of breathing may be judged as labored, difficult, or painful.

Sounds of respiration include **snoring**, **wheezing**, **crowing** (birdlike sounds), and **gurgling** (sounds like breaths are passing through water).

You should count respirations as soon as you have determined the pulse rate. Count the number of breaths taken by the patient during 30 seconds and multiply by 2 to obtain the breaths per minute. While you are counting breaths, note the rhythm, depth, ease of breathing, and sounds of respiration.

Blood Pressure.—The measurement of the pressure blood exerts against the wall of blood vessels is known as blood pressure. The pressure created in the arteries when the heart pumps blood out into circulation (heart beat) is called the **systolic** blood pressure. The pressure remaining in the arteries when the heart is relaxed (between beats) is called the **diastolic** blood pressure. The systolic pressure is always reported first and the diastolic pressure second (e.g., 120 over 80).

Blood pressure varies from one person to another and is measured with a stethoscope and a sphygmomanometer (BP cuff). Low blood pressure (**hypotension**) is considered to exist when the systolic pressure falls below 90 millimeters of mercury (mm Hg) and/or the diastolic falls below 60. "Millimeters of mercury" refers to the units of the BP cuff's gauge. High blood pressure (**hypertension**) exists once the pressure rises above 150/90 mm Hg. Keep in mind that patients may exhibit a temporary rise in blood pressure during emergency situations. More than one reading will be necessary to determine if a high or low reading is only temporary. If a patient's blood pressure drops, the patient may be going into shock. You should report major changes in blood pressure immediately to medical facility personnel.

Temperature.—Body temperatures are determined by the measurement of oral, rectal, axillary (armpit), and aural (ear) temperatures. In emergency situations, taking a traditional body temperature may not be indicated, so a relative skin temperature may be done. A relative skin temperature is a quick assessment of skin temperature and condition. To assess skin temperature and condition, feel the patient's forehead with the back of your hand. In doing this, note if the patient's skin feels normal, warm, hot, cool, or cold. At the same time, see if the skin is dry, moist, or clammy. Also check for "goose pimples," indicating chills.

BASIC LIFE SUPPORT

LEARNING OBJECTIVE: *Recall basic life support techniques for upper airway obstruction, respiratory failure, and cardiac arrest.*

Basic life support is the emergency technique for recognizing and treating upper airway obstruction and failures of the respiratory system and heart. The primary emphasis should be on the **ABC**s of basic life support: maintaining an open **airway** to counter upper airway obstruction; restoring **breathing** to counter respiratory arrest; and restoring **circulation** to counter cardiac arrest.

UPPER AIRWAY OBSTRUCTION

The assurance of breathing takes precedence over all other emergency measures. The reason for this is simple: If a person cannot breathe, he cannot survive.

Many factors may cause a person's airway to become fully or partially obstructed. A very common cause of obstruction with both adults and children is improperly chewed food that becomes lodged in the airway (an event commonly referred to as a "cafe coronary"). Additionally, children have a disturbing tendency to swallow foreign objects while at play. Another cause for upper airway obstruction occurs during unconsciousness, when the tongue may fall back and block the pharynx (fig. 4-1). When the upper airway is obstructed, the heart will normally continue to beat until oxygen deficiency becomes acute. Periodic checks of the carotid artery must be made to ensure that circulation is being maintained.

Partial Airway Obstruction

The signs of partial airway obstruction include unusual breath sounds, cyanosis, or changes in breathing pattern. Conscious patients will usually make clutching motions toward their neck, even when the obstruction does not prevent speech. Encourage conscious patients with apparent partial obstructions

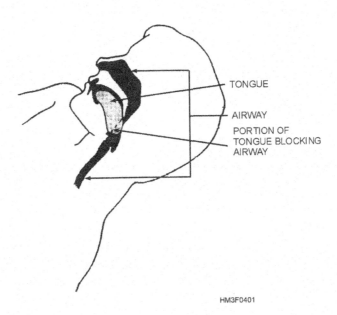

TONGUE

AIRWAY

PORTION OF TONGUE BLOCKING AIRWAY

HM3F0401

Figure 4-1.—Tongue blocking airway.

to cough. If the patient is unable to cough, begin to treat the patient as if this were a complete obstruction. (This also applies to patients who are cyanotic.)

Complete Airway Obstruction

Conscious patients will attempt to speak but will be unable to do so. Nor will they be able to cough. Usually, patients will display the universal distress signal for choking by clutching their neck. The unconscious patient with a complete airway obstruction exhibits none of the usual signs of breathing: rise and fall of the chest and air exchange through the nose and/or mouth. A complete blockage is also indicated if a correctly executed attempt to perform artificial ventilation fails to instill air into the lungs.

Opening the Airway

Many problems of airway obstruction, particularly those caused by the tongue, can be corrected simply by repositioning the head and neck. If repositioning does not alleviate the problem, more aggressive measures must be taken.

POSITIONING THE PATIENT.—When a patient is unresponsive, you must determine if he is breathing. This assessment requires the patient to be positioned properly with the airway opened.

Before repositioning patients, it is imperative that you remember to check them for possible spinal injuries. If there is no time to immobilize these injuries and the airway cannot be opened with the victim in the present position, then great care must be taken when repositioning. The head, neck, and back must be moved as a single unit. To do this, adhere to the following four steps (see figure 4-2).

Step 1—Kneel to the side of the victim in line with the victim's shoulders, but far enough away so that the victim's body will not touch yours when it is rolled toward you. Straighten the victim's legs, gently but quickly. Then move the victim's closer arm along the floor until it reaches straight out past the head.

Step 2—Support the back of the victim's head with one hand while you reach over with the other hand to grasp under the distant armpit.

Step 3—Pull the patient toward you while at the same time keeping the head and neck in a natural straight line with the back. Resting the head on the extended arm will help you in this critical task.

Step 4—Roll the patient onto his back and reposition the extended arm.

Once the patient is supine with the arms alongside the body, you should position yourself at the patient's side. By positioning yourself at the patient's side, you can more easily assess whether the patient is breathing. If the patient is not breathing, you are already positioned to perform artificial respirations (also referred to as rescue breathing) and chest compressions.

Either one of two maneuvers—the head tilt-chin lift maneuver or the jaw-thrust maneuver—may be used to open an obstructed airway. When performing these maneuvers, you may discover foreign material or vomitus in the mouth that needs to be removed. Do not spend very much time to perform this task. Liquids or semiliquids should be wiped out with the index and middle finger covered by a piece of cloth. Solid material should be extracted with a hooked index finger.

HEAD TILT-CHIN LIFT MANEUVER.—The head tilt-chin lift maneuver is the primary method used to open the airway. To perform the head tilt-chin lift maneuver, place one of your hands on the patient's forehead and apply gentle, firm, backward pressure using the palm of your hand. Place the fingers of the other hand under the bony part of the chin. Lift the chin forward and support the jaw, helping to tilt the head back. See figure 4-3. This maneuver will lift the patient's tongue away from the back of the throat and provide an adequate airway.

PRECAUTIONS: When performing the head tilt-chin lift maneuver, do not press too deeply into the soft tissue under the chin. Undue pressure in this location may obstruct the airway. In addition, make sure the mouth is kept open so exhalation and inhalation are not hindered.

JAW-THRUST MANEUVER.—The jaw-thrust maneuver is considered an alternate method for opening the airway. This maneuver is accomplished by kneeling near the top of the victim's head, grasping the angles of the patient's lower jaw, and lifting with both hands, one on each side. This will displace the mandible (jawbone) forward while tilting the head backward. Figure 4-4 illustrates the jaw-thrust maneuver. If the lips close, retract the lower lip with your thumb. If mouth-to-mouth breathing is necessary, close the nostrils by placing your cheek tightly against them.

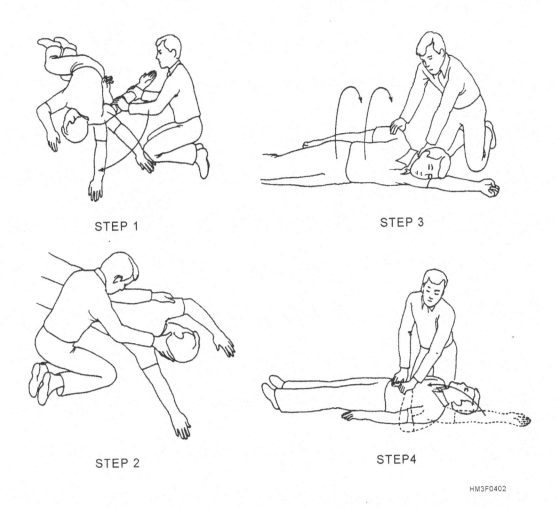

STEP 1

STEP 3

STEP 2

STEP4

HM3F0402

Figure 4-2.—The four steps to reposition the victims of spinal injuries.

NOTE: The jaw-trust technique without head tilt is considered the safest approach to opening the airway of patients with suspected neck injuries because it usually can be done without extending the neck.

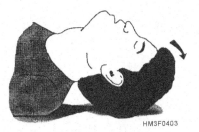

HM3F0403

Figure 4-3.—Head tilt-chin lift maneuver.

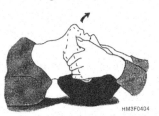

HM3F0404

Figure 4-4.—Jaw-thrust maneuver.

Foreign-Body Airway Obstruction Management

Foreign-body airway obstruction should be considered in any victim—especially a younger victim—who suddenly stops breathing, becomes cyanotic, or loses consciousness for no apparent reason.

The **Heimlich maneuver** (subdiaphragmatic abdominal thrusts) is recommended for relieving foreign-body airway obstruction. By elevating the diaphragm, the Heimlich maneuver can force air from the lungs to create an artificial cough intended to expel a foreign body obstructing the airway. Each individual thrust should be administered with the intent of relieving the obstruction. It may be necessary to repeat the thrust several times to clear the airway. Five thrusts per sequence is recommended.

When you perform this maneuver, you should guard against damage to internal organs, such as rupture or laceration of abdominal or thoracic viscera. To minimize this possibility, your hands should never be placed on the xiphoid process of the sternum or on the lower margins of the rib cage. They should be below this area but above the navel and in the midline.

Regurgitation may occur as a result of abdominal thrusts. Be prepared to position the patient so aspiration does not occur.

HEIMLICH MANEUVER WITH VICTIM STANDING OR SITTING.—To perform the Heimlich maneuver with victim standing or sitting, stand behind the victim, wrap your arms around the victim's waist, and proceed as follows:

Step 1—Make a fist with one hand.

Step 2—Place the thumb side of the fist against the victim's abdomen, in the midline slightly above the navel and well below the tip of the xiphoid process.

Step 3—Grasp the fist with the other hand and press the fist into the victim's abdomen with a quick upward thrust. See figure 4-5.

Step 4—Repeat the thrusts and continue until the object is expelled from the airway or the patient becomes unconscious. Each new thrust should be a separate and distinct movement.

HEIMLICH MANEUVER WITH VICTIM LYING DOWN.—To perform the Heimlich maneuver with victim lying down, proceed as follows:

Step 1—Place the victim in the supine position (face up).

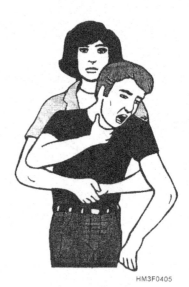

HM3F0405

Figure 4-5.—Administering the Heimlich maneuver to a conscious victim who is standing.

Step 2—Kneel astride the victim's thighs and place heel of one hand against the victim's abdomen, in the midline slightly above the navel and well below the tip of the xiphoid.

Step 3—Place the second hand directly on top of the first.

Step 4—Press into the abdomen with a quick upward thrust. See figure 4-6.

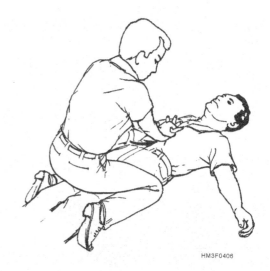

HM3F0406

Figure 4-6.—Administering the Heimlich maneuver to an unconscious victim who is lying down.

If you are in the correct position, you will have a natural midabdominal position and are unlikely to direct the thrust to the right or left. A rescuer too short to reach around the waist of an unconscious victim can use this technique. The rescuer can use their body weight to perform the maneuver.

CHEST THRUSTS WITH VICTIM STANDING OR SITTING.—This technique is used only in the late stages of pregnancy or in the markedly obese victim. To perform chest thrusts with victim standing or sitting, proceed as follows:

Step 1—Stand behind the victim, with your arms directly under the victim's armpits, and encircle the victim's chest.

Step 2—Place the thumb side of your fist on the middle of the victim's sternum (breastbone), taking care to avoid the xiphoid process and the margins of the rib cage.

Step 3—Grab your fist with the other hand and perform backward thrust until the foreign body is expelled or the victim becomes unconscious. See figure 4-7.

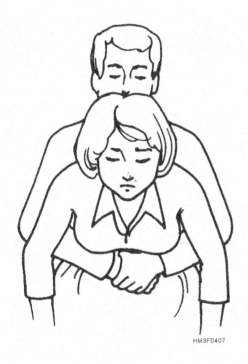

HM3F0407

Figure 4-7.—Administering the chest thrust to a conscious victim who is standing.

CHEST THRUSTS WITH VICTIM LYING DOWN.—Chest thrusts should be used only for victims in the late stages of pregnancy and when the Heimlich maneuver cannot be applied effectively to the unconscious, markedly obese victim. To perform chest thrusts with victim lying down, proceed as follows:

Step 1—Place the victim on his back and kneel close to the victim's side.

Step 2—Place the heel of your hand on the lower portion of the sternum (in the same manner as you would when performing chest compressions).

Step 3—Deliver each thrust firmly and distinctly, with the intent of relieving the obstruction.

MANUAL REMOVAL OF FOREIGN BODY.—A foreign body can be removed by performing a "finger sweep." This procedure, however, **must be performed on unconscious victims only** (though not on seizure victims). To perform a finger sweep, proceed as follows:

Step 1—With the victim's face up, open the victim's mouth by grasping both the tongue and lower jaw between the thumb and fingers and lifting the jaw. This action draws the tongue away from the back of the throat and away from a foreign body that may be lodged there. This step alone may partially relieve the obstruction.

Step 2—Insert the index finger of the other hand down along the inside of the cheek and deeply into the throat to the base of the tongue.

Step 3—Use a hooking action to dislodge the foreign body and maneuver it into the mouth so that it can be removed. See figure 4-8.

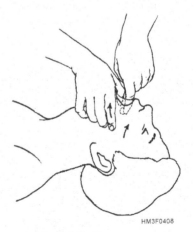

HM3F0408

Figure 4-8.—Finger sweep.

It is sometimes necessary to use the index finger to push a foreign body against the opposite side of the throat to dislodge and remove it. Be careful not to force the object deeper into the airway. If the foreign body comes within reach, grasp and remove it.

BREATHING

The second aspect of basic life support is to restore breathing in cases of respiratory arrest. Failure of the breathing mechanism may be caused by various factors. They include complete airway obstruction, insufficient oxygen in the air, inability of the blood to carry oxygen (e.g., carbon monoxide poisoning), paralysis of the breathing center of the brain, and external compression of the body. Respiratory arrest is usually but not always immediately accompanied by cardiac arrest. Periodic checks of the carotid pulse must be made, and you must be prepared to start cardiopulmonary resuscitation (CPR).

Signs of respiratory arrest are an absence of respiratory effort, a lack of detectable air movement through the nose or mouth, unconsciousness, and a cyanotic discoloration of the lips and nail beds.

Determining Breathlessness

To assess the presence or absence of breathing (fig. 4-9), you should use the following procedures:

Step 1—Place your ear over the patient's mouth and nose, while maintaining an open airway.

Step 2—While observing the patient's chest,

- **look** for the chest to rise and fall,

- **listen** for air escaping during exhalation, and

- **feel** for the flow of air.

Recovery Position

If the patient is unresponsive, has no evidence of trauma, and is obviously breathing adequately, place the patient in the "recovery position." See figure 4-10. In the recovery position, the airway is more likely to remain open, and an unrecognized airway obstruction caused by the tongue is less likely to occur. It is important to continue close observation of the patient who has been placed in the recovery position until he becomes responsive.

To place a patient in the recovery position, roll the patient onto his side so that the head, shoulders, and

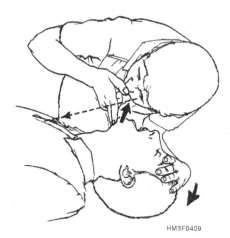

HM3F0409

Figure 4-9.—Determining breathlessness.

torso move simultaneously without twisting. If the patient has sustained trauma or trauma is suspected, the patient should NOT be moved.

Artificial Ventilation

If a patient is in respiratory arrest, artificial ventilations must be started immediately. Any delay could result in brain damage or death. The purpose of artificial ventilation is to provide air exchange until natural breathing is re-established. Artificial ventilation should be given only when natural breathing has been suspended; **it must not be given to a person who is breathing naturally**. Do not assume that a person's breathing has stopped merely because the person is unconscious or has been rescued from water, from poisonous gas, or from contact with an electric wire.

Techniques of artificial ventilation include **mouth-to-mouth, mouth-to-nose, mouth-to-stoma**, and **mouth-to-mask**. These techniques as they apply to adult patients are discussed in the following sections.

MOUTH-TO-MOUTH.—Artificial ventilation with the mouth-to-mouth technique is a quick, effective way to provide oxygen to the patient. The exhaled air contains enough oxygen to supply the patient's needs.

To perform mouth-to-mouth ventilation, the airway must be open. To open the airway, perform the head tilt-chin lift or jaw-thrust maneuver. If there is no spontaneous breathing, start artificial ventilation by pinching the nose closed with your thumb and index

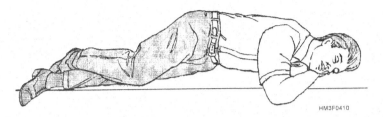

Figure 4-10.—A patient in the recovery position.

finger. Take a deep breath and seat your lips around the patient's mouth (creating an airtight seal), and give two slow ventilations (1 ½ to 2 seconds per breath). See figure 4-11. Allow enough time for the lungs to deflate between ventilations. If the patient still does not respond, continue mouth-to-mouth ventilations at the rate of 10 to 12 ventilations per minute or one breath every 5 seconds. Periodically, check the pupils for reaction to light; constriction is a sign of adequate oxygenation.

NOTE: When performing artificial ventilation and the lungs cannot be inflated adequately, repeat head tilt-chin lift or jaw-thrust maneuver, and again attempt ventilation. If the lungs still do not inflate adequately, assume the airway is obstructed by a foreign object.

MOUTH-TO-NOSE.—Mouth-to-nose ventilation is effective when the patient's mouth cannot be opened (lockjaw), extensive facial or dental injuries occur, or an airtight seal of the mouth cannot be achieved. Figure 4-12 shows an example of this procedure.

To administer this technique, tilt the head back with one hand on the patient's forehead and use the other hand to lift the jaw (as in the head tilt-chin lift maneuver). Close the victim's mouth. Take a deep

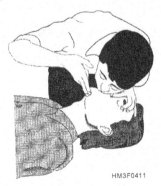

Figure 4-11.—Mouth-to-mouth ventilation.

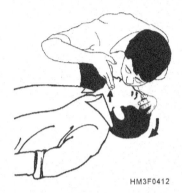

Figure 4-12.—Mouth-to-nose ventilation.

breath, seal your lips around the patient's nose, and give two ventilations. Allow the victim's lungs to deflate passively after each ventilation. If the victim does not respond, then you must fully inflate the lungs at the rate of 10 to 12 ventilations per minute or one breath every 5 seconds until the victim can breathe spontaneously.

MOUTH-TO-STOMA.—A casualty who has had surgery to remove part of the windpipe will breathe through an opening in the front of the neck called a stoma. Cover the casualty's mouth with your hand, take a deep breath, and seal your mouth over the stoma. Breathe slowly, using the procedures for mouth-to-mouth breathing. Do not tilt the head back. (In some situations, a person may breathe through the stoma as well as his nose and mouth. If the casualty's chest does not rise, cover his mouth and nose, and continue breathing through the stoma.)

MOUTH-TO-MASK.—The mouth-to-mask breathing device includes a transparent mask with a one-way valve mouth piece. The one-way valve directs the rescuer's breath into the patient's airway while diverting the patients's exhaled air away from the rescuer. Some devices have an oxygen adaptor that permits the administration of supplemental oxygen.

Mouth-to-mask is a reliable form of ventilation since it allows the rescuer to use two hands to create a seal. Follow the steps below to perform the mouth-to-mask technique.

Step 1—Place the mask around the patient's mouth and nose, using the bridge of the nose as a guide for correct position. Proper positioning of the mask is critical because gaps between the mask and the face will result in air leakage.

Step 2—Seal the mask by placing the heel and thumb of each hand along the border of the mask and compressing firmly to provide a tight seal around the margin of the mask.

Step 3—Place your remaining fingers along the bony margin of the jaw and lift the jaw while performing a head tilt.

Step 4—Give breaths in the same sequence and at the same rate as in mouth-to-mouth resuscitation; observe the chest for expansion.

Gastric Distention

Sometimes during artificial ventilation, air is forced into the stomach instead of into the lungs. The stomach becomes distended (bulges), indicating that the airway is blocked or partially blocked, or that ventilations are too forceful. This problem is more common in children but can occur with adults as well. A slight bulge is of little worry, but a major distention can cause two serious problems. First, it reduces lung volume: the distended stomach forces the diaphragm up. Second, there is a strong possibility of vomiting.

The best way to avoid gastric distention is to position the head and neck properly and/or limit the volume of ventilations delivered.

NOTE: THE AMERICAN RED CROSS (ARC) STATES THAT NO ATTEMPT SHOULD BE MADE TO FORCE AIR FROM THE STOMACH UNLESS SUCTION EQUIP- MENT IS ON HAND FOR IMMEDIATE USE.

If suction equipment is ready and the patient has a marked distention, you can turn the patient on his side facing away from you. With the flat of your hand, apply gentle pressure between the navel and the rib cage. Be prepared to use suction should vomiting occur.

CIRCULATION

Cardiac arrest is the complete stoppage of heart function. If the patient is to live, action must be taken immediately to restore heart function. The symptoms of cardiac arrest include absence of carotid pulse, lack of heartbeat, dilated pupils, and absence of breathing.

A rescuer knowing how to administer cardiopulmonary resuscitation (CPR) greatly increases the chances of a victim's survival. CPR consists of external heart compression and artificial ventilation. External heart compression is performed on the outside of the chest, and the lungs are ventilated by the mouth-to-mouth, mouth-to-nose, mouth-to-stoma, or mouth-to-mask techniques. To be effective, CPR must be started within 4 minutes of the onset of cardiac arrest. The victim should be supine on a firm surface.

CPR should not be attempted by a rescuer who has not been properly trained. If improperly done, CPR can cause serious damage. It must never be practiced on a healthy individual. For training purposes, use a training aid instead. To learn this technique, see your medical education department or an American Heart Association- or American Red Cross-certified Hospital Corpsman, nurse, or physician.

One-Rescuer CPR

The rescuer must not assume that a cardiac arrest has occurred solely because the victim is lying on the floor and appears to be unconscious. First, try to rouse the victim by gently shaking the shoulders and trying to obtain a response (e.g., loudly ask: "Are you OK?"). If there is no response, place the victim supine on a firm surface. **Always assume neck injuries in unconscious patients.** Kneel at a right angle to the victim, and open the airway using the head tilt-chin lift or jaw-thrust methods described previously. Attempt to ventilate. If unsuccessful, reposition the head and again attempt to ventilate. If still unsuccessful, deliver five abdominal thrusts (Heimlich maneuver) or chest thrusts to open the airway. Repeat the thrust sequence until the obstruction is removed.

DETERMINING PULSELESSNESS.—Once the airway has been opened, check for the carotid pulse. The carotid artery is most easily found by locating the larynx at the front of the neck and then sliding two fingers down the side of the neck toward you (fig. 4-13). The carotid pulse is felt in the groove between the larynx and the sternocleidomastoid muscle. If the pulse is present, ventilate as necessary. If the pulse is absent, locate the sternum and begin chest compressions.

PROPER POSITIONING OF HANDS ON STERNUM.—To locate the sternum, use the middle and index fingers of your lower hand to locate the lower margin of the victim's rib cage on the side closest to you (fig. 4-14). Then move your fingers up along the edge of the rib cage to the notch where the ribs meet the sternum in the center of the lower chest. Place your middle finger on the notch and your index finger next to it. Place the heel of your other hand along the midline of the sternum next to your index finger. Remember to keep the heel of your hand off the xiphoid (tip of the sternum). A fracture in this area may damage the liver, causing hemorrhage and death.

CHEST COMPRESSIONS.—Place the heel of one hand directly on the sternum and the heel of the other on top of the first. Interlock your fingers or extend them straight out and **KEEP THEM OFF THE VICTIM'S CHEST!** Effective compression is

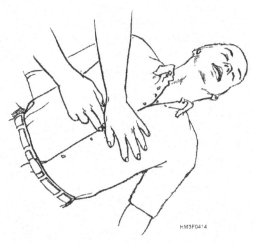

Figure 4-14.—Proper position of hands on the sternum for chest compressions.

accomplished by locking your elbows into position, straightening your arms, and positioning your shoulders directly over hands so that the thrust for each chest compression is straight down on the sternum. See figure 4-15. The sternum should be depressed approximately 1 ½ to 2 inches (for adults). Release chest compression pressure between each compression to allow blood to flow into the chest and heart. When releasing chest compression pressure, remember to keep your hands in place on the chest.

Not only will you feel less fatigue if you use the proper technique, but a more effective compression

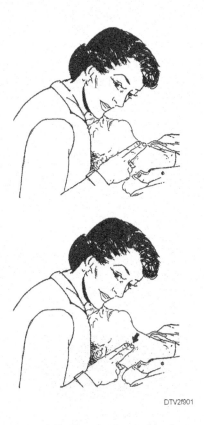

Figure 4-13.—Locating the carotid pulse.

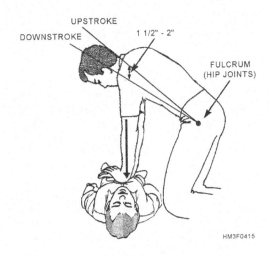

Figure 4-15.—Proper position of the rescuer.

will also result. Ineffective compression occurs when the elbows are not locked, the rescuer is not directly over the sternum, or the hands are improperly placed on the sternum.

PERFORMANCE AND REASSESSMENT OF CPR.—When one rescuer performs CPR, the ratio of compressions to ventilations is 15 to 2, and it is performed at a rate of 80 to 100 compressions per minute. Vocalize: "one and, two and, three and,...." until you reach 15. After 15 compressions, you must give the victim two slow ventilations (1 ½ to 2 seconds). Continue for four full cycles. Quickly check for the carotid pulse and spontaneous breathing. If there are still no signs of recovery, continue CPR with compressions. Reassess the patient every few minutes thereafter.

If a periodic check reveals a return of pulse and respiration, discontinue CPR and place the victim in the recovery position. Continue monitoring the victim and be prepared to restart CPR .

Two-Rescuer CPR

If there are two people trained in CPR on the scene, one should perform chest compressions while the other performs ventilations. The compression rate for two-rescuer CPR is the same as it is for one-rescuer CPR: 80 to 100 compressions per minute. However, the compression-ventilation ratio is 5 to 1, with a pause for ventilation of 1 ½ to 2 seconds consisting primarily of inspiration. Exhalation occurs during chest compressions.

Two-rescuer CPR should be performed with one rescuer positioned at the chest area and the other positioned beside the victim's head. The rescuers should be on opposite sides of the victim to ease position changes when one rescuer gets tired. Changes should be made on cue without interrupting the rhythm.

The victim's condition must be monitored to assess the effectiveness of the rescue effort. The person ventilating the patient assumes the responsibility for monitoring pulse and breathing. To assess the effectiveness of the partner's chest compressions, the rescuer should check the pulse during compressions. To determine if the victim has resumed spontaneous breathing and circulation, chest compressions must be stopped for 5 seconds at the end of the first minute (20 cycles) and every few minutes thereafter.

NOTE: Although it has fallen out to favor with some agencies, two-person CPR remains a viable method of resuscitation.

CPR for Children and Infants

CPR for children (1 to 8 years old) is similar to that for adults. The primary differences are that the heel of only one hand is used to apply chest compressions, and ventilations are increased to a rate of 20 breaths per minute (once every 3 seconds). Chest compressions are performed on the lower half of the sternum (between the nipple line and the notch). The chest should be depressed approximately one-third to one-half (about 1 to 1 ½ inches) the total depth of the chest.

For infants (under 1 year old), CPR is performed with the infant supine on a hard, flat surface. The hard surface may be the rescuer's hand or arm, although using the arm to support the infant during CPR enables the rescuer to transport the infant more easily while continuing CPR. See figure 4-16. Once the infant is positioned on a hard surface, the airway should be opened using the head tilt-chin lift or jaw-thrust maneuver. Both maneuvers, however, must be performed very carefully and gently to prevent hyperextension of the infant's neck. Pulselessness is determined by palpating the brachial artery (fig. 4-17). If the infant has no pulse and is not breathing, CPR must be started immediately.

To perform CPR on an infant, place your mouth over the infant's nose and mouth, creating a seal. Give two slow breaths (1 to 1 ½ seconds per breath) to the infant, pausing after the first breath to take a breath. Pausing to take a breath after the first breath of each pair of breaths maximizes oxygen content and

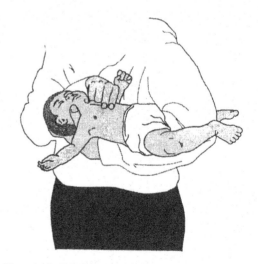

Figure 4-16.—Infant supported on rescuer's arm, and proper placement of fingers for chest compressions.

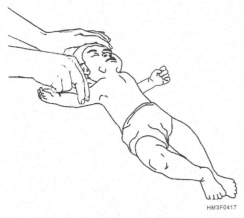

Figure 4-17.—Palpating brachial artery pulse in an infant.

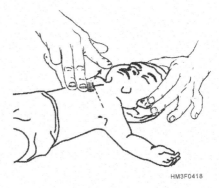

Figure 4-18.—Locating proper finger position to perform chest compressions in infants.

minimizes carbon dioxide concentration in the delivered breaths. Perform chest compressions by using two fingers to depress the middle of the sternum approximately ½ to 1 inch. See figures 4-16 and 4-18 for proper finger positioning for chest compressions.

For both infants and children, the compression rate should be at least 100 compressions per minute. Compressions must be coordinated with ventilations at a 5-to-1 ratio. The victim should be reassessed after 20 cycles of compressions and ventilations (approximately 1 minute) and every few minutes thereafter for any sign of resumption of spontaneous breathing and pulse. If the child or infant resumes effective breathing, place the victim in the recovery position.

SHOCK

> **LEARNING OBJECTIVE:** *Recognize the signs and symptoms of shock, and determine treatment by the type of shock presented.*

Shock is the collapse of the cardiovascular system, characterized by circulatory deficiency and the depression of vital functions. There are several types of shock:

- **Hypovolemic shock**–caused by the loss of blood and other body fluids.

- **Neurogenic shock**–caused by the failure of the nervous system to control the diameter of blood vessels.

- **Cardiogenic shock**–caused by the heart failing to pump blood adequately to all vital parts of the body.

- **Septic shock**–caused by the presence of severe infection.

- **Anaphylactic shock**–caused by a life-threatening reaction of the body to a substance to which a patient is extremely allergic.

Multiple types of shock may be present in varying degrees in the same patient at the same time. The most frequently encountered and most important type for the Hospital Corpsman to understand is **hemorrhagic shock**, a type of hypovolemic shock which will be discussed later in this chapter.

Shock should be expected in all cases of major injury, including gross hemorrhage, abdominal or chest wounds, crash or blast injuries, extensive large-muscle damage (particularly of the extremities), major fractures, traumatic amputations, or head injuries, or in burns involving more than 10 percent of the body surface area.

SYMPTOMS OF SHOCK

The symptoms of shock vary from patient to patient and even within an individual during the course of illness. Evaluation of the whole situation is more important than one particular sign or symptom.

Degrees of Shock

Table 4-2 provides a generalized overview of the degrees of shock and their symptoms correlated to the approximate volume deficit.

Table 4-2.—Correlation of Magnitude of Volume Deficit and Clinical Presentation

Approximate Deficit (ml)	Decrease in Blood Volume %	Degree	Signs
0-500	0-10	None	None
500-1200	10-25	Mild	Slight tachycardia Postural changes in blood pressure Mild peripheral vasoconstriction Increased respirations
1200-1800	25-35	Moderate	Thready pulse 100-120 Systolic blood pressure 90-100 Marked vasoconstriction Labored breathing Diaphoresis (profuse perspiration) Anxiety and restlessness Decreased urine output
1800-2500	35-50	Severe	Thready pulse > 120 Systolic blood pressure < 60 Weakened respirations Increased diaphoresis Changes in levels of consciousness No urine output

Shock Control and Prevention

The essence of shock control and prevention is to recognize the onset of the condition and to start treatment before the symptoms fully develop. The following are general signs and symptoms of the development of shock (see figure 4-19):

- Restlessness and apprehension are early symptoms, often followed by apathy.

- Eyes may be glassy and dull. Pupils may be dilated. (These are also the symptoms of morphine use.)

- Breathing may be rapid or labored, often of the gasping, "air hunger" type. In the advanced stages of shock, breathing becomes shallow and irregular.

- The face and skin may be very pale or ashen gray; in the dark complexioned, the mucous membranes may be pale. The lips are often cyanotic.

- The skin feels cool and is covered with clammy sweat. The skin's coolness is related to a decrease in the peripheral circulation.

- The pulse tends to become rapid, weak, and thready. If the blood pressure is severely lowered, the peripheral pulse may be absent. The pulse rate in hemorrhagic shock may reach 140 or higher. In neurogenic shock, however, the pulse rate is slowed, often below 60.

- The blood pressure is usually lowered in moderately severe shock; the systolic pressure drops below 100, while the pulse rises above 100. The body is compensating for circulatory fluid loss by peripheral vasoconstriction. This process tends to maintain the blood pressure at a nearly normal level despite a moderately severe loss of circulating blood volume. A point comes, however, when decompensation occurs, and a small amount of additional blood loss will produce a sudden, alarming fall in blood pressure.

- There may be nausea, vomiting, and dryness of the mouth, lips, and tongue.

- Surface veins may collapse. Veins normally visible at the front of the elbow, forearms,

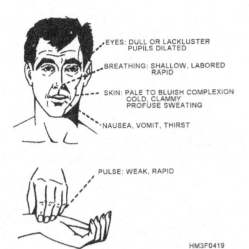

EYES: DULL OR LACKLUSTER
PUPILS DILATED

BREATHING: SHALLOW, LABORED
RAPID

SKIN: PALE TO BLUISH COMPLEXION
COLD, CLAMMY
PROFUSE SWEATING

NAUSEA, VOMIT, THIRST

PULSE: WEAK, RAPID

HM3F0419

Figure 4-19.—Symptoms of shock.

and the back of the hands will be hard to distinguish.

- There are frequent complaints of thirst. Even the severely wounded may complain of thirst rather than pain.

- The kidneys may shut down. Urine formation either ceases or greatly diminishes if the systolic blood pressure falls below 80 for long periods of time.

- The person may faint from inadequate venous blood return to the heart. This may be the result of a temporary gravitational pooling of the blood associated with standing up too quickly.

HYPOVOLEMIC SHOCK

Hypovolemic shock is also known as oligemic or hematogenic shock. The essential feature of all forms of hypovolemic shock is loss of fluid from the circulating blood volume, so that adequate circulation to all parts of the body cannot be maintained.

Hemorrhagic Shock

In cases where there is internal or external hemorrhage due to trauma (hemorrhagic shock), there is a loss of whole blood, including red blood cells. The diminished blood volume causes a markedly lessened cardiac output and reduced peripheral circulation. This results in reduction of oxygen transported to the tissues (hypoxia); reduction of perfusion, the circulation of blood within an organ; and reduction of

waste products transported away from the tissue cells. Under these conditions, body cells are able to carry on their normal functions for only a short period of time. The body tries to restore the circulatory volume by supplying fluid from the body tissues. The result is a progressive fall in the hematocrit (ratio of red blood cells to plasma) and in the red blood cell count.

Burn Shock

In burn shock, on the other hand, there is a progressive increase in the hematocrit and red blood cell count. This increase is due to hemoconcentration from loss of the plasma fraction of the blood into and through the burned area.

NEUROGENIC SHOCK

Neurogenic shock, sometimes called vasogenic shock, results from the disruption of autonomic nervous system control over vasoconstriction. Under normal conditions, the autonomic nervous system keeps the muscles of the veins and arteries partially contracted. At the onset of most forms of shock, further constriction is signaled. However, the vascular muscles cannot maintain this contraction indefinitely. A number of factors, including increased fluid loss, central nervous system trauma, or emotional shock, can override the autonomic nervous system control. The veins and arteries immediately dilate, drastically expanding the volume of the circulatory system, with a corresponding reduction of blood pressure.

Simple fainting (syncope) is a variation of neurogenic shock. It often is the result of a temporary gravitational pooling of the blood as a person stands up. As the person falls, blood again rushes to the head, and the problem is solved. Neurogenic shock may also be induced by fear or horror, which will override the autonomic nervous system control.

Shell shock and bomb shock are other variations of neurogenic shock that are important to the Hospital Corpsman. These are psychological adjustment reactions to extremely stressful wartime experiences and do not relate to the collapse of the cardiovascular system. Symptoms range from intense fear to complete dementia and are manifestations of a loss of nervous control. Care is limited to emotional support of the patient and his evacuation to the care of a psychiatrist or psychologist.

CARDIOGENIC SHOCK

Cardiogenic shock is caused by inadequate functioning of the heart, not by loss of circulating blood volume. If the heart muscle is weakened by disease or damaged by trauma or lack of oxygen (as in cases of pulmonary disease, suffocation, or myocardial infarction), the heart will no longer be able to maintain adequate circulatory pressure, even though the volume of fluid is unchanged. Shock will develop as the pressure falls. Heart attack is an extreme medical emergency all Hospital Corpsmen must be ready to handle. It will be discussed in greater detail in the "Common Medical Emergencies" section of this chapter.

SEPTIC SHOCK

Septic shock usually does not develop for 2 to 5 days after an injury and the patient is not often seen by the Corpsman in a first aid situation. Septic shock may appear during the course of peritonitis caused by penetrating abdominal wounds or perforation of the appendix. Gross wound contamination, rupture of an ulcer, or complications from certain types of pneumonia may also cause septic shock. Septic shock is the result of vasodilation of small blood vessels in the wound area, or general vasodilation if the infection enters the bloodstream. In addition to increasing circulatory system volume, the walls of the blood vessels become more permeable, which allows fluids to escape into the tissues. This type of shock carries a poor prognosis and should be treated under the direct supervision of a medical officer.

ANAPHYLACTIC SHOCK

Anaphylactic shock occurs when an individual is exposed to a substance to which his body is particularly sensitive. In the most severe form of anaphylactic shock, the body goes into an almost instantaneous violent reaction. A burning sensation, itching, and hives spread across the skin. Severe edema affects body parts and the respiratory system. Blood pressure drops alarmingly, and fainting or coma may occur.

The causative agent may be introduced into the body in a number of ways. The injection of medicines (especially penicillin and horse- or egg-cultured serums) is one route. Another method is the injection of venoms by stinging insects and animals. The inhalation of dusts, pollens, or other materials to which a person is sensitive is a third route. Finally, a slightly slower but no less severe reaction may develop from the ingestion of certain foods and medications. Specific treatment of venoms and poisons will be discussed in chapter 5, "Poisoning, Drug Abuse, and Hazardous Material Exposure."

GENERAL TREATMENT PROCEDURES

Intravenous fluid administration is the most important factor in the treatment of all types of shock except cardiogenic shock. Ringer's lactate is the best solution to use, although normal saline is adequate until properly cross-matched whole blood can be administered. The electrolyte solutions replace not only the lost blood volume, but also lost extracellular fluid that has been depleted. If the shock is severe enough to warrant immediate administration of intravenous fluids, or if transportation to a medical facility will be delayed and a medical officer is not available to write an administrative order, be conservative: Start the intravenous fluids and let them run at a slow rate of 50 to 60 drops per minute. If intravenous solutions are unavailable or transportation to a medical treatment facility will be delayed, and there are no contraindications (such as gastrointestinal bleeding or unconsciousness), you may give the patient an electrolyte solution by mouth. An electrolyte solution may be prepared by adding a teaspoon of salt and half a teaspoon of baking soda to a quart or liter of water. Allow the patient to sip the solution.

Other treatment procedures for shock are as follows:

- Maintain an open airway. Oxygen may also be administered if proper equipment is available.

- Control hemorrhages.

- Check for other injuries that may have been sustained. Remove the victim from the presence of identifiable causative agents.

- Place the victim in a supine position, with the feet slightly higher than the head (shock position). Certain problems, such as breathing difficulties or head injuries, may require other positioning.

- Reduce pain by splinting fractures, providing emotional support, and attending to the victim's comfort. Unless contraindicated, aspirin may be dispensed.

- Conserve the patient's body heat.

- Avoid rough handling of the victim, and transport to a medical treatment facility.

- If transportation to a definitive care facility will be lengthy or delayed, seek the radio or phone advice of a medical officer on whether to give fluids by mouth or to start an intravenous line. If this consultation is impossible, use your own judgment. In the case of cardiogenic shock, DO NOT start intravenous fluids since blood volume is sufficient and only function is impaired.

- Constantly monitor the patient and record vital signs every 15 minutes so that you are able to keep track of the patient's progress.

PNEUMATIC COUNTER-PRESSURE DEVICES (MAST)

Commonly known as Medical Anti-Shock Trousers or Military Anti-Shock Trousers (MAST), pneumatic counter-pressure devices are designed to correct or counteract certain internal bleeding conditions and hypovolemia. The garment does this by developing an encircling pressure up to 120 mm Hg around both lower extremities, the pelvis, and the abdomen. The pressure created

- slows or stops venous and arterial bleeding in areas of the body enclosed by the pressurized garment;

- forces available blood from the lower body to the heart, brain, and other vital organs;

- prevents pooling of blood in the lower extremities; and

- stabilizes fractures of the pelvis and lower extremities.

Some indications for use of the pneumatic counter-pressure devices are when

- systolic blood pressure is less than 80 mm Hg,

- systolic blood pressure is less than 100 mm Hg and the patient exhibits the classic signs of shock, or

- fracture of the pelvis or lower extremities is present.

Although the only absolute contraindication in the use of these devices is in the case of pulmonary edema, other conditional contraindications include congestive heart failure, heart attack, stroke, pregnancy, abdominal evisceration, massive bleeding into the thoracic cavity, and penetrating wounds where the object is still impaled in the victim.

Application of the anti-shock garment is a simple procedure, but it requires some important preliminary steps. When the garment is laid out flat, ensure that there are no wrinkles. If the patient is to remain clothed, remove all sharp and bulky objects from the patient's pockets. Take vital signs before applying the MAST garment. When applying the garment, inflate sufficiently so the patient's systolic blood pressure is brought to and maintained at 100 mm Hg. Once the garment is inflated, take the patient's vital signs every 5 minutes. The garment should be removed only under the direct supervision of a physician.

BREATHING AIDS

LEARNING OBJECTIVE: *Recognize breathing aids and their uses.*

As a Hospital Corpsman, you should become familiar with the breathing aids that may be available to help you maintain an open airway and to restore breathing in emergency situations. Breathing aids include oxygen, artificial airways, bag-valve mask ventilator, pocket face mask, and suction devices.

USE OF OXYGEN (O_2)

In an emergency situation, you will probably have a size E, 650-liter cylinder of oxygen available. The oxygen cylinder is usually fitted with a yoke-style pressure-reducing regulator, with gauges to show tank pressure and flow rate (adjustable from 0 to 15 liters per minute). A humidifier can be attached to the flowmeter nipple to help prevent tissue drying caused by the water-vapor-free oxygen. An oxygen line can be connected from the flowmeter nipple or humidifier to a number of oxygen delivery devices that will be discussed later.

When available, oxygen should be administered, as described below, to cardiac arrest patients and to self-ventilating patients who are unable to inhale enough oxygen to prevent **hypoxia** (oxygen deficiency). Hypoxia is characterized by tachycardia, nervousness, irritability, and finally cyanosis. It develops in a wide range of situations, including poisoning, shock, crushing chest injuries, cerebrospinal accidents, and heart attacks.

Oxygen must never be used near open flames since it supports burning. Oxygen cylinders must be handled carefully since they are potentially lethal missiles if punctured or broken.

ARTIFICIAL AIRWAYS

The oropharyngeal and nasopharyngeal airways are primarily used to keep the tongue from occluding (closing) the airway.

Oropharyngeal Airway

The oropharyngeal airway can be used only on unconscious victims because a conscious person will gag on it. This airway comes in various sizes for different age groups and is shaped to rest on the contour of the tongue and extend from the lips to the pharynx. Selecting the correct size oropharyngeal airway is very important to its effectiveness. An airway of proper size will extend from the corner of the patient's mouth to the tip of the earlobe on the same side of the patient's face.

One method of insertion is to depress the tongue with a tongue blade and slide the airway in. Another method is to insert the airway upside down into the victim's mouth; then rotate it 180° as it slides into the pharynx (fig. 4-20).

Nasopharyngeal Airway

The nasopharyngeal airway may be used on conscious victims since it is better tolerated because it generally does not stimulate the gag reflex. Since it is made of flexible material, it is designed to be lubricated and then gently passed up the nostril and down into the pharynx. If the airway meets an obstruction in one nostril, withdraw it and try to pass it up the other nostril. See figure 4-21 for proper insertion of the nasopharyngeal airway.

BAG-VALVE MASK VENTILATOR

The bag-valve mask ventilator (fig. 4-22) is designed to help ventilate an unconscious victim for long periods while delivering high concentrations of oxygen. This system can be useful in extended CPR attempts because, when using external cardiac compressions, the cardiac output is cut to 25 to 30 percent of the normal capacity, and artificial ventilation does not supply enough oxygen through the circulatory system to maintain life for a long period.

Various types of bag-valve-mask systems that come in both adult and pediatric sizes are in use in the Navy. Essentially, they consist of a self-filling ventilation bag, an oxygen reservoir, plastic face masks of various sizes, and tubing for connecting to an oxygen supply.

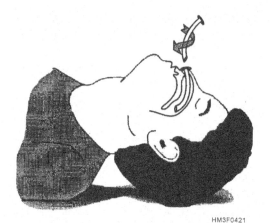

HM3F0421

Figure 4-21.—Proper insertion of a nasopharyngeal airway.

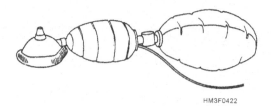

HM3F0422

Figure 4-22.—Bag-valve mask ventilator.

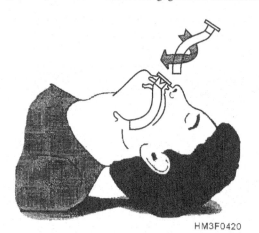

HM3F0420

Figure 4-20.—The rotation method of inserting an oropharyngeal airway.

Limitations of the Bag-Valve Mask Ventilator

The bag-valve mask ventilator is difficult to use unless the user has had sufficient practice with it. It must not be used by inexperienced individuals. The system can be hard to clean and reassemble properly; the bagging hand can tire easily; and an airtight seal at the face is hard to maintain, especially if a single rescuer must also keep the airway open. In addition, the amount of air delivered to the victim is limited to the volume that the hand can displace from the bag (approximately 1 liter per compression).

Procedures for Operating the Bag-Valve Mask Ventilator

To use the bag-valve mask ventilator, hook the bag up to an oxygen supply and adjust the flow in the range of 10 to 15 liters per minute, depending on the desired concentration (15 liters per minute will deliver an oxygen concentration of 90 percent). After opening the airway or inserting an oropharyngeal airway, place the mask over the face and hold it firmly in position with the index finger and thumb, while keeping the jaw tilted upward with the remaining fingers (fig. 4-23). Use the other hand to compress the bag once every 5 seconds. Observe the chest for expansion. If none is observed, the face mask seal may not be airtight, the airway may be blocked, or some component of the bag-valve mask ventilator may be malfunctioning.

POCKET FACE MASK

A pocket face mask designed with an oxygen-inlet flow valve for mouth-to-mask ventilation can be used to give oxygen-enriched artificial ventilation. Although a pocket face mask system cannot achieve oxygen concentrations as high as the bag-valve mask system, it has the advantages of providing greater air volume (up to 4 liters per breath) and of being much easier to use (since both hands are free to maintain the airway and keep the mask firmly in place). See figure 4-24. The pocket face mask also acts as a barrier device. It prevents the rescuer from coming in contact with the patient's body fluids and breath, which are possible sources of infection.

To use the pocket face mask, stand behind the head of the victim, and open the airway by tilting the head backward. Place the mask over the victim's face (for adults, the apex goes over the bridge of the nose; for infants, the apex fits over the chin, with the base resting on the bridge of the nose). Form an airtight seal between the mask and the face, and keep the airway open by pressing down on the mask with both thumbs while using the other fingers to lift the jaw up and back. Ventilate into the open chimney of the mask.

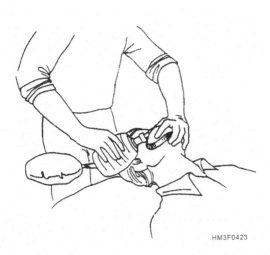

HM3F0423

Figure 4-23.—Bag-valve mask ventilator in use.

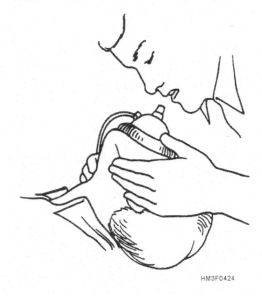

HM3F0424

Figure 4-24.—Providing mouth-to-mask ventilations with pocket face mask.

Oxygen can be added by hooking the valve up to an oxygen supply. Since the rescuer's breath dilutes the oxygen flow in artificial ventilation, adjust the flow rate to increase oxygen concentration. At 5 liters per minute, the oxygen concentration will be approximately 50 percent. At 15 liters per minute, this concentration will increase to 55 percent.

The mask has an elastic strap so it can be used on conscious, self-ventilating patients to increase oxygen concentration.

SUCTION DEVICES

The patient's airway must be kept clear of foreign materials, blood, vomitus, and other secretions. Materials that remain in the airway may be forced into the trachea and eventually into the lungs. This will cause complications ranging from severe pneumonia to a complete airway obstruction. Use suction to remove such materials.

In the field, a Hospital Corpsman may have access to a fixed (installed) suction unit or a portable suction device. Both types of suction devices are equipped with flexible tubing, suction tips and catheters, and a non-breakable collection container.

Maintenance of suction devices consists of testing the suction pressure regularly and cleaning the device after each use.

Before using a suction device, always test the apparatus. Once the suction pressure has been tested, attach a suction catheter or tip. Position the patient on his side, and open the patient's mouth. This position permits secretions to flow from the patient's mouth while suction is being delivered. Use caution in patients with suspected neck or spinal injuries. If the patient is fully and securely immobilized on a backboard, the backboard may be tilted to place the patient on his side. If you suspect such injuries but the patient is not immobilized, suction as best you can without turning the patient. Carefully insert the suction tip or catheter at the top of the throat (fig. 4-25). DO NOT push the tip down into the throat or into the larynx. Apply suction, but for no more than a few seconds, since supplemental oxygen or ventilations cease while suctioning, keeping oxygen from the patient. Suction may be repeated after a few breaths.

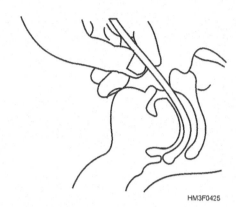

HM3F0425

Figure 4-25.—Proper insertion of suction tip.

CRICOTHYROIDOTOMY

A cricothyroidotomy, often called an emergency tracheotomy, consists of incising the cricothyroid membrane, which lies just beneath the skin between the thyroid cartilage and the cricoid cartilage. In most cases, the cricothyroid membrane can be easily located by hyperextending the neck so that the thyroid notch (Adam's apple) becomes prominent anteriorly. Identify the position of the thyroid notch with the index finger. This finger descends in the midline to the prominence of the cricoid cartilage. The depression of the cricothyroid membrane is identified above the superior margin of the cricoid cartilage (fig. 4-26). Make a small lateral incision at the base of the thyroid cartilage to expose the cricothyroid membrane. Excise this membrane (taking care not to go too deeply) and insert a small-bore air line into the trachea.

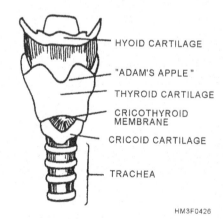

HYOID CARTILAGE

"ADAM'S APPLE"

THYROID CARTILAGE

CRICOTHYROID MEMBRANE

CRICOID CARTILAGE

TRACHEA

HM3F0426

Figure 4-26.—Anatomical structures of the neck to identify the cricothyroid membrane.

An alternate method is to use a 12- to 16-gauge intercatheter. Locate the cricothyroid membrane as described above and insert the needle into the trachea. Immediately upon penetration of the cricothyroid membrane, thread the plastic catheter into the trachea and remove the needle. Then connect the catheter to an oxygen line for translaryngeal oxygen jet insufflation.

Do not attempt a cricothyroidotomy except as a last resort when other methods of opening the airway have been unsuccessful.

SOFT TISSUE INJURIES

LEARNING OBJECTIVE: *Recognize the different types of wounds, and determine management and treatment procedures for open and internal soft-tissue injuries.*

The most common injuries seen by the Corpsman in a first aid setting are soft tissue injuries with the accompanying hemorrhage, shock, and danger of infection. Any injury that causes a break in the skin, underlying soft tissue structures, or body membranes is known as a **wound**. This section will discuss the classification of wounds, the general and specific treatment of soft tissue injuries, the use of dressings and bandages in treating wounds, and the special problems that arise because of the location of wounds.

CLASSIFICATION OF WOUNDS

Wounds may be classified according to their general condition, size, location, the manner in which the skin or tissue is broken, and the agent that caused the wound. It is usually necessary for you to consider these factors to determine what first aid treatment is appropriate for the wound.

General Condition of the Wound

If the wound is fresh, first aid treatment consists mainly of stopping the flow of blood, treating for shock, and reducing the risk of infection. If the wound is already infected, first aid consists of keeping the victim quiet, elevating the injured part, and applying a warm wet dressing. If the wound contains foreign objects, first aid treatment may consist of removing the objects if they are not deeply embedded. DO NOT remove objects embedded in the eyes or the skull, and **do not** remove impaled objects. Stabilize impaled

objects with a bulky dressing before transporting the victim.

Size of the Wound

In general, since large wounds are more serious than small ones, they usually involve more severe bleeding, more damage to the underlying organs or tissues, and a greater degree of shock. However, small wounds are sometimes more dangerous than large ones since they may become infected more readily due to neglect. The depth of the wound is also important because it may lead to a complete perforation of an organ or the body, with the additional complication of entrance and exit wounds.

Location of the Wound

Since a wound may involve serious damage to the deeper structures, as well as to the skin and the tissue immediately below it, the location of the wound is important. For example, a knife wound to the chest may puncture a lung and cause interference with breathing. The same type of wound in the abdomen may result in a dangerous infection in the abdominal cavity, or it might puncture the intestines, liver, kidneys, or other vital organs. A knife wound to the head may cause brain damage, but the same wound in a less vital spot (such as an arm or leg) might be less important.

Types of Wounds

When you consider the manner in which the skin or tissue is broken, there are six general kinds of wounds: abrasions, incisions, lacerations, punctures, avulsions, and amputations. Many wounds, of course, are combinations of two or more of these basic types.

ABRASIONS.—Abrasions are made when the skin is rubbed or scraped off. Rope burns, floor burns, and skinned knees or elbows are common examples of abrasions. This kind of wound can become infected quite easily because dirt and germs are usually embedded in the tissues.

INCISIONS.—Incisions, commonly called cuts, are wounds made by sharp cutting instruments such as knives, razors, and broken glass. Incisions tend to bleed freely because the blood vessels are cut cleanly and without ragged edges. There is little damage to the surrounding tissues. Of all classes of wounds, incisions are the least likely to become infected, since the free flow of blood washes out many of the microorganisms (germs) that cause infection.

LACERATIONS.—These wounds are torn, rather than cut. They have ragged, irregular edges and masses of torn tissue underneath. These wounds are usually made by blunt (as opposed to sharp) objects. A wound made by a dull knife, for instance, is more likely to be a laceration than an incision. Bomb fragments often cause lacerations. Many of the wounds caused by accidents with machinery are lacerations; they are often complicated by crushing of the tissues as well. Lacerations are frequently contaminated with dirt, grease, or other material that is ground into the tissue. They are therefore very likely to become infected.

PUNCTURES.—Punctures are caused by objects that penetrate into the tissues while leaving a small surface opening. Wounds made by nails, needles, wire, and bullets are usually punctures. As a rule, small puncture wounds do not bleed freely; however, large puncture wounds may cause severe internal bleeding. The possibility of infection is great in all puncture wounds, especially if the penetrating object has tetanus bacteria on it. To prevent anaerobic infections, primary closures are not made in the case of puncture wounds.

AVULSIONS.—An avulsion is the tearing away of tissue from a body part. Bleeding is usually heavy. In certain situations, the torn tissue may be surgically reattached. It can be saved for medical evaluation by wrapping it in a sterile dressing and placing it in a cool container, and rushing it—along with the victim—to a medical facility. Do not allow the avulsed portion to freeze, and do not immerse it in water or saline.

AMPUTATIONS.—A traumatic amputation is the nonsurgical removal of the limb from the body. Bleeding is heavy and requires a tourniquet (which will be discussed later) to stop the flow. Shock is certain to develop in these cases. As with avulsed tissue, wrap the limb in a sterile dressing, place it in a cool container, and transport it to the hospital with the victim. Do not allow the limb to be in direct contact with ice, and do not immerse it in water or saline. The limb can often be successfully reattached.

Causes of Wounds

Although it is not always necessary to know what agent or object has caused the wound, it is helpful. Knowing what has caused the wound may give you some idea of the probable size of the wound, its general nature, the extent to which it is likely to become

contaminated with foreign matter, and what special dangers must be guarded against. Of special concern in a wartime setting is the velocity of wound-causing missiles (bullets or shrapnel). A low-velocity missile damages only the tissues it comes into contact with. On the other hand, a high-velocity missile can do enormous damage by forcing the tissues and body parts away from the track of the missile with a velocity only slightly less than that of the missile itself. These tissues, especially bone, may become damage-causing missiles themselves, thus accentuating the destructive effects of the missile.

Having classified the wound into one or more of the general categories listed, the Corpsman will have a good idea of the nature and extent of the injury, along with any special complications that may exist. This information will aid in the treatment of the victim.

MANAGEMENT OF OPEN SOFT-TISSUE INJURIES

There are three basic rules to be followed in the treatment of practically all open soft tissue injuries: to control hemorrhage, to treat the victim for shock, and to do whatever you can to prevent infection. These will be discussed, along with the proper application of first aid materials and other specific first aid techniques.

Hemorrhage

Hemorrhage is the escape of blood from the vessels of the circulatory system. The average adult body contains about 5 liters of blood. Five hundred milliliters of blood, the amount given by blood donors, can usually be lost without any harmful effect. The loss of 1 liter of blood usually causes shock, but shock may develop if small amounts of blood are lost rapidly, since the circulatory system does not have enough time to compensate adequately. The degree of shock progressively increases as greater amounts of blood escape. Young children, sick people, or the elderly may be especially susceptible to the loss of even small amounts of blood since their internal systems are in such delicate balance.

Capillary blood is usually brick red in color. If capillaries are cut, the blood oozes out slowly. Blood from the veins is dark red. Venous bleeding is characterized by a steady, even flow. If an artery near the surface is cut, the blood, which is bright red in color, will gush out in spurts that are synchronized with the heartbeats. If the severed artery is deeply buried, however, the bleeding will appear to be a steady stream.

In actual practice, you might find it difficult to decide whether bleeding is venous or arterial, but the distinction is not usually important. The important thing to know is that all bleeding must be controlled as quickly as possible.

External hemorrhage is of greatest importance to the Corpsman because it is the most frequently encountered and the easiest to control. It is characterized by a break in the skin and visible bleeding. Internal hemorrhage (which will be discussed later) is far more difficult to recognize and to control.

Control of Hemorrhage

The best way to control external bleeding is by applying a compress to the wound and exerting pressure directly to the wound. If direct pressure does not stop the bleeding, pressure can also be applied at an appropriate pressure point. At times, elevation of an extremity is also helpful in controlling hemorrhage. The use of splints in conjunction with direct pressure can be beneficial. In those rare cases where bleeding cannot be controlled by any of these methods, you must use a tourniquet.

If bleeding does not stop after a short period, try placing another compress or dressing over the first and securing it firmly in place. If bleeding still will not stop, try applying direct pressure with your hand over the compress or dressing.

Remember that in cases of severe hemorrhage, it is less important to worry too much about finding appropriate materials or about the dangers of infection. The most important problem is to stop rapid exsanguination. If no material is available, simply thrust your hand into the wound. In most situations, direct pressure is the first and best method to use in the control of hemorrhage.

Pressure Points

Bleeding can often be temporarily controlled by applying hand pressure to the appropriate pressure point. A pressure point is the spot where the main artery to an injured part lies near the skin surface and over a bone. Apply pressure at this point with the fingers (digital pressure) or with the heel of the hand. No first aid materials are required. The object of the pressure is to compress the artery against the bone, thus shutting off the flow of blood from the heart to the wound.

There are 11 principal points on each side of the body where hand or finger pressure can be used to stop hemorrhage. These points are shown in figure 4-27. If bleeding occurs on the face below the level of the eyes, apply pressure to the point on the mandible. This is shown in figure 4-27A. To find this pressure point, start at the angle of the jaw and run your finger forward along the lower edge of the mandible until you feel a small notch. The pressure point is in this notch.

If bleeding is in the shoulder or in the upper part of the arm, apply pressure with the fingers behind the clavicle. You can press down against the first rib or forward against the clavicle; either kind of pressure will stop the bleeding. This pressure point is shown in figure 4-27B.

Bleeding between the middle of the upper arm and the elbow should be controlled by applying digital pressure to the inner (body) side of the arm, about halfway between the shoulder and the elbow. This compresses the artery against the bone of the arm. The application of pressure at this point is shown in figure 4-27C. Bleeding from the hand can be controlled by pressure at the wrist, as shown in figure 4-27D. If it is possible to hold the arm up in the air, the bleeding will be relatively easy to stop.

Figure 4-27E shows how to apply digital pressure in the middle of the groin to control bleeding from the thigh. The artery at this point lies over a bone and quite close to the surface, so pressure with your fingers may be sufficient to stop the bleeding.

Figure 4-27F shows the proper position for controlling bleeding from the foot. As in the case of bleeding from the hand, elevation is helpful in controlling the bleeding.

If bleeding is in the region of the temple or the scalp, use your finger to compress the main artery to the temple against the skull bone at the pressure point just in front of the ear. Figure 4-27G shows the proper position.

If the neck is bleeding, apply pressure below the wound, just in front of the prominent neck muscle. Press inward and slightly backward, compressing the main artery of that side of the neck against the bones of the spinal column. The application of pressure at this point is shown in figure 4-27H. Do not apply pressure at this point unless it is absolutely essential, since there

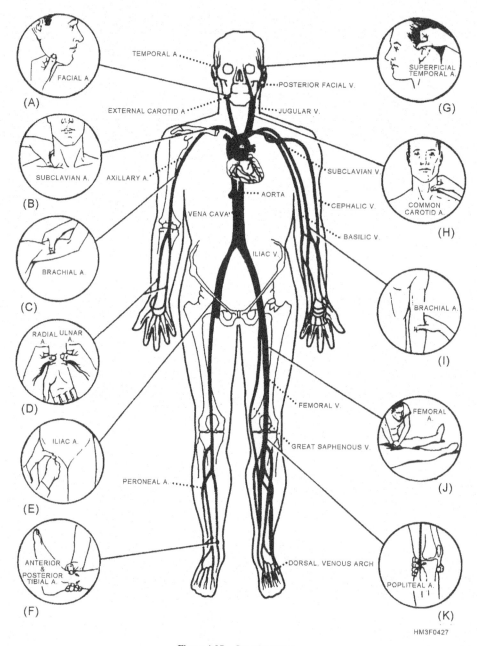

Figure 4-27.—Pressure points.

HM3F0427

is a great danger of pressing on the windpipe, thereby choking the victim.

Bleeding from the lower arm can be controlled by applying pressure at the elbow, as shown in figure 4-27I.

As mentioned before, bleeding in the upper part of the thigh can sometimes be controlled by applying digital pressure in the middle of the groin, as shown in figure 4-27E. Sometimes, however, it is more effective to use the pressure point of the upper thigh, as shown in figure 4-27J. If you use this point, apply pressure with the closed fist of one hand and use the other hand to give additional pressure. The artery at this point is deeply buried in some of the heaviest muscle tissue in the body, so a great deal of pressure must be exerted to compress the artery against the bone.

Bleeding between the knee and the foot may be controlled by firm pressure at the knee. If pressure at the side of the knee does not stop the bleeding, hold the front of the knee with one hand and thrust your fist hard against the artery behind the knee, as shown in figure 4-27K. If necessary, you can place a folded compress or bandage behind the knee, bend the leg back, and hold it in place by a firm bandage. This is a most effective way of controlling bleeding, but it is so uncomfortable for the victim that it should be used only as a last resort.

You should memorize these pressure points so that you will know immediately which point to use for controlling hemorrhage from a particular part of the body. Remember, the correct pressure point is that which is (1) **nearest the wound**, and (2) **between the wound and the main part of the body**.

It is very tiring to apply digital pressure, and it can seldom be maintained for more than 15 minutes. Pressure points are recommended for use while direct pressure is being applied to a serious wound by a second rescuer. Using the pressure-point technique is also advised after a compress, bandage, or dressing has been applied to the wound, since this method will slow the flow of blood to the area, thus giving the direct pressure technique a better chance to stop the hemorrhage. The pressure-point system is also recommended as a stopgap measure until a pressure dressing or a tourniquet can be applied.

Elevation

The elevation of an extremity, where appropriate, can be an effective aid in hemorrhage control when used in conjunction with other methods of control, especially direct pressure. This is because the amount of blood entering the extremity is decreased by the uphill gravitational effect. Do not elevate an extremity until it is certain that no bones have been broken or until broken bones are properly splinted.

Splints

Another effective method of hemorrhage control in cases of bone fractures is splinting. The immobilization of sharp bone ends reduces further tissue trauma and allows lacerated blood vessels to clot. In addition, the gentle pressure exerted by the splint helps the clotting process by giving additional support to compresses or dressings already in place over open fracture sites.

Later in this chapter we will go into the subject of splinting in greater detail.

Tourniquets

A tourniquet is a constricting band that is used to cut off the supply of blood to an injured limb. Use a tourniquet **only as a last resort** and if the control of hemorrhage by other means proves to be difficult or impossible. A tourniquet must always be applied **above** the wound (i.e., toward the trunk), and it must be applied as close to the wound as practical.

Basically, a tourniquet consists of a pad, a band, and a device for tightening the band so that the blood vessels will be compressed. It is best to use a pad, compress, or similar pressure object, if one is available. The pressure object goes under the band and must be placed directly over the artery or it will actually decrease the pressure on the artery, allowing a greater flow of blood. If a tourniquet placed over a pressure object does not stop the bleeding, there is a good chance that the pressure object is in the wrong place. If placement is not effective, shift the object around until the tourniquet, when tightened, will control the bleeding.

Any long flat material may be used as the band. It is important that the band be flat: belts, stockings, flat strips of rubber, or neckerchiefs may be used; however, rope, wire, string, or very narrow pieces of cloth should not be used because they can cut into the flesh. A short stick may be used to twist the band, tightening the tourniquet. Figure 4-28 shows the proper steps in applying a tourniquet.

To be effective, a tourniquet must be tight enough to stop the arterial blood flow to the limb. Be sure, therefore, to draw the tourniquet tight enough to stop the bleeding. Do not make it any tighter than necessary, though, since a tourniquet that is too tight can lead to loss of the limb the tourniquet is applied to.

After you have brought the bleeding under control with the tourniquet, apply a sterile compress or dressing to the wound and fasten it in position with a bandage.

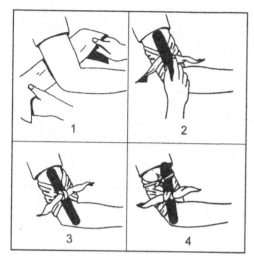

HM3F0428

Figure 4-28.—Applying a tourniquet.

Here are the points to remember about using a tourniquet:

1. **Use a tourniquet only as a last resort!** Don't use a tourniquet unless you can't control the bleeding by any other means.

2. Don't use a tourniquet for bleeding from the head, face, neck, or trunk. Use it only on the limbs.

3. Always apply a tourniquet **above the wound** and as close to the wound as possible. As a general rule, do not place a tourniquet below the knee or elbow except for complete amputations. In certain distal areas of the extremities, nerves lie close to the skin and may be damaged by the compression. Furthermore, rarely does one encounter bleeding distal to the knee or elbow that requires a tourniquet.

4. Be sure you draw the tourniquet tight enough to stop the bleeding, but don't make it any tighter than necessary. The pulse beyond the tourniquet should disappear.

5. **Don't loosen a tourniquet after it has been applied.** Transport the victim to a medical facility that can offer proper care.

6. Don't cover a tourniquet with a dressing. If it is necessary to cover the injured person in some way, **make sure** that all the other people concerned with the case know about the

tourniquet. Using crayon, skin pencil, or blood, mark a large "T" and the time the tourniquet was applied on the victim's forehead or on a medical tag attached to the wrist.

MANAGEMENT OF INTERNAL SOFT-TISSUE INJURIES

Internal soft-tissue injuries may result from deep wounds, blunt trauma, blast exposure, crushing accidents, bone fracture, poison, or sickness. They may range in seriousness from a simple contusion to life-threatening hemorrhage and shock.

Visible Indications

Visible indications of internal soft-tissue injury include the following:

- Hematemesis (vomiting bright red blood)
- Hemoptysis (coughing up bright red blood)
- Melena (excretion of tarry black stools)
- Hematochezia (excretion of bright red blood from the rectum)
- Hematuria (passing of blood in the urine)
- Nonmenstrual (vaginal bleeding)
- Epistaxis (nosebleed)
- Pooling of the blood near the skin surface

Other Symptoms

More often than not, however, there will be no visible signs of injury, and the Corpsman will have to infer the probability of internal soft-tissue injury from other symptoms such as the following:

- Pale, moist, clammy skin
- Subnormal temperature
- Rapid, feeble pulse
- Falling blood pressure
- Dilated, slowly reacting pupils with impaired vision
- Tinnitus
- Syncope
- Dehydration and thirst
- Yawning and air hunger
- Anxiety, with a feeling of impending doom

Immediate Treatment

There is little that a Corpsman can do to correct internal soft-tissue injuries since they are almost always surgical problems. The Hospital Corpsman's goal must be to obtain the greatest benefit from the victim's remaining blood supply. The following steps should be taken:

1. Treat for shock.

2. Keep the victim warm and at rest.

3. Replace lost fluids with a suitable blood volume expander. DO NOT give the victim anything to drink until the extent of the injury is known for certain.

4. Give oxygen, if available.

5. Splint injured extremities.

6. Apply cold compresses to identifiable injured areas.

7. Transport the victim to a medical treatment facility as soon as possible.

SPECIAL CONSIDERATIONS IN WOUND TREATMENT

There are special considerations that should be observed when treating wounds. The first of these is immediate treatment to prevent shock. Next, infection should be a concern: Look for inflammation and signs of abscess. Hospital Corpsmen should be aware of these conditions and have the knowledge to treat them.

Shock

Shock is likely to be severe in a person who has lost a large amount of blood or suffered any serious wound. The causes and treatment of shock are explained earlier in this chapter.

Infection

Although infection may occur in any wound, it is a particular danger in wounds that do not bleed freely, in wounds in which torn tissue or skin falls back into place and prevents the entrance of air, and in wounds that involve the crushing of tissues. Incisions (in which there is a free flow of blood and relatively little crushing of tissues) are the least likely to become infected.

Battle wounds are especially likely to become infected. They present the problem of devitalized (dead or dying) tissue; extravasated blood (blood that has escaped its natural boundaries); foreign bodies such as missile fragments, bits of cloth, dirt, dust; and a variety of bacteria. The devitalized tissue proteins and extravasated blood provide a nutritional medium for the support of bacterial growth and thus are conducive to the development of serious wound infection. Puncture wounds are also likely to become infected by the germs causing tetanus.

COMMON INFECTION-CAUSING BACTERIA.— There are two types of bacteria that commonly cause infection in wounds: aerobic and anaerobic. Aerobic bacteria live and multiply in the presence of air or free oxygen, while anerobic bacteria live and multiply only in the absence of air.

Aerobic Bacteria.—The principal aerobic bacteria that cause infection, inflammation, and septicemia (blood poisoning) are streptococci and staphylococci, some varieties of which are hemolytic (destroy red blood cells). The staphylococci and streptococci may be introduced at the time of infliction, or they may be introduced to the wound later (at the time of first aid treatment or in the hospital if nonsterile instruments or dressings are employed).

Anaerobic Bacteria.—Anaerobic bacteria are widespread in soil (especially manured soil). While not invasive, anaerobic bacteria contribute to disease by producing toxins and destructive enzymes, often leading to necrosis and/or gangrene of the infected area.

MINOR WOUND CLEANING AND DRESSING.—Wash minor wounds immediately with soap and clean water; then dry and paint them with a mild, nonirritating antiseptic. Apply a dressing if necessary. In the first aid environment, do not attempt to wash or clean a large wound, and do not apply an antiseptic to it since it must be cleaned thoroughly at a medical treatment facility. Simply protect it with a large compress or dressing, and transport the victim to a medical treatment facility. After an initial soap and water cleanup, puncture wounds must also be directed to a medical treatment facility for evaluation.

Inflammation

Inflammation is a local reaction to irritation. It occurs in tissues that are injured, but not destroyed. Symptoms include redness, pain, heat, swelling, and sometimes loss of motion.

The body's physiologic response to the irritation is to dilate local blood vessels, which increases the blood supply to the area. The increased blood flow, in turn, causes the skin to appear red and warmer. As the blood vessels dilate, their injured walls leak blood serum into surrounding tissues, causing edema and pain from increased pressure on nerve endings. In addition, white blood cells increase in the area and act as scavengers (phagocytes) in destroying bacteria and ingesting small particles of dead tissue and foreign matter.

Inflammation may be caused by trauma or mechanical irritation; chemical reaction to venom, poison ivy, acids, or alkalies; heat or cold injuries; microorganism penetration; or other agents such as electricity or solar radiation.

Inflammation should be treated by the following methods:

- Remove the irritating cause.

- Keep the inflamed area at rest and elevated.

- Apply cold for 24 to 48 hours to reduce swelling. Once swelling is reduced, apply heat to soft tissues, which hastens the removal of products of inflammation.

- Apply wet dressings and ointments to soften tissues and to rid the area of the specific causal bacteria.

Abscesses

An abscess is a localized collection of pus that forms in cavities created by the disintegration of tissue. Abscesses may follow injury, illness, or irritation. Most abscesses are caused by staphylococcal infections and may occur in any area of the body, but they are usually on the skin surface.

A **furuncle** (boil) is an abscess in the true skin caused by the entry of microorganisms through a hair follicle or sweat gland. A **carbuncle** is a group of furuncular abscesses having multiple sloughs, often interconnected under the true skin. When localized, there are several "heads." Symptoms begin with localized itching and inflammation, followed by swelling, fever, and pain. Redness and swelling localize, and the furuncle or carbuncle becomes hard and painful. Pus forms into a cavity, causing the skin to become taut and discolored.

Treatment for furuncles and carbuncles includes the following:

- **DO NOT** squeeze! Squeezing may damage surrounding healthy tissue and spread the infection.

- Use aseptic techniques when handling.

- Relieve pain with aspirin.

- Apply moist hot soaks/dressings (110°F) for 40 minutes, three to four times per day.

- Rest and elevate the infected body part.

- Antibiotic therapy may be ordered by a physician.

- Abscesses should be incised after they have localized (except on the face) to establish drainage. Abscesses in the facial triangle (nose and upper lip) should be seen by a physician.

SPECIAL WOUNDS AND THEIR TREATMENT

LEARNING OBJECTIVE: *Recall medical precautions and wound-treatment procedures for the following list of wounds: animal bites, eye wounds, head wounds, facial wounds, abdominal wounds, crushing injuries, and the removal of foreign objects.*

As a Hospital Corpsman, you should find most general wounds very easy to diagnose and treat. There are other wounds, however, that require special consideration and treatment. They are discussed below.

Eye Wounds

Many eye wounds contain foreign objects. Dirt, coal, cinders, eyelashes, bits of metal, and a variety of other objects may become lodged in the eye. Since even a small piece of dirt is intensely irritating to the eye, the removal of such objects is important. However, the eye is easily damaged. Impairment of vision (or even total loss of vision) can result from fumbling, inexpert attempts to remove foreign objects from the eye. The following precautions **must** be observed:

- **DO NOT** allow the victim to rub the eye.

- **DO NOT** press against the eye or manipulate it in any way that might cause the object to become embedded in the tissues of the eye. Be very gentle; roughness is almost sure to cause injury to the eye.

- **DO NOT** use such things as knives, toothpicks, matchsticks, or wires to remove the object.

- **DO NOT UNDER ANY CIRCUMSTANCES ATTEMPT TO REMOVE AN OBJECT THAT IS EMBEDDED IN THE EYEBALL OR THAT HAS PENETRATED THE EYE!** If you see a splinter or other object sticking out from the eyeball, leave it alone! Only specially trained medical personnel can hope to save the victim's sight if an object has actually penetrated the eyeball.

Small objects that are lodged on the surface of the eye or on the membrane lining the eyelids can usually be removed by the following procedures:

1. Try to wash the eye gently with lukewarm, sterile water. A sterile medicine dropper or a sterile syringe can be used for this purpose. Have the victim lie down, with the head turned slightly to one side as shown in figure 4-29. Hold the eyelids apart. Direct the flow of water to the **inside** corner of the eye, and let it run down to the **outside** corner. Do not let the water fall directly onto the eyeball.

2. Gently pull the lower lid down, and instruct the victim to look up. If you can see the object, try to remove it with the corner of a clean handkerchief or with a small moist cotton swab. You can make the swab by twisting cotton around a wooden applicator, not too tightly, and moistening it with sterile water.

   CAUTION: Never use **dry** cotton anywhere near the eye. It will stick to the eyeball or to the inside of the lids, and you will have the problem of removing it as well as the original object.

3. If you cannot see the object when the lower lid is pulled down, turn the upper lid back over a smooth wooden applicator. Tell the victim to look down. Place the applicator lengthwise across the center of the upper lid. Grasp the lashes of the upper lid gently but firmly. Press gently with the applicator. Pull up on the eyelashes, turning the lid back over the applicator. If you can see the object, try to

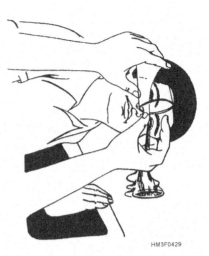

Figure 4-29.—Irrigating the eye.

remove it with a moist cotton swab or with the corner of a clean handkerchief.

4. If the foreign object cannot be removed by any of the above methods, **DO NOT MAKE ANY FURTHER ATTEMPTS TO REMOVE IT.** Instead, place a small, thick gauze dressing over both eyes and hold it in place with a **loose** bandage. This limits movement of the injured eye.

5. Get medical help for the victim at the earliest opportunity.

Head Wounds

Head wounds must be treated with particular care, since there is always the possibility of brain damage. The general treatment for head wounds is the same as that for other fresh wounds. However, certain special precautions must be observed if you are giving first aid to a person who has suffered a head wound.

- **NEVER GIVE ANY MEDICATIONS**.

- Keep the victim lying flat, with the head at the level of the body. Do not raise the feet if the face is flushed. If the victim is having trouble breathing, you may raise the head slightly.

- If the wound is at the back of the head, turn the victim on his side.

- Watch closely for vomiting and position the head to avoid aspiration of vomitus or saliva into the lungs.

- Do not use direct pressure to control hemorrhage if the skull is depressed or obviously fractured.

Facial Wounds

Wounds of the face are treated, in general, like other fresh wounds. However, in all facial injuries make sure neither the tongue nor injured soft tissue blocks the airway, causing breathing obstruction. Keep the nose and throat clear of any obstructing materials, and position the victim so that blood will drain out of the mouth and nose.

Facial wounds that involve the eyelids or the soft tissue around the eye must be handled carefully to avoid further damage. If the injury does not involve the eyeball, apply a sterile compress and hold it in place with a **firm** bandage. If the eyeball appears to be injured, use a **loose** bandage. (Remember that you must **NEVER** attempt to remove any object that is embedded in the eyeball or that has penetrated it; just apply a dry, sterile compress to cover both eyes, and hold the compress in place with a **loose bandage**).

Any person who has suffered a facial wound that involves the eye, the eyelids, or the tissues around the eye must receive medical attention as soon as possible. Be sure to keep the victim lying down. Use a stretcher for transport.

Chest Wounds

Since chest injuries may cause severe breathing and bleeding problems, all chest injuries must be considered as serious conditions. Any victim showing signs of difficulty in breathing without signs of airway obstruction must be inspected for chest injuries. The most serious chest injury that requires immediate first aid treatment is the **sucking chest wound**. This is a penetrating injury to the chest that produces a hole in the chest cavity. The chest hole causes the lung to collapse, preventing normal breathing functions. This is an extremely serious condition that will result in death if not treated quickly.

Victims with open chest wounds gasp for breath, have difficulty breathing out, and may have a bluish skin color to their face. Frothy-looking blood may bubble from the wound during breathing.

The proper treatment for a sucking chest wound is as follows:

1. Immediately seal the wound with a hand or any airtight material available (e.g., ID card). The material must be large enough so that it cannot be sucked into the wound when the victim breathes in.

2. Firmly tape the material in place with strips of adhesive tape and secure it with a pressure dressing. It is important that the dressing is airtight. If it is not, it will not relieve the victim's breathing problems. The object of the dressing is to keep air from going in through the wound.

   NOTE: If the victim's condition suddenly deteriorates when you apply the seal, remove it **immediately**.

3. Give the victim oxygen if it is available and you know how to use it.

4. Place the victim in a Fowler's or semi-Fowler's position. This makes breathing a little easier. During combat, lay the victim on a stretcher on the affected side.

5. Watch the victim closely for signs of shock, and treat accordingly.

6. Do not give victims with chest injuries anything to drink.

7. Transport the victim to a medical treatment facility immediately.

Abdominal Wounds

A deep wound in the abdomen is likely to constitute a major emergency since there are many vital organs in this area. Abdominal wounds usually cause intense pain, nausea and vomiting, spasm of the abdominal muscles, and severe shock. Immediate surgical treatment is almost always required; therefore, the victim must receive medical attention at once, or the chances of survival will be poor. Give only the most essential first aid treatment, and concentrate your efforts on getting the victim to a medical treatment facility. The following first aid procedures may be of help to a person suffering from an abdominal wound:

- Keep the victim in a supine position. If the intestine is protruding or exposed, the victim may be more comfortable with the knees drawn up. Place a coat, pillow, or some other bulky cloth material under the knees to help maintain this position. **DO NOT ATTEMPT TO PUSH THE INTESTINES BACK IN OR TO MANIPULATE THEM IN ANY WAY!**

- If bleeding is severe, try to stop it by applying direct pressure.

- If the intestines are not exposed, cover the wound with a dry sterile dressing. If the intestines are exposed, apply a sterile compress moistened with sterile water. If no sterile water is available, clean sea water or any water that is fit to drink may be used to moisten the compress. Figure 4-30 shows an abdominal wound with the intestine protruding. Figure 4-31 shows the application of compresses large enough to cover the wound and the surrounding area. The compress should be held in place by a bandage. Fasten the bandage firmly so that the compress will not slip around, but do not apply any more pressure than is necessary to hold the compress in position. Large battle dressings are ideal.

- Treat for shock, but do not waste any time doing it. The victim must be transported to a hospital at the earliest possible opportunity. However, you can minimize the severity of shock by making sure that the victim is comfortably warm and kept in the supine position. **DO NOT GIVE ANYTHING TO DRINK**. If the victim is

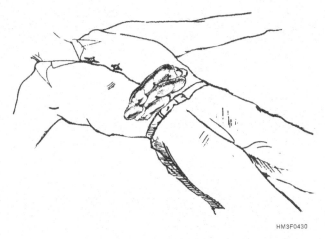

Figure 4-30.—Protruding abdominal wounds.

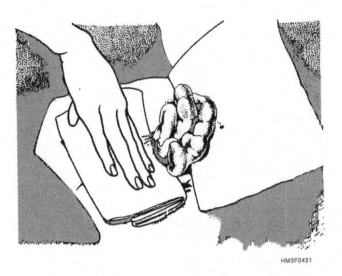

Figure 4-31.—Applying compresses to a protruding abdominal wound.

thirsty, moisten the mouth with a small amount of water, but do not allow any liquid to be swallowed.

- Upon the direction of a medical officer, start an intravenous line.

Crush Injuries

Force can be transmitted from the body's exterior to its interior structure, leaving the skin intact, with a simple bruise as the only external evidence of trauma. This force can cause internal organs to be crushed or to rupture and bleed. When this happens, it is called a **crush injury**. Organs such as the liver and spleen contain a lot of blood. When crushed, these organs bleed severely, and this severe internal bleeding can cause shock. Contents of hollow organs (e.g., urine or digested food) can leak into the body cavities, causing severe inflammation and tissue damage. Bones can also be broken along with muscles, and nerves damaged. Assessment and treatment for the Hospital Corpsman can be difficult when a crush injury is involved. Treat symptomatically and evacuate to the nearest medical treatment facility as soon as possible.

Removing Foreign Objects

Many wounds contain foreign objects. Wood or glass splinters, bullets, metal fragments, bits of wire, fishhooks, nails, tacks, cinders, and small particles from grinding wheels are examples of the variety of objects or materials that are sometimes found in wounds. When such objects are near the surface and exposed, first aid treatment includes their removal. However, first aid treatment does not include the removal of deeply embedded objects, powdered glass, or any widely scattered material of this nature. You should never attempt to remove bullets, but you should try to find out whether the bullet remains in the victim. Look for both entrance and exit wounds. The general rule to remember is this: Remove foreign objects from a wound when you can do so easily and without causing further damage; but **NEVER HUNT FOR OR ATTEMPT TO REMOVE DEEPLY BURIED OR WIDELY SCATTERED OBJECTS OR MATERIALS,** except in a definitive care environment.

The following procedure may be used to remove a small object from the skin or tissues if the object is near the surface and clearly visible:

1. Cleanse the skin around the object with soap and water and paint with any available skin antiseptic solution.

2. If necessary, pierce the skin with a sharp instrument (a needle, razor, or sharp knife that has been sterilized by passing it through a flame several times).

3. Grasping the object at the end, remove it. Tweezers, small pincers, or forceps may be used for this purpose. (Whatever instrument you use should first be sterilized by boiling if at all possible.)

4. If the wound is superficial, apply gentle pressure to encourage bleeding.

5. Cover the wound with a dry, sterile dressing.

If the foreign object is under a fingernail or toenail, you may have to cut a V-shaped notch in the nail so that the object can be grasped by the forceps. Do not try to dig the object out from under the nail with a knife or similar instrument.

A curved or barbed object (such as a fishhook) may present special problems. Figure 4-32 shows one method of removing a fishhook that has become embedded in the flesh. As you can see from figure 4-32A, the barb on the hook prevents its direct removal. However, if you push the hook forward through the skin, as shown in figure 4-32B, you can clip off the barb with a wire cutter or similar tool, as shown in figure 4-32. The remainder of the fishhook

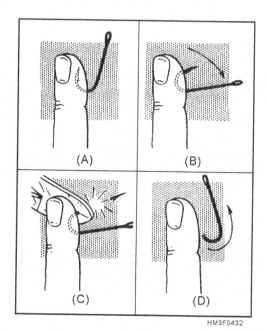

HM3F0432

Figure 4-32.—Removing a fishhook.

can then be withdrawn in the manner indicated in figure 4-32D.

Animal Bites

A special kind of infection that must be guarded against in case of animal bites is rabies (sometimes called "hydrophobia"). This disease is caused by a virus that is present in the saliva of infected animals. The disease occurs most commonly in wild animals, but it has been found in domestic animals and household pets. In fact, it is probable that all mammals are susceptible to it. The virus that causes rabies is ordinarily transmitted by a bite, but it can be transmitted by the saliva of an infected animal coming in contact with a fresh wound or with the thin mucous membrane of the lips or nose. The virus does not penetrate normal unbroken skin. If the skin is broken, **DO NOT** attempt wound closure.

If rabies develops in man, it is usually fatal. A preventive treatment is available and it is very effective, but only if it is started shortly after the bite. This treatment is outlined in BUMEDINST 6220.6. Since the vaccine can be obtained only at a medical treatment facility or a major ship, any person bitten by an animal **must** be transferred quickly to the nearest treatment facility for evaluation, along with a complete report of the circumstances surrounding the incident. Remember, prevention is of utmost importance.

Immediate local treatment of the wound should be given. Wash the wound and the surrounding area carefully, using sterile gauze, soap, and sterile water. Use sterile gauze to dry the wound, and then cover the wound with a sterile dressing. **DO NOT** use any chemical disinfectant. Do not attempt to cauterize the wound in any way.

All of the animal's saliva must be removed from the victim's skin to prevent further contamination of the wound.

CAUTION: DO NOT allow the animal's saliva to come in contact with open sores or cuts on your hands.

When a person has been bitten by an animal, every effort must be made to catch the animal and to keep it confined for a minimum of 8 to 10 days. **DO NOT** kill it if there is any possible chance of catching it alive. The symptoms of rabies are not always present in the animal at the time the bite occurs, but the saliva may nevertheless contain the rabies virus. It is essential, therefore, that the animal is kept under observation until a diagnosis can be made. The rabies treatment is given if the animal develops any definite symptoms, if it dies during the observation period, or if for any reason the animal cannot be kept under observation.

Remember that any animal bite is dangerous and **MUST** be evaluated at a treatment facility.

WOUND CLOSURE

LEARNING OBJECTIVE: *Recognize the different types of suture material and their uses; recall topical, local infiltration and nerve-block anesthetic administration procedures; and identify the steps in wound suturing and suture removal.*

The care of the wound is largely controlled by the tactical situation, facilities available, and the length of time before proper medical care may be available. Normally, the advice to the Corpsman regarding the suturing of wounds is **DO NOT ATTEMPT IT**. However, if days are expected to elapse before the patient can be seen by a surgeon, the Corpsman should know how to use the various suture procedures and materials, and how to select the most appropriate of both.

Before discussing the methods of coaptation (bringing together), some of the contraindications to wound closing should be described.

- If there is reddening and edema of the wound margins, infection manifested by the discharge of pus, and persistent fever or toxemia, **DO NOT CLOSE THE WOUND**. If these signs are minimal, the wound should be allowed to "clean up." The process may be hastened by warm, moist dressings, and irrigations with sterile saline. These aid in the liquefaction of necrotic wound materials and the removal of thick exudates and dead tissues.

- If the wound is a puncture wound, a large gaping wound of the soft tissue, or an animal bite, leave it unsutured. Even under the care of a surgeon, it is the rule **not** to close wounds of this nature until after the fourth day. This is called "delayed primary closure" and is performed upon the indication of a healthy appearance of the wound. Healthy muscle tissue that is viable is evident by its color, consistency, blood supply, and contractibility. Muscle that is dead or dying is comparatively dark and mushy; it does not contract when pinched, nor does it bleed when cut. If this type of tissue is evident, do not close the wound.

- If the wound is deep, consider the support of the surrounding tissue; if there is not enough support to bring the deep fascia together, do not suture because dead (hollow) spaces will be created. In this generally gaping type of wound, muscles, tendons, and nerves are usually involved. Only a surgeon should attempt to close this type of wound.

NOTE: To a certain extent, firm pressure dressings and immobilization can obliterate hollow spaces. If tendons and nerves do not seem to be involved, absorbable sutures may be placed in the muscle. Be careful to suture muscle fibers end-to-end and to correctly appose them. Close the wound in layers. This is extremely delicate surgery, and the Corpsman should weigh carefully the advisability of attempting it–and then only if he has observed and assisted in numerous surgical operations.

If the wound is small, clean, and free from foreign bodies and signs of infection, steps should be taken to close it. All instruments should be checked, cleaned, and thoroughly sterilized. Use a good light and position the patient on the table so that access to the wound will be unhampered.

The area around the wound should be cleansed and then prepared with an antiseptic. The wound area should be draped, whenever possible, to maintain a sterile field in which the Corpsman will work. The Corpsman should wear a cap and mask, scrub his hands and forearms, and wear sterile gloves.

Suture Materials

In modern surgery, many kinds of ligature and suture materials are used. All can be grouped into two classes: nonabsorbable sutures and absorbable sutures.

NONABSORBABLE SUTURES.—These are sutures that cannot be absorbed by the body cells and fluids in which they are embedded during the healing process. When used as buried sutures, these sutures become surrounded or encapsulated in fibrous tissue and remain as innocuous foreign bodies. When used as skin sutures, they are removed after the skin has healed. The most commonly used sutures of this type and the characteristics associated with each are listed below.

- **Silk**—frequently reacts with tissue and can be "spit" from the wound.

- **Cotton**—loses tensile strength with each autoclaving.

- **Linen**—is better than silk or cotton but is more expensive and not as readily available.

- **Synthetic materials** (e.g., nylon, dermalon)—are excellent, particularly for surface use. They cause very little tissue reaction. Their only problem seems to be the tendency for the knots to come untied. (Because of this tendency, most surgeons tie 3 to 4 square knots in each such suture.) Nylon is preferred over silk for face and lip areas because silk too often causes tissue reactions.

- **Rust-proof metal** (usually stainless steel wire)—has the least tissue reaction of all suture materials and is by far the strongest. The primary problems associated with it are that it is more difficult to use because it kinks and that it must be cut with wire cutters.

ABSORBABLE SUTURES.—These are sutures that are absorbed or digested during and after the healing processes by the body cells and tissue fluids in which they are embedded. It is this characteristic that enhances their use beneath the skin surfaces and on mucous membranes.

Surgical gut fulfills the requirements for the perfect suture—ease of manufacture, tensile strength, and variety available—more often than any other material.

- **Manufacture of catgut**: Though it is referred to as "catgut," surgical gut is derived from the submucosal connective tissue of the first one-third (about 8 yards) of the small intestine of healthy government-inspected sheep. The intestine of the sheep has certain characteristics that make it especially adaptable for surgical use. Among these characteristics is its uniformly fine-grained tissue structure and its great tensile strength and elasticity.

- **Tensile strength of catgut**: This suture material is available in sizes of 6-0 to 0 and 1 to 4, with 6-0 being the smallest diameter and 4 being the largest. The tensile strength increases with the diameter of the suture.

- **Varieties of catgut**: Surgical gut varies from plain catgut (the raw gut that has been gauzed, polished, sterilized, and packaged) to chromic catgut (that has undergone various intensities of tanning with one of the salts of chromic acid to delay tissue absorption time). Some examples of these variations and their absorption times follow in table 4–3.

Suture Needles

Suture needles may be straight or curved, and they may have either a tapered round point or a cutting edge point. They vary in length, curvature, and diameter for various types of suturing. Specific characteristics of suture needles are listed below.

- **Size**: Suture needles are sized by diameter and are available in many sizes.

- **Taper point**: Most often used in deep tissues, this type **needle causes minimal amounts of tissue damage.**

- **Cutting edge point:** This type needle is preferred for suturing the skin because of the needle's ability to penetrate the skin's toughness.

- **Atraumatic (atraloc, wedged)**: These needles may either have a cutting edge or a taper point. Additionally, the suture may be fixed on the end of the needle by the manufacturer to cause the least tissue trauma.

Preparation of Casualty

Before suturing the wound(s) of any victim, the following steps should be taken to prepare the casualty.

1. Examine the casualty carefully to determine what materials are needed to properly close the wound.

    a. Select and prepare sterile instruments, needles, and suture materials.

Table 4-3.—Absorption Times of Various Types of Surgical Gut

Type Gut	Absorption Time
A: Plain	10 days
B: Mild chromic	20 days
C: Medium chromic	30 days
D: Extra chromic	40 days

b. Position the patient securely so that access to the wound and suture tray is optimal. It is usually not necessary to restrain patients for suturing.

c. Make sure a good light is available.

2. Strictly observe aseptic wound preparation. Use mask, cap, and gloves. Thorough cleaning and proper draping are essential.

3. Select an anesthetic with care. Consider the patient's tolerance to pain, time of injury, medications the patient is taking or has been given, and the possible distortion of the tissue when the anesthetic are infiltrated.

SELECTION OF ANESTHESIA.—The most common local anesthetic used is Xylocaine®, which comes in various strengths (0.5%, 1%, 2%) and with or without epinephrine. Injectables containing epinephrine must never be used on the fingers, toes, ears, nose—any appendage with small vessels—because of the vasoconstricting effect of the epinephrine. Epinephrine is also contraindicated in patients with hypertension, diabetes, or heart disease.

The three methods of anesthestia administration are topical, local infiltration, and nerve block. Topical anesthetics are generally reserved for ophthalmic or plastic surgery, and nerve blocks are generally accomplished by an anesthesiologist or anesthetist for the surgical patient. For a Corpsman, topical anesthesia is limited to the instillation of eye drops for mild corneal abrasions after all foreign bodies have been removed. **DO NOT** attempt to remove embedded foreign bodies. Nerve blocks are limited to digital blocks wherein the nerve trunks that enervate the fingers or toes are anesthetized. The most common method of anesthesia used by a Corpsman is the infiltration of the anesthetizing agent around a wound or minor surgical site.

ADMINISTRATION OF ANESTHESIA.— Performing a digital block is a fairly simple procedure, but it should not be attempted except under the supervision of a medical officer or after a great deal of practice. The first step is cleansing the injection site with an antiseptic solution. The anesthetizing agent is then infiltrated into the lateral and medial aspects at the base of the digit with a small bore needle (25- or 26-gauge), taking care not to inject into the veins or arteries. Proper placement of the anesthesia should result in a loss of sensitivity in a few minutes. This is tested by asking the patient if he can distinguish a sharp sensation or pain when a sharp object is gently applied to the skin.

Administering local anesthesia is similar except you are anesthetizing nerves immediately adjacent to where you will be working instead of nerve trunks. There are two generally accepted methods of infiltrating the anesthesia. One is through the skin surrounding the margin of the wound and the other is through the wound into the surrounding tissue. In either case, sufficient quantities must be infiltrated to effect anesthesia approximately ½ inch around the wound, taking care not to inject into a vein or artery.

CAUTION: The maximum recommended amount of Xylocaine to be used is 50 cc for a 1% solution or the equivalent.

General Principles of Wound Suturing

Wounds are closed either primarily or secondarily. A **primary closure** takes place within a short time of when the wound occurs, and it requires minimal cleaning and preparation. A **secondary closure**, on the other hand, occurs when there is a delay of the closure for up to several days after the wound's occurrence. A secondary closure requires a more complex procedure. Wounds 6 to 14 hours old may be closed primarily if they are not grossly contaminated and are meticulously cleaned. Wounds 14 to 24 hours old should not be closed primarily. When reddening and edema of the wound margins, discharge of pus, persistent fever, or toxemia are present, do not close the wound.

Do not use a primary closure for a large, gaping, soft-tissue wound. This type of wound will require warm dressings and irrigations, along with aseptic care for 3 to 7 days to clear up the wound. Then a secondary wound closure may be performed.

The steps to perform a delayed wound closure are outlined below.

1. Debride the wound area and convert circular wounds to elliptical ones before suturing. Circular wounds cannot be closed with satisfactory cosmetic results.

2. Try to convert a jagged laceration to one with smooth edges before suturing it. Make sure that not too much skin is trimmed off; that would make the wound difficult to approximate.

3. Use the correct technique for placing sutures. The needle holder is applied at approximately one-quarter of the distance from the blunt end of the needle. Suturing with a curved needle is done toward the person doing the suturing. Insert the needle into the skin at a 90° angle, and sweep it through in an arclike motion, following the general arc of the needle.

4. Carefully avoid bruising the skin edges being sutured. Use Adson forceps and very lightly grasp the skin edges. It is improper to use dressing forceps while suturing. Since there are no teeth on the grasping edges of the dressing forceps, the force required to hold the skin firmly may be enough to cause necrosis.

5. Do not put sutures in too tightly. Gentle approximation of the skin is all that is necessary. Remember that postoperative edema will occur in and about the wound, making sutures tighter. Figure 4-33 illustrates proper wound-closure techniques.

6. If there is a significant chance that the sutured wound may become infected (e.g., bites, delayed closure, gross contamination), place an iodoform (anti-infective) in the wound. Or place a small rubber drain in the wound, and remove the drain in 48 hours.

7. When suturing, the best cosmetic effect is obtained by using numerous interrupted simple sutures placed 1/8 inch apart. Where cosmetic result is not a consideration, sutures may be slightly farther apart. Generally, the distance of the needle bite from the wound edges should be equal to the distance between sutures.

8. When subcutaneous sutures are needed, it is proper to use 4-0 chromic catgut.

9. When deciding the type of material to use on skin, use the finest diameter that will satisfactorily hold the tissues. Table 4-4 provides guidance as to the best suture to use in selected circumstances.

10. When cutting sutures, subcutaneous catgut should have a 1/16-inch tail. Silk skin sutures should be cut as short as is practical for removal on the face and lip. Elsewhere, skin sutures may have longer tails for convenience. A tail over ¼ inch is unnecessary, however, and tends to collect exudate.

11. The following general rules can be used in deciding when to remove sutures:

    a. **Face**: As a general rule, 4 or 5 days. Better cosmetic results are obtained by removing every other suture and any suture with redness around it on the third day and the remainder on the fifth day.

b. **Body and scalp**: 7 days.

c. **Soles, palms, back, or over joints**: 10 days, unless excess tissue reaction is apparent around the suture, in which case they should come out sooner.

d. Any suture with pus or infection around it should be removed immediately, since the suture's presence will make the infection worse.

e. When wire is used, it may be left in safely for 10 to 14 days.

ORTHOPEDIC INJURIES

Many kinds of accidents cause injuries to bones, joints, or muscles. In giving first aid or emergency treatment to an injured person, you must always look for signs of fractures (broken bones), dislocations, sprains, strains, and contusions.

An essential part of the emergency treatment for fractures consists of immobilizing the injured part with splints so that the sharp ends of broken bones will not move around and cause further damage to nerves, blood vessels, or vital organs. Splints are also used to immobilize severely injured joints or muscles and to prevent the enlargement of extensive wounds. You must have a general understanding of the use of splints before going on to learn the detailed first aid treatment for injuries to bones, joints, and muscles.

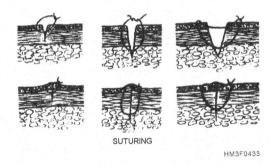

SUTURING

HM3F0433

Figure 4-33.—Suturing.

Table 4-4.—Suture Guide

Wound	Suture Material/Size
Children under 3 years	6-0
All other faces	5-0
Body	4-0
Feet, elbows, knees	#34 or #36 wire, or 4-0
Child's scalp	4-0
Adult's scalp	3-0
Lip	6-0 or 5-0

SPLINTS

LEARNING OBJECTIVE: *Recognize the different types of splints that are available, and determine how and when they should be used.*

In an emergency, almost any firm object or material will serve as a splint. Thus, umbrellas, canes, rifles, tent pegs, sticks, oars, wire mesh, boards, corrugated cardboard, and folded newspapers can be used as splints. A fractured leg may sometimes be splinted by fastening it securely to the uninjured leg. Whenever available, use manufactured splints such as pneumatic splints or traction splints.

Requirements

Splints, whether manufactured or improvised, must fulfill certain requirements. They should be lightweight, strong, fairly rigid, and long enough to reach past the joints above and below the fracture. They should be wide enough so that the bandages used to hold them in place will not pinch the injured part. Splints must be well padded on the sides touching the body; if they are not properly padded, they will not fit well and will not adequately immobilize the injured part. If you have to improvise the padding for a splint, you may use clothing, bandages, cotton, blankets, or any other soft material. If the victim is wearing heavy clothes, you may be able to apply the splint on the outside, allowing the clothing to serve as at least part of the required padding. Fasten splints in place with bandages, strips of adhesive tape, clothing, or other suitable materials. If possible, one person should hold the splints in position while another person fastens them.

Application

Although splints should be applied snugly, they should **never** be tight enough to interfere with the circulation of the blood. When you are applying splints to an arm or a leg, try to leave the fingers or toes exposed. If the tips of the fingers or toes become blue or cold, you will know that the splints or bandages are too tight. You should examine a splinted part approximately every half hour and loosen the fastenings if the circulation appears to be impaired. Remember that any injured part is likely to swell, and splints or bandages that are otherwise applied correctly may later become too tight.

MANAGEMENT OF BONE INJURIES

LEARNING OBJECTIVE: *Select the appropriate stabilization and treatment procedure for the management of bone injuries.*

A break in a bone is called a **fracture**. There are two main kinds of fractures. A **closed fracture** is one in which the injury is entirely internal; the bone is broken but there is no break in the skin. An **open fracture** is one in which there is an open wound in the tissues and the skin. Sometimes the open wound is made when a sharp end of the broken bone pushes out through the flesh; sometimes it is made by an object such as a bullet that penetrates from the outside.

Figure 4-34 shows closed and open fractures.

Open fractures are more serious than closed fractures. They usually involve extensive damage to the tissues and are quite likely to become infected. Closed fractures are sometimes turned into open fractures by rough or careless handling of the victim.

It is not always easy to recognize a fracture. All fractures, whether closed or open, are likely to cause severe pain and shock; but the other symptoms may vary considerably. A broken bone sometimes causes the injured part to be deformed or to assume an unnatural position. Pain, discoloration, and swelling may be localized at the fracture site, and there may be a

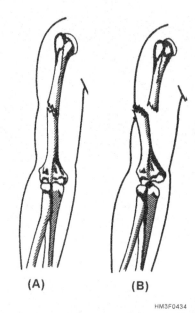

(A)   (B)

HM3F0434

Figure 4-34.—Fractures: A. Closed; B. Open.

wobbly movement if the bone is broken clear through. It may be difficult or impossible for the victim to move the injured part; if able to move it, there may be a grating sensation (crepitus) as the ends of the broken bone rub against each other. However, if a bone is cracked rather than broken through, the victim may be able to move the injured part without much difficulty. An open fracture is easy to recognize if an end of the broken bone protrudes through the flesh. If the bone does not protrude, however, you might see the external wound but fail to recognize the broken bone.

General Guidelines

If you are required to give first aid to a person who has suffered a fracture, you should follow these general guidelines:

- If there is any possibility that a fracture has been sustained, treat the injury as a fracture until an X-ray can be made.

- Get the victim to a definitive care facility at the first possible opportunity. All fractures require medical treatment.

- Do not move the victim until the injured part has been immobilized by splinting (unless the move is necessary to save life or to prevent further injury).

- Treat for shock.

- Do not attempt to locate a fracture by grating the ends of the bone together.

- Do not attempt to set a broken bone unless a medical officer will not be available for many days.

- When a long bone in the arm or leg is fractured, the limb should be carefully straightened so that splints can be applied, unless it appears that further damage will be caused by such a maneuver. Never attempt to straighten the limb by applying force or traction with any improvised device. Pulling gently with your hands along the long axis of the limb is permissible and may be all that is necessary to get the limb back into position.

- Apply splints. If the victim is to be transported only a short distance, or if treatment by a medical officer will not be delayed, it is probably best to leave the clothing on and place emergency splinting over it. However, if the victim must be transported for some distance, or if a considerable period of time will elapse before treatment by a medical officer, it may be better to remove enough clothing so that you can apply well padded splints directly to the injured part. If you decide to remove clothing over the injured part, cut the clothing or rip it along the seams. In any case, **be careful**! Rough handling of the victim may convert a closed fracture into an open fracture, increase the severity of shock, or cause extensive damage to the blood vessels, nerves, muscles, and other tissues around the broken bone.

- If the fracture is open, you must take care of the wound before you can deal with the fracture. Bleeding from the wound may be profuse, but most bleeding can be stopped by direct pressure on the wound. Other supplemental methods of hemorrhage control are discussed in the section on wounds of this chapter. Use a tourniquet as a last resort. After you have stopped the bleeding, treat the fracture.

Now that we have seen the general rules for treating fractures, we turn to the symptoms and emergency treatment of specific fracture sites.

Forearm Fracture

There are two long bones in the forearm, the radius and the ulna. When both are broken, the arm usually appears to be deformed. When only one is broken, the other acts as a splint and the arm retains a more or less natural appearance. Any fracture of the forearm is likely to result in pain, tenderness, inability to use the forearm, and a kind of wobbly motion at the point of injury. If the fracture is open, a bone will show through.

If the fracture is open, stop the bleeding and treat the wound. Apply a sterile dressing over the wound. Carefully straighten the forearm. (Remember that rough handling of a closed fracture may turn it into an open fracture.) Apply a pneumatic splint if available; if not, apply two well-padded splints to the forearm, one on the top and one on the bottom. Be sure that the splints are long enough to extend from the elbow to the wrist. Use bandages to hold the splints in place. Put the forearm across the chest. The palm of the hand should be turned in, with the thumb pointing upward. Support the forearm in this position by means of a wide sling and a cravat bandage, as shown in figure 4-35. The hand should be raised about 4 inches above the level of the elbow. Treat the victim for shock and evacuate as soon as possible.

Upper Arm Fracture

The signs of fracture of the upper arm include pain, tenderness, swelling, and a wobbly motion at the point

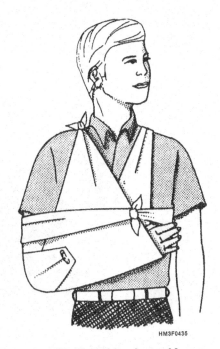

HM3F0435

Figure 4-35.—First aid for a fractured forearm.

of fracture. If the fracture is near the elbow, the arm is likely to be straight with no bend at the elbow.

If the fracture is open, stop the bleeding and treat the wound before attempting to treat the fracture.

NOTE: Treatment of the fracture depends partly upon the location of the break.

If the fracture is in the upper part of the arm near the shoulder, place a pad or folded towel in the armpit, bandage the arm securely to the body, and support the forearm in a narrow sling.

If the fracture is in the middle of the upper arm, you can use one well-padded splint on the outside of the arm. The splint should extend from the shoulder to the elbow. Fasten the splinted arm firmly to the body and support the forearm in a narrow sling, as shown in figure 4-36.

Another way of treating a fracture in the middle of the upper arm is to fasten two wide splints (or four narrow ones) about the arm and then support the forearm in a narrow sling. If you use a splint between the arm and the body, be very careful that it does not extend too far up into the armpit; a splint in this position can cause a dangerous compression of the blood vessels and nerves and may be extremely painful to the victim.

If the fracture is at or near the elbow, the arm may be either bent or straight. No matter in what position you find the arm, **DO NOT ATTEMPT TO STRAIGHTEN IT OR MOVE IT IN ANY WAY**. Splint the arm as carefully as possible in the position in

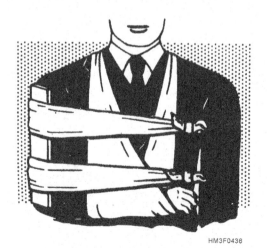

HM3F0436

Figure 4-36.—Splint and sling for a fractured upper arm.

which you find it. This will prevent further nerve and blood vessel damage. The only exception to this is if there is no pulse distal to the fracture, in which case gentle traction is applied and then the arm is splinted. Treat the victim for shock and get him under the care of a medical officer as soon as possible.

Thigh Fracture

The femur is the long bone of the upper part of the leg between the kneecap and the pelvis. When the femur is fractured through, any attempt to move the limb results in a spasm of the muscles and causes excruciating pain. The leg has a wobbly motion, and there is complete loss of control below the fracture. The limb usually assumes an unnatural position, with the toes pointing outward. By actual measurement, the fractured leg is shorter than the uninjured one because of contraction of the powerful thigh muscles. Serious damage to blood vessels and nerves often results from a fracture of the femur, and shock is likely to be severe.

If the fracture is open, stop the bleeding and treat the wound before attempting to treat the fracture itself. Serious bleeding is a special danger in this type of injury, since the broken bone may tear or cut the large artery in the thigh.

Carefully straighten the leg. Apply two splints, one on the outside of the injured leg and one on the inside. The outside splint should reach from the armpit to the foot. The inside splint should reach from the crotch to the foot. The splints should be fastened in five places: (1) around the ankle; (2) over the knee; (3) just below the hip; (4) around the pelvis; and (5) just below the armpit (fig. 4-37). The legs can then be tied together to support the injured leg as firmly as possible.

It is essential that a fractured thigh be splinted before the victim is moved. Manufactured splints, such as the Hare or the Thomas half-ring traction splints, are best, but improvised splints may be used. Figure 4-37 shows how boards may be used as an emergency splint for a fractured thigh. Remember, **DO NOT MOVE THE VICTIM UNTIL THE INJURED LEG HAS BEEN IMMOBILIZED**. Treat the victim for shock, and evacuate at the earliest possible opportunity.

Lower Leg Fracture

When both bones of the lower leg are broken, the usual signs of fracture are likely to be present. When only one bone is broken, the other one acts as a splint and, to some extent, prevents deformity of the leg. However, tenderness, swelling, and pain at the point of

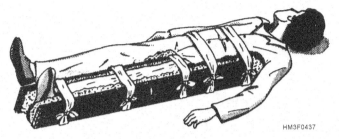

Figure 4-37.—Splint for a fractured femur.

fracture are almost always present. A fracture just above the ankle is often mistaken for a sprain. If both bones of the lower leg are broken, an open fracture is very likely to result.

If the fracture is open, stop the bleeding and treat the wound. Carefully straighten the injured leg. Apply a pneumatic splint if available; if not, apply **three** splints, one on each side of the leg and one underneath. Be sure that the splints are well padded, particularly under the knee and at the bones on each side of the ankle.

A pillow and two side splints work very well for treatment of a fractured lower leg. Place the pillow beside the injured leg, then carefully lift the leg and place it in the middle of the pillow. Bring the edges of the pillow around to the front of the leg and pin them together. Then place one splint on each side of the leg (over the pillow), and fasten them in place with strips of bandage or adhesive tape. Treat the victim for shock and evacuate as soon as possible. When available, you may use the Hare or Thomas half-ring traction splints.

Kneecap Fracture

The following first aid treatment should be given for a fractured kneecap (patella):

Carefully straighten the injured limb. Immobilize the fracture by placing a padded board under the injured limb. The board should be at least 4 inches wide and should reach from the buttock to the heel. Place extra padding under the knee and just above the heel, as shown in figure 4-38. Use strips of bandage to fasten the leg to the board in four places: (1) just below the knee; (2) just above the knee; (3) at the ankle; and (4) at the thigh. **Do not cover the knee itself.** Swelling is likely to occur very rapidly, and any bandage or tie fastened over the knee would quickly become too tight. Treat the victim for shock and evacuate as soon as possible.

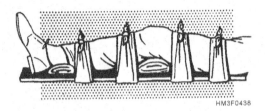

Figure 4-38.—Immobilization of a fractured patella.

Clavicle Fracture

A person with a fractured clavicle usually shows definite symptoms. When the victim stands, the injured shoulder is lower than the uninjured one. The victim is usually unable to raise the arm above the level of the shoulder and may attempt to support the injured shoulder by holding the elbow of that side in the other hand. This is the characteristic position of a person with a broken clavicle. Since the clavicle lies immediately under the skin, you may be able to detect the point of fracture by the deformity and localized pain and tenderness.

If the fracture is open, stop the flow of blood and treat the wound before attempting to treat the fracture. Then apply a sling and swathe splint as described below (and illustrated in figure 4-39).

Bend the victim's arm on the injured side, and place the forearm across the chest. The palm of the hand should be turned in, with the thumb pointed up. The hand should be raised about 4 inches above the level of the elbow. Support the forearm in this position by means of a wide sling. A wide roller bandage (or any wide strip of cloth) may be used to secure the victim's arm to the body (see figure 4-35). A figure-eight bandage may also be used for a fractured clavicle. Treat the victim for shock and evacuate to a definitive care facility as soon as possible.

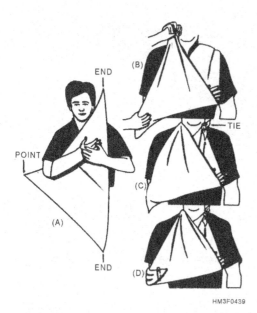

Figure 4-39.—Sling for immobilizing fractured clavicle.

Rib Fracture

If a rib is broken, make the victim comfortable and quiet so that the greatest danger—the possibility of further damage to the lungs, heart, or chest wall by the broken ends—is minimized.

The common finding in all victims with fractured ribs is pain localized at the site of the fracture. By asking the patient to point out the exact area of the pain, you can often determine the location of the injury. There may or may not be a rib deformity, chest wall contusion, or laceration of the area. Deep breathing, coughing, or movement is usually painful. The patient generally wishes to remain still and may often lean toward the injured side, with a hand over the fractured area to immobilize the chest and to ease the pain.

Ordinarily, rib fractures are **not** bound, strapped, or taped if the victim is reasonably comfortable. However, they may be splinted by the use of external support. If the patient is considerably more comfortable with the chest immobilized, the best method is to use a swathe (fig. 4-40) in which the arm on the injured side is strapped to the chest to limit motion. Place the arm on the injured side against the chest, with the palm flat, thumb up, and the forearm

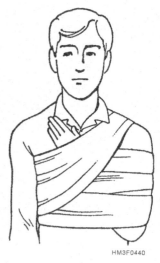

Figure 4-40.—Swathe bandage of fractured rib victim.

raised to a 45° angle. Immobilize the chest, using wide strips of bandage to secure the arm to the chest.

Do not use wide strips of adhesive plaster applied directly to the skin of the chest for immobilization since the adhesive tends to limit the ability of the chest to expand (interfering with proper breathing). Treat the victim for shock and evacuate as soon as possible.

Nose Fracture

A fracture of the nose usually causes localized pain and swelling, a noticeable deformity of the nose, and extensive nosebleed.

Stop the nosebleed. Have the victim sit quietly, with the head tipped slightly backward. Tell the victim to breathe through the mouth and not to blow the nose. If the bleeding does not stop within a few minutes, apply a cold compress or an ice bag over the nose.

Treat the victim for shock. Ensure the victim receives a medical officer's attention as soon as possible. Permanent deformity of the nose may result if the fracture is not treated promptly.

Jaw Fracture

A person who has a fractured jaw may suffer serious interference with breathing. There is likely to be great difficulty in talking, chewing, or swallowing. Any movement of the jaw causes pain. The teeth may be out of line, and there may be bleeding from the gums. Considerable swelling may develop.

One of the most important phases of emergency care is to clear the upper respiratory passage of any obstruction. If the fractured jaw interferes with breathing, pull the lower jaw and the tongue well **forward** and keep them in that position.

Apply a four-tailed bandage, as shown in figure 4-41. Be sure that the bandage pulls the lower jaw **forward**. Never apply a bandage that forces the jaw backward, since this might seriously interfere with breathing. The bandage must be firm so that it will support and immobilize the injured jaw, but it must not press against the victim's throat. Be sure that the victim has scissors or a knife to cut the bandage in case of vomiting. Treat the victim for shock and evacuate as soon as possible.

Skull Fracture

When a person suffers a head injury, the greatest danger is that the brain may be severely damaged; whether or not the skull is fractured is a matter of secondary importance. In some cases, injuries that fracture the skull do not cause serious brain damage; but brain damage can—and frequently does—result from apparently slight injuries that do not cause damage to the skull itself.

It is often difficult to determine whether an injury has affected the brain because the symptoms of brain damage vary greatly. A person suffering from a head injury must be handled very carefully and given immediate medical attention.

Some of the symptoms that may indicate brain damage are listed below. However, you must remember that all of these symptoms are not always present in any one case and that the symptoms that do occur may be greatly delayed.

- Bruises or wounds of the scalp may indicate that the victim has sustained a blow to the head. Sometimes the skull is depressed (caved in) at the point of impact. If the fracture is open, you may find glass, shrapnel, or other objects penetrating the skull.

- The victim may be conscious or unconscious. If conscious, the victim may feel dizzy and weak, as though about to faint.

- Severe headache sometimes (but not always) accompanies head injuries.

- The pupils of the eyes may be unequal in size and may not react normally to light.

- There may be bleeding from the ears, nose, or mouth.

- The victim may vomit.

- The victim may be restless and perhaps confused and disoriented.

- The arms, legs, face, or other parts of the body may be partially paralyzed.

- The victim's face may be very pale, or it may be unusually flushed.

- The victim is likely to be suffering from shock, but the symptoms of shock may be disguised by other symptoms.

It is not necessary to determine if the skull is fractured when you are giving first aid to a person who has suffered a head injury. The treatment is the same in either case, and the primary intent is to prevent further damage to the brain.

Keep the victim lying down. If the face is flushed, raise the head and shoulders slightly. If the face is pale, have the victim lie so that the head is level with, or slightly lower than, the body. Watch carefully for vomiting. If the victim begins to vomit, position the head to prevent choking on the vomitus.

If there is serious bleeding from the wounds, try to control that bleeding by the application of direct pressure, using caution to avoid further injury to the skull or brain. Use a donut-shaped bandage to gently surround protruding objects. Never manipulate those objects.

- Be very careful about moving or handling the victim. Move the victim no more than is

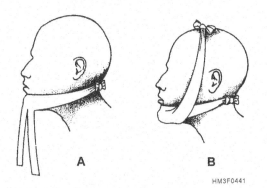

A   B

HM3F0441

Figure 4-41.—Four-tailed bandage for the jaw.

necessary. If transportation is necessary, keep the victim lying down.

- In any significant head or facial injury, assume injury to the cervical spine. Immobilization of the cervical spine is indicated.

- Be sure that the victim is kept comfortably warm, but not too warm.

- **Do not** give the victim anything to drink. **DO NOT GIVE ANY MEDICATIONS**. See that the victim receives a medical officer's attention as soon as possible.

Spinal Fractures

If the spine is fractured at any point, the spinal cord may be crushed, cut, or otherwise damaged so severely that death or paralysis will result. However, if the fracture occurs in such a way that the spinal cord is not seriously damaged, there is a very good chance of complete recovery, **provided** that the victim is properly cared for. Any twisting or bending of the neck or back—whether due to the original injury or carelessness from handling later—is likely to cause irreparable damage to the spinal cord.

The primary symptoms of a fractured spine are pain, shock, and paralysis. **Pain** is likely to be acute at the point of fracture. It may radiate to other parts of the body. **Shock** is usually severe, but (as in all injuries) the symptoms may be delayed for some time. **Paralysis** occurs if the spinal cord is seriously damaged. If the victim cannot move the legs, feet, or toes, the fracture is probably in the back; if the fingers will not move, the neck is probably broken. Remember that a spinal fracture does not always injure the spinal cord, so the victim is not always paralyzed. Any person who has an acute pain in the back or the neck following an injury should be treated as though there is a fractured spine, even if there are no other symptoms.

Emergency treatment for all spinal fractures, whether of the neck or of the back, has two primary purposes: (1) to minimize shock, and (2) to prevent further injury to the spinal cord. Keep the victim comfortably warm. Do not attempt to keep the victim in the position ordinarily used for the treatment of shock, because it might cause further damage to the spinal cord. Just keep the victim lying flat and do **NOT** attempt to lower the head.

To avoid further damage to the spinal cord, **DO NOT MOVE THE VICTIM UNLESS IT IS ABSOLUTELY ESSENTIAL!** If the victim's life is threatened in the present location or transportation is necessary to receive medical attention, then, of course, you must move the victim. However, if movement is necessary, be sure that you do it in a way that will cause the least possible damage. **DO NOT BEND OR TWIST THE VICTIM'S BODY, DO NOT MOVE THE HEAD FORWARD, BACKWARD, OR SIDEWAYS, AND DO NOT UNDER ANY CIRCUMSTANCES ALLOW THE VICTIM TO SIT UP**.

If it is necessary to transport a person who has suffered a fracture of the spine, follow these general rules:

- If the spine is broken at the **neck**, the victim must be transported lying on the back, **face up.** Place pillows or sandbags beside the head so that it cannot turn to either side. **DO NOT** put pillows or padding under the neck or head.

- If you suspect that the spine is fractured but do not know the location of the break, treat the victim as though the neck is broken (i.e., keep the victim supine). If both the neck and the back are broken, keep the victim supine.

- No matter where the spine is broken, **use a firm support in transporting the victim.** Use a rigid stretcher, or a door, shutter, wide board, etc. Pad the support carefully, and put blankets both under and over the victim. Use cravat bandages or strips of cloth to secure the victim firmly to the support.

- When placing the victim on a spineboard, one of two acceptable methods may be used. However, **DO NOT ATTEMPT TO LIFT THE VICTIM UNLESS YOU HAVE ADEQUATE ASSISTANCE**. Remember: Any bending or twisting of the body is almost sure to cause serious damage to the spinal cord. Figure 4-42 shows the straddle-slide method. One person lifts and supports the head while two other persons each lift at the shoulders and hips, respectively. A fourth person slides the spineboard under the patient. Figure 4-43 shows the proper procedure in performing the log-roll method. The victim is rolled as a single unit towards the rescuers, the spineboard is positioned, and the victim is rolled back onto the spineboard and secured in place. If there are at least four (preferably six) people present to help lift the victim, they can accomplish the job without too much movement of the victim's

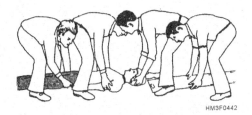

Figure 4-42.—Straddle-slide method of moving spinal cord injury victim onto a backboard.

body. **NEVER** attempt to lift the victim, however, with fewer than four people.

• Evacuate the victim very carefully.

Pelvic Fracture

Fractures in the pelvic region often result from falls, heavy blows, and accidents that involve crushing. The great danger in a pelvic fracture is that the organs enclosed and protected by the pelvis may be seriously damaged when the bony structure is fractured. In particular, there is danger that the bladder will be ruptured. There is also danger of severe internal bleeding; the large blood vessels in the pelvic region may be torn or cut by fragments of the broken bone.

The primary symptoms of a fractured pelvis are severe pain, shock, and loss of ability to use the lower part of the body. The victim is unable to sit or stand. If the victim is conscious, there may be a sensation of "coming apart." If the bladder is injured, the victim's urine may be bloody.

Do not move the victim unless ABSOLUTELY necessary. The victim should be treated for shock and

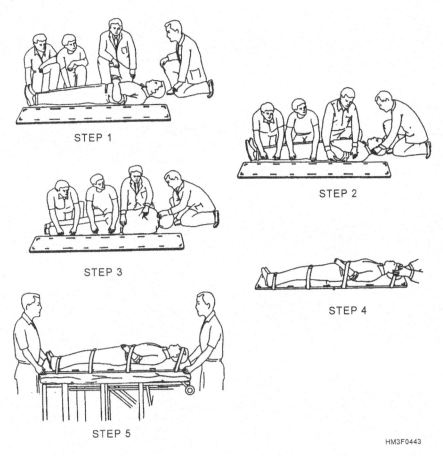

Figure 4-43.—Log-roll method of moving spinal cord injury victim onto a backboard.

4-53

kept warm but should not be moved into the position ordinarily used for the treatment of shock.

If you must transport the victim to another place, do it with the utmost care. Use a rigid stretcher, a padded door, or a wide board. Keep the victim supine. In some cases, the victim will be more comfortable if the legs are straight, while in other cases the victim will be more comfortable with the knees bent and the legs drawn up. When you have placed the victim in the most comfortable position, immobilization should be accomplished. Fractures of the hip are best treated with traction splints. Adequate immobilization can also be obtained by placing pillows or folded blankets between the legs as shown in figure 4-44 and using cravats, roller bandages, or straps to hold the legs together, or through the use of MAST garments. Fasten the victim securely to the stretcher or improvised support, and evacuate very carefully.

MANAGEMENT OF JOINT AND MUSCLE INJURIES

LEARNING OBJECTIVE: *Select the appropriate stabilization and treatment procedure for the management of joint and muscle injuries.*

Injuries to joints and muscles often occur together, and it is sometimes difficult to tell whether the primary injury is to a joint or to the muscles, tendons, blood vessels, or nerves near the joint. Sometimes it is difficult to distinguish joint or muscle injuries from fractures. In case of doubt, **always** treat any injury to a bone, joint, or muscle as though it were a fracture.

In general, joint and muscle injuries may be classified under four headings: (1) dislocations, (2) sprains, (3) strains, and (4) contusions (bruises).

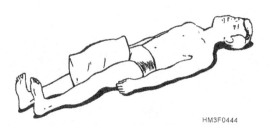

HM3F0444

Figure 4-44.—Immobilizing a fractured pelvis.

Dislocations

When a bone is forcibly displaced from its joint, the injury is known as a **dislocation**. In some cases, the bone slips back quickly into its normal position, but at other times it becomes locked in the new position and remains dislocated until it is put back into place. Dislocations are usually caused by falls or blows but occasionally by violent muscular exertion. The most frequently dislocated joints are those of the shoulder, hip, fingers, and jaw.

A dislocation is likely to bruise or tear the muscles, ligaments, blood vessels, tendons, and nerves near a joint. Rapid swelling and discoloration, loss of ability to use the joint, severe pain and muscle spasms, possible numbness and loss of pulse below the joint, and shock are characteristic symptoms of dislocations. The fact that the injured part is usually stiff and immobile, with marked deformation at the joint, will help you distinguish a dislocation from a fracture. In a fracture, there is deformity **between** joints rather than **at** joints, and there is generally a wobbly motion of the broken bone at the point of fracture.

As a general rule, you should **not** attempt to reduce a dislocation—that is, put a dislocated bone back into place—unless you know that a medical officer cannot be reached within 8 hours. Unskilled attempts at reduction may cause great damage to nerves and blood vessels or actually fracture the bone. Therefore, except in great emergencies, you should leave this treatment to specially trained medical personnel and concentrate your efforts on making the victim as comfortable as possible under the circumstances.

The following emergency measures will be helpful:

1. Loosen the clothing around the injured part.

2. Place the victim in the most comfortable position possible.

3. Support the injured part by means of a sling, pillows, bandages, splints, or any other device that will make the victim comfortable.

4. Treat the victim for shock.

5. Get medical help as soon as possible.

You should **NEVER** attempt to reduce the more serious dislocations, such as those of the hip. However, if it is probable that the victim cannot be treated by a medical officer within a **reasonable time**, you should make a careful effort to reduce certain dislocations (such as those of the jaw, finger, or shoulder) if there is no arterial or nerve involvement (pulse will be palpable and there will be no numbness below the joint). Treat all other dislocations as fractures, and evacuate the victim to a definitive care facility.

DISLOCATION OF THE JAW.—When the lower jaw is dislocated, the victim cannot speak or close the mouth. Dislocation of the jaw is usually caused by a blow to the mouth; sometimes it is caused by yawning or laughing. This type of dislocation is not always easy to reduce, and there is considerable danger that the operator's thumbs will be bitten in the process. For your own protection, wrap your thumbs with a handkerchief or bandage. While facing the victim, press your thumbs down just behind the last lower molars and, at the same time, lift the chin up with your fingers. The jaw should snap into place at once. You will have to remove your thumbs quickly to avoid being bitten. No further treatment is required, but you should warn the victim to keep the mouth closed as much as possible during the next few hours. Figure 4-45 shows the position you must assume to reduce a dislocated jaw.

DISLOCATION OF THE FINGER.—The joints of the finger are particularly susceptible to injury, and even minor injuries may result in prolonged loss of function. Great care must be used in treating any injury of the finger.

To reduce a dislocation of the finger, grasp the finger firmly and apply a steady pull in the same line as the deformity. If it does not slip into position, try it again, but if it does not go into position on the third attempt, **DO NOT TRY AGAIN**. In any case, and whether or not the dislocation is reduced, the finger should be strapped, slightly flexed, with an aluminum splint or with a roller gauze bandage over a tongue blade. Figure 4-46 shows how a dislocated finger can be immobilized by strapping it to a flat, wooden stick, such as a tongue depressor.

DISLOCATION OF THE SHOULDER.—Before reduction, place the victim in a supine position. After putting the heel of your foot in the victim's armpit, grasp the wrist and apply steady traction by pulling gently and increasing resistance gradually. Pull the arm in the same line as it is found. After several minutes of steady pull, flex the victim's elbow slightly. Grasp the arm below the elbow, apply traction from the point of the elbow, and gently rotate the arm into the external or outward position. If three reduction attempts fail, carry the forearm across the chest and apply a sling and swathe. An alternate method involves having the patient lie face down on an examining table with the injured arm hanging over the side. Apply prolonged, firm, gentle traction at the wrist with gentle external rotation. A water bucket with a padded handle placed in the crook of the patient's elbow may be substituted. Gradually add sand or water to the bucket to increase traction. Grasping the wrist and using the elbow as a pivot point, gently rotate the arm into the external position.

Sprains

Sprains are injuries to the ligaments and soft tissues that support a joint. A sprain is caused by the violent wrenching or twisting of the joint beyond its normal limits of movement and usually involves a momentary dislocation, with the bone slipping back into place of its own accord. Although any joint may

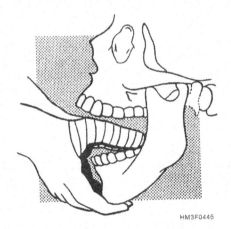

HM3F0445

Figure 4-45.—Position for reducing a dislocated jaw.

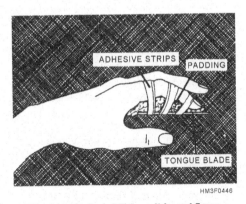

HM3F0446

Figure 4-46.—Immobilizing a dislocated finger.

be sprained, sprains of the ankle, wrist, knee, and finger are most common.

Symptoms of a sprain include pain or pressure at the joint, pain upon movement, swelling and tenderness, possible loss of movement, and discoloration. Treat all sprains as fractures until ruled out by X-rays.

Emergency care for a sprain includes application of cold packs for the first 24 to 48 hours to reduce swelling and to control internal hemorrhage; elevation and rest of the affected area; application of a snug, smooth, figure-eight bandage to control swelling and to provide immobilization (basket weave adhesive bandages can be used on the ankle); a follow-up examination by a medical officer; and X-rays to rule out the presence of a fracture.

NOTE: Check bandaged areas regularly for swelling that might cause circulation impairment and loosen bandages if necessary.

After the swelling stops (24 to 48 hours), moist heat can be applied for short periods (15 to 30 minutes) to promote healing and reduce swelling. Moist heat can be warm, wet compresses, warm whirlpool baths, etc.

CAUTION: Heat should not be applied until 24 hours after the last cold pack.

Strains

Injuries caused by the forcible overstretching or tearing of muscles or tendons are known as **strains**. Strains may be caused by lifting excessively heavy loads, sudden or violent movements, or any other action that pulls the muscles beyond their normal limits.

The chief symptoms of a strain are pain, lameness or stiffness (sometimes involving knotting of the muscles), moderate swelling at the place of injury, discoloration due to the escape of blood from injured blood vessels into the tissues, possible loss of power, and a distinct gap felt at the site.

Keep the affected area elevated and at rest. Apply cold packs for the first 24 to 48 hours to control hemorrhage and swelling. After the swelling stops, apply mild heat to increase circulation and aid in healing. As in sprains, heat should not be applied until 24 hours after the last cold pack. Muscle relaxants, adhesive straps, and complete immobilization of the area may be indicated. Evacuate the victim to a medical facility where X-rays can be taken to rule out the presence of a fracture.

Contusions

Contusions, commonly called bruises, are responsible for the discoloration that almost always accompanies injuries to bones, joints, and muscles. Contusions are caused by blows that damage bones, muscles, tendons, blood vessels, nerves, and other body tissues. They do not necessarily break the skin.

The symptoms of a contusion or bruise are familiar to everyone. There is immediate pain when the blow is received. Swelling occurs because blood from the broken vessels leaks into the soft tissue under the skin. At first the injured place is reddened due to local skin irritation from the blow. Later the characteristic "black and blue" marks appear. Perhaps several days later, the skin turns yellowish or greenish before normal coloration returns. The bruised area is usually very tender.

As a rule, slight bruises do not require treatment. However, if the victim has severe bruises, treat for shock. Immobilize the injured part, keep it at rest, and protect it from further injury. Sometimes the victim will be more comfortable if the bruised area is bandaged firmly with an elastic or gauze bandage. If possible, elevate the injured part. A sling may be used for a bruised arm or hand. Pillows or folded blankets may be used to elevate a bruised leg.

ENVIRONMENTAL INJURIES

LEARNING OBJECTIVE: *Recall the classification and evaluation process for burns, and determine the appropriate treatment for each type of burn.*

Under the broad category of environmental injuries, we will consider a number of emergency problems. Exposure to extremes of temperature, whether heat or cold, causes injury to skin, tissues, blood vessels, vital organs, and, in some cases, the whole body. In addition, contact with the sun's rays, electrical current, or certain chemicals causes injuries similar in character to burns.

THERMAL BURNS

True burns are generated by exposure to extreme heat that overwhelms the body's defensive mechanisms. Burns and scalds are essentially the same injury: Burns are caused by dry heat, and scalds are caused by moist heat. The seriousness of the injury can be estimated by the depth, extent, and location of the burn, the age and health of the victim, and other medical complications.

Classification of Severity

Burns are classified according to their depth as first-, second-, and third-degree burns (as shown in figure 4-47).

FIRST-DEGREE BURN.—With a first-degree burn, the epidermal layer is irritated, reddened, and tingling. The skin is sensitive to touch and blanches with pressure. Pain is mild to severe, edema is minimal, and healing usually occurs naturally within a week.

SECOND-DEGREE BURN.—A second-degree burn is characterized by epidermal blisters, mottled appearance, and a red base. Damage extends into—but not through—the dermis. Recovery usually takes 2 to 3 weeks, with some scarring and depigmentation. This condition is painful. Body fluids may be drawn into the injured tissue, causing edema and possibly a "weeping" fluid (plasma) loss at the surface.

THIRD-DEGREE BURN.—A third-degree burn is a full-thickness injury penetrating into muscle and fatty connective tissues, or even down to the bone. Tissues and nerves are destroyed. Shock, with blood in the urine, is likely to be present. Pain will be absent at the burn site if all the area nerve endings are destroyed, and the surrounding tissue (which is less damaged)

will be painful. Tissue color will range from white (scalds) to black (charring burns). Although the wound is usually dry, body fluids will collect in the underlying tissue. If the area has not been completely cauterized, significant amounts of fluids will be lost by plasma "weeping" or by hemorrhage, thus reducing circulation volume. There is considerable scarring and possible loss of function. Skin grafts may be necessary.

Rule of Nines

Of greater importance than the depth of the burn in evaluating the seriousness of the condition is the extent of the burned area. A first-degree burn over 50 percent of the body surface area (BSA) may be more serious than a third-degree burn over 3 percent. The **Rule of Nines** is used to give a rough estimate of the surface area affected. Figure 4-48 shows how the rule is applied to adults.

Other Factors

A third factor in burn evaluation is the location of the burn. Serious burns of the head, hands, feet, or genitals will require hospitalization.

The fourth factor is the presence of any other complications, especially respiratory tract injuries or other major injuries or factors.

FIRST DEGREE
PARTIAL THICKNESS

SECOND DEGREE
PARTIAL THICKNESS

THIRD DEGREE
FULL THICKNESS

EPIDERMIS

DERMIS

FAT

MUSCLE

SKIN REDDENED   BLISTERS   CHARRING   HM3f0447

Figure 4-47.—Classification of burns.

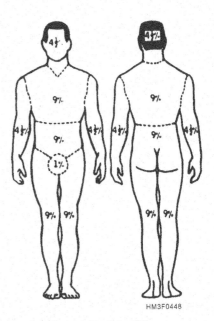

HM3F0448

Figure 4-48.—Rule of Nines.

The Corpsman must take all these factors into consideration when evaluating the condition of the burn victim, especially in a triage situation.

First Aid

After the victim has been removed from the source of the thermal injury, first aid should be kept to a minimum.

- Maintain an open airway.

- Control hemorrhage, and treat for shock.

- Remove constricting jewelry and articles of clothing.

- Protect the burn area from contamination by covering it with clean sheets or dry dressings. **DO NOT** remove clothing adhering to a wound.

- Splint fractures.

- For all serious and extensive burns (over 20 percent BSA), and in the presence of shock, start intravenous therapy with an electrolyte solution (Ringer's lactate) in an unburned area.

- Maintain intravenous treatment during transportation.

- Relieve mild pain with aspirin. Relieve moderate pain with cool, wet compresses or ice water immersion (for burns of less than 20 percent BSA). Severe pain may be relieved with morphine or demerol injections. Pain resulting from small burns may be relieved with an anesthetic ointment if the skin is not broken.

Aid Station Care

Once the victim has arrived at the aid station, observe the following procedures.

- Continue to monitor for airway patency, hemorrhage, and shock.

- Continue intravenous therapy that is in place, or start a new one under a medical officer's supervision to control shock and replace fluid loss.

- Monitor urine output.

- Shave body hair well back from the burned area, and then cleanse the area gently with disinfectant soap and warm water. Remove dirt, grease, and nonviable tissue. Apply a sterile dressing of dry gauze. Place bulky dressings around the burned parts to absorb serous exudate.

- All major burn victims should be given a booster dose of tetanus toxoid to guard against infection. Administration of antibiotics may be directed by a medical officer or an Independent Duty Corpsman.

- If evacuation to a definitive care facility will be delayed for 2 to 3 days, start topical antibiotic therapy after the patient stabilizes and following debridement and wound care. Gently spread a 1/16-inch thickness of Sulfamylon® or Silvadene® over the burn area. Repeat the application after 12 hours, and then after daily debridement. Treat minor skin reactions with antihistamines.

SUNBURN

Sunburn results from prolonged exposure to the ultraviolet rays of the sun. First- and second-degree burns similar to thermal burns result. Treatment is essentially the same as that outlined for thermal burns. Unless a major percentage of the body surface is affected, the victim will not require more than first aid attention. Commercially prepared sunburn lotions and ointments may be used. Prevention through education and the proper use of sun screens is the best way to avoid this condition.

ELECTRICAL BURNS

Electrical burns may be far more serious than a preliminary examination may indicate. The entrance and exit wounds may be small, but as electricity penetrates the skin it burns a large area below the surface, as indicated in figure 4-49. A Corpsman can do little for these victims other than monitoring the basic life functions, delivering CPR, treating for shock if necessary, covering the entrance and exit wounds with a dry, sterile dressing, and transporting the victim to a medical treatment facility.

Before treatment is started, ensure that the victim is no longer in contact with a live electrical source. Shut the power off or use a nonconducting rope or stick to move the victim away from the line or the line away from the victim. See figure 3-26.

CHEMICAL BURNS

When acids, alkalies, or other chemicals come in contact with the skin or other body membranes, they

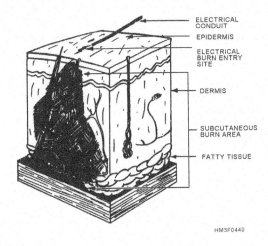

ELECTRICAL
CONDUIT

EPIDERMIS

ELECTRICAL
BURN ENTRY
SITE

DERMIS

SUBCUTANEOUS
BURN AREA

FATTY TISSUE

HM3F0449

Figure 4-49.—Electrical burns.

may cause injuries that are generally referred to as chemical burns. For the most part, these injuries are not caused by heat but by direct chemical destruction of body tissues. Areas most often affected are the extremities, mouth, and eyes. Alkali burns are usually more serious than acid burns because alkalies penetrate deeper and burn longer.

When such burns occur, the following emergency procedures must be carried out immediately:

1. Quickly flush the area with large amounts of water, using a shower or hose, if available. Do not apply water too forcefully. Flood the area while the clothing (including shoes and socks) is being removed and continue often removal.

NOTE: There are two exceptions to the above: (1) In alkali burns caused by dry lime, the mixing of water and lime creates a very corrosive substance. Dry lime should be **brushed** away from the skin and clothing, unless large amounts of water are available for rapid and complete flushing. (2) In acid burns caused by phenol (carbolic acid), wash the affected area with alcohol because phenol is not water soluble; then wash with water. If alcohol is not available, flushing with water is better than no treatment at all.

2. After thorough washing, neutralize any chemical remaining on the affected area.

WARNING: DO NOT attempt to neutralize a chemical unless you know exactly what it is and what substance will neutralize it. Further damage may be done by a neutralizing agent that is too strong or incorrect.

For acid burns, make a solution of 1 teaspoon of baking soda to a pint of water and flush it over the affected area. For alkali burns, mix 1 or 2 teaspoons of vinegar to a pint of water and flush it over the affected area.

3. Flush the area again with water and gently pat dry with a sterile gauze. Do not rub the area.

4. Transport the victim to a medical treatment facility.

When treating chemical burns to the eye, the one and only emergency treatment is to flush the eye(s) immediately with large amounts of water or a sterile saline solution. Irrigate acid burns to the eyes for at least 5 to 10 minutes with at least 2000 ml of water. Irrigate alkali burns to the eyes for at least 20 minutes. Because of the intense pain, the victim may be unable to open the eyes. If this occurs, hold the eyelids apart so that water can flow across the eye.

A drinking fountain or field "water buffalo" may be used to supply a steady stream of water. Hold the victim's head in a position that allows water to flow from the inside corner of the eye toward the outside. Do not allow the water to fall directly on the eye, and do not use greater force than is necessary to keep the water flowing across the eye.

CAUTION: Never use any chemical antidotes such as baking soda or alcohol in treating burns of the eye, and do not try to neutralize chemical agents.

After thorough irrigation, loosely cover both eyes with a clean dressing. This prevents further damage by decreasing eye movement.

The aftercare for all chemical burns is similar to that for thermal burns: Cover the affected area and get the victim to a medical treatment facility as soon as possible.

WHITE PHOSPHORUS BURNS

A special category of burns that may affect military personnel in a wartime or training situation is that caused by exposure of white phosphorus (WP or Willy Peter). First aid for this type of burn is complicated by the fact that white phosphorus particles ignite upon contact with air.

Superficial burns caused by simple skin contact or burning clothes should be flushed with water and treated like thermal burns. Partially embedded white phosphorus particles must be continuously flushed with water while the first aid provider removes them with whatever tools are available (i.e., tweezers, pliers, forceps). Do this quickly, but gently. Firmly or deeply embedded particles that cannot be removed by the first aid provider must be covered with a saline-soaked dressing, and this dressing must be kept wet until the victim reaches a medical treatment facility. The wounds containing embedded phosphorus particles may then be rinsed with a dilute, freshly mixed 1% solution of copper sulfate. This solution combines with phosphorus on the surface of the particles to form a blue-black cupric phosphite covering, which both impedes further oxidation and facilitates identification of retained particles. **Under no circumstances** should the copper sulfate solution be applied as a wet dressing. Wounds must be flushed thoroughly with a saline solution following the copper sulfate rinse to prevent absorption of excessive amounts of copper. (Copper has been associated with extensive intravascular hemolysis.) An adjunct to the management of phosphorus burn injuries is the identification of the retained phosphorescent particles in a darkened room during debridement.

> **NOTE**: Combustion of white phosphorus results in the formation of a severe pulmonary irritant. The ignition of phosphorus in a closed space (such as the BAS tent or sickbay) may result in the development of irritant concentrations sufficient to cause acute inflammatory changes in the tracheobronchial tree. The effects of this gas, especially during debridement, can be minimized by placing a moist cloth over the nose and mouth to inactivate the gas and by ventilating the tent.

HEAT EXPOSURE INJURIES

> **LEARNING OBJECTIVE:** *Identify the signs, symptoms, and emergency treatment of heat cramps, heat exhaustion, and heat stroke.*

Excessive heat affects the body in a variety of ways. When a person exercises or works in a hot environment, heat builds up inside the body. The body automatically reacts to get rid of this heat through the sweating mechanism. This depletes water and electrolytes from the circulating volume. If they are not adequately replaced, body functions are affected, and, initially, heat cramps and heat exhaustion develop. If the body becomes too overheated or water or electrolytes too depleted, the sweat-control mechanism of the body malfunctions and shuts down. The result is heat stroke (sunstroke). Heat exposure injuries are a threat in any hot environment, but especially in desert or tropical areas and in the boiler rooms of ships. Under normal conditions, it is a preventable injury. Individual and command awareness of the causes of heat stress problems should help eliminate heat exposure injuries.

Heat Cramps

Excessive sweating may result in painful cramps in the muscles of the abdomen, legs, and arms. Heat cramps may also result from drinking ice water or other cold drinks either too quickly or in too large a quantity after exercise. Muscle cramps are often an early sign of approaching heat exhaustion.

To provide first aid treatment for heat cramps, move the victim to a cool place. Since heat cramps are caused by loss of salt and water, give the victim plenty of cool (not cold) water to drink, adding about one teaspoon of salt to a liter or quart of water. Apply manual pressure to the cramped muscle, or gently massage it to relieve the spasm. If there are indications of anything more serious, transport the victim immediately to a medical treatment facility.

Heat Exhaustion

Heat exhaustion (heat prostration or heat collapse) is the most common condition caused by working or exercising in hot environments. In heat exhaustion, there is a serious disturbance of blood flow to the brain, heart, and lungs. This causes the victim to experience weakness, dizziness, headache, nausea, and loss of appetite. The victim may faint but will probably regain consciousness as the head is lowered, which improves the blood supply to the brain. Signs and symptoms of heat exhaustion are similar to those of shock; the victim will appear ashen gray, the skin cool, moist, and clammy and the pupils may be dilated (fig. 4-50). The vital signs usually are normal; however, the victim may have a weak pulse, together with rapid and shallow breathing. Body temperature may be below normal.

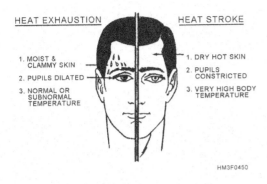

HEAT EXHAUSTION   HEAT STROKE

1. MOIST & CLAMMY SKIN   1. DRY HOT SKIN

2. PUPILS DILATED   2. PUPILS CONSTRICTED

3. NORMAL OR SUBNORMAL TEMPERATURE   3. VERY HIGH BODY TEMPERATURE

HM3F0450

Figure 4-50.—Heat exhaustion and heat stroke.

Treat heat exhaustion as if the victim were in shock. Move the victim to a cool or air-conditioned area. Loosen the clothing, apply cool wet cloths to the head, axilla, groin, and ankles, and fan the victim. Do not allow the victim to become chilled. (If this does occur, cover with a light blanket and move into a warmer area.) If the victim is conscious, give a solution of 1 teaspoon of salt dissolved in a liter of cool water. If the victim vomits, do not give any more fluids. Transport the victim to a medical treatment facility as soon as possible. Intravenous fluid infusion may be necessary for effective fluid and electrolyte replacement to combat shock.

Heat Stroke

Sunstroke is more accurately called heat stroke since it is not necessary to be exposed to the sun for this condition to develop. It is a less common but far more serious condition than heat exhaustion, since it carries a 20 percent mortality rate. The most important feature of heat stroke is the extremely high body temperature (105°F, 41°C or higher) accompanying it. In heat stroke, the victim suffers a breakdown of the sweating mechanism and is unable to eliminate excessive body heat build up while exercising. If the body temperature rises too high, the brain, kidneys, and liver may be permanently damaged.

Sometimes the victim may have preliminary symptoms such as headache, nausea, dizziness, or weakness. Breathing will be deep and rapid at first, later shallow and almost absent. Usually the victim will be flushed, very dry, and very hot. The pupils will be constricted (pinpoint) and the pulse fast and strong (fig. 4-50). Compare these symptoms with those of heat exhaustion.

When providing first aid for heat stroke, remember that this is a true life-and-death emergency. The longer the victim remains overheated, the more likely irreversible brain damage or death will occur. First aid is designed to reduce body heat fast.

Reduce heat immediately by dousing the body with cold water or by applying wet, cold towels to the whole body. Move the victim to the coolest place available and remove as much clothing as possible. Maintain an open airway. Place the victim on his back, with the head and shoulders slightly raised. If cold packs are available, place them under the arms, around the neck, at the ankles, and in the groin. Expose the victim to a fan or air conditioner, since drafts will promote cooling. Immersing the victim in a cold water bath is also very effective. If the victim is conscious, give cool water to drink. **Do not give any hot drinks or stimulants.** Discontinue cooling when the rectal temperature reaches 102°F; watch for recurrence of temperature rise by checking every 10 minutes. Repeat cooling if temperature reaches 103°F rectally.

Get the victim to a medical facility as soon as possible. Cooling measures must be continued while the victim is being transported. Intravenous fluid infusion may be necessary for effective fluid and electrolyte replacement to combat shock.

Prevention of Heat Exposure Injuries

LEARNING OBJECTIVE: *Determine the steps needed to prevent heat exposure injuries.*

The prevention of heat exposure injuries is a command responsibility, but the medical department plays a role in it by educating all hands about the medical dangers, monitoring environmental health, and advising the commanding officer.

On the individual level, prevention centers on water and salt replacement. Sweat must be replaced ounce for ounce; in a hot environment, water consumption must be drastically increased. Salt should be replaced by eating well-balanced meals, three times a day, salted to taste. In the field, "C" rations contain enough salt to sustain a person in most situations. **DO NOT** use salt tablets unless specified by a physician. **DO NOT** consume alcoholic beverages.

At the command level, prevention centers on an awareness of the environment. The Wet Bulb Globe

Temperature (WBGT) must be monitored regularly, and the results interpreted with the Physiological Heat Exposure Limit (PHEL) chart before work assignments are made. In addition, unnecessary heat sources, especially steam leaks, must be eliminated, and vents and exhaust blowers must be checked for adequate circulation. The results will be a happier, healthier, and more productive crew.

COLD EXPOSURE INJURIES

LEARNING OBJECTIVE: *Identify the signs, symptoms, and emergency treatment of each type of cold exposure injury.*

When the body is subjected to extremely cold temperatures, blood vessels constrict, and body heat is gradually lost. As the body temperature drops, tissues are easily damaged or destroyed.

The cold injuries resulting from inadequate response to the cold in military situations have spelled disaster for many armies—those of Napoleon and Hitler in their Russian campaigns, for example. The weather (i.e., temperature, humidity, precipitation, and wind) is the predominant influence in the development of cold injuries. Falling temperature interacting with high humidity, a wet environment, and rising wind accelerates the loss of body heat.

Other factors that influence the development of cold injuries are the individual's level of dehydration, the presence of other injuries (especially those causing a reduction in circulatory flow), and a previous cold injury (which increases susceptibility by lowering resistance). In addition, the use of any drug (including alcohol) that modifies autonomic nervous system response or alters judgment ability can drastically reduce an individual's chance for survival in a cold environment.

Like heat exposure injuries, cold exposure injuries are preventable. Acclimatization, the availability of warm, layered clothing, and maintenance of good discipline and training standards are important factors. These are command—not medical—responsibilities, but the Corpsman plays a crucial role as a monitor of nutritional intake and personal hygiene (with emphasis on foot care) and as an advisor to the commanding officer. A Corpsman is also responsible for acquainting the troops with the dangers of cold exposure and with preventive measures.

Two major points must be stressed in the management of all cold injuries: Rapid rewarming is

of primary importance, and all unnecessary manipulations of affected areas must be avoided. More will be said about these points later.

In military operations the treatment of cold injuries is influenced by the tactical situation, the facilities available for the evacuation of casualties, and the fact that most cold injuries are encountered in large numbers during periods of intense combat when many other wounded casualties appear. Highly individualized treatment under these circumstances may be impossible because examination and treatment of more life-endangering wounds must be given priority. In a high-casualty situation, shelter cold-injury victims, and try to protect them from further injury until there is sufficient time to treat them.

All cold injuries are similar, varying only in the degree of tissue damage. Although the effects of cold can, in general, be divided into two types—general cooling of the entire body and local cooling of parts of the body—cold injuries are seldom strictly of one type or the other; rather, these injuries tend to be a combination of both types. Each type of cooling, however, will be discussed separately in the sections that follow.

General Cooling (Hypothermia)

General cooling of the whole body is caused by continued exposure to low or rapidly falling temperatures, cold moisture, snow, or ice. Those exposed to low temperatures for extended periods may suffer ill effects, even if they are well protected by clothing, because cold affects the body systems slowly, almost without notice. As the body cools, there are several stages of progressive discomfort and disability. The first symptom is shivering, which is an attempt to generate heat by repeated contractions of surface muscles. This is followed by a feeling of listlessness, indifference, and drowsiness. Unconsciousness can follow quickly. Shock becomes evident as the victim's eyes assume a glassy stare, respiration becomes slow and shallow, and the pulse is weak or absent. As the body temperature drops even lower, peripheral circulation decreases and the extremities become susceptible to freezing. Finally, death results as the core temperature of the body approaches 80°F.

The steps for treatment of hypothermia are as follows:

1. Carefully observe respiratory effort and heart beat; CPR may be required while the warming process is underway.

2. Rewarm the victim as soon as possible. It may be necessary to treat other injuries before the victim can be moved to a warmer place. Severe bleeding must be controlled and fractures splinted over clothing before the victim is moved.

3. Replace wet or frozen clothing and remove anything that constricts the victim's arms, legs, or fingers, interfering with circulation.

4. If the victim is inside a warm place and is conscious, the most effective method of warming is immersion in a tub of warm (100° to 105°F or 38° to 41°C) water. The water should be warm to the elbow—never hot. Observe closely for signs of respiratory failure and cardiac arrest (rewarming shock). Rewarming shock can be minimized by warming the body trunk before the limbs to prevent vasodilation in the extremities with subsequent shock due to blood volume shifts.

5. If a tub is not available, apply external heat to both sides of the victim. Natural body heat (skin to skin) from two rescuers is the best method. This is called "buddy warming." If this is not practical, use hot water bottles or an electric rewarming blanket. Do not place the blanket or bottles next to bare skin, however, and be careful to monitor the temperature of the artificial heat source, since the victim is very susceptible to burn injury. Because the victim is unable to generate adequate body heat, placement under a blanket or in a sleeping bag is not sufficient treatment.

6. If the victim is conscious, give warm liquids to drink. Never give alcoholic beverages or allow the victim to smoke.

7. Dry the victim thoroughly if water is used for rewarming.

8. As soon as possible, transfer the victim to a definitive care facility. Be alert for the signs of respiratory and cardiac arrest during transfer, and keep the victim warm.

Local Cooling

Local cooling injuries, affecting individual parts of the body, fall into two categories: freezing and nonfreezing injuries. In the order of increasing seriousness, they include chilblain, immersion foot, superficial frostbite, and deep frostbite. The areas most commonly affected are the face and extremities.

CHILBLAIN.—Chilblain is a mild cold injury caused by prolonged and repeated exposure for several hours to air temperatures from above freezing 32°F (0°C) to as high as 60°F (16°C). Chilblain is characterized by redness, swelling, tingling, and pain to the affected skin area. Injuries of this nature require no specific treatment except warming of the affected part (if possible use a water bath of 90°F to 105°F), keeping it dry, and preventing further exposure.

IMMERSION FOOT.—Immersion foot, which also may occur in the hands, results from prolonged exposure to wet cold at temperatures ranging from just above freezing to 50°F (10°C). Immersion foot is usually seen in connection with limited motion of the extremities and water-soaked protective clothing.

Signs and symptoms of immersion foot are tingling and numbness of the affected areas; swelling of the legs, feet, or hands; bluish discoloration of the skin; and painful blisters. Gangrene may occur. General treatment for immersion foot is as follows:

1. Get the victim off his feet as soon as possible.

2. Remove wet shoes, socks, and gloves to improve circulation.

3. Expose the affected area to warm, dry air.

4. Keep the victim warm.

5. **Do not** rupture blisters or apply salves and ointments.

6. If the skin is not broken or loose, the injured part may be left exposed; however, if it is necessary to transport the victim, cover the injured area with loosely wrapped fluff bandages of sterile gauze.

7. If the skin is broken, place a sterile sheet under the extremity and gently wrap it to protect the sensitive tissue from pressure and additional injury.

8. Transport the victim as soon as possible to a medical treatment facility as a litter patient.

FROSTBITE.—Frostbite occurs when ice crystals form in the skin or deeper tissues after exposure to a temperature of 32°F (0°C) or lower. Depending upon the temperature, altitude, and wind speed, the exposure time necessary to produce frostbite varies from a few minutes to several hours.

The areas most commonly affected are the face and extremities.

The symptoms of frostbite are progressive. Victims generally incur this injury without being acutely aware of it. Initially, the affected skin reddens and there is an uncomfortable coldness. With continued heat loss, there is a numbness of the affected area due to reduced circulation. As ice crystals form, the frozen extremity appears white, yellow-white, or mottled blue-white, and is cold, hard, and insensitive to touch or pressure. Frostbite is classified as superficial or deep, depending on the extent of tissue involvement.

Superficial Frostbite.—In superficial frostbite the surface of the skin will feel hard, but the underlying tissue will be soft, allowing it to move over bony ridges. This is evidence that only the skin and the region just below it are involved. General treatment for superficial frostbite is as follows:

1. Take the victim indoors.

2. Rewarm hands by placing them under the armpits, against the abdomen, or between the legs.

3. Rewarm feet by placing them in the armpit or against the abdomen of the buddy.

4. Gradually rewarm the affected area by warm water immersion, skin-to-skin contact, or hot water bottles.

5. Never rub a frostbite area.

Deep Frostbite.—In deep frostbite, the freezing reaches into the deep tissue layers. There are ice crystals in the entire thickness of the extremity. The skin will not move over bony ridges and will feel hard and solid.

The objectives of treatment are to protect the frozen areas from further injury, to rapidly thaw the affected area, and to be prepared to respond to circulatory or respiratory difficulties.

1. Carefully assess and treat any other injuries first. Constantly monitor the victim's pulse and breathing since respiratory and heart problems can develop rapidly. Be prepared to administer CPR if necessary.

2. Do not attempt to thaw the frostbitten area if there is a possibility of refreezing. It is better to leave the part frozen until the victim arrives at a medical treatment facility equipped for long-term care. Refreezing of a thawed extremity causes severe and disabling damage.

3. Treat all victims with injuries to the feet or legs as litter patients. When this is not possible, the victim may walk on the frozen limb, since it has been proven that walking will not lessen the chances of successful treatment as long as the limb has not thawed out.

4. When adequate protection from further cold exposure is available, prepare the victim for rewarming by removing all constricting clothing such as gloves, boots, and socks. Boots and clothing frozen on the body should be thawed by warm-water immersion before removal.

5. Rapidly rewarm frozen areas by immersion in water at 100°F to 105°F (38°C to 41°C). Keep the water warm by adding fresh hot water, but do not pour the water directly on the injured area. Ensure that the frozen area is completely surrounded by water; do not let it rest on the side or bottom of the tub.

6. After rewarming has been completed, pat the area dry with a soft towel. Later it will swell, sting, and burn. Blisters may develop. These should be protected from breaking. Avoid pressure, rubbing, or constriction of the injured area. Keep the skin dry with sterile dressings and place cotton between the toes and fingers to prevent their sticking together.

7. Protect the tissue from additional injury and keep it as clean as possible (use sterile dressings and linen).

8. Try to improve the general morale and comfort of the victim by giving hot, stimulating fluids such as tea or coffee. Do not allow the victim to smoke or use alcoholic beverages while being treated.

9. Transfer to a medical treatment facility as soon as possible. During transportation, slightly elevate the frostbitten area and keep the victim and the injured area warm. Do not allow the injured area to be exposed to the cold.

LEARNING OBJECTIVE: *Determine the steps needed for the later management of cold-exposure injuries.*

When the patient reaches a hospital or a facility for definitive care, the following treatment should be employed:

1. Maintain continued vigilance to avoid further damage to the injured tissue. In general, this is accomplished by keeping the patient at bed rest with the injured part elevated (on surgically clean sheets) and with sterile pieces of cotton separating the toes or fingers. Expose all lesions to the air at normal room temperature. Weight bearing on injured tissue must be avoided.

2. Whirlpool baths, twice daily at 98.6°F (37°C) with surgical soap added, assist in superficial debridement, reduce superficial bacterial contamination, and make range of motion exercises more tolerable.

3. Analgesics may be required in the early post-thaw days but will soon become unnecessary in uncomplicated cases.

4. Encourage the patient to take a nutritious diet with adequate fluid intake to maintain hydration.

5. Perform superficial debridement of ruptured blebs, and remove suppurative scabs and partially detached nails.

MORPHINE USE FOR PAIN RELIEF

LEARNING OBJECTIVE: *Recall morphine dosage, administration routes, indications, contraindications, and casualty marking procedures.*

As a Corpsman, you may be issued morphine for the control of shock through the relief of severe pain. You will be issued this controlled drug under very strict accountability procedures. Possession of this drug is a medical responsibility that must not be taken lightly. Policies pertaining to morphine administration are outlined in BUMEDINST 6570.2, *Morphia Dosage and Casualty Marking.*

Morphine is the most effective of all pain-relieving drugs. It is most commonly available in premeasured doses in syrettes or tubexes. Proper administration in selected patients relieves distressing pain and assists in preventing shock. The adult dose of morphine is 10 to 20 mg, which may be repeated, if necessary, in no less than 4 hours.

Morphine has several undesirable effects, however, and a Corpsman must thoroughly understand these effects. Morphine

- is a severe respiratory depressant and must not be given to patients in moderate or severe shock or in respiratory distress.

- increases intracranial pressure and may induce vomiting. These effects may be disastrous in head injury cases.

- causes constriction of the pupils (pinpoint pupils). This effect prevents the use of the pupillary reactions for diagnosis in head injuries.

- is cardiotoxic and a peripheral vasodilator. Small doses of morphine may cause profound hypotension in a patient in shock.

- poisoning is always a danger. There is a narrow safety margin between the amounts of morphine that may be given therapeutically and the amounts that produce death.

- causes considerable mental confusion and interferes with the proper exercise of judgment. Therefore, morphine should not be given to ambulatory patients.

- is a highly addictive drug. Morphine should not be given trivially and must be rigidly accounted for. Only under emergency circumstances should the Corpsman administer morphine.

Rigidly control morphine administration to patients in shock or with extensive burns. Because of the reduced peripheral circulation, morphine administration by subcutaneous or intramuscular routes may not be absorbed into the bloodstream, and pain may persist. When pain persists, the uninformed often give additional doses, hoping to bring about relief. When resuscitation occurs and the peripheral circulation improves, the stored quantities of morphine are released into the system, and an extremely serious condition (morphine poisoning) results.

When other pain-relieving drugs are not available and the patient in shock or with burns is in severe pain, 20 mg of morphine may be given intramuscularly (followed by massage of the injection site). Resist the temptation to give more, however. Unless otherwise ordered by a medical officer, doses should not be repeated more than twice, and then at least 4 hours apart.

If the pain from a wound is severe, morphine may be given when examination of the patient reveals no

- head injury;

- chest injury, including sucking and nonsucking wounds;

- wounds of the throat, nasal passages, oral cavity, or jaws wherein blood might obstruct the airway;

- massive hemorrhage;

- respiratory impairment, including chemical burns of the respiratory tract (any casualty having fewer than 16 respirations per minute should not be given morphine);

- evidence of severe or deepening shock; or

- loss of consciousness.

CASUALTY MARKING

Morphine overdose is always a danger. For this reason, plainly identify every casualty who has received morphine. Write the letter "M" and the hour of injection on the patient's forehead (e.g., M0830) with a skin pencil or semi-permanent marking substitute. Attach the empty morphine syrette or tubex to the patient's shirt collar or another conspicuous area of the clothing with a safety pin or by some other means. This action will alert others that the drug has been administered. If a Field Medical Card is prepared, record the dosage, time, date, and route of administration.

COMMON MEDICAL EMERGENCIES

LEARNING OBJECTIVE: *Choose the appropriate treatment and management techniques for the common medical emergencies.*

This section of the chapter deals with relatively common medical emergencies a Hospital Corpsman may face. Generally speaking, these particular problems are the result of previously diagnosed medical conditions; so, at least for the victim, they do not come as a complete surprise. Many of these victims wear a medical identification device (necklace or bracelet), or carry a medical identification card that specifies the nature of the medical condition or the type of medications being taken. In all cases of sudden illness, search the victim for a medical identification device.

SYNCOPE

Uncomplicated syncope (fainting) is the result of blood pooling in dilated veins, which reduces the amount of blood being pumped to the brain. Causes of syncope include getting up too quickly, standing for long periods with little movement, and stressful situations. Signs and symptoms that may be present are dizziness; nausea; visual disturbance from pupillary dilation; sweating; pallor; and a weak, rapid pulse. As the body collapses, blood returns to the head, and consciousness is quickly regained. Revival can be promoted by carefully placing the victim in the shock position or in a sitting position with the head between the knees. Placing a cool, wet cloth on the patient's face and loosening their clothing can also help.

Syncope may also result from an underlying medical problem such as diabetes, cerebrovascular accident (stroke), heart condition, or epilepsy.

DIABETIC CONDITIONS

Diabetes mellitus is an inherited condition in which the pancreas secretes an insufficient amount of the protein hormone insulin. Insulin regulates carbohydrate metabolism by enabling glucose to enter cells for use as an energy source. Diabetics almost always wear a medical identification device.

Diabetic Ketoacidosis

Diabetic ketoacidosis most often results either from forgetting to take insulin or from taking too little insulin to maintain a balanced condition. Diabetics may suffer from rising levels of glucose in the blood stream (hyperglycemia). The rising levels of glucose result in osmotic diuresis, an increased renal excretion of urine. Serious dehydration (hypovolemia) may result. Concurrently, the lack of glucose in the cells leads to an increase in metabolic acids in the blood (acidosis) as other substances, such as fats, are metabolized as energy sources. The result is gradual central nervous system depression, starting with symptoms of confusion and disorientation, and leading to stupor and coma. Blood pressure falls, and the pulse rate becomes rapid and weak. Respirations are deep, and a sickly sweet acetone odor is present on the breath. The skin is warm and dry.

NOTE: Diabetic victims are often mistakenly treated as if intoxicated since the signs and symptoms presented are similar to those of alcohol intoxication.

The diabetic under treatment tries to balance the use of insulin against glucose intake to avoid the above problems. The victim or the victim's family may be able to answer two key questions:

1. Has the victim eaten today?

2. Has he taken the prescribed insulin?

If the answer is yes to the first and no to the second question, the victim is probably in a diabetic coma.

Emergency first aid centers around ABC support, administration of oral or intravenous fluids to counter shock, and rapid evacuation to a medical officer's supervision.

Insulin Shock

Insulin shock results from too little sugar in the blood (hypoglycemia). This type of shock develops when a diabetic exercises too much or eats too little after taking insulin. Insulin shock is a very serious condition because glucose is driven into the cells to be metabolized, leaving too little glucose in circulation to support the brain. Brain damage develops quickly. Signs and symptoms of insulin shock include

- pale, moist skin;

- dizziness and headache;

- strong, rapid pulse; and

- fainting, seizures, and coma.

Treatment is centered on getting glucose into the system quickly to prevent brain damage. Placing sugar cubes under the tongue or administering oral liquid glucose are the most beneficial treatments. Transport the victim to a medical treatment facility as soon as possible.

NOTE: If you are in doubt as to whether the victim is in insulin shock or a ketoacidotic state, give them sugar. Brain damage develops very quickly in insulin shock and must be reversed immediately. If the victim turns out to be ketoacidotic, a condition that progresses

slowly, the extra sugar will do no appreciable harm.

CEREBROVASCULAR ACCIDENT

A cerebrovascular accident, also known as **stroke** or **apoplexy**, is caused by an interruption of the arterial blood supply to a portion of the brain. This interruption may be caused by arteriosclerosis or by a clot forming in the brain. Tissue damage and loss of function result.

Onset of a cerebrovascular accident is sudden, with little or no warning. The first signs include weakness or paralysis on the side of the body opposite the side of the brain that has been injured. Muscles of the face on the affected side may be involved. The patient's level of consciousness varies from alert to unresponsive. Additionally, motor functions— including vision and speech—on the affected side are disturbed, and the throat may be paralyzed.

Emergency treatment for a cerebrovascular accident is mainly supportive. Special attention must be paid to the victim's airway, since he may not be able to keep it clear. Place the victim in a semi-reclining position or on the paralyzed side.

- Be prepared to use suction if the victim vomits.

- Act in a calm, reassuring manner, and keep any onlookers quiet since the victim may be able to hear what is going on.

- Administer oxygen to combat cerebral hypoxia.

- Carefully monitor the victim's vital signs and keep a log. Pay special attention to respirations, pulse strength and rate, and the presence or absence of the bilateral carotid pulse.

- Transport the victim to a medical treatment facility as soon as possible.

ANAPHYLACTIC REACTION

This condition, also called **anaphylaxis** or **anaphylactic shock**, is a severe allergic reaction to foreign material. The most frequent causes are probably penicillin and the toxin from bee stings, although foods, inhalants, and contact substances can also cause a reaction. Anaphylaxis can happen at any time, even to people who have taken penicillin many times before without experiencing any problems. This condition produces severe shock and cardiopulmonary failure of a very rapid onset. Because of the rapidity and severity of the onset of symptoms, immediate intervention is necessary. The general treatment for severe anaphylaxis is the subcutaneous injection of 0.3 cc of epinephrine and supportive care.

The most characteristic and serious symptoms of an anaphylactic reaction are loss of voice and difficulty breathing. Other typical signs are giant hives, coughing, and wheezing. As the condition progresses, signs and symptoms of shock develop, followed by respiratory failure. Emergency management consists of maintaining vital life functions. Summon the medical officer immediately.

POISONS/DRUG ABUSE/HAZARDOUS MATERIALS

As a Hospital Corpsman, you could encounter special situations that include poisoning, suspected drug abuse, or exposure to hazardous materials. Knowledge of these conditions—along with the ability to assess and treat them—is essential. These situations are discussed in detail in chapter 5, "Poisoning, Drug Abuse, and Hazardous Material Exposure."

HEART CONDITIONS

A number of heart conditions are commonly referred to as heart attacks. These conditions include **angina pectoris**, **acute myocardial infarction**, and **congestive heart failure**. Together these heart conditions are the cause of at least half a million deaths per year in our country. Heart conditions occur more commonly in men in the 50-to-60-year age group. Predisposing factors are the lack of physical conditioning, high blood pressure and blood cholesterol levels, smoking, diabetes, and a family history of heart disease.

Angina Pectoris

Angina pectoris, also known simply as **angina**, is caused by insufficient oxygen being circulated to the heart muscle. This condition results from a spasm of the coronary artery, which allows the heart to function adequately at rest but does not allow enough oxygen-enriched blood to pass through the heart to support sustained exercise. When the body exerts itself, the heart muscle becomes starved for oxygen. The result of this condition is a squeezing, substernal pain that may radiate to the left arm and to the jaw.

Angina is differentiated from other forms of heart problems because the pain results from exertion and

subsides with rest. Many people who suffer from angina pectoris carry nitroglycerin tablets. If the victim of a suspected angina attack is carrying a bottle of these pills, place one pill under the tongue. Relief will be almost instantaneous. Other first aid procedures include providing supplemental oxygen, reassurance, comfort, monitoring vital signs, and transporting the victim to a medical treatment facility.

Acute Myocardial Infarction

Acute myocardial infarction results when a coronary artery is severely occluded by arteriosclerosis or completely blocked by a clot. The pain associated with myocardial infarction is similar to that of angina pectoris but is longer in duration, not related to exertion or relieved by nitroglycerin, and leads to death of heart-muscle tissue. Other symptoms are sweating, weakness, and nausea. Additionally, although the patient's respirations are usually normal, his pulse rate increases and may be irregular, and his blood pressure falls. The victim may have an overwhelming feeling of doom. Death may result.

First aid for an acute myocardial infarction includes

- reassurance and comfort while placing the victim in a semi-sitting position;

- loosening of all clothing;

- carefully maintaining a log of vital signs, and recording the history and general observations;

- continuously monitoring vital signs and being prepared to start CPR;

- starting a slow intravenous infusion of 5% dextrose solution in water;

- administering oxygen; and

- quickly transporting the victim to a medical treatment facility.

Congestive Heart Failure

A heart suffering from prolonged hypertension, valve disease, or heart disease will try to compensate for decreased function by increasing the size of the left ventricular pumping chamber and increasing the heart rate. This condition is known as congestive heart failure. As blood pressure increases, fluid is forced out of the blood vessels and into the lungs, causing pulmonary edema. Pulmonary edema leads to rapid shallow respirations, the appearance of pink frothy bubbles at the nose and mouth and distinctive rattling sounds (known as **rales**) in the chest. Increased blood pressure may also cause body fluids to pool in the extremities.

Emergency treatment for congestive heart failure is essentially the same as that for acute myocardial infarction. Do not start CPR unless the patient's heart function ceases. If an intravenous line is started, it should be maintained at the slowest rate possible to keep the vein open since an increase in the circulatory volume will make the condition worse. Immediately transport the patient to a medical treatment facility.

CONVULSIONS

Convulsions, or seizures, are a startling and often frightening phenomenon. Convulsions are characterized by severe and uncontrolled muscle spasms or muscle rigidity. Convulsive episodes occur in one to two percent of the general population.

Although epilepsy is the most widely known form of seizure activity, there are numerous forms of convulsions that are classified as either central nervous system (CNS) or non-CNS in origin. It is especially important to determine the cause in patients who have no previous seizure history. This determination may require an extensive medical workup in the hospital. Since epilepsy is the most widely known form of seizure activity, this section will highlight epileptic seizure disorders.

Epilepsy, also known as seizures or fits, is a condition characterized by an abnormal focus of activity in the brain that produces severe motor responses or changes in consciousness. Epilepsy may result from head trauma, scarred brain tissue, brain tumors, cerebral arterial occlusion, fever, or a number of other factors. Fortunately, epilepsy can often be controlled by medications.

Grand mal seizure is the more serious type of epilepsy. Grand mal seizure may be—but is not always—preceded by an aura. The victim soon comes to recognize these auras, which allows him time to lie down and prepare for the seizure's onset. A burst of nerve impulses from the brain causes unconsciousness and generalized muscular contractions, often with loss of bladder and bowel control. The primary dangers in a grand mal seizure are tongue biting and injuries resulting from falls. A period of sleep or mental confusion follows this type of seizure. When full consciousness returns, the victim will have little or no recollection of the attack.

Petit mal seizure is of short duration and is characterized by an altered state of awareness or partial loss of consciousness, and localized muscular contractions. The patient has no warning of the seizure's onset and little or no memory of the attack after it is over.

First aid treatment for both types of epileptic seizure consists of protecting the victim from self-injury. Additional methods of seizure control may be employed under a medical officer's supervision. In all cases, be prepared to provide suction to the victim since the risk of aspiration is significant. Transport the patient to a medical treatment facility once the seizure has ended.

DROWNING

Drowning is a suffocating condition in a water environment. Water seldom enters the lungs in appreciable quantities because, upon contact with fluid, laryngeal spasms occur, and these spasms seal the airway from the mouth and nose passages. To avoid serious damage from the resulting hypoxia, quickly bring the victim to the surface and immediately—even before the victim is pulled to shore—start artificial ventilation. Do not interrupt artificial ventilation until the rescuer and the victim are ashore. Once on dry ground, quickly administer an abdominal thrust (Heimlich maneuver) to empty the lungs, and then immediately restart the ventilation until spontaneous breathing returns. Oxygen enrichment is desirable if a mask is available.

Remember that an apparently lifeless person who has been immersed in cold water for a long period of time may be revived if artificial ventilation is started immediately.

PSYCHIATRIC EMERGENCIES

A psychiatric emergency is defined as a sudden onset of behavioral or emotional responses that, if not responded to, will result in a life-threatening situation. Probably the most common psychiatric emergency is the suicide attempt. A suicide attempt may range from verbal threats and suicidal gestures to a successful suicide. Always assume that a suicide threat is real; do not leave the patient alone. In all cases, the prime consideration for a Hospital Corpsman is to keep patients from inflicting harm to themselves and to get them under the care of a trained psychiatric professional. When dealing with suicidal gestures or attempts, treat any self-inflicted wounds appropriately.

In the case of ingested substances, do not induce vomiting in a patient who is not awake and alert. For specific treatment of ingested substances, refer to the section on poisons in chapter 5.

There are numerous other psychiatric conditions that would require volumes to expound upon. In almost all cases, appropriate first aid treatment consists of a calm, professional, understanding demeanor that does not aggravate or agitate the patient. With an assaultive or hostile patient, a "show of force" may be all that is required. Almost all cases of psychiatric emergencies will present with a third party—]often the family or friend of the patient—who has recognized a distinct change in the behavior pattern of the patient and who is seeking help for them.

DERMATOLOGIC EMERGENCIES

Most dermatologic cases that present as emergencies are not real emergencies. The patient perceives them as such because of the sudden presentation and/or repulsive appearance or excessive discomfort. Treat most dermatologic conditions symptomatically. The major exception to symptomatic treatment is **toxic epidermal necrolysis** (TEN).

Toxic epidermal necrolysis is a condition characterized by sudden onset, excessive skin irritation, painful erythema (redness of skin produced by congestion of the capillaries), **bullae** (large blisters), and exfoliation of the skin in sheets. TEN is also known as the **scalded skin syndrome** because of its appearance. TEN is thought to be caused by a staphylococcal infection in children and by a toxic reaction to medications in adults.

Since skin is the largest single organ of the body and serves as a barrier to infection, prevention of secondary skin infection is very important. Treatment of skin infections consists of isolation techniques, silver nitrate compresses, aggressive skin care, intravenous antibiotic therapy and, in drug-induced cases, systemic steroids.

EMERGENCY CHILDBIRTH

Every Hospital Corpsman must be prepared to handle the unexpected arrival of a new life into the world. If the Corpsman is fortunate, a prepackaged sterile delivery pack will be available. This pack will contain all the equipment needed for the normal delivery of a healthy baby. If the pack is not available,

a Hospital Corpsman will require imaginative improvisation of clean alternatives.

When faced with an imminent childbirth, the Hospital Corpsman must first determine whether there will be time to transport the expectant mother to a hospital. To help make this determination, the Corpsman should try to find out

- if this will be the woman's first delivery (first deliveries usually take much longer than subsequent deliveries);

- the time between contractions (if less than 3 minutes, delivery is approaching);

- if the mother senses that she has to move her bowels (if so, then the baby's head is well advanced down the birth canal);

- if there is crowning (bulging) of the orifice (crowning indicates that the baby is ready to present itself); and

- how long it will take to get to the hospital.

The Corpsman must weigh the answers to these questions and decide if it will be safe to transport the patient to the hospital.

Prior to childbirth, a Corpsman must quickly "set the stage." The mother must not be allowed to go to the bathroom since straining may precipitate delivery. Do not try to inhibit the natural process of childbirth. The mother should lie back on a sturdy table, bed, or stretcher with a folded sheet or blanket placed under her buttocks for absorption and comfort. Remove all the patient's clothing below the waist, bend the knees, move the thighs apart, and drape her lower extremities with clean towels or sheets. Don sterile gloves, or, if these are not available, rewash your hands.

In a normal delivery, your calm professional manner and sincere reassurance to the mother will reduce her anxiety and make the delivery easier for everyone. Help the woman rest and relax as much as possible between contractions. During a contraction, deep, open-mouth breathing will relieve some pain and straining. As the child's head reaches the area of the rectum, the mother will feel an urgent need to defecate. Reassurance that this is a natural feeling and a sign that the baby will be born soon will help alleviate her apprehension.

Watch for the presentation of the top of the baby's head. Once the head appears, take up your station at the foot of the bed and gently push against the head to keep it from emerging too quickly. Allow it to come out slowly. As more of the head appears, check to be sure that the umbilical cord is not wrapped around the neck. If it is, either gently try to untangle the cord, or move one section over the baby's shoulder. If neither of these actions is possible, clamp the cord in two places, 2 inches apart, and cut it. Once the baby's chin emerges, support the head with one hand and use the bulb syringe from the pack to suction the nostrils and mouth. Before placing the bulb in the baby's mouth or nose, compress it; otherwise, a forceful aspiration into the lungs will result. The baby will now start a natural rotation to the left or right, away from the face-down position. As this rotation occurs, keep the baby's head in a natural relationship with the back. The shoulders appear next, usually one at a time.

NOTE: From this point on, it is essential to remember that the baby is VERY slippery, and great care must be taken so that you do not drop it. The surface beneath the mother should extend at least 2 feet out from her buttocks so that the baby will not be hurt if it does slip out of your hands. Keep one hand beneath the baby's head, and use the other hand to support its emerging body.

Once the baby has been born, suction the nose and mouth again if breathing has not started. Wipe the baby's face, nose, and mouth clean with sterile gauze. Your reward will be the baby's hearty cry.

Clamp the umbilical cord as the pulsations cease. Use two clamps from the prepackaged sterile delivery pack, 2 inches apart, with the first clamp 6 to 8 inches from the navel. Cut the cord between the clamps. For safety, use gauze tape to tie the cord 1 inch from the clamp toward the navel. Secure the tie with a square knot. Wrap the baby in a warm, sterile blanket, and log its time of arrival.

The **placenta** (afterbirth) will deliver itself in 10 to 20 minutes. Massaging the mother's lower abdomen can aid this delivery. Do not pull on the placenta. Log the time of the placenta's delivery, and wrap it up for hospital analysis.

Place a small strip of tape (½ -inch wide), folded and inscribed with the date, time of delivery, and mother's name, around the baby's wrist.

COMPLICATIONS IN CHILDBIRTH

Unfortunately, not all deliveries go smoothly. The following sections cover various complications in childbirth.

Breech Delivery

A breech delivery occurs when the baby's legs and buttocks emerge first. Follow the steps for a normal delivery, and support the lower extremities with one hand. If the head does not emerge within 3 minutes, try to maintain an airway by gently pushing fingers into the vagina. Push the vagina away from the baby's face and open its mouth with one finger. Get medical assistance immediately.

Prolapsed Cord

If the cord precedes the baby, protect it with moist, sterile wraps. If a physician cannot be reached quickly, place the mother in an extreme shock position. Give the mother oxygen, if available, and gently move your gloved hand into the vagina to keep its walls and the baby from compressing the cord. Get medical assistance immediately.

Excessive Bleeding

If the mother experiences severe bleeding, treat her for shock and give her oxygen, if available. Place sanitary napkins over the vaginal entrance and rush her to a hospital.

Limb Presentation

If a single limb presents itself first, immediately get the mother to a hospital.

SUMMARY

A medical emergency can occur at anytime. You must be prepared to act expeditiously and confidently, whether you are in a combat situation, on board a naval vessel, or at the Navy Exchange. This chapter covers the preliminary steps you should follow when managing sick or injured patients. The preliminary emergency steps include triage, patient assessment, and, when needed, basic life support. Other related topics covered in this chapter are breathing aids, shock, diagnosis and emergency treatment procedures for medical conditions and injuries, morphine use for pain relief, and other common emergencies. In the following chapters, diagnosis and emergency treatment procedures for medical conditions and injuries will be discussed.

CHAPTER 5

POISONING, DRUG ABUSE, AND HAZARDOUS MATERIAL EXPOSURE

As a Hospital Corpsman, you may encounter patients as the result of poisoning, drug overdose, or exposure to hazardous materials. Such patients may initially present with no symptoms or with varying degrees of overt intoxication. The asymptomatic patient may have been exposed to or ingested a lethal dose of a substance but not exhibit any manifestations of toxicity. A patient with mild symptoms may deteriorate rapidly, so observe them closely. Potentially significant exposures should be observed in an acute care facility whenever possible. Remember, though: We are not always in a hospital environment, and we must be prepared to deal with each situation when and wherever it should present itself.

In this chapter, we will discuss the assessment and treatment for ingested, inhaled, absorbed, and injected poisons. Drug abuse assessment and treatment procedures, patient handling techniques, and the recognition of hazardous material (HAZMAT) personal safety guidelines and information sources will also be covered. The last part of the chapter will cover rescue, patient care, and decontamination procedures for patients exposed to HAZMAT.

NOTE: Prior to deployments and operational commitments, commands are strongly recommended to contact the area Environmental Preventive Medicine Unit (EPMU) for current, specific, medical intelligence, and surveillance data. With this information at hand, the local preventive medicine authority can identify, prevent, and treat conditions not common to the homeport area. The cognizant EPMU will provide data through MEDIC, (*Medical, Environmental, Diagnosis, Intelligence and Counter-measure*). Formally called a *Disease Risk Assessment Profile* (DISRAP), MEDIC is a comprehensive, constantly updated management tool. MEDIC is an invaluable aid for identifying at-risk communicable diseases, immunization requirements, and—as applies especially to this chapter—local pests and environmental dangers.

POISONING

LEARNING OBJECTIVE: *Recall assessment and treatment procedures for ingested, inhaled, absorbed, and injected poisons*

A **poison** is a substance that, when introduced into the body, produces a harmful effect on normal body structures or functions. Poisons come in solid, liquid, and gaseous forms, and they may be ingested, inhaled, absorbed, or injected into the system.

Every chemical in a sufficient dose can cause toxic effects in a human—or in any organism. The amount or concentration of a chemical and the duration of exposure to it are what determine the chemical's dose and toxicity. A 16th century quotation from Paracelsus states, "Dose alone makes a poison. . . .All substances are poisons, there is none which is not a poison. The right dose differentiates a poison and a remedy."

A **poisoning** is defined as the presence of signs or symptoms associated with exposure or contact with a substance. If there are no clinical manifestations or toxic effects, the incident is simply an "exposure" or a contact with a potentially poisonous substance. Just being exposed to a chemical does not mean that a poisoning has or will occur. It is a matter of dose and a few other variables (e.g., age, sex, individual resistance, or state of health) that determine if, or what, toxic effects will occur.

ASSESSMENT AND TREATMENT OF PATIENT

In most cases, ASSESSMENT AND TREATMENT OF THE PATIENT IS MORE IMPORTANT THAN EFFORT TO IDENTIFY AND TREAT A SPECIFIC POISON. Supportive therapy—managing the **ABCs (Airway, Breathing,** and **Circulation)** of basic life support and treating the signs and symptoms—is safe and effective in the vast majority of poisonings. Extraordinary means to enhance elimination of the poison (hemodialysis and hemoperfusion) are seldom needed. Except for agents with a delayed onset of toxicity (such as acetaminophen), most ingested poisons produce signs and symptoms in less than 4 hours, and most efforts to decontaminate the gut (remove an ingested poison) have little value more than 1 hour after ingestion.

In acute poisonings, prompt treatment is indicated. After the patient has been evaluated and stabilized, general poison management can be initiated. There are six steps in the initial evaluation and follow-on poison management:

1. **Stabilization**, which consists of a brief evaluation and assessment directed toward identifying the measures required to maintain life and prevent further deterioration of the patient.

   - Observe the **ABC + D & E** (**D**rug-induced central nervous system (CNS) depression, and undressing/uncovering to **E**xpose the patient for disabilities (injuries) to ensure areas of contact or exposure to a chemical can be seen.)

   - Check the pupils for size and reactivity to light, and do a basic neurologic exam.

   - Administer oxygen as needed, IV line for fluids.

   - Watch for signs and symptoms of anaphylaxis.

2. **Evaluation**, which must be performed once the patient is stabilized.

   - Include a full history, physical exam, and ordering of appropriate tests (i.e., labs, EKG, x-rays) directed toward identification of toxic agent, evaluating the severity of toxic effects, and searching for trauma and complications.

   - Periodically reassess the patient. Look for changes. Monitor vital signs, urine output, and cardiac rhythm.

   - Record your findings (including time), and respond to important changes appropriately.

3. **Prevention or limitation of absorption**, through skin decontamination, flushing of eyes, ventilation, stomach emptying, administration of charcoal and cathartics, and whole bowel irrigation.

4. **Elimination enhancement,** through serially administered activated charcoal, ion-trapping (pH adjustment of the urine to promote excretion of certain poisons), hemodialysis, and hemoperfusion (similar to hemodialysis, but used for larger size molecules).

5. **Administration of specific antidotes.** Less than 5 percent of poisons have specific antidotes. All patients who present should receive glucose, thiamine, and naloxone. Consider supplemental oxygen.

6. **Continuing care and disposition,** including a period of observation and education (i.e., poison prevention) or psychiatric counseling. Establish follow-up.

THE DIAGNOSIS OF POISONING

In most situations, the treatment of a poisoning victim will be under the direction of a medical officer. However, in isolated situations, a Hospital Corpsman must be ready to treat the victim.

Poisoning should be suspected in all cases of sudden, severe, and unexpected illness. You should investigate such situations by ascertaining, as quickly and thoroughly as possible, the answers to the following questions:

- What are the signs and symptoms of the illness?

- What was happening before the illness occurred? (Remember, there may have been a chronic exposure over time with the signs and symptoms just becoming apparent.)

- What substances were in use? Could more than one substance have been involved?

- Is there a container of the suspected substance? If so, how much was there initially, and how much is there now? (If possible, bring the container to the treatment facility. The label will often identify the contents and the recommended precautions and treatment. The label may also list a contact number for emergency advice. Remember, though, that other people— including you—may become contaminated through contact with the container. Handle it carefully.)

- What was the duration of exposure? When did it happen?

- What is the location of the bite or injury (if applicable)?

- Has this happened before?

- Are there other people involved?

- Does the patient have a significant past medical history?

- Is the patient's condition improving/deteriorating?

The presence of a toxic syndrome or **toxidrome** can help establish that a poison has been involved by suggesting the class of poison(s) to which the patient may have been exposed. Table 5-1 provides a list of commonly encountered toxidromes, their sources and symptoms.

The "non-syndrome syndrome" is of special importance. The only method to recognize the potential for a delayed onset poisoning to occur is to suspect the possibility from the history or presentation of a person. In some cases, the individual's affect or behavior may provide a clue. In other cases, the examiner must rely on clinical experience or even a hunch.

GENERAL TREATMENT

Once poisoning has been established, the general rule is to quickly remove as much of the toxic substance from the victim as possible. The method of removal of the poison varies depending upon how the poison was introduced:

- **Ingested poisons**: There is a choice between emetics and gastric lavage, followed by adsorbents and cathartics.

- **Inhaled poisons**: Oxygen ventilation is the method of choice.

- **Absorbed poisons**: Removal of the poison is primarily attained by cleansing the skin.

- **Injected poisons**: Antidotal medications are recommended.

INGESTED POISONS

Ingested poisons are those poisons which have been consumed, whether accidentally or intentionally, by the victim. Ingestion is the most common route of exposure to toxic materials in the home.

The local actions of an ingested poison can have irritant, acidic (corrosive), or basic (caustic) effects at the site of contact.

Table 5-1.—Commonly Encountered Toxidromes

Syndrome	Sources	Signs & Symptoms
narcotic	opiates, benzodiazepines, barbiturates	"beady eyes," sunglasses, decreased blood pressure, CNS and respiratory depression
withdrawal	alcohol, barbiturates, benzodiazepines, narcotics, sedative-hypnotics	diarrhea, dilated pupils, goose bumps, increased heart rate, tearing, yawning, stomach cramps, hallucinations
sympathomimetic	theophylline, caffeine, LSD, PCP, amphetamine, cocaine, decongestants	CNS excitation (confusion, incoordination, agitation, hallucination, delirium, seizures), increased blood pressure and heart rate
anticholinergic	antihistamines, atropine, scopolamine, antidepressants, anti-Parkinson R, antipsychotics, antispasmodics, mushrooms, hallucinogens, antidepressants	dry skin, increased heart rate, dilated pupils, fever, urinary retention, decreased bowel sounds, CNS excitation
cholinergic	organophosphates, carbamates, physostigmine, neostigmine, endrophonium	"**SLUDGE**": increased **salivation, lacrimation, urination, defecation, GI** cramping, **emesis**; CNS (headache, restless, anxiety, confusion, coma, seizures); muscle weakness and fasciculations
non-syndrome syndrome	various chemicals with delayed onset due to biotransformation, depletion of natural detoxifying agent, accumulation of dose or effect	from "nothing" to minor complaints that initially appear to be trivial

Ingested substances can be absorbed into the body and transported to a distant site with systemic action(s). In such situations, the poisonous substance may cause few effects—or even no effect—at the site of contact or absorption, but it may have severe systemic effects.

Ingestion of substances that do not produce local effects can be divided into two types:

- nontoxic substances (latex paint, dirt, silica gel, spider plant), and

- potentially toxic substances (poisonous fish, medications, heavy metals (lead, mercury), pesticides, and personal care products).

Episodes involving the ingestion of non-toxic substances do not require decontamination of the gut. (Swallowing a non-toxic foreign body, however, like a coin or button battery in a child, may result in choking and require prompt medical intervention.)

The toxicity range of absorbed poisons extends from essentially non-toxic to extremely toxic (remember Paracelsus' "dose"). Ingestion of substances with a low order of toxicity may result in the production of only minor systemic effects (nausea, vomiting, diarrhea), effects that are mild, self-limiting, and do not require significant medical intervention.

NOTE: Do not induce unnecessary vomiting to discourage a patient from repeating a voluntary ingestion again.

Table 5-2.—Common Stomach Irritants and Possible Sources of Contact

Irritant	Sources of Contact
Arsenic	Dyes, insecticides, paint, printer's ink, wood preservatives
Copper	Antifoulant paint, batteries, canvas preservative, copper plating, electro-plating, fungicides, insecticides, soldering, wood preservatives
Iodine	Antiseptics
Mercury	Bactericides, batteries, dental supplies and appliances, disinfectants, dyes, fungicides, ink, insecticides, laboratories, photography, wood preservatives
Phosphorus	Incendiaries, matches, pesticides, rat poison
Silver nitrate	Batteries, cleaning solutions, ink, photographic film, silver polish, soldering
Zinc	Disinfectants, electroplating, fungicides, galvanizing, ink, insecticides, matches, metal plating and cutting, paint, soldering, wood preservatives

Noncorrosives

The many different noncorrosive substances have the common characteristic of irritating the stomach. They produce nausea, vomiting, convulsions, and severe abdominal pain. The victim may complain of a strange taste, and the lips, tongue, and mouth may look different than normal. Shock may also occur. Examples of noncorrosives are listed in table 5-2.

First aid for most forms of noncorrosive poisoning centers on quickly emptying the stomach of the irritating substance. The following steps are suggested:

1. Maintain an open airway. Be prepared to give artificial ventilation.

2. Dilute the poison by having the conscious victim drink one to two glasses of water or milk.

3. Empty the stomach using emetic, gastric lavage, adsorbent, and/or cathartic.

    a. Giving an emetic is a preferred method for emptying the contents of the stomach. It is quick and—except in cases of caustic or petroleum distillate poisoning, or when an antiemetic has been ingested—can be used in almost every situation when the victim is conscious. In most situations, a Hospital Corpsman will have access to syrup of Ipecac. This emetic acts locally by irritating the gastric mucosa and centrally by stimulating the medullary vomiting center in the brain. The usual adult dose is 15-30 cc, and the dose for a child (age 1 to 12 years) is 15 cc. The dosage should be followed immediately by a glass of water. Most people will vomit within 30 minutes. The amount of stomach contents (and poison) recovered will vary. In an emergency room, the medical officer can rapidly induce vomiting by the injection of various medications. If nothing else is available, tickle the back of the victim's throat with your finger or a blunt object. This procedure should induce vomiting.

b. Trained personnel may use gastric lavage by itself or after two doses of Ipecac syrup has failed to induce vomiting. After passing a large—caliber nasogastric tube, aspirate the stomach contents. Next, instill 100 ml of normal saline into the stomach, then aspirate it out again. Continue this flushing cycle until the returning fluid is clear. Gastric lavage is preferred when the victim is unconscious or—as in the case of strychnine poisoning—is subject to seizures.

c. Activated charcoal (AC) adsorbs many substances in the gut and prevents absorption into the body. After the substance is adsorbed to the AC, the bound substance moves through the gut and is eliminated with the production of a charcoal-black bowel movement. AC may be administered after emesis or lavage, or it may be used alone.

d. A cathartic (magnesium sulfate or sorbitol) may be used to "speed" the movement of the bound substance and minimize absorption.

4. Collect the vomitus for laboratory analysis.

5. Soothe the stomach with milk or milk of magnesia.

6. Transport the victim to a definitive care facility if symptoms persist.

Corrosives

Acids and alkalies (bases) produce actual chemical burning and corrosion of the tissues of the lips, mouth, throat, and stomach. Acids do most of their damage in the acidic stomach environment, while alkalies primarily destroy tissues in the mouth, throat, and esophagus. Stains and burns around the mouth, and the presence of characteristic odors provide clues as to an acid or base ingestion. Swallowing and breathing may be difficult, especially if any corrosive was aspirated into the lungs. Stridor, a high-pitched sound coming from the upper airway, may be heard. The abdomen may be tender and swollen with gas, and perforation of the esophagus or stomach may occur. **NEVER ATTEMPT TO TREAT AN ACID OR BASE INGESTION BY ADMINISTERING A NEUTRALIZING SOLUTION BY MOUTH. GIVE WATER ONLY, UNLESS DIRECTED BY A POISON CONTROL CENTER (PCC) OR MEDICAL OFFICER.** Monitor the **ABC+D&Es**, and watch for signs of shock.

Examples of corrosive agents and sources of contact are listed in table 5-3.

When providing treatment for the above poisons, **DO NOT INDUCE VOMITING**. The damage to the mouth and esophagus will be compounded. In addition, the threat of aspiration during vomiting is too great. Gastric lavage could cause perforation of the esophagus or stomach. Therefore, use it only on a doctor's order. First aid consists of diluting the corrosive and keeping alert for airway potency and shock. If spontaneous vomiting occurs, administer an antiemetic.

Irritants

Substances such as automatic dishwasher detergent, diluted ammonia, and chlorine bleach can produce local irritation to the mucous membranes and potentially cause mild chemical burns. The pH of irritants may be slightly acidic or basic. If a person has ingested an irritant, direct the patient to spit the product out and rinse the mouth repeatedly with water. Spit the rinse water out also. Do **NOT** administer anything other than water unless directed by a PCC or medical officer.

Petroleum Distillates or Hydrocarbons

Volatile petroleum products (such as kerosene, gasoline, turpentine, and related petroleum products

Agent		Sources of Contact
ACIDS	Hydrochloric	Electroplating, metal cleaners, photoengraving
	Nitric	Industrial cleaners, laboratories, photoengraving, rocket fuels
	Oxalic	Cleaning solutions, paint and rust removers, photo developer
	Sulfuric	Auto batteries, detergents, dyes, laboratories, metal cleaners
ALKALIES	Ammonia	Galvanizers, household cleaners, laboratories, pesticides, rocket fuels
	Lime	Brick masonry, cement, electroplating, insecticides, soap, water treatment
	Lye	Bleaches, degreasers, detergents, laboratories, paint and varnish removers
	Carbolic	Disinfectants, dry batteries, paint removers, photo materials, wood preservatives
PHENOLS	Creosol	Disinfectants, ink, paint and varnish removers, photo developer, stainers
	Creosote	Asbestos, carpentry, diesel engines, electrical shops, furnaces, lens grinders, painters, waterproofing, wood preservatives

like red furniture polish) usually cause severe chemical pneumonia as well as other toxic effects in the body. Symptoms include abdominal pain, choking, gasping, vomiting, and fever. Often these products may be identified by their characteristic odor. Mineral oil and motor oil are not as serious since they usually do nothing more than cause diarrhea.

When providing treatment for the ingestion of petroleum distillates, **DO NOT INDUCE VOMITING** unless told to do so by a physician or poison control center. Vomiting may cause additional poison to enter the lungs. However, the quantity of poison swallowed or special petroleum additives may make gastric lavage or the use of cathartics advisable. If a physician or poison control center cannot be reached, give the victim 30 to 60 ml of vegetable oil. Transport the victim immediately to a medical treatment facility.

Food Poisoning

Food poisoning can occur from ingesting animal or plant materials, or even from the chemicals that are used in raising, processing, or preserving crops and livestock. Although illness associated with a contaminated water supply could be considered a type of food poisoning, this issue will not be addressed.

Most bacterial and viral food poisonings appear within 8 hours of ingesting food. The signs and symptoms of poisoning include nausea, vomiting, diarrhea, muscle aches, and low-grade fever. The general treatment is supportive and directed at preventing dehydration through the administration of fluids. If diarrhea persists more than 24 hours, or if the patient is unable to keep fluids down, further definitive medical care is necessary. Food poisoning can also occur from ingestion of parasites.

Marine food-borne illnesses from ingesting fish and shellfish is a concern especially when traveling to new destinations. Wherever you are in the world, you should learn which local seafood is known to be safe and which present the potential for harm. Table 5-4 lists some of toxins found in fish and shellfish and their potential sources.

Mussels, clams, oysters, and other shellfish often become contaminated with bacteria during the warm months of March through November (in the northern hemisphere). Numerous varieties of shellfish should not be eaten at all. Therefore, wherever you are in the world, you should learn which local seafoods are known to be safe and which present the potential for harm.

Table 5-4.—Examples of Toxins from Fish Known to be Poisonous

Toxin	Source
Ciguatoxin (cholinergic effects)	tends to be found in fish from coral reefs, including barracuda, grouper, red snapper, parrot fish
Scombrotoxin (histamine-like reaction)	tuna, bonito, skipjack, mackerel, mahi mahi
Saxitoxin (neurologic effects)	bivalve shellfish (mussels, clams, scallops) accumulate toxin from dinoflagellate during red tides causing "paralytic shellfish poisoning"
***Tetrodotoxin** (neurotoxin)	bacteria found in puffer fish, California newt, eastern salamander
***Neurotoxin**	Moray eel

* toxic at all times

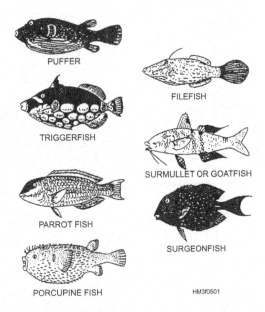

Figure 5-1.—Poisonous fish.

Most fish poisonings occur from eating fish that normally are considered to be safe to eat. However, fish can become poisonous at different times of the year because of their consumption of poisonous algae and plankton (red tide) that occur in certain locations. The signs and symptoms of red tide paralytic shellfish poisoning are tingling and numbness of the face and mouth, muscular weakness, nausea and vomiting, increased salivation, difficulty in swallowing, and respiratory failure. Primary treatment is directed at evacuating the stomach contents as soon as possible. If the patient has not vomited, select the appropriate method to remove the stomach contents by either syrup of Ipecac or gastric lavage. If respiratory failure develops, support ventilation and other life-sustaining systems as needed.

Examples of fish that are known to be poisonous **AT ALL TIMES** are shown in figure 5-1.

The symptoms of shellfish and fish poisoning are tingling and numbness of the face and mouth, muscular weakness, nausea and vomiting, increased salivation, difficulty in swallowing, and respiratory failure.

Primary treatment is directed toward evacuating the stomach contents. If the victim has not vomited, cause him to do so. Use syrup of Ipecac, gastric lavage, or manual stimulation; then administer a cathartic. If respiratory failure develops, give artificial ventilation and treat for shock.

INHALATION POISONS

In the Navy, and in other industrial settings in general, inhalation is the most common route of exposure to toxic substances. The irritants and corrosives mentioned in tables 5-2 and 5-3 are more often a source of poisoning by means of inhalation rather than by ingestion. An inhaled poison can act directly on the upper respiratory tract or lungs with immediate, delayed, or chronic effects, or the substance can use the pulmonary system to gain entry into the body, be absorbed into the blood, and cause toxic effects (systemic toxicity) at a distant site of action.

The handling of large quantities of petroleum products (fuel oil and gasoline, in particular) constitutes a special hazard, since all of these products give off hazardous vapors. Other poisonous gases are by-products of certain operations or processes: exhaust fumes from internal combustion engines; fumes or vapors from materials used in casting, molding, welding, or plating; gases associated with bacterial decomposition in closed spaces; and gases that accumulate in voids, double bottoms, empty fuel tanks, and similar places. Some sources of inhalation chemical poisoning are listed in table 5-5.

NOTE: Inhaled substances can cause **olfactory fatigue.** After a few minutes of exposure, the smell is no longer detected, fooling the individual into believing the substance is no longer there and, thus, no longer a danger.

Table 5-5.—Sources of Inhalation Poisoning

Inhaled Substance	Source of Exposure
Acetone, isopropyl alcohol, amyl acetate	Nail polish remover
Aliphatic hydrocarbons	Fuels, Stoddard solvent, PD-680, mineral spirits, naphtha
Butane	"Throw-away" lighters
Carbon dioxide	Fire suppression/fighting, evaporation of dry ice, wells and sewers
Carbon monoxide	Fires, lightning, heating and fuel exhausts
Chlorinated hydrocarbons	Shoe polish
Chlorine	Water purification, sewage treatment
Chlorofluorocarbons (CFCs)	Refrigerants, degreasers, propellants (old)
Hydrogen sulfide	Sewer, decaying materials, CHT system
Methylethylketone	Paint
Methylene chloride	Paint stripper, solvent, dyes
N-hexane	Rubber cement
Nitrous oxide	Aerosol can propellant
Tetrachloroethylene (perchloroethylene)	Dry cleaning
Toluene	Plastic adhesive, acrylic paint, shoe polish
Trichloroethane (methylchloroform)	Solvent, degreaser

Carbon monoxide is the most common agent of gas poisoning. It is present in exhaust gases of internal combustion engines as well as in sewer gas, lanterns, charcoal grills, and in manufactured gas used for heating and cooking. It gives no warning of its presence since it is completely odorless and tasteless. The victim may lose consciousness and suffer respiratory distress with no warning other than slight dizziness, weakness, and headache. The lips and skin of a victim of carbon monoxide poisoning are characteristically cherry red. Death may occur within a few minutes.

Most inhalation poisoning causes shortness of breath and coughing. The victim's skin will turn blue. If the respiratory problems are not corrected, cardiac arrest may follow.

Inhaling fine metal fumes can cause a special type of acute or delayed poisoning. These metal fumes are generated from heating metal to boiling and evaporation during hot metal work in such operations as metal cutting or welding. The resulting illness is called **metal fume fever (MFF).** In the Navy, the most common cause of MFF is the inhalation of vaporized zinc found in the galvanized covering of iron/steel. Proper local and general ventilation and/or the use of respiratory protection are necessary to prevent this illness.

The first stage of treatment for an inhalation poisoning is to remove the victim from the toxic atmosphere immediately. **WARNING**: Never try to remove a victim from the toxic environment if you do not have the proper protective mask or breathing apparatus, or if you are not trained in its use. Too often, well-intentioned rescuers become victims. If help is not immediately available, and if you know you can reach and rescue the victim, take a deep breath, hold it, enter the area, and pull the victim out. Next,

1. start basic life support (the ABC+D&Es);

2. remove or decontaminate the clothing (if chemical warfare agents or volatile fuels were the cause);

3. keep the victim quiet, treat for shock, and administer oxygen; and

4. transport the victim to a medical treatment facility for further treatment.

ABSORBED POISONS

Some substances may cause tissue irritation or destruction by contact with the skin, eyes, and lining of the nose, mouth, and throat. These substances include acids, alkalies, phenols, and some chemical warfare agents. Direct contact with these substances will cause inflammation or chemical burns in the affected areas. Consult the "Chemical Burns" section of chapter 4 and the "Chemical Agents" section of chapter 8 of this manual for treatment.

INJECTED POISONS AND ENVENOMATIONS

Injection of venom by stings and bites from various insects and arthropods, while not normally life-threatening, can cause acute allergic reaction that can be fatal. Poisons may also be injected by snakes and marine animals.

Bee, Wasp, and Fire Ant Stings

Stings from bees, wasps, and ants account for more poisonings than stings from any other insect group. Fortunately, they rarely result in death. The vast majority of stings cause a minor local reaction at the injection site, with pain, redness, itching, and swelling. These symptoms usually fade after a short time. A small percentage of these stings can cause an allergic victim severe anaphylactic reactions, presenting with itching, swelling, weakness, headache, difficulty breathing, and abdominal cramps. Shock may follow quickly, and death may occur.

The following first aid measures are recommended for all but minor, local reactions to bites or stings:

1. Closely monitor vital signs (and the whole patient), and remove all rings, bracelets, and watches.

2. Remove stingers without squeezing additional venom (remaining in poison sacs attached to stingers) into the victim. To do this, scrape along the skin with a **dull** knife (as if you were shaving the person). The dull blade will catch the stinger and pull it out.

3. Place an ice cube or analgesic-corticosteroid cream or lotion over the wound site to relieve pain. Do **NOT** use "tobacco juice," saliva, or other concoctions.

4. For severe allergic reactions (generalized itching or swelling, breathing difficulty, feeling faint or clammy, unstable pulse or blood pressure), immediately give the victim a subcutaneous injection of 1:1000 aqueous solution of epinephrine. Dosage is 0.5 cc for adults and ranges from 0.1 to 0.3 cc for children.

5. Patients with severe allergic reactions should be evacuated immediately to a medical facility.

Scorpion Stings

About 40 species of scorpions (fig. 5-2) exist in America. *Centruroides exilicauda* may cause severe effects. Most dangerous species are found from North Africa to India. Scorpion stings vary in severity, depending on the species of the scorpion and the amount of poison actually injected. They cause severe pain in the affected area.

Mild reactions may include local swelling, skin discoloration, swollen lymph nodes near the sting area, itching, paresthesias ("pins and needles," numbness), and even nausea and vomiting. The duration of symptoms is less than 24 hours.

The following first aid treatment should be given for scorpion stings:

1. Place ice over the sting site (cool the area for up to 2 hours). Do **NOT** use tobacco juice, saliva, or other concoctions.

2. Elevate the affected limb to approximately heart level.

3. Give acetaminophen for minor pain.

4. Calcium gluconate, 10 ml of 10 percent solution, may be given intravenously to relieve muscle spasms.

5. Valium may be used to control excitability and convulsions.

6. An antivenom is available for severe bites by *Centruroides exilicauda* (also called "bark scorpion," it is the scorpion found in Mexico and the American southwest). It is available from the Antivenom Production Laboratory, Arizona State University, Tempe, Arizona 85281, phone (602) 965-6443 or (602) 965-1457, and from Poison Control in Phoenix, phone (602) 253-3334.

CAUTION: Morphine and meperidine hydrochloride may worsen the respiratory depression from the venom of *Centruroides exilicauda.*

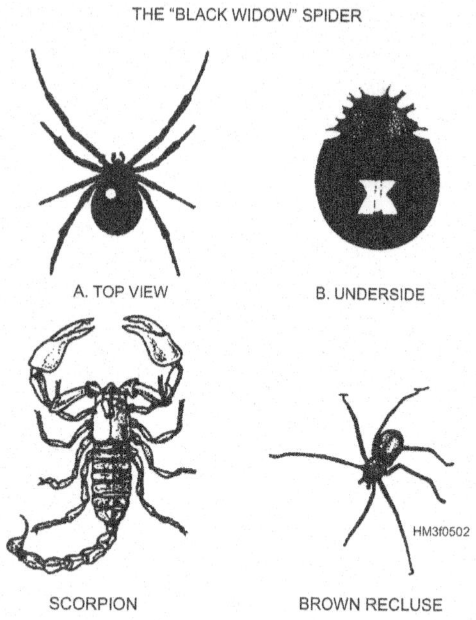

THE "BLACK WIDOW" SPIDER

A. TOP VIEW   B. UNDERSIDE

SCORPION   BROWN RECLUSE

HM3f0502

Figure 5-2.—Black widow and brown recluse spiders and scorpion.

Spider Bites

Spiders in the United States are generally harmless, with several exceptions. The most notable are the black widow (*Latrodectus mactans*) and brown recluse (*Loxosceles reclusa*, also found in South America) spiders. Their bites are serious but rarely fatal. Wandering spiders (*Phoneutria* species, found in South America), funnel web spiders (*Atrax* species, found in Australia), and more widely distributed spiders of the *Chiracanthium* species may also cause moderate to severe human reactions. Check current MEDIC CD-ROM for management of specific situations and venues.

The female black widow spider is usually identified by the red hourglass-shaped spot on its belly (fig. 5-2). Its bite causes a dull, numbing pain, which gradually spreads from the region of the bite to the muscles of the entire torso. The pain becomes severe, and a board-like rigidity of the abdominal muscles is common. Nausea, vomiting, headache, dizziness, difficulty in breathing, edema, rash, hypertension, and anxiety are frequently present. The bite site can be very hard to locate (there is little or no swelling at the site), and the victim may not be immediately aware of having been bitten. The buttocks and genitalia should be carefully examined for a bite site if the suspected victim has recently used an outside latrine. The following first aid treatment steps are suggested:

1. Place ice over the bite to reduce pain.

2. Hospitalize victims who are under 16 or over 65 (for observation).

3. Be prepared to give antivenom in severe cases.

The brown recluse spider (fig. 5-2) is identified by its violin-shaped marking. Its bite may initially go unnoticed, but after several hours, a bleb develops over the site, and rings of erythema begin to surround the bleb. Other symptoms include skin rash, fever and chills, nausea and vomiting, and pain. A progressively enlarging necrotic (dead tissue) ulcerating lesion (with a crusty black scab) eventually develops. Intravascular hemolysis (breakdown of the blood) is most often seen in children and may be fatal. Antivenom is not currently available.

Treatment for brown recluse spider bites includes the following:

- Debridement of lesion, followed by peroxide cleansing and Burrow's solution soaks

- Application of polymyxin-bacitracin-neomycin ointment and sterile dressing

- Dapsone 50-100 mg twice a day is used to promote healing in some cases, **but only after screening for G6PD deficiency.** Other antibiotics may be used to treat infection, and steroids to reduce inflammation

NOTE: Glucose-6-phosphate dehydrogenase (G6PD) deficiency is a common human enzyme deficiency. A G6PD deficiency can cause a harmful reaction to a number of medications, including dapsone.

- Based upon medical consultation, excision of the lesion and optional commencement of corticosteroid therapy

Centipede Bites

Centipedes can attain sizes of over one foot in length! Their bite, though rare, leaves two tiny red marks and causes redness and swelling. Severe pain, swelling, and inflammation may follow, and there may be headache, dizziness, vomiting, irregular pulse, muscle spasm, and swollen lymph nodes. No long-term effects are usually seen. Treat discomfort with acetaminophen, cool packs, and elevation of the affected limb to heart level.

Snakebites

Poisonous snakes are found throughout the world, with the exception of certain islands and the Antarctic. There are five venomous families of snakes.

- **Viperidae**–includes rattlesnakes, moccasins, South American lance-headed vipers and bushmaster, Asian pit vipers, African and Asian vipers and adders, the European adder, and saw-scaled viper (Middle-eastern). Kills mainly by coagulopathy (a blood clotting disorder) and shock.

- **Elapidae**–Includes cobras, kraits, mambas, and coral snakes. Kills from neurotoxic venom that can cause respiratory failure, paralysis, and cardiac failure.

- **Hydrophidae**–Includes sea snakes and venomous snakes from the islands of the southern Pacific Ocean, including Australia, New Zealand, and New Guinea. Also kills from neurotoxic venom.

- **Colubridae**–Includes most of the common nonvenomous species, as well as the boomslang, and vine/twig/bird snake (Africa); Japanese yamakagashi; Southeast Asian red-necked callback. Venom's method of toxic action varies according to type of snake.

- **Atractaspididae**–Includes the burrowing asps/mole vipers, stiletto snakes, and adders. Venom's method of toxic action varies according to type of snake.

Within the United States, poisonous snakes are Crotalids (rattlesnakes, copperheads, and moccasins) and the Elapids (coral snakes).

CROTALIDS.—Crotalids are of the *Viperidae* (viper) family and are called "pit vipers" because of the small, deep pits between the nostrils and the eyes (fig. 5-3). They have two long, hollow fangs. These fangs are normally folded against the roof of the mouth, but they can be extended when the snake strikes. Other identifying features of the Crotalids include thick bodies; slit-like pupils of the eyes; and flat, triangular heads. The most identifying feature of a pit viper is the relative width of the snake's head compared to the thickness of the body. The head will be much wider than the body, giving the appearance of an arrowhead. The difference in size is so obvious that identification of a snake as a pit viper can usually be made from a safe distance.

Further identification can be made by examining the wound for signs of fang entry in the bite pattern. Pit viper bites leave two puncture marks (sometimes only one, and sometimes more). Nonvenomous snakes (for example, garter snakes) leave a series, often in a curve or semi-circle, of tiny scratches or punctures. Individual identifying characteristics include rattles on the tails of most rattlesnakes, and the cotton-white interior of the mouths of moccasins.

ELAPIDS.—Coral snakes are of the family *Elipidae* and related to the cobra, kraits, and mamba snakes in other parts of the world (fig. 5-4). Corals, which are found in the Southeastern United States, are comparatively thin snakes with small bands of red, black, and yellow (or almost white). Some

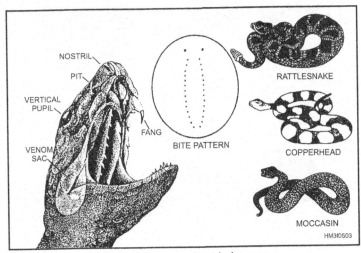

Figure 5-3.—American pit vipers.

nonpoisonous snakes have similar coloring, but in the North American coral snake, the red band always touches the yellow band, and the bands go all the way around the body. (In some of the nonvenomous, similarly colored varieties, the bands are only on the back and sides, not the belly.) There is an old saying that only applies to **NORTH** American coral snakes: "Red on yellow, kill a fellow; red on black, venom lack." The coral snake has short, hollow fangs that chew into its victim and introduce the poison. Coral snake venom is dangerous, so **if the skin is broken, give antivenom before envenomation is evidenced by symptoms or findings**.

Venom, which is stored in sacs in the snake's head, is introduced into a victim through hollow or grooved fangs. An important point to remember, however, is that a bitten patient has not necessarily received a dose of venom. The snake can control whether or not it will release the poison and how much it will inject. As a result, while symptoms in a poisonous snakebite incident may be severe, they may also be mild or not develop at all.

SIGNS AND SYMPTOMS OF SNAKE-BITE.— In a snakebite situation, every reasonable effort should be made to positively identify the culprit, since treatment of a nonpoisonous bite is far simpler and less dangerous to the victim than treatment of a poisonous bite. However, unless the snake can be

POSITIVELY identified as nonpoisonous, **CONSIDER ALL SNAKEBITES AS POISONOUS! SEEK CONSULTATION FROM EXPERT SOURCE.**

Signs and symptoms of venomous snakebite may include

- a visible bite on the skin (possibly no more than a local discoloration);

- pain and swelling in the bite area (may develop slowly, from 30 minutes to several hours);

- continued bleeding from site of bite (often seen with viper bites);

- rapid pulse;

- labored breathing;

- progressive weakness;

- dim or blurred vision;

- nausea and vomiting;

- seizures; or

- drowsiness (or loss of consciousness).

Usually enough symptoms present themselves within an hour of a poisonous snakebite to erase any doubt as to the victim's having been envenomated or

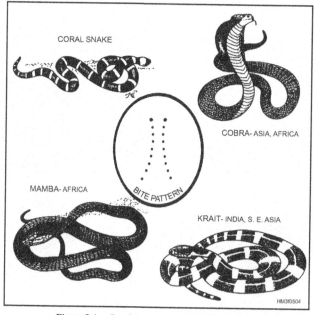

Figure 5-4.—Corals, cobras, kraits, and mambas.

not. The victim's condition provides the best information as to the seriousness of the situation.

The aims of first aid for envenomated snakebites are to reduce—**not stop**—the circulation of blood through the bite area, delay absorption of venom, prevent aggravation of the local wound, maintain vital signs, and transport the victim as soon as possible to an MTF with minimum movement.

TREATMENT OF SNAKEBITES.—The proper steps in the treatment of snakebites are listed below.

1. Try to identify the snake. Positive identification is important to selecting the correct antivenom for the treatment of the patient.

NOTE: Do not risk further injury by trying to kill the snake.

2. Certain suction extractors have benefit (for example, the Sawyer extractor), especially if used within the first 3 minutes. If available immediately, use the extractor and leave it on for 30 minutes. The cups may fill up. Empty and re-use them as necessary.

3. GENTLY wash the wound with soap and water (it may remove some of the venom). Do **NOT** rub vigorously, as it may cause the venom to be absorbed more rapidly.

4. Place the victim in a comfortable position.

5. Tell the patient to remove any jewelry (especially rings and bracelets, as these may impede blood flow if there is swelling of the extremities). Assist, if necessary.

6. Start an IV line.

7. Monitor vital signs (including ABC+D&Es) closely, responding appropriately as necessary.

8. Until evacuation or treatment is possible, ensure the victim lies quietly and does not move any more than necessary.

9. Do not allow the victim to smoke, eat, or drink any fluids. (Water is permissible if you anticipate more than several hours will pass before arriving at a hospital and being able to establish an IV line.)

10. Transport the victim to a hospital or other appropriate facility.

11. Place a **lymphatic** (light) constriction on the extremity (if the bite is on an extremity). The goal is to obstruct lymphatic—not blood-flow. (See instructions below.) **DO NOT USE A TOURNIQUET!**

LYMPHATIC CONSTRICTION INSTRUCTIONS

An appropriate lymphatic constriction device is a blood pressure cuff, inflated to the diastolic blood pressure (so the blood can be felt flowing past the cuff). Other devices may be used, but **IT IS IMPORTANT THAT BLOOD CIRCULA-TION TO THE BITE AREA BE MAINTAINED.**

Constriction should be fully released every 30 minutes for 15 seconds. If the constriction pressure cannot be carefully controlled, **THE MAXIMUM TOTAL TIME OF USE OF THE CONSTRICTION DEVICE IS 2 HOURS.** (Thus, three 15-second breaks, and the fourth time the cuff, belt, or band remains **OFF**.)

NOTE: If you use a blood pressure cuff (or device that you **KNOW** is not constricting more than an Ace® bandage on a sprain), you may continue to apply constriction until the patient reaches a hospital.

---

12. Splint the extremity at the level of the body (heart). **DO NOT ELEVATE THE EXTREMITY!**

13. Hospitalize and observe all snakebites for at least 24 hours.

In the case of spitting cobras (found in Africa, Thailand, Malaysia, Indonesia, and the Philippines), which attempt to spray venom into victims' eyes, rinse the eyes with large volumes of water (neither a blast nor a trickle, and not with hot water). Apply antibacterial (tetracycline or chloramphenicol) eye ointment, and apply a patch with just enough pressure to keep the eyelid from blinking.)

Other aid will be mainly supportive:

- Check pulse and respiration frequently. Give artificial ventilation, if necessary.

- Treat for shock, including IV fluids (normal saline or lactated Ringer's solution).

- When possible, clean the area of the bite with soap and water, and cover the wound to prevent further contamination.

- Give acetaminophen for pain if delay in hospital treatment is anticipated.

Antivenom.—Antivenom (also called antivenin) is available for many snakes, and is indicated for severe envenomations by *Viperidae* family snakes and most envenomations by snakes of the other poisonous families. Antivenom is best given as soon as possible after an envenomation, but may be of value up to a few days after a bite.

If possible, antivenom specific to the snake should be used. Otherwise, a "polyspecific" antivenom may be used. READ THE PACKAGE INSERT OF THE ANTIVENOM FOR VALUABLE INFORMATION. Epinephrine and diphenhydramine must be available, as allergic reactions (including anaphylaxis) to antivenom have occurred (they are often prepared from horse serum, which some people are allergic to).

Antivenom is diluted (for example, 1:10) and given at 5 ml/minute IV, and the dose is based on stopping the progression of signs and symptoms, not the victim's body weight (the children's dose is the same as the adult dose). For neurotoxic snakebites, if there is no improvement in 30 minutes, the dose should be repeated. For *Viperidae* (which can cause bleeding disorders), spontaneous bleeding should stop after sufficient antivenom is given; continue giving antivenom until bleeding stops and progression of swelling is retarded. Because you may need to administer antivenom a number of times, one vial may not be enough to treat a patient.

Antivenom is available via PCCs and hospitals. It may also be available at zoos and embassies.

The "Don'ts" of Snakebite Treatment.—The following are the "don'ts" when it comes to treatment of snakebite.

- **DO NOT** use any ice or cooling on the bite.

- **DO NOT** use a tourniquet. Obstructing blood flow can make local tissue injury much worse.

- **DO NOT** use electric shock.

- **DO NOT** make any cuts or incisions in the wound. Cuts at the bite site may impede circulation and promote infection and make local tissue injury much worse.

- **DO NOT** give victim alcohol or narcotics.

Further information may be obtained on an emergent basis from a PCC or from Arizona Poison Control, (520) 626-6016.

Bites, Stings, and Punctures from Sea Animals

A number of sea animals are capable of inflicting painful wounds by biting, stinging, or puncturing. Except under rare circumstances, these stings and puncture wounds are not fatal. Major wounds from sharks, barracuda, moray eels, and alligators can be treated by controlling the bleeding, preventing shock, giving basic life support, splinting the injury, and transporting the victim to a medical treatment facility. Minor injuries inflicted by turtles and stinging corals require only that the wound be thoroughly cleansed and the injury splinted.

JELLYFISH INJURIES.—Other sea animals inflict injury by means of stinging cells located in tentacles. This group includes the jellyfish and the Portuguese man-of-war (fig. 5-5). The tentacles (which may be impossible to see, even in relatively clear water) release poison or tiny stingers through which poison is injected into the victim. Jellyfish stings may cause symptoms ranging from minor irritation (pain and itching) to death. Contact with the tentacles produces burning pain, a rash with small hemorrhage in the skin, and, on occasion, shock, muscular cramping, nausea, vomiting, and respiratory and cardiac distress. Treatment for minor jellyfish injuries consists of pouring sea water over the injured area and then removing the tentacles with a towel or gloves. Next, pour rubbing alcohol, formalin, vinegar, meat tenderizer, or diluted ammonia over the affected area to neutralize any remaining nematocysts (minute stinging structures). Finally, cover the area with any dry powder (to which the last nematocysts will

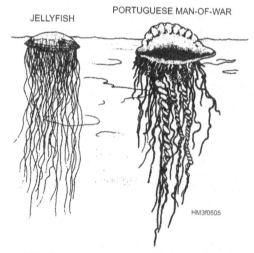

JELLYFISH   PORTUGUESE MAN-OF-WAR

HM3f0505

Figure 5-5.—Jellyfish and Portuguese Man-of-war.

adhere), and then scrape off with a dull knife. Apply cool packs and hydrocortisone cream.

Some jellyfish (notably, the Portuguese man-of-war, the box jellyfish, and certain jellyfish from northeastern Australia) may cause serious injuries and even have the potential to be lethal. In cases where the kind of jellyfish that caused the sting is either unknown or is known to have been from a box jellyfish or Portuguese man-of-war, the injury should be treated as a serious one, regardless of initial symptoms. The following steps should be taken in the case of serious jellyfish stings.

1. Retrieve the victim from the water if necessary.

2. Send others for an ambulance and antivenom. (Antivenom is available for box jellyfish stings. It is from sheep, and should be given in all serious stings.)

3. Pour vinegar liberally (2 liters) over the sting area for at least 30 seconds to inactivate stinging cells that may remain.

4. Remove any remaining tentacles carefully. (Excessive manipulation may cause rupture of nematocysts and further poison release.) Carefully (and gently) use a towel if necessary, or use a dull knife edge (as described above to remove arthropod stingers).

5. Apply a compression bandage to stings covering more than half of one limb or causing altered consciousness.

6. Start an IV.

7. Remain with the victim, and monitor vital signs (the ABCs and consciousness, responding appropriately (possibly including CPR) and as necessary).

8. Transport the patient to a hospital as quickly as possible.

9. Opiate analgesics (morphine or meperidine) may be necessary for pain relief.

"SPINE" INJURIES.—Spiny fish, stingrays, urchins, and cone shells inject their venom by puncturing with spines (fig. 5-6). General signs and symptoms include swelling, nausea, vomiting, generalized cramps, diarrhea, muscular paralysis, and shock. General emergency care consists of prompt flushing with cold sea water to remove the venom and to constrict hemorrhaging blood vessels. Next, debride the wound of any remaining pieces of the spine's venom-containing integumentary sheath. Soak

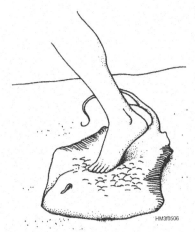

Figure 5-6.—Stingray sting.

the wound area in very hot water (110°F/43° C) for 30 to 60 minutes to neutralize the venom. Finally, completely debride the wound, control hemorrhage, suture, provide tetanus prophylaxis and a broad-spectrum antibiotic, and elevate the extremity. For minor injuries, a steroid cream to the wound area may relieve discomfort. For serious injuries—wounds that are deep, very painful, or causing the patient distress—stabilize the patient and transport immediately to a hospital.

In the case of contact with stonefish, scorpionfish, zebra, or lionfish, immerse the wound in very hot water for a **minimum** of 30 minutes until the pain is decreased. Inject emetine hydrochloride directly into the wound within 30 minutes, and provide meperidine (or other opiate) for pain. Monitor the victim's vital signs closely. Obtain antivenom (from local zoos or aquariums) for all serious cases.

SEA SNAKE INJURIES.—Sea snakes are found in the warm water areas of the Pacific and Indian Oceans. Their venom is **VERY** poisonous, but their fangs are only 1/4 inch long. The first aid outlined for land snakes also applies to sea snakes.

DRUG ABUSE

LEARNING OBJECTIVE: *Recall drug abuse assessment and treatment procedures and patient handling techniques.*

Drug abuse is the use of drugs for purposes or in quantities for which they were not intended. Drugs of abuse may be swallowed, inhaled, snorted (or by nose drops), injected, or even absorbed through the skin, rectum, or vagina. When abused, therapeutic drugs become a source of "poison" to the body. Drug abuse can lead to serious illness, dependency, and death. Death is usually because of acute intoxication or overdoses.

Drugs of abuse can be classified in many different ways. This chapter will classify drugs of abuse based on the symptoms they produce: CNS depression, CNS stimulation, and hallucinations. The CNS depressants include narcotics, ethanol, barbiturates, non-barbiturate sedative-hypnotics (including benzo-diazepines). The CNS stimulants include caffeine, nicotine, amphetamines, and cocaine. The hallucinogens include LSD, PCP, and marijuana.

Table 5-6 lists many of the most frequently abused drugs with their recognizable trade names, some commonly used street names, and observable symptoms of abuse.

The following sections contain specific information about commonly abused drugs, as classified in table 5-6, including availability and methods of administration.

NARCOTIC INTOXICATION

Unfortunately, narcotic abuse is common, although it is rare among military personnel. This group of drugs includes the most effective and widely used pain killers in existence. Prolonged use of narcotic drugs, even under medical supervision, inevitably leads to physical and psychological dependence. The more commonly known drugs within this group are opium, morphine, heroin, codeine, and methadone (a synthetic narcotic). In addition, Darvon 7 and Talwin7 are included in this group because of their narcotic-like action. Next to cocaine (discussed later), heroin is the most popular narcotic drug because of its intense euphoria and long-lasting effect. It is far more potent than morphine but has no legitimate use in the United States. Heroin appears as a white, gray, or tan fluffy powder. The most common method of using heroin is by injection directly into the vein, although it can be sniffed. Codeine, although milder than heroin and morphine, is sometimes abused as an ingredient in cough syrup preparations. Symptoms of narcotic drug abuse include slow, shallow breathing; possible unconsciousness; constriction (narrowing) of the pupils of the eyes to pinpoint size; drowsiness; confusion; and slurred speech.

The narcotic user, suddenly withdrawn from drugs, may appear as a wildly disturbed person who is agitated, restless, and possibly hallucinating. Initial symptoms start within 2 to 48 hours and peak at about 72 hours. Although these signs and symptoms are not life-threatening, most users will state that they feel so bad they wish they were dead. The signs and symptoms of withdrawal immediately stop upon re-administering a narcotic and withdrawing the drug by tapering the dose over several days.

ALCOHOL INTOXICATION

Alcohol is the most widely abused drug today. Alcohol intoxication is so common that it often fails to receive the attention and respect it deserves. Although there are many other chemicals that are in the chemical grouping of "alcohols," the type consumed by people as a beverage (in wines, beers, and distilled liquors) is known as ethyl alcohol, ethanol, grain alcohol, or just "alcohol." It is a colorless, flammable, intoxicating liquid, classed as a drug because it depresses the central nervous system, affecting physical and mental activities.

Alcohol affects the body of the abuser in stages. Initially, there is a feeling of relaxation and well-being, followed by confusion with a gradual disruption of coordination, resulting in inability to accurately and efficiently perform normal activities and skills. Continued alcohol consumption leads to a stuporous state of inebriation that results in vomiting, an inability to walk or stand, and impaired consciousness (sleep or stupor). Excessive consumption can cause loss of consciousness, coma, and even—in extreme cases — death from alcohol poisoning.

The potential for physical and psychological addiction is very high when alcohol is abused. The severely intoxicated individual must be closely monitored to avoid inhalation of vomit (aspiration) and adverse behavioral acts to the patient or others. Withdrawal from alcohol is considered to be life-threatening and should be appropriately treated in a healthcare facility. Individuals withdrawing from alcohol are at a greater risk of serious complications or death than those withdrawing from narcotics. The effects of alcohol withdrawal include severe agitation, anxiety, confusion, restlessness, sleep disturbances, sweating, profound depression, delirium tremens ("DTs," a particular type of confusion and shaking), hallucinations, and seizures.

Table 5-6.—Classification of Abused Drugs

A. NARCOTICS

Agent	Trade Name	Some Street Names	Symptoms of Abuse
Morphine	....	"H", Miss Emma, smack	•Lethargy •Drowsiness
Diacetylmorphine	Heroin	"H", horse, junk, smack, stuff, whack	•Confusion •Euphoria
Codeine	....		•Slurred speech •Flushing of the skin on face, neck, and chest
Meperidine	Demerol		•Nausea and vomiting
Methadone	Dolphine	Dolly	•Pupils constricted to pinpoint size
Propoxyphene	Darvon		
Pentazocine	Talwin		

B. ALCOHOL
(Ethyl)

Agent	Trade Name	Some Street Names	Symptoms of Abuse
Alcohol (ethyl)	Ethanol	Liquors, beer, wines	•Slurred speech •Incoordination •Confusion •Tremors •Drowsiness •Agitation •Nausea and vomiting •Respiratory depression •Hallucinations •Possible coma

C. STIMULANTS
(Uppers)

Agent	Trade Name	Some Street Names	Symptoms of Abuse
Amphetamine	Benzedrine	Bennies, pep pills, ups, cartwheels	•Excitability •Rapid and unclear speech
Cocaine	....	Crack, coke, snow, gold dust, rock, freebase, snort, hubba hubba, flake	•Restlessness •Tremors •Sweating
Dextroamphetamine	Dexadrine	Dexies	•Dry lips and mouth •Dilated pupils
Methamphetamine	Methadrine	Speed, meth, crystal, diet pills, crank	•Loss of consciousness •Coma
Methylphenidate	Ritalin		•Hallucinations

D. BARBITURATES
(Downers, dolls, barbs, rainbows)

Agent	Trade Name	Some Street Names	Symptoms of Abuse
Phenobarbital	....	Goofballs, phennies	Same as those noted in alcohol intoxication, plus pupils may be dilated.
Amobarbital	Amytal	Blues, blue birds, blue devils, downers	
Pentobarbital	Nembutal	Yellows, yellow jackets	
Secobarbital	Seconal	Reds, red devils, seggy	

Table 5-6.—Classification of Abused Drugs—Continued

E.   OTHER SEDATIVES & HYPNOTICS
(Downers)

Agent	Trade Name	Some Street Names	Symptoms of Abuse
Glutethimide	Doriden	Goofers	
Chlordiazepoxide	Librium		Same as those noted in alcohol and barbiturate intoxication.
Meprobamate	Miltown, Equanil		
Methaqualone	Quaalude, Sopor	Ludes, sopors	

F.   HALLUCINOGENS

Agent	Trade Name	Some Street Names	Symptoms of Abuse
Lysergic acid diethylamide	....	LSD, acid, sunshine	•Trance-like state
Mescaline	....	Peyote, mesc	•Anxiety •Confusion
Phencyclidine (PCP)		Angel dust, hog, peace pills	•Tremors •Euphoria
Psilocin, psilocybin	Peyote	Buttons, mesc, magic mushrooms	•Depression •Hallucinations •Psychotic manifestations •Suicidal or homicidal tendencies

G.   CANNABIS

Agent	Trade Name	Some Street Names	Symptoms of Abuse
Cannabis	Marijuana	Pot, grass, weed, joint, tea, reefer, rope, Jane, hay, dope	•Euphoria •Excitability •Increased appetite •Dryness of mouth •Odor of burned rope on breath •Intoxication •Laughter •Mood swings •Increase in heart rate •Reddening of eyes •Loss of memory •Distortion of time and spatial perception

H.   INHALANTS

Agent	Trade Name	Some Street Names	Symptoms of Abuse
Amyl nitrate		Snappers, poppers	•Dazed, temporary loss of contact with reality
Butyl nitrate		Locker room, rush	•Possible coma •Swollen membranes in mouth and nose
Other volatile chemicals: Cleaning fluid, furniture polish, gasoline, glue, hair spray, nail polish remover, paint thinner, correction fluid			•"Funny numb feeling" •"Tingling" inside the head •Changes in heart rhythm •Possible death

BARBITURATE INTOXICATION

Benzodiazepines have largely replaced barbiturates, or "downers," as sedatives, hypnotics (sleeping pills), or anxiolytic (anti-anxiety) agents. Barbiturates are still used to treat various seizure disorders. They are classified based on their duration of action: ultra-short acting, short acting, intermediate acting, and long acting. Barbiturate use classically causes various degrees of CNS depression with nystagmus (eyes moving up and down, or side-to-side involuntarily), vertigo (sensation of the room spinning), slurred speech, lethargy, confusion, ataxia (difficulty walking) and respiratory depression. Severe overdose may result in coma, shock, apnea (stopped breathing), and hypothermia. In combination with ethanol or other CNS depressants, there are additive CNS and respiratory depression effects.

Prolonged use of barbiturates can lead to a state of physical and psychological dependence. Upon discontinued use, the dependant person may go into withdrawal. Unlike narcotic (opiate) withdrawal, barbiturate withdrawal is **LIFE THREATENING!** Depending on type of barbiturate, signs and symptoms start within 24 hours. The withdrawal syndrome includes nausea, vomiting, sweating, tremors (trembling or shaking), weakness, insomnia, and restlessness. These clinical findings progress to apprehension, acute anxiety, fever, increased blood pressure, and increased heart rate. If untreated, severe and life-threatening effects include delirium, hallucinations, and seizures. The signs and symptoms will stop upon re-administration of the barbiturate and by tapering the dose slowly over several days.

NONBARBITURATE SEDATIVE-HYPNOTIC INTOXICATION

Nonbarbiturate sedative-hypnotics (a "hypnotic" is a sleeping pill) have actions very similar to the barbiturates. However, they have a higher margin of safety; overdose and addiction require larger doses and addiction requires a longer time period to occur. Like the barbiturates, when combined with ethanol or other depressants, there are addictive CNS- and respiratory-depression effects. Most of the traditional, nonbarbiturate sedative-hypnotics are either no longer available (Methaquaalone, Ethchlorovynol, Glutethimide) or rarely used today (chloral hydrate) because of their profound "hangover effect." Newer sedative-hypnotics are emerging for the temporary treatment of insomnia. Benzodiazepines are widely used to treat seizure disorders, anxiety, muscle spasms, and insomnia.

STIMULANT INTOXICATION

The stimulants ("uppers") directly affect the central nervous system by increasing mental alertness and combating drowsiness and fatigue. One group of stimulants, called amphetamines, is legitimately used in the treatment of conditions such as mild depression, obesity, and narcolepsy (sleeping sickness).

Amphetamines are also commonly abused. Usually referred to as stimulants, speed, or uppers, amphetamines can be taken orally, intravenously, or smoked as "ice." Amphetamines directly affect the central nervous system by increasing mental alertness and combating drowsiness and fatigue. They are abused for their stimulant effect, which lasts longer than cocaine.

Amphetamines cause central nervous system stimulation with euphoria, increased alertness, intensified emotions, aggressiveness, altered self-esteem, and increased sexuality. In higher doses, unpleasant CNS effects of agitation, anxiety, hallucinations, delirium, psychosis, and seizures can occur. When stimulants are combined with alcohol ingestion, patients have increased psychological and cardiac effects.

Signs and symptoms associated with amphetamine use include mydriasis (dilated pupils), sweating, increased temperature, tachycardia (rapid pulse), and hypertension. Patients seeking medical attention usually complain of chest pain, palpitations, and shortness of breath.

"Heavy use" (involving large quantities) of amphetamines is physically addicting, and even "light use" (involving small amounts) can cause psychological dependence. Tolerance to increasingly higher doses develops and withdrawal can occur from these levels. Abruptly stopping chronic amphetamine use does not cause seizures or present a life-threatening situation. The withdrawal is typically characterized by apathy, lethargy, muscle aches, stomachaches, increased appetite, anxiety, sleep disturbances, and depression with suicidal tendencies.

Cocaine, although classified as a narcotic, acts as a stimulant and is commonly abused. It is relatively ineffective when taken orally; therefore, the abuser either injects it into the vein or "snorts" it through the nose. Its effect is much shorter than that of amphetamines, and occasionally the abuser may inject or snort cocaine every few minutes in an attempt to maintain a constant stimulation and prevent depression experienced during withdrawal (come-down). Overdose is very possible, often resulting in convulsion and death.

The physical symptoms observed in the cocaine abuser will be the same as those observed in the amphetamine abuser.

HALLUCINOGEN INTOXICATION

The group of drugs that affect the central nervous system by altering the user's perception of self and environment are commonly known as hallucinogens. Included within this group are lysergic acid diethylamide (LSD), mescaline, dimethoxymethyl-amphetamine (STP), phencyclidine (PCP), and psilocybin. They appear in several forms: crystals, powders, and liquids.

The symptoms of hallucinogenic drugs include dilated pupils, flushed face, increased heartbeat, and a chilled feeling. In addition, the person may display a distorted sense of time and self, show emotions ranging from ecstasy to horror, and experience changes in visual depth perception.

Although no deaths have resulted from the drugs directly, hallucinogen-intoxicated persons have been known to jump from windows, walk in front of automobiles, or injure themselves in other ways because of the vivid but unreal perception of their environment.

Even though no longer under the direct influence of a hallucinogenic drug, a person who has formerly used one of the drugs may experience a spontaneous recurrence (flashback) of some aspect of the drug experience. The most common type of flashback is the recurrence of perceptual distortion; however, victims of flashback may also experience panic or disturbing emotion. Flashback may be experienced by heavy or occasional users of hallucinogenic drugs, and its frequency is unpredictable and its cause unknown.

CANNABIS INTOXICATION

Cannabis sativa, commonly known as marijuana, is widely abused and may be classified as a mild hallucinogen. The most common physical appearance of marijuana is as ground, dried leaves, and the most common method of consumption is smoking, but it can be taken orally. A commercially prepared product of the active ingredient in marijuana, tetrahydro-cannabinol (THC), is dronabinol (Marinol R) available in the U.S. as a controlled Schedule II drug. Dronabinol is used for the treatment of nausea and vomiting in chemotherapy patients. It may also be useful in the treatment of acute glaucoma, asthma, and nausea and vomiting from other chronic illnesses. The individual response to the recreational use of marijuana varies and depends on the dose, the personality and expectation of the user, and the setting. Unexpected ingestion, emotional stress, or underlying psychiatric disorders can increase the possibility of an unfavorable reaction.

After a single inhaled dose of marijuana, a subjective "high" begins in several minutes and is gone within four hours. Marijuana causes decreased pupil size and conjunctivitis (reddening of the white of the eye). Smoking marijuana can increase the heart rate (tachycardia) for about two hours. It can slightly increase systolic blood pressure in low doses and can lower blood pressure in high doses. An increased appetite and dry mouth are common complaints after marijuana use.

Social setting influences the psychological effects associated with "usual doses" of marijuana smoking. Smoking in a solitary setting may produce euphoria, relaxation, and sleep. In a group setting, increased social interaction, friendliness, and laughter or giddiness may be produced. Subjectively, time moves slower, images appear more vivid, and hearing seems keener. High doses can cause lethargy, depersonali-zation, pressured speech, paranoia, hallucinations, and manic psychosis (imagining everything is wonderful in a way that is out of reality).

INHALANT INTOXICATION

Inhalants are potentially dangerous, volatile chemicals that are not meant for human consumption. They are found in consumer, commercial, and industrial products intended for use in well-ventilated areas. The vapors they produce can be extremely dangerous when inhaled inadvertently or by design.

Substances in this category include adhesives (synthetic "glues"), paint, wet markers, lighter fluids, solvents, and propellants in aerosol spray cans, and air fresheners. Inhalants can be abused by "sniffing" (inhaling through the nose directly over an open container), "bagging" (holding an open bag or container over the head), or "huffing" (pouring or spraying material on a cloth that is held over the mouth and inhaling through the mouth). These methods usually use a bag or other container to concentrate and retain the propellant thereby producing a quick "high" for the abuser.

Persons who regularly abuse inhalants risk permanent and severe brain damage and even sudden death. The vapors from these volatile chemicals can react with the fatty tissues in the brain and literally dissolve them. Additionally, inhalants can reduce the availability and use of oxygen. Acute and chronic damage may also occur to the heart, kidneys, liver, peripheral nervous system, bone marrow, and other organs. Sudden death can occur from respiratory arrest or irregular heart rhythms that are often difficult to treat even if medical care is quickly available.

Signs and symptoms of inhalant abuse closely resemble a combination of alcohol and marijuana intoxication. Acute symptoms are very short-lived and are completely gone within two hours. Physical symptoms of withdrawal from inhalants include hallucinations, nausea, excessive sweating, hand tremors, muscle cramps, headaches, chills and delirium tremens. Thirty to forty days of detoxification is required, and relapse is frequent.

HANDLING DRUG-INTOXICATED PERSONS

As in any emergency medical situation, priorities of care must be established. Conditions involving respiratory or cardiac failure must receive immediate attention before specific action is directed to the drug abuse symptom. General priorities of care are outlined below:

- The **ABCs + D & E**: check for adequacy of airway, breathing, and circulation, signs of drug/chemical (**"D"**) induced altered mental status, and hidden injuries or contact with a poison revealed by exposing (**"E"**) parts of the body covered with clothing or other articles. Watch for shock! Give appropriate treatment.

- If the victim cannot be aroused, place him on his side so secretions and vomitus can drain from the mouth and not be aspirated into the lungs.

- All adult patients with an altered mental status should receive dextrose after blood sugar testing, thiamine, naloxone, and oxygen.

- If recommended by the PCC or medical officer, place the patient on a cardiac monitor and/or obtain specimens for comprehensive laboratory work-up (blood and urine).

- If recommended by the PCC or medical officer, decontaminate the gut. (This decontamination should be accomplished ONLY if the victim is conscious and the drug was RECENTLY TAKEN ORALLY.)

- Prevent the victim from self-injury while highly excited or lacking coordination. Use physical restraints only if absolutely necessary (i.e., upon failure of chemical restraints).

- Calm and reassure the excited patient by "talking them down" in a quiet, relaxed, and sympathetic manner.

- Gather materials and information to assist in identifying and treating the suspected drug problem. Spoons, paper sacks, eyedroppers, hypodermic needles, and vials are excellent identification clues.

- The presence of capsules, pills, drug containers, needle marks (tracks) on the patient's body, or paint or other substance around the mouth and nose, are also important findings of substance abuse.

- A personal history of drug use from the patient or those accompanying the patient is very important and may reveal how long the victim has been abusing drugs, approximate amounts taken, and time between doses. Knowledge of past medical problems, including history of convulsions (with or without drugs) is also important.

- Transport the patient and the materials collected to a medical treatment facility.

- Inform MTF personnel and present the materials collected at the scene upon arrival at the facility.

HAZARDOUS MATERIAL EXPOSURE

LEARNING OBJECTIVE: *Recognize hazardous material personal safety guidelines and hazardous material information sources.*

Hazardous materials are substances with the potential of harming people or the environment. Hazardous materials can be gaseous, liquid, or solid, and can include chemical or radioactive materials. (Radiological exposure will be covered in depth in chapter 8 of this manual. Radioactive materials are regulated by specific instructions/directives.) The most common substances involved in incidents of hazardous material (HAZMAT) exposure are volatile organic compounds, pesticides, ammonia, chlorine, petroleum products, and acids.

Your initial action at the scene of a hazardous materials incident must be to assess the situation, since your safety—as well as that of the public and any patients—is of primary concern. You must first determine the nature of the HAZMAT, then establish a safety zone. Only after these things have been accomplished can a victim who has been exposed to hazardous materials be rescued, transported to an appropriate facility, and properly decontaminated.

The Department of Transportation (DOT) publication, *Emergency Response Guidebook* (ERG series, published every four years), RSPA P5800.8, is a useful tool for first responders during the initial phase of a hazardous materials/dangerous goods incident. ERG series addresses labeling, identification, toxicity, safety/contamination zones, and decontamination procedures. **IT IS IMPERATIVE THAT ALL PERSONNEL INVOLVED WITH HAZMAT INCIDENT RESPONSE BE FAMILIAR WITH THIS PUBLICATION.** It is also available on the Internet at http://hazmat.dot.gov/gydebook.htm.

DETERMINING THE NATURE OF THE HAZARDOUS MATERIAL

When an incident involving the exposure of hazardous material occurs, it is of prime importance to any rescue operation to determine the nature of the substance(s) involved. All facilities that produce HAZMAT are required by law to prominently display this information, as is any vehicle transporting it. Any carton or box containing such material must also be properly labeled. The name of the substance may also be displayed, along with a required four-digit identification number (sometimes preceded by the letters **UN** or **NA**).

The various kinds of hazardous materials usually have different labels to assist in their identification. These are generally diamond-shaped signs that have specific colors to identify the type of HAZMAT involved. Table 5-7 provides a list of the Department of Transportation (DOT)-mandated classifications of hazardous materials.

The ERG series provides a list of hazardous materials and appropriate emergency response actions. The Guidebook is primarily a tool to enable first responders to quickly identify the specific or generic classification of the material(s) involved in the incident, and to protect themselves and the general public during the initial phase of the incident.

SAFETY GUIDELINES

Your first objective should be to try to read the labels and identification numbers **FROM A DISTANCE**. If necessary, use binoculars. **DO NOT** go into the area unless you are absolutely certain that has been no hazardous spill. Relay any and all information available to your dispatch center where it can be used to identify the HAZMAT.

Once the HAZMAT has been identified, it can be classified as to the danger it presents (i.e., toxicity level). Based on this classification, the appropriate specialized equipment (known as personal protective equipment, or PPE) can be determined to provide adequate protection (i.e., protection level) from

Table 5-7.—Hazardous Materials Warning Labels

HAZMAT Type	Label Description
Explosives	solid orange color
Nonflammable gases	solid green color
Flammable liquids	solid red color
Flammable solids	white and red stripes
Oxidizers & peroxides	solid yellow color
Poisons & biohazards	solid white color
Radioactive materials	half white/half yellow with black radiation symbol
Corrosives	half white/half black
Other	usually white

secondary contamination to rescue personnel and healthcare providers.

Toxicity Levels

The National Fire Protection Association (NFPA) has developed a system for indicating the health, flammability, and reactivity hazards of chemicals. It is called the **NFPA 704 Labeling System** and is made up of symbols arranged in squares to comprise a diamond-shaped label (fig. 5-7). Each of the four hazards is indicated by a different colored square:

- **Red** indicates the flammability.
- **Yellow** indicates the reactivity.
- **White** indicates any special hazards.
- **Blue** indicates health hazards.
- The health hazard levels are
- **4** - deadly,
- **3** - extreme danger,
- **2** - hazardous,
- **1** - slightly hazardous, and
- **0** - normal material.

Protection Levels

The protection levels, B, C, and D—indicate the type and amount of protective equipment required in a given hazardous circumstance, with level A being the most hazardous.

- **Level A** - positive pressure-demand, full-face piece self-contained breathing apparatus (SCBA) or positive pressure-demand supplied air respirator with escape SCBA; fully encapsulating, chemical-resistant suit; inner chemical-resistant gloves; chemical-resistant safety boots/shoes; and two-way radio communication.

- **Level B** - positive pressure-demand, full-face piece SCBA or positive pressure-demand supplied air respirator with escape SCBA; chemical-resistant clothing (overalls and long-sleeved jacket with hooded one- or two-piece chemical splash suit or disposable chemical-resistant one-piece suit); chemical-resistant safety boots/shoes; hard hat; and two-way communication.

- **Level C** - full-face piece, air-purifying canister-equipped respirator; chemical-resistant clothing (overalls and long-sleeved jacket with hooded one- or two-piece chemical splash suit or disposable chemical-resistant one-piece suit); inner and outer chemical-resistant gloves; chemical-resistant safety boots/shoes; hard hat; and two-way communication.

- **Level D** - Coveralls, safety boots/shoes, safety glasses or chemical splash goggles, and hard hat.

You are required to wear gloves at all four protection levels. If the correct type of glove to be used is not known, use neoprene or rubber, and avoid using latex or vinyl. In any instance, contact with HAZMAT should be avoided or minimized, and proper

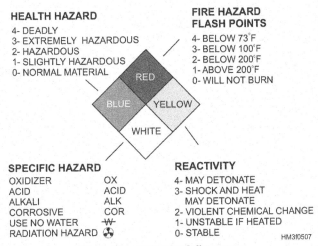

HEALTH HAZARD
4- DEADLY
3- EXTREMELY HAZARDOUS
2- HAZARDOUS
1- SLIGHTLY HAZARDOUS
0- NORMAL MATERIAL

FIRE HAZARD FLASH POINTS
4- BELOW 73°F
3- BELOW 100°F
2- BELOW 200°F
1- ABOVE 200°F
0- WILL NOT BURN

SPECIFIC HAZARD
OXIDIZER	OX
ACID	ACID
ALKALI	ALK
CORROSIVE	COR
USE NO WATER	W
RADIATION HAZARD	

REACTIVITY
4- MAY DETONATE
3- SHOCK AND HEAT MAY DETONATE
2- VIOLENT CHEMICAL CHANGE
1- UNSTABLE IF HEATED
0- STABLE

HM3f0507

Figure 5-7.—NFPA 704 labeling system.

decontamination should be performed promptly. Protect feet from contact with chemical by using a disposable boot/shoe cover made from appropriate material.

Site Control

For management purposes, site control is divided up into three sections.

- **Exclusion Zone (Hot Zone):** The area where the contamination has occurred. The outer boundary of the exclusion zone should be marked either by lines, placards, hazard tape and/or signs, or enclosed by physical barriers. Access control points should be established at the periphery of the exclusion zone to regulate the flow of personnel and equipment. Remember also to remain **upwind** of the danger area, and avoid low areas where toxic gases/vapors may tend to settle.

- **Contamination-Reduction Zone (Warm Zone):** The transition area between the contaminated area and the clean area. This zone is designed to prevent the clean support zone from becoming contaminated or affected by other site hazards. Decontamination of personnel/equipment takes place in a designated area within the contamination-reduction zone called the "contamination-reduction corridor."

- **Support Zone:** The location of the administrative and other support functions needed to keep the operations in the exclusion and contamination-reduction zones running smoothly. The command post supervisor should be present in the support zone. Personnel may wear normal work clothes within this zone.

Figure 5-8 shows the three management sections of a hazard zone.

RESCUE AND PATIENT CARE PROCEDURES

LEARNING OBJECTIVE: *Recall rescue, patient care, and decontamination procedures for patients exposed to hazardous material.*

After a safety zone has been established—and regardless of your level of training—you should follow the procedures outlined below:

- Help isolate the incident site and keep the area clear of unauthorized and unprotected personnel.

- Establish and maintain communications with your dispatcher.

- Stay upwind and upgrade from the site, and monitor wind and weather changes.

- Don't breathe any smoke, vapors, or fumes.

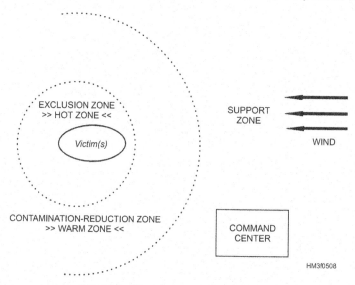

Figure 5-8.—Hazard zone management sections

- Don't touch, walk, or drive through the spilled materials, since these will increase the area of the spill.

- Don't eat, drink, or smoke at the site; don't touch your face, nose, mouth, or eyes. (These are all direct routes of entry into your body.)

- Eliminate any possible source of ignition (e.g., flares, flames, sparks, smoking, flashes, flashlights, engines, portable radios).

- Notify your dispatcher and give your location. Request the assistance of the HAZMAT response team.

- If possible, identify the hazardous material and report it to the dispatcher.

- Observe all safety precautions and directions given by the on-site HAZMAT expert. **All orders should be given and received face to face.**

- Stay clear of restricted areas until the on-site HAZMAT expert declares them to be safe.

Rescue from Exclusion Zone (Hot Zone)

The most dangerous element of any HAZMAT incident—both to the exposed victims and the rescuers—is the rescue from the hot zone. Rescue operations should always be performed using appropriate protective equipment (PPE). **You must never enter the area unless you have been appropriately trained to do so.** Let the experts handle this aspect of the rescue, but be prepared to provide supportive care once the victim is clear of the contaminated area.

As soon as the patient has been removed to safety, you should follow normal primary and secondary survey procedures, including interviews of the patient and bystanders. Observe the patient and provide basic life support. Give the patient supplemental oxygen, and monitor vital signs closely.

Patient Decontamination Procedures

Decontamination is the process of removing or neutralizing and properly disposing of contaminants that have accumulated on personnel and equipment. Decontamination protects site personnel by minimizing the transfer of contaminants, helps to prevent the mixing of incompatible chemicals, and protects the community by preventing uncontrolled

transportation of contaminants from the site. All personnel, clothing, and equipment that leave the contamination area (exclusion zone) must be decontaminated to remove any harmful chemicals that may have adhered to them. Some decontamination methods include those listed below.

- **Dilution**: the flushing of the contaminated person or equipment with water.

- **Absorption**: the use of special filters and chemicals to absorb the hazardous material.

- **Chemical washes**: specific chemicals used to neutralize the hazardous material.

- **Disposal and isolation**: the proper disposal of contaminated materials instead of attempting to decontaminate them.

Dilution is the most frequently appropriate method of decontamination.

Decontamination requires the use of PPE, although the level of protection required may be less once the victim is out of the hot zone. A victim who is exposed to a gas may not require actual "decontamination" after rescue and only require cessation of exposure and an opportunity to breathe fresh air. However, if a victim is soaked with a liquid, the HAZMAT may pose an ongoing risk to the victim and to the rescuers or medical personnel. **IT IS IMPORTANT TO ALWAYS ASSUME THAT THE VICTIM HAS BEEN CONTAMINATED WITH SOMETHING THAT COULD HARM YOU AND OTHERS UNTIL DETERMINED OTHERWISE.** Do not be foolish or bold and presume that you or others will not be exposed and harmed!

Once the victim is medically evaluated, carefully remove any solid material that remains on the patient's clothing. Be alert not to get any on yourself. If the material is dry, immediately remove the victim's clothing while avoiding or minimizing contact with the HAZMAT or loss of the HAZMAT from the clothing. Unless specifically contraindicated by the hazardous nature of the HAZMAT and directed by the incident commander or the supporting medical advisor, flush the patient's skin, clothing, and eyes with water. To the maximum extent possible, control or retain the runoff (which is contaminated) which will be containerized for proper disposal. Remove all of the victim's clothing, shoes, and jewelry. Place everything that may have contacted the HAZMAT in a special container. Mark the container as contaminated. Continue flushing the skin with water for at least 20 minutes. Again, try to retain the runoff. Using available items like towels or clean rags, mechanically remove the HAZMAT by wiping; avoid rubbing the skin too vigorously. Dry the skin and provide uncontaminated dry clothing or coverings.

The nature of the HAZMAT involved and the threat to the health of others (rescue team, other victims, medical personnel, transport crew) determines the degree of decontamination necessary before treatment or transporting the patient. Generally, it is preferred that decontamination be accomplished before treatment or transport. However, the patient's immediate medical condition may be more serious than the contamination itself. For example, ingested HAZMAT may pose little immediate threat to nearby personnel, but be an imminent threat to the victim's life. Therefore, the consequences of delaying the emergency care of the patient's injuries to accomplish gut decontamination must be carefully evaluated. In some cases, decontamination and emergency medical care can be carried out simultaneously. In rare instances of great urgency, the victim may require transportation to the hospital before decontamination. In these unusual cases, notify both the hospital and transportation crew of the patient's medical condition and contamination. Depending on the situation, the transportation crew will have to appropriately prepare to carry and care for the contaminated victim; otherwise, the crew themselves could be contaminated and/or be affected by the contamination. For example, the transport crew may need to wear level A or B suits and/or respirators. Remember, if the victim is contaminated and the transport requires personal protective devices, it is likely that the vehicle will be contaminated and require appropriate decontamination. There is also a potential to contaminate the receiving medical facility and its staff.

Diagnosis, Treatment, and Transport

As soon as the victim has been removed to safety, follow normal primary and secondary survey procedures, including interviews of the patient and bystanders. Observe the patient and provide the ABCs of basic life support (airway, breathing, circulation) and add "D" and "E" for disability and exposure. Look for signs of trauma and provide proper exposure (i.e., remove clothing) to fully assess the victim. Monitor vital signs and the victim closely! As a guideline, give the patient supplemental oxygen (4 to 6 liters per minute), and start an IV at an area of skin not exposed to the hazardous material (or at least that has been thoroughly decontaminated).

If the HAZMAT victim has swallowed a known or identified toxic material, treat the victim as a poisoned patient using the information provided above. Dress wounds and prepare the patient for transport to a medical treatment facility.

Finally, transport the victim to a medical treatment facility for complete medical evaluation and treatment. Care should be taken during transport to stabilize the victim by maintaining normal body temperature, administering oxygen, and treating shock.

SUMMARY

In this chapter, we discussed the assessment and treatment for poisoning, drug abuse, and hazardous material exposure, along with the rescue and decontamination procedures for patients exposed to HAZMAT. In our rapidly changing environment, we must be up to date on the latest changes in assessment and treatment for these conditions. You may stay informed through contact with the local Poison Control Center, MEDIC releases, or via the World Wide Web on the Internet.

CHAPTER 6

PHARMACY AND TOXICOLOGY

As you advance in rate, you will become more and more involved in the administration of medicines. Although drugs and their dosages are prescribed by medical officers and other authorized prescribers, you, as the Hospital Corpsman, are involved in their administration. It is necessary for you to learn drug sources, composition, methods of preparation and administration, and physiologic and toxicologic action. This chapter covers pharmacology, toxicology, medication calculations, pharmaceutical preparations, and prescriptions.

PHARMACOLOGY

LEARNING OBJECTIVE: *Recall the subsciences of pharmacology, drug standards, medication administration methods, and factors that affect dosage.*

Pharmacology is the science that deals with the origin, nature, chemistry, effects, and uses of drugs. The subsciences of pharmacology and their specific areas of concentration are as follows:

- **PHARMACOGNOSY**—the branch of pharmacology that deals with biological, biochemical, and economic features of natural drugs and their constituents.

- **PHARMACY**—the branch of pharmacology that deals with the preparation, dispensing, and proper use of drugs.

- **POSOLOGY**—the science of dosages.

- **PHARMACODYNAMICS**—the study of drug action on living organisms.

- **PHARMACOTHERAPEUTICS**—the study of the uses of drugs in the treatment of disease.

- **TOXICOLOGY**—the study of poisons, their actions, their detection, and the treatment of the conditions produced by them.

The science of treating disease by any method that will relieve pain, cure disease, or prolong life is called **therapeutics**. Therapeutics does not deal solely with giving or taking medicine. This field also includes many other methods, such as radiological treatment, diathermy, and hydrotherapy.

DRUG STANDARDS

The texts dealing with pharmaceutical preparations include the *United States Pharmacopeia and National Formulary (USP-NF)*, which provides standards for drugs of therapeutic usefulness and pharmaceutical necessity. Inclusion of drugs into this compendium is based on therapeutic effectiveness and popularity. The USP-NF provides tests for drug identity, quality, strength, and purity.

Drug Facts and Comparisons and the *Physicians' Desk Reference (PDR)* have multiple indexes of commercially available drugs. Both are used as advertising outlets for various drug manufacturers. A comprehensive description of each pharmaceutical preparation (including composition, action and use, administration and dosage, precautions and side effects, dosage forms available, and the common (generic) drug names) is provided in both publications. These two publications are used as references for in-depth information on pharmaceutical products by healthcare providers and pharmacy personnel.

Remington: The Science and Practice of Pharmacy is probably the most widely used text/reference in American pharmacies. It contains all areas relevant to the art/science of pharmacy. The *Pharmacological Basis of Therapeutics* (Goodman and Gilman) is a textbook of pharmacology, toxicology, and therapeutics. This work is known as the "blue bible" of pharmacology.

MEDICATION ADMINISTRATION

The quantity and frequency of a drug's administration to a patient depend on several factors, as does the method of that medication's administration. This section will cover some of the factors affecting dosage calculations and methods of administration.

Dosage

The amount of medication to be administered is referred to as the **dose**. The study of dosage and the criteria that influence it is called **posology**. The doses given in the *United States Pharmacopeia and National Formulary (USP-NF)* are average therapeutic doses and are known as "usual adult doses." The following terms are used in connection with doses.

THERAPEUTIC DOSE.—Therapeutic dose is also referred to as the normal adult dose, the usual dose or average dose. It is the amount needed to produce the desired therapeutic effect. This therapeutic dose is calculated on an average adult of 24 years who weighs approximately 150 pounds.

DOSAGE RANGE.—Dosage range is a term that applies to the range between the minimum and maximum amounts of a given drug required to produce the desired effect. Many drugs (such as penicillin) require large initial doses that are later reduced to smaller amounts. Closely associated with "dosage range" are the terms **minimum dose** (the least amount of drug required to produce a therapeutic effect), **maximum dose** (the largest amount of drug that can be given without reaching the toxic effect), and **toxic dose** (the least amount of drug that will produce symptoms of poisoning).

MINIMUM LETHAL DOSE.—Minimum lethal dose is the least amount of drug that can produce death.

Factors Affecting Dosage

The two primary factors that determine or influence the dosage of a medication are the age and weight of the patient.

AGE.—Age is the most common factor that influences the amount of drug to be given. An infant requires a lower dose than an adult. Elderly patients may require a higher or lower dose than the average dose, depending upon the action of the drug and the condition of the patient.

The rule governing calculation of pediatric (child's) doses, **Young's Rule**, is expressed as follows:

$$\frac{\text{age in years}}{\text{age in years} + 12} \times \text{adult dose} = \text{child's dose}$$

The age in years of the child is the numerator, and the age plus 12 is the denominator. This fraction is multiplied by the normal adult dose.

> **Example:** The adult dose of aspirin is 650 mg. What is the dose for a 3-year-old child?
>
> $$\frac{3}{3+12} \times \frac{650 \text{ mg}}{15} = 130 \text{ mg}$$

WEIGHT.—In the calculation of dosages, weight has a more direct bearing on the dose than any other factor, especially in the calculation of pediatric doses. The rule governing calculation of pediatric doses based on weight is **Clark's Rule**, expressed as follows:

$$\frac{\text{weight in pounds}}{150} \times \text{adult dose} = \text{child's dose}$$

The child's weight in pounds is the numerator, and the average adult weight (150 pounds) is the denominator. This fraction is multiplied by the adult dose.

> **Example:** The adult dose of aspirin is 650 mg. What is the dose for a child weighing 60 pounds?
>
> $$\frac{60 \text{ lbs}}{150 \text{ lbs}} \times 650 \text{ mg} = 260 \text{ mg}$$

OTHER FACTORS THAT INFLUENCE DOSAGE.—Other factors that influence dosage include the following:

- **Sex**—Females usually require smaller doses than males.

- **Race**—Black individuals usually require larger doses, and Asians require smaller doses than Caucasians.

- **Occupation**—Persons working in strenuous jobs may require larger doses than those who sit at a desk all day.

- **Habitual use**—Some patients must take medications continuously, causing their bodies to build up tolerance to the drug. This tolerance may require larger doses than their initial doses to obtain the same therapeutic effect.

- **Time of administration**—Therapeutic effect may be altered depending upon time of administration (e.g., before or after meals).

- **Frequency of administration**—Drugs given frequently may need a smaller dose than if administered at longer intervals.

- **Mode of administration**—Injections may require smaller doses than oral medications.

Methods of Administering Drugs

Drugs may be introduced into the body in several ways, each method serving a specific purpose.

ORAL.—Oral administration of medications is the most common method. Among the advantages of administering medication orally (as opposed to other methods) are the following:

- Oral medications are convenient.

- Oral medications are cheaper.

- Oral medications do not have to be pure or sterile.

- A wide variety of oral dosage forms is available.

Oral medication administration may be disadvantageous for the following reasons:

- Some patients may have difficulty swallowing tablets or capsules.

- Oral medications are often absorbed too slowly.

- Oral medications may be partially or completely destroyed by the digestive system.

Other methods of administration closely associated with oral administration are **sublingual** and **buccal**. Sublingual drugs are administered by placing the medication under the tongue. The medication is then rapidly absorbed directly into the blood stream. An example of a sublingual drug is nitroglycerin sublingual tablets (for relief of angina pectoris).

Buccal drugs are administered by placing the medication between the cheek and gum. Buccal drugs, like sublingual drugs, are quickly absorbed directly into the blood stream. An example of a drug that may be given buccally is the anesthetic benzocaine.

PARENTERAL.—Parenteral medications are introduced by injection. All drugs used by this route must be pure, sterile, pyrogen-free (pyrogens are products of the growth of microorganisms), and in a liquid state. There are several methods of parenteral administration, including subcutaneous, intradermal, intramuscular, intravenous, and intrathecal or intraspinal.

Subcutaneous.—The drug is injected just below the skin's cutaneous layers. **Example:** Insulin.

Intradermal.—The drug is injected within the dermis layer of the skin. **Example:** Purified protein derivative (PPD).

Intramuscular.—The drug is injected into the muscle. **Example:** Procaine penicillin G.

Intravenous.—The drug is introduced directly into the vein. **Example:** Intravenous fluids.

Intrathecal or Intraspinal.—The drug is introduced into the subarachnoid space of the spinal column. **Example:** Procaine hydrochloride.

INHALATION.—Inhalation is a means of introducing medications through the respiratory system in the form of a gas, vapor, or powder. Inhalation is divided into three major types: vaporization, gas inhalation, and nebulization.

Vaporization.—Vaporization is the process by which a drug is changed from a liquid or solid to a gas or vapor by the use of heat (such as in steam inhalation).

Gas Inhalation.—Gas inhalation is almost entirely restricted to anesthesia.

Nebulization.—Nebulization is the process by which a drug is converted into a fine spray by the use of compressed gas.

TOPICAL.—Topical drugs are applied to a surface area of the body. Topically applied drugs serve two purposes:

- **Local effect**: The drug is intended to relieve itching, burning, or other skin conditions without being absorbed into the bloodstream.

- **Systemic effect**: The drug is absorbed through the skin into the bloodstream.

Examples of topical preparations are ointments, creams, lotions, and shampoos.

RECTAL.—Drugs are administered rectally by inserting them into the rectum. The rectal method is preferred to the oral route when there is danger of vomiting or when the patient is unconscious, uncooperative, or mentally incapable. Examples of rectal preparations are suppositories and enemas.

VAGINAL.—Drugs are inserted into the vagina to produce a local effect. Examples of vaginal preparations are suppositories, creams, and douches.

DRUG CLASSIFICATIONS

LEARNING OBJECTIVE: *Recall drug groups, the generic and trade names of drugs listed in each drug group, and recognize each drug's use.*

The definition of a drug is any chemical substance that has an effect on living tissue but is not used as a food. Drugs are administered to humans or animals as an aid in the diagnosis, treatment, or prevention of disease or other abnormal condition; for the relief of pain or suffering; and to control or improve any physiologic or pathologic condition. Drugs are classified according to set criteria and fall into three specific areas: general, chemical, and therapeutic.

- **General**—Drugs are grouped according to their source, whether animal, vegetable, or mineral in origin.

- **Chemical**—Drugs are grouped by their chemical characteristics.

- **Therapeutic (Pharmacological)**—Drugs are grouped according to their action on the body.

  NOTE: Some drugs may have more than one action.

Drug Nomenclature

Drugs normally have three names: chemical, generic, and trade (brand).

- **Chemical name** relates to the chemical and molecular structure. An example is 2,4,7-triamino-6-phenylpteridine.

- **Generic name** is often derived from the chemical name. Generic name is the common name of the drug. An example is triamterene. (Note the underlining of the chemical name above.)

- **Trade name** is the proprietary name given by the manufacturer. Trade name is referred to as the brand name. An example is Dyrenium®, a brand of triamterene made by SmithKline Beecham.

Drug Groups

The types of drugs discussed in this chapter and the correlating drugs in common use described in appendix IV are grouped according to pharmacological classes. Only a brief summary is possible here, and the Corpsman who desires a more complete description of each drug should refer to the *USP-NF, Drug Facts and Comparisons*, the *Physicians' Desk Reference*, or other drug reference books.

ASTRINGENTS.—Astringents are drugs that cause shrinkage of the skin and mucous membranes. Astringents are mainly used to stop seepage, weeping, or discharge from mucous membranes. (See appendix IV, page 1.)

EMOLLIENTS.—Emollients are bland or fatty substances that may be applied to the skin to make it more pliable and soft. They may also serve as vehicles for application of other medicinal substances. Emollients are available as ointments, creams, or lotions. (See appendix IV, page 1.)

EXPECTORANTS AND ANTITUSSIVES.—Expectorants and antitussives are commonly used in the symptomatic treatment of the common cold or bronchitis. (See appendix IV, page 1.) **Expectorants** are more accurately known as bronchomucotropic agents. These agents assist in the removal of secretions or exudate from the trachea, bronchi, or lungs. They act by liquefying viscid mucous or mucopurulent exudates. Therefore, they are used in the treatment of coughs to help expel these exudates and secretions. **Antitussives** are agents that inhibit or suppress the act of coughing. Other cold and allergy relief preparations are discussed later in this chapter.

NASAL DECONGESTANTS.—Nasal decongestants reduce congestion and the swelling of mucous membranes. They are used for the temporary relief of nasal congestion due to the common cold, nasal congestion associated with sinusitis, and to promote nasal or sinus drainage. Nasal decongestants are also used to relieve eustachian tube congestion. Nasal decongestants are often combined with antihistamines, antitussives, and expectorants to relieve the symptoms of colds, allergies, and sinusitis. Some of the more frequently used drug combinations are covered in appendix IV, page 2.

ANTIHISTAMINES.—Antihistamines are used to counteract the physical symptoms that histamines cause. Histamine, a substance released by mast cells distributed in connective tissues usually near blood vessels, promotes some of the reactions associated with inflammation and allergies, such as asthma and hay fever. Antihistamines may cause drowsiness, so patients should be warned against driving or operating machinery while taking this type of medication. (See appendix IV, page 2.)

HISTAMINE H₂ RECEPTOR ANTAGONISTS.— Histamine H_2 receptor antagonists block histamines that cause an increase of gastric acid secretion in the stomach. Histamine H_2 receptor antagonists are effective in preventing complications of peptic ulcer disease and alleviating symptoms of this disease. (See appendix IV, page 2.)

ANTACIDS.—Antacids are drugs used to counteract hyperacidity in the stomach. Normally, there is a certain degree of acidity in the stomach. An excess of acid can irritate the mucous membranes and is commonly known as indigestion, heartburn, or dyspepsia. In some disease states, the gastrointestinal tract may become excessively acidic (very low pH), causing diarrhea or leading to peptic ulcer formation. Antacids may interfere with the body's ability to use many drugs. For this reason, oral drugs normally should not be taken within 2 hours of taking an antacid. (See appendix IV, page 3.)

NOTE: It is important for you to be aware of the significance of the sodium content of most antacids, particularly for cardiac patients or patients on a low-sodium diet.

ANTISEPTICS, DISINFECTANTS, AND GERMICIDES.—These agents are primarily intended for the prevention of infections by destroying bacteria or preventing their growth. The differences among them are based primarily on degree of activity and how they are used. **Antiseptics** suppress the growth of microorganisms. **Germicides** kill susceptible organisms. **Disinfectants** are agents used to disinfect inanimate objects and are primarily germicidal in their action. All of these agents are for external use only, unless otherwise indicated. (See appendix IV, pages 3 and 4.)

SULFONAMIDES.—Sulfonamides were the first effective chemotherapeutic agents to be available in safe therapeutic dosage ranges. They were the mainstay of therapy of bacterial infections in humans before the introduction of the penicillins in 1941. Sulfonamides are synthetically produced and are effective against both gram-positive and gram-negative organisms. (See appendix IV, page 5.)

PENICILLINS.—Penicillin is one of the most important antibiotics. It is derived from a number of *Penicillium* molds commonly found on breads and fruits. The mechanisms of action for the penicillins is the inhibition of cell wall synthesis during the reproductive phase of bacterial growth. It is one of the most effective and least toxic of the antimicrobial agents. (See appendix IV, page 5.)

CEPHALOSPORINS.—The cephalosporins are a group of semisynthetic derivatives of *cephalosporin C*, an antimicrobial agent of fungal origin. They are structurally and pharmacologically related to the penicillins. Because the cephalosporins are structurally similar to the penicillins, some patients allergic to penicillin may also be allergic to cephalosporin drugs. The incidence of cross-sensitivity is estimated to be 5 to 16 percent.

This family of antibiotics is generally divided into generations:

- First generation — cefazolin sodium (Ancef®, Kefzol®)

- Second generation — cefoxitin sodium (Mefoxin®)

- Third generation — cefotaxime sodium (Claforan®)

The main differences among the groups is the change in the antibacterial spectrum. The third generation agents have a much broader gram-negative spectrum than the earlier generations.

Examples of various cephalosporins are listed in appendix IV, page 6.

TETRACYCLINES.—Tetracyclines, introduced in 1948, were the first truly broad-spectrum antibiotics. They include a large group of drugs with a common basic structure and chemical activity. The most important mechanism of action of the tetracyclines is the blocking of the formation of polypeptides used in protein synthesis. Because of their broad spectrum of activity, tetracyclines are most valuable to treat mixed infection, such as chronic bronchitis and peritonitis; however, they are drugs of choice for only a few bacterial infections. Tetracycline is also used as a topical preparation to treat acne.

The tetracyclines are relatively nontoxic, the most common side effects being mild gastrointestinal disturbances. Allergic reactions and anaphylaxis are rare. Administration to children and pregnant women is not indicated because it may produce discoloration of the teeth and depress bone marrow growth. The major hazard of tetracycline therapy is the overgrowth of resistant organisms, especially *Candida* and staphylococci.

Tetracyclines should not be administered with milk, milk products, antacids or iron preparations; they combine with metal ions to form nonabsorbable compounds.

Examples of tetracyclines in common use are listed in appendix IV, page 6.

AMINOGLYCOSIDES.—Aminoglycosides are a group of drugs that share chemical, antimicrobial, pharmacologic, and toxic characteristics, and that are effective against most gram-positive and gram-negative organisms. Their method of action is by inhibiting protein synthesis. Aminoglycosides can cause varying degrees of ototoxicity and nephrotoxicity, depending on the particular agent and the dose. Toxicity is more prevalent in the very young or old, in the presence of renal impairment or dehydration, or with the use of diuretics. Because of their high toxicity, aminoglycosides are not recommended when the infective organism is susceptible to less toxic preparations.

Examples of several aminoglycosides are listed in appendix IV, page 7.

MACROLIDES.—Macrolide antibiotics constitute a large group of bacteriostatic agents that inhibit protein synthesis. They are effective against gram-positive cocci, *Neisseria*, *Hemophilus*, and mycobacteria. All are similar to penicillin in their antibacterial spectra, and are often used in patients who are sensitive to penicillin. (See appendix IV, pages 7 and 8.)

ANTIFUNGALS.—Antifungal agents inhibit or suppress the growth systems of fungi, dermatophytes, or *Candida*. Antifungals have not been developed to the same degree as antibacterial agents. Most fungi are completely resistant to the action of chemicals at concentrations that can be tolerated by the human cell. Since there are only a few available for internal use, most antifungal agents are topical. The antifungal agents that are available for systemic use generally produce hepatic or renal dysfunction or other serious side effects. Because of these side effects, systemic antifungals should be limited to serious or potentially fatal conditions. Therapy that includes topical preparations may be provided in conjunction with oral or parenteral antifungal agents.

Examples of several antifungal agents are listed in appendix IV, page 8.

ANTIPARASITICS.—Antiparasitics are agents that are destructive to parasites. Parasitic infections or infestations account for the largest number of chronic disabling diseases known. They are especially prevalent in the tropics or subtropics and in lesser-developed countries where overcrowding and poor sanitation exist. Parasitic infections include protozoal infections (malaria, amebiasis, and to a lesser extent, trichomoniasis), helminthic infections (intestinal worms), and **ectopara- sites**. Ectoparasites, such as head lice and crab lice, although not disabling, are considered a nuisance and can transmit disease.

Examples of antiparasitics in common use are listed in appendix IV, page 9.

LAXATIVES.—Laxatives are drugs that facilitate the passage and elimination of feces from the colon and rectum. They are indicated to treat simple constipation and to clean the intestine of any irritant or toxic substances (catharsis). Laxatives may also be used to soften painfully hard stools and to lessen straining of certain cardiac patients when defecating. They are contraindicated in certain inflammatory conditions of the bowel, bowel obstruction, and abdominal pain of unknown origin, and should not be used in the presence of nausea and vomiting. Laxatives are classified as irritant, bulk, emollient, or stool softeners. Frequent or prolonged use of any laxative may result in dependence. (See appendix IV, pages 9 and 10.)

ANTIDIARRHEALS.—Antidiarrheals are drugs that are effective in combating diarrhea. Diarrhea is defined as an abnormal frequency and liquidity of fecal discharge. This condition may result from food poisoning, parasitic infestation of the bowel, and gastrointestinal diseases. (See appendix IV, page 10.)

DIURETICS.—The kidney is the primary organ that excretes water-soluble substances (urine) from the body. Diuretics are agents that increase the rate of urine formation. These agents are useful in treating hypertension and edematous conditions, such as congestive heart failure and acute pulmonary edema. However, loss body fluids due to use of diuretics can seriously deplete electrolytes from the system, and care should be taken to monitor and replenish lost sodium and potassium through diet and supplement therapy. (See appendix IV, page 10 and 11)

NON-NARCOTIC ANALGESICS, ANTI-PYRETICS, AND ANTI-INFLAMMATORY AGENTS.—**Non-narcotic analgesics** are drugs that relieve pain without producing unconsciousness or impairing mental capacities. **Antipyretics** relieve or reduce fevers. **Anti-inflammatory agents** counteract or suppress inflammation or the inflammatory process. Many of the drugs discussed in appendix IV, page 11, were developed with two or more of these properties.

CENTRAL NERVOUS SYSTEM STIMU-LANTS.—Certain drugs stimulate the activity of various portions of the central nervous system (CNS). The *Manual of the Medical Department* (MANMED) is explicit as to the usage of these drugs in the Navy. Primary indications for this class of drugs are narcolepsy, hyperkinesis, and attention deficit disorders in children. Central nervous system stimulants are generally contraindicated in patients with hypertension, arteriosclerosis, symptomatic cardiovascular disorders, agitated states, glaucoma, or history of drug abuse. (See appendix IV, page 12.)

CENTRAL NERVOUS SYSTEM DEPRES-SANTS.—Central nervous system (CNS) depressants range in depressive action from mild sedation to deep coma, differing mainly in rapidity, degree, and duration of action. Any of these CNS depressants may, in sufficient doses, cause respiratory depression. Alcohol use while taking CNS depressants should be avoided. Many of the central nervous system depressants are controlled medications. Refer to the MANMED for control, custody, and accountability guidelines for controlled substances.

Barbiturates comprise a widely used group of CNS depressants. They are used mainly as sedative-hypnotics, anticonvulsants, anesthetics for short anesthesia, and may be used in combination with analgesics to enhance their analgesic effect.

NOTE: Barbiturates may be habit forming.

See appendix IV, page 12, for examples of central nervous system depressants.

OPIUM AND OPIUM ALKALOIDS.—The activity of opium is primarily due to its morphine content. The major medical use of opium has been for its antiperistaltic activity, particularly in diarrhea. Opium alkaloids, e.g., morphine and codeine, have replaced opium in medical use. Members of this drug group are used as analgesics, cough sedatives, and for certain types of diarrhea. (See appendix IV, pages 12 and 13.)

NOTE: Warn patients taking opium or opium alkaloids that drowsiness, dizziness, and blurring of vision may occur. For this reason, they should not drive or perform other tasks that require alertness. Also, caution patients against consuming alcohol and other CNS depressants. Patients should notify their physician immediately if shortness of breath or difficulty in breathing occurs.

PSYCHOTHERAPEUTIC AGENTS.—Tranquilizers and mood modifiers are the two primary groups of psychotherapeutic agents. Psychotherapeutic agents are classified as **major tranquilizers**, **minor tranquilizers**, and **mood modifiers**. The mood modifiers have replaced amphetamines as treatment of choice for depressive states. (See appendix IV, pages 13 and 14.)

SKELETAL MUSCLE RELAXANTS.—Skeletal muscle relaxants are used in connection with the treatment of muscle spasm due to various conditions. They may also be used to produce muscular relaxation during surgical anesthesia. Skeletal muscle relaxants may cause drowsiness and impair performance of tasks that require alertness. (See appendix IV, page 14.)

CARDIOVASCULAR AGENTS.—Cardio-vascular agents affect the action of the circulatory system. Most of these agents are highly specialized. (See appendix IV, pages 14 and 15.)

VASOCONSTRICTORS.—Vasoconstrictors produce constriction of the blood vessels with consequent rise in blood pressure. (See appendix IV, page 15.)

ANTICOAGULANTS.—Anticoagulants delay or prevent blood coagulation. Before an anticoagulant agent is prescribed and its dosage determined, laboratory testing of the patient's blood-clotting capabilities should be performed.

Examples of commonly used anticoagulants are listed in appendix IV, page 15.

VITAMINS.—Vitamins are unrelated organic substances that occur in many foods and are necessary for the normal metabolic functioning of the body. Vitamins may be **water-soluble** or **fat-soluble**. The majority of vitamins are water-soluble. Water-soluble vitamins are excreted in the urine and are not stored in the body in appreciable quantities. The fat-soluble vitamins (A, D, E, and K) are soluble in fat solvents and are absorbed along with dietary fats. Fat-soluble vitamins are not normally excreted in the urine and tend to be stored in the body in moderate amounts.

See appendix IV, page 16, for a listing of several of the major vitamins and their respective properties.

GENERAL AND LOCAL ANESTHETICS.—Generally speaking, anesthesia means "without feeling." Consequently, we apply the word to drugs that produce insensibility to pain. The field of anesthesia is a highly specialized one.

General anesthetics are usually gas or vapor and are administered by inhalation. Anesthesiology is a highly specialized field, and the administration of a general anesthetic should never be undertaken without the supervision of a medical officer. There may be times, however, when you, as a Hospital Corpsman, are called upon to assist by administering general anesthesia. You should, therefore, acquaint yourself with the most commonly used general anesthetics and their respective properties.

Local anesthetics produce loss of sensation to pain in a specific area or locality of the body, without loss of consciousness or mental capacity. The majority of these drugs are administered parenterally or topically.

See appendix IV, pages 17 and 18, for a listing of several of the most commonly used anesthetics.

OXYTOCICS.—Oxytocics are drugs that produce a rhythmic contraction of the uterus. Their action is selective for the uterus, although other smooth muscles are affected. (See appendix IV, page 18.)

Biological Agents

Biological agents are prepared from living organisms or their products. The chief purpose served by these preparations in the Navy is the immunization of personnel against infectious disease. They may, however, be used in the treatment of disease or act in a diagnostic capacity. Dosage and routes of administration are described in BUMEDINST 6320.1.

Biologicals include serums, viruses, toxins, antitoxins, antigens, and bacterial vaccines.

Manufacturers of these products must be licensed by the Secretary of the Treasury. Their products are monitored by the U.S. Public Health Service.

The label that must be placed on each package will bear the name, address, and license number of the manufacturer. It will also list the name of the product, lot number, date of manufacture (or expiration), period of potency, and the minimum potency (or the fact that there is no standard of potency).

FACTORS TO BE REMEMBERED CONCERNING BIOLOGICALS.—Most immunizing agents that are used in routine procedures may be obtained through normal supply channels. (Yellow fever vaccine must be ordered from activities that have been designated as supply points for this biological.) Biologicals must be stored in a cool, dry, and preferably dark place. (Yellow fever vaccine must be maintained in a frozen state until prepared for use.) All biological products should be examined periodically, and a thorough examination for deterioration will be held immediately preceding their use.

EXAMINATIONS OF PARENTERAL SOLUTIONS.—Solutions are examined at least three times at the activity at which they are ultimately used:

1. Upon receiving the solution.

2. Periodically while in storage.

3. Immediately preceding use. Parenteral solutions, unless the label states otherwise, must be free of turbidity or undissolved material. All solutions should be inverted and gently swirled to bring any sediment or particulate matter into view. A well-illuminated black or white background will facilitate this examination.

Parenteral solutions may be unfit for use because of

- deterioration from prolonged storage,

- accidental contamination occurring upon original packaging, or

- defects that may develop in containers or seals.

There is no set rule that can be applicable in regards to any of these factors. Therefore, to ensure suitability for use, a regimented program of inspection is necessary.

IMMUNIZING AGENTS.—Following is a descriptive list of the most common immunizing agents used by the U.S. armed forces to inoculate military personnel against disease.

Diphtheria Antitoxin.—Diphtheria antitoxin is a transparent or slightly opalescent liquid, nearly colorless, and has a very slight odor due to its preservative. It is a sterile solution of antitoxic substances obtained from the blood serum or plasma of a healthy horse immunized against diphtheria toxin.

Tetanus Antitoxin.—Tetanus antitoxin is a sterile solution of antitoxic substances that are usually obtained from the blood serum or plasma of a healthy horse that has been immunized against tetanus toxin or toxoid. Tetanus antitoxin contains not more than 0.4 percent cresol or 0.5 percent phenol as a preservative. It is slightly opalescent with a yellow, brown, or greenish color, depending upon the manufacturer. There will be a slight odor of the preservative used.

Tetanus Toxoid.—Tetanus toxoid is a sterile solution of the growth of the tetanus bacillus,

Clostridium tetani, which has been treated with formaldehyde. It is a brownish yellow or slightly turbid liquid, usually having the distinctive odor of formaldehyde.

Alum Precipitated Diphtheria and Tetanus Toxoids and Pertussis Vaccines Combined (DPT).— This is a markedly turbid, whitish liquid. It is nearly odorless or may have a slight odor of the preservative. It is a sterile suspension of the precipitate obtained by treating the mixture of diphtheria toxoid, tetanus toxoid, and pertussis vaccine with alum and combining in such proportions as to ensure an immunizing dose of each in the total dosage as listed on the label.

Cholera Vaccine.—Cholera vaccine is a suspension of killed cholera, *Vibrio comma*, in a suitable diluent, usually normal saline. The vaccine presents a turbid appearance, and there may be a slight odor due to the preservative. On storage, autolysis may occur so that the vaccine may become almost as clear as water.

Poliovirus Vaccine.—There are two kinds of polio vaccine: Inactivated poliovirus vaccine (**IPV**), which is the shot recommended in the United States today, and a live, oral polio vaccine (**OPV**), which consists of drops that are swallowed. Until recently, OPV was recommended for most children in the United States. OPV helped us rid the country of polio, and it is still used in many parts of the world.

Both vaccines give immunity to polio, but OPV is better at keeping the disease from spreading to other people. However, for a few people (about one in 2.4 million), OPV actually causes polio. Since the risk of getting polio in the United States is now extremely low, experts believe that using oral polio vaccine is no longer worth the slight risk, except in limited circumstances.

Inactivated poliovirus vaccine (IPV) must be stored between 2°C and 8°C (24°F and 46°F). The vaccine is clear and colorless, and it should be administered intramuscularly or subcutaneously.

ORAL POLIOVIRUS VACCINE MUST NEVER BE ADMINISTERED PARENTERALLY. To maintain potency, OPV must be stored in the freezer compartment of the refrigerator. It should be noted that certain forms of this vaccine will remain fluid at temperatures above -14°C. If frozen, after thawing, agitate the vaccine to ensure homogeneity of its contents before use. Once the temperature rises above 0°C, the vaccine MUST BE USED WITHIN 7 DAYS. During this period, it must be stored below 10°C.

Yellow Fever Vaccine.—This vaccine is a dull, light orange, flaky or crust-like desiccated mass that requires rehydration immediateley before use. It must be stored at or below 0°C until rehydration is effected with sterile sodium chloride injection USP.

Plague Vaccine.—The vaccine for plague is a sterile suspension of killed plague bacilli in an isotonic solution. The strain of bacilli used has been selected for its high antigenic efficiency. The vaccine is a turbid, whitish liquid with little or no odor. The presence of any precipitate is reason to suspect contamination.

Influenza Virus Vaccine.—The influenza virus vaccine is prepared from the allantoic fluid of incubated fertile hen eggs. It is a slightly hazy fluid, the result of minute amounts of egg protein. Its color varies from gray to very faint red, depending upon the method of manufacture.

The duration of immunity is probably no longer than a few months, which necessitates repeating the inoculation before the expected seasonal occurrence.

Do not inoculate individuals who are known to be sensitive to eggs or egg products, or personnel suffering from upper respiratory infections.

Dried Smallpox Vaccine.—This vaccine is prepared directly from calf lymph, purified, concentrated, stabilized, and dried by lyophilization. Dried smallpox vaccine is much more stable than the conventional liquid. When stored at or below 25°C, it retains its full potency for 18 months. When reconstituted and stored below 4°C (preferably 0°C), it retains its full potency for 3 months.

Smallpox is no longer considered to be a threat to world health, and immunizations against it are no longer required. However, a general knowledge of the disease and its prevention is important.

Anthrax Vaccine.—The anthrax vaccine for humans licensed for use in the United States is a cell-free filtrate vaccine (using dead as opposed to live bacteria). Inspect the vaccine visually for particulate matter and discoloration before administration. Anthrax vaccine should be stored between 2°C and 8°C (refrigerator temperature); it must not be frozen. Do not use the vaccine if the expiration date listed on the package has expired.

The vaccine should be administered only to healthy men and women from 18 to 65 years of age. It should **NOT** be administered to pregnant women.

The immunization consists of three subcutaneous injections given 2 weeks apart, followed by three additional subcutaneous injections given at 6, 12, and 18 months. Annual booster injections of the vaccine are required to maintain immunity.

TOXICOLOGY

LEARNING OBJECTIVE: *Identify how poisons are introduced into the body and the factors that affect their toxicity.*

Toxicology is the science of poisons, their actions, their detection, and the treatment of the conditions produced by them. A **poison** is a substance that, when inhaled, swallowed, absorbed, applied to the skin, or injected into the body in relatively small amounts, may cause damage to structures or disturbances of function. Poisons act by changing the normal metabolism of cells or by actually destroying them.

The effects of poisons may be local or remote, and in some instances, poisons can produce both effects. A **local effect** is produced when a poison only affects the area in which it is applied. A **remote effect** is produced when a poison affects parts of the body that are remote to the site of application or point of introduction. Poisons sometimes show no effect—or only a slight effect—until several doses have been taken. Then, suddenly, an effect is produced that nearly equals that produced by taking the whole amount at one time. This is known as a **cumulative effect**.

The toxicity of poisons depends upon their method of introduction into the body and how fast they are absorbed by the body. For example, snake venom taken into the mouth or into the stomach during first aid treatment of snakebite is not ordinarily harmful, but snake venom injected parenterally is extremely poisonous.

Various conditions affect an individual's reaction and susceptibility to poisons. For instance, some individuals by nature are unusually sensitive to certain poisons (such as venom from bee stings), while others possess a natural tolerance. Additionally, the age of the victim can affect the severity of the poisoning. Young children, for example, are normally more susceptible to poisons than adults. Habitual use of certain poisons, such as narcotics, may cause individuals to become accustomed to a poison's effects, even though the amount taken by these individuals would ordinarily be considered lethal. This habitual use of poisons, however, may result in a sudden hypersensitivity that could be deadly. The actions of poisons may also be considerably modified by disease, some diseases increasing and others lessening the action of poisons.

Poisons are eliminated from the body by way of the kidneys, liver, gastrointestinal tract, and skin. Poisons are eliminated either unchanged or in the form of other compounds. These compounds are the result of chemical changes made in various body organs and tissues.

For a more in-depth understanding of the various types of poisoning and their emergency treatment procedures, see chapter 5, "Poisoning, Drug Abuse, and Hazardous Material Exposure."

PHARMACY

LEARNING OBJECTIVE: *Recall the various pharmaceutical weight and measurement systems, and determine medication dosage by using the conversion process or the percentage and ratio calculations.*

As you progress in your career as a Hospital Corpsman, you will be assigned duties in specialized departments throughout the hospital and especially aboard ship. Not only will your responsibilities increase, but your training will become more and more diversified.

One of the departments to which you may be assigned is the pharmacy, where you will assist in preparing and dispensing medicines. This section will give you a basic introduction to the field of pharmacy and help prepare you for these responsibilities.

METROLOGY AND CALCULATION

Metrology, called the arithmetic of pharmacy, is the science of weights and measures and its application to drugs, their dosage, preparation, compounding, and dispensing.

It is absolutely vital for Hospital Corpsmen to thoroughly understand the principles and applications of metrology in pharmacy. Errors in this area endanger the health—even the life—of the patient.

The Metric System

The metric system is the official system of weights and measures used by Navy Pharmacy Departments for weighing and calculating pharmaceutical preparations. The metric system is becoming the accepted system throughout the world. Hospital Corpsmen need to be concerned primarily with the divisions of weight, volume, and linear measurement of the metric system. Each of these divisions has a primary or basic unit and is listed below:

- Basic unit of weight is the **gram**, abbreviated "g"
- Basic unit of volume is the **liter**, abbreviated "l"
- Basic linear unit is the **meter**, abbreviated "m"

By using the prefixes **deka**, **hecto**, and **kilo** for multiples of, respectively, ten, one hundred, and one thousand basic units, and the prefixes **micro**, **milli**, **centi**, and **deci** for one-ten thousandth, one-thousandth, one-hundredth, and one-tenth, respectively, you have the basic structure of the metric system. By applying the appropriate basic unit to the scale of figure 6-1, you can readily determine its proper terms. For example, using the gram as the basic unit of weight, we can readily see that 10 g equals 1 dekagram, 100 g equals 1 hectogram, and 1000 g is referred to as a kilogram. Conversely, going down the scale, 0.1 g is referred to as a decigram, 0.01 g is called a centigram, and 0.001 g is a milligram.

The Apothecary System

Although fast becoming obsolete, the apothecary system for weighing and calculating pharmaceutical preparations is still used and must be taken into consideration. It has two divisions of measurement: weight and volume. In this system, the basic unit of weight is the **grain** (abbreviated "gr"), and the basic unit of volume is the **minim** (abbreviated "m").

The Avoirdupois System

The avoirdupois system is a system used in the United States for ordinary commodities. The basic units of the avoirdupois system are dram (27.344 grains), ounce (16 drams), and pound (16 ounces).

Table of Weights and Measures

See table 6-1, a table of weights and measures; study it thoroughly.

Converting Weights and Measures

Occasionally, there are times when it will be necessary to convert weights and measures from one system to another, either metric to apothecary or vice versa. Since patients can hardly be expected to be familiar with either system, always translate the dosage directions on the prescription into a household equivalent that they can understand. Household measurements are standardized, on the assumption that the utensils are common enough to be found in any home. Table 6-2 is a table of household measures, with their metric and apothecary equivalents.

> **CAUTION:** For the conversion of specific quantities in a prescription or in converting a pharmaceutical formula from one system to another, exact equivalents must be used.

CONVERSION

As stated earlier, in the practice of pharmacy it may be necessary to convert from one system to another to dispense in their proper amounts the substances that have been ordered. Although the denominations of the metric system are not the same as the common systems, the Bureau of International Standards has established conversion standards that will satisfy the degree of accuracy required in almost any practical situation. Ordinary pharmaceutical procedures generally require something between two- and three-figure accuracy, and the following tables of conversion (tables 6-3 and 6-4) are more than sufficient for practical use. Naturally, if potent agents are involved, you must use a more precise conversion factor for purposes of calculation.

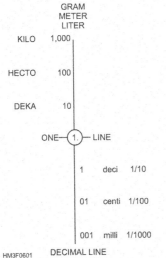

Figure 6-1.—Graph comparing the metric system with the decimal equivalent.

Table 6-1.—Measuring Equivalents

Systems of Weights	Systems of Volume Measures	Linear Measure

AVOIRDUPOIS

Primary unit of weight is the grain.

437.5 grains   = 1 ounce
               (av. oz.)
16.0 ounces   = 1 pound
               (av. lb.)

APOTHECARY

Primary unit of weight is the grain.

20 grains (gr) = 1 scruple (℈)
3 scruples   = 1 dram (ʒ)
8 drams   = 1 ounce (℥)
(480 gr)
12 ounces   = 1 pound (lb)

METRIC

Primary unit of weight is the gram.

1000.000 grams = 1 kilogram (kg)
100.000 grams = 1 hectogram (hg)
10.000 grams = 1 dekagram (dkg)
1.000 gram = 1 gram (gm)
0.1 gram   = 1 decigram (dg)
0.01 gram   = 1 centigram (cg)
0.001 gram = 1 milligram (mg)

APOTHECARY

Smallest unit of volume is the minim.

60 minims (m) = 1 fluid dram (ʒ)
8 fluid drams = 1 fluid ounce (℥)
16 fluid ounces = 1 pint (0)
2 pints   = 1 quart (qt.)
4 quarts   = 1 gallon (Cong. or
                       gal.)

METRIC

Primary unit of volume is the liter.

1000.000 liters = 1 kiloliter (kl)
100.000 liters = 1 hectoliter (hl)
10.000 liters = 1 dekaliter (dkl)
1.000 liter = 1 liter (l)
0.1 liter   = 1 deciliter (dl)
0.01 liter   = 1 centiliter (cl)
0.001 liter = 1 milliliter (ml)

METRIC

Primary unit of linear measure is the meter.

1000.000 meters = 1 kilometer (km)
100.000 meters = 1 hectometer (hm)
10.000 meters = 1 dekameter (dkm)
1.000 meter = 1 meter (m)
0.1 meter   = 1 decimeter (dm)
0.01 meter   = 1 centimeter (cm)
0.001 meter = 1 millimeter (mm)

NOTE: The relationship of the basic units in the Metric System should be noted. The meter, which is 1/40,000,000 of the earth's polar circumference, is the natural standard. The volume contained in 1/10 of a meter cubed is 1 liter. The weight of 1 cubic centimeter of distilled water is 1 gram. Grams of water are approximately equivalent at all temperature ranges. Current usage prefers that ml rather than cc be used since it has been found that 1000 cc do not equal exactly 1 liter.

HM3t0601

Table 6-2.—Table of Metric Doses with Approximate Equivalents

Metric	Apothecary	Household
5 ml	1 fl dr	1 teaspoonful*
10 ml	2 fl dr	1 dessertspoonful
15 ml	4 fl dr	1 tablespoonful (½ fl oz)
30 ml	8 fl dr	2 tablespoons (1 fl oz)
60 ml	2 fl oz	1 wineglassful
120 ml	4 fl oz	1 teacupful
240 ml	8 fl oz	1 tumblerful
480 ml	16 fl oz	1 pint
960 ml	32 fl oz	1 quart
*Official U.S.P. teaspoonful is 5 ml.		

Table 6-3.—Conversion Table for Weights and Liquid Measures

Conversion Table for Weights and Liquid Measures
1 grain = 0.065 gram or 65 milligrams
1 gram = 15.432 grains
1 milliliter = 16.23 minims
1 fluid ounce = 29.57 milliliters

Table 6-4.—Examples of Weight and Liquid Conversions

Examples of Weight and Liquid Conversions	
gr to **g**	gr/15.432 = g
ml to **fl oz**	ml/29.57 = fl oz
minims to **ml**	minims/16.23 = ml
mg to **gr**	mg/65 = gr
g to **gr**	g x 15.432 = gr
fl oz to **ml**	fl oz x 29.57 = ml
ml to **minims**	ml x 16.23 = minims
gr to **mg**	gr x 65 = mg

PERCENTAGE CALCULATIONS

Percentage means "parts per hundred" or the expression of fractions with denominators of 100. Thus, a 10 percent solution may be expressed as 10%, 10/100, 0.10, or 10 parts per 100 parts.

It is often necessary for the pharmacist to compound solutions of a desired percentage strength. Percentage in that respect means **parts of active ingredient per 100 parts of total preparation**.

Following are the three basic rules to remember in solving percentage problems:

1. **To find the amount of the active ingredient when the percentage strength and the total quantity are known,** multiply the total weight or volume by the percent (expressed as a decimal fraction).

Example: Substance X contains 38% fat. How many grams of fat are required to prepare 120 g of substance X?

Solution: 38% is expressed as a decimal fraction (0.38) and multiplied by the amount of the finished product required.

$$\begin{array}{r} 120\ g \\ \times .38 \\ \hline 960 \\ 360 \\ \hline \mathbf{45.60\ g} \end{array}$$, the weight of fat needed.

2. **To find the total quantity of a mixture when the percentage strength and the amount of the active ingredient are known**, divide the weight or volume of the active ingredient by the percent (expressed as a decimal fraction).

Example: If a mixture contains 20% of substance Y, how many grams of the 20% mixture would contain 8 g of Y?

Solution: 20% is expressed as a decimal fraction (0.20). Divide the weight (8 g) by the percent, thus:

$$
\begin{array}{r}
\underline{40.0 \text{ g}} \\
.20\,)\,8.00 \\
\underline{8\,0} \\
00
\end{array}
$$

the weight of 20% mixture that would contain 8 g of substance Y.

---

3. **To find the percentage strength when the amount of the active ingredient and the total quantity of the mixture are known**, divide the weight or volume of the active ingredient by the total weight or volume of the mixture. Then multiply the resulting answer by 100 to convert the decimal fraction to percent.

Example: Find the percentage strength of Z if 300 g of a mixture contains 90 g of substance Z.

Solution:

$$
\begin{array}{r}
\underline{0.3 \text{ g}} \\
300\,)\,90.00 \\
\underline{90} \\
00
\end{array}
$$

is the percent of Z expressed as a decimal fraction

0.3 x 100(%) = **30%** of Z in the mixture

ALTERNATE METHODS FOR SOLVING PERCENTAGE PROBLEMS

The alternate method for solving percentage problems, illustrated below, incorporates the three rules discussed above into one equation. This method is often preferred since it eliminates errors that may result from misinterpreting the values given in the problem.

% strength = $\dfrac{\text{Amt of active ingredient x 100(\%)}}{\text{Total amt of preparation}}$

Example #1: Calculate the percent of A in a solution if 120 g of that solution contains 6 g of A.

Solution: Substitute the known values in the equation and use X for the percent (the unknown factor).

$$ X = 6/120 \text{ x } 100(\%) = 5 \ (\%) $$

Therefore, **X = 5**, which is the percent strength of the solution.

Example #2: Calculate the amount of active ingredient in 300 g of a 5% mixture of active ingredient B.

Solution: Convert 5% to a decimal fraction (0.05). Substitute the known values in the equations, and use X for the amount of the unknown ingredient.

$$ 0.05 = X/300 \qquad\qquad X = 15 \text{ g} $$

A variation of the alternate percentage equation, illustrated below, uses "parts per hundred" instead of percent, with X used as the unknown.

$$ \frac{\text{Amt of active ingredient}}{\text{Amt of total preparation}} = \frac{\text{Parts of active ingredient}}{\text{100 parts (total mixture)}} $$

Example: Ascertain the percent B in a mixture of 600 g that contains 15 g of B.

Solution:

$$ \frac{15}{600} = \frac{X}{100} \qquad = \qquad 600X = 1500 $$

$$ X = \frac{1500}{600} $$

X = 2.5, the parts of active ingredient per 100 parts of total mixture, or **2.5%**

RATIO AND PROPORTION CALCULATIONS

Ratio is the relationship of one quantity to another quantity of like value. Example ratios are 5:2, 4:1. These ratios are expressed as "5 to 2" and "4 to 1," respectively. A ratio can exist only between values of the same kind, as the ratio of percent to percent, grams to grams, dollars to dollars. In other words, the denominator must be constant.

Proportion is two equal ratios considered simultaneously. An example proportion is

$$1:3::3:9$$

This proportion is expressed as "1 is to 3 as 3 is to 9." Since the ratios are equal, the proportion may also be written $1:3 = 3:9$

Terms of Proportion

The first and fourth terms (the terms on the ends) are called the **extremes**. The second and third terms (middle terms) are called the **means**.

In a proportion, the product of the means equals the product of the extremes; therefore, when three terms are known, the fourth (or unknown) term may be determined.

Application of Proportion

The important factor when working proportions is to put the right values in the right places within the proportion. By following a few basic rules, you can accomplish this without difficulty and solve the problem correctly.

In numbering the four positions of a proportion from left to right (i.e., first, second, third, and fourth, observe the following rules):

- Let X (the unknown value) always be in the fourth position.

- Let the unit of like value to X be the third position.

- If X is smaller than the third position, place the smaller of the two leftover values in the second position; if X is larger, place the larger of the two values in the second position.

- Place the last value in the first position. When the proportion is correctly placed, multiply the extremes and the means and determine the value of X, the unknown quantity.

Example #1: What is the percent strength of 500 ml of 70% alcohol to which 150 ml of water has been added?

Solution: When adding 150 ml to 500 ml, the total quantity will be 650 ml; consequently, our four values will be **500 ml, 650 ml, 70%,** and **X** (the unknown percent). Following the rules stated above, the problem will appear as follows:

4th position: X (%)

3rd position: 70% (like value to X)

When we add water to a solution, the strength is diluted; consequently, the 70% strength of this solution will be lessened when we add the extra 150 ml of water. Therefore, of the two remaining given quantities (650 ml and 500 ml), the smaller (500 ml) will be placed in the second position, leaving the quantity 650 ml to be placed in the first position:

2nd position: 500 ml

1st position: 650 ml

The proportion appears as follows:

$$650 : 500 :: 70 : X$$

Multiplying the extremes and the means, we arrive at:

$$650X = 35,000, \quad \text{or} \quad \mathbf{X = 53.8}$$

When 150 ml of water is added to 500 ml of 70% alcohol, the result is 650 ml of 53.8% solution.

Example #2: When 1000 ml of 25% solution is evaporated to 400 ml, what is the percent strength?

Solution:

4th position: X(%)

3rd position: 15% (like value to X)

When we evaporate a solution, it becomes stronger. Therefore, the larger of the two remaining given values (1000 ml and 400 ml), will be placed in the second position, leaving the quantity 400 ml to be placed in the first position:

2nd position: 1000 ml

1st position: 400 ml

The proportion appears as follows:

$$400 : 1000 :: 15 : X$$

Multiplying the extremes and the means, we arrive at:

$$400X = 25,000, \quad \text{or} \quad \mathbf{X = 62.5}$$

When 1000 ml of water is evaporated to 400 ml, the result is a 62.5% solution.

Ratio Solutions

Ratio solutions are usually prepared in strengths as follows: 1:10, 1:150, 1:1000, 1:25000, etc., using even numbers to simplify the calculations. When a solution is made by this method, the first term of the ratio expresses the part of the solute (the substance dissolved in a solvent), while the second term expresses the total amount of the finished product.

Rules for solving ratio-solution problems are as follows:

W/W (weight/weight) solution: Divide the total weight (grams) of solution desired by the larger number of the ratio, and the quotient will be the number of grams of the solute to be used.

Example: How many grams of $KMNO_4$ are needed to make 500 g of a 1:2000 solution?

Solution:

$500 \div 2000$ =   **0.25** g of drug needed

$500 - 0.25$ = **499.75** g of solvent needed

            500.00 g total solution

W/V (weight/volume) solution: Divide the total volume (in milliliters) of solution desired by the larger number of the ratio, and the quotient will be the number of grams of the solute needed.

Example: How many grams of bichloride of mercury are needed to prepare 500 ml of a 1:1000 solution?

Solution:

    $500 \div 1000$ =   **0.50** g of drug needed

Add sufficient solvent to make 500 ml of solution.

V/V (volume/volume) Solution: Divide the total volume (in milliliters) of the solution desired by the larger number of the ratio, and the quotient will be the number of milliliters of the drug to be used.

Example: How many milliliters of HCl are needed to prepare a 1:250 solution with a total volume of 500 ml?

Solution:

    $500 \div 250$ = **2.0** ml of drug needed

Percentage solutions from stock and/or ratio solutions:

Example: From a 1:10 solution of silver nitrate in water, prepare 60 ml of a 1.5% solution of the same ingredients.

Solution: A 1:10 (W/V) solution contains 1 g of solute and enough solvent to total 10 ml of solution (finished product). Therefore, 1 ml of the solution would contain 0.1 g of the solute. Since it is required that 0.9 g of the solute be used to prepare 60 ml of the required strength, use 9 ml of the stock solution and enough solvent (water) to make the total volume measure 60 ml.

PHARMACEUTICAL PREPARATIONS

LEARNING OBJECTIVE: *Recall the composition and physical characteristics of commonly used pharmaceutical preparations.*

While assigned to a pharmacy or naval vessel, you may be required to make pharmaceutical preparations. The following sections will acquaint you with the composition and physical characteristics of some of these preparations.

Elixirs

Elixirs are aromatic, sweetened hydroalcoholic solutions containing medicinal substances. The color of elixirs varies according to the nature of the ingredients; some are artificially colored.

Suspensions

Suspensions are coarse dispersions comprised of finely divided insoluble material suspended in a liquid medium. To keep the insoluble material suspended, a third agent, called a suspending agent, is required. The process of mixing or combining the ingredients to form a suspension is called **reconstitution**.

Ointments

Ointments are semisolid, fatty, or oily preparations of medicinal substances. These preparations are of such a consistency as to be easily applied to the skin and gradually liquefy or melt at body temperature. Ointments vary in color according to their ingredients. The base of an ointment is generally greasy in texture, and the medicinal substances combined with it are always intended to be very fine particles, uniformly distributed.

Suppositories

Suppositories are solid bodies intended to introduce medicinal substances into the various orifices of the body (rectum, vagina, and urethra). The ingredients are incorporated in a base that melts at body temperature.

Capsules

Capsules are gelatin shells containing solid or liquid medicinal substances to be taken orally. A common type of capsule contains medicine in the form of a dry powder that is enclosed in transparent cases made of gelatin. Capsules are sized by universally designated numbers: 5, 4, 3, 2, 1, 0, 00, 000. The number 5 has the capacity of about 65 mg of powder (such as aspirin) and the number 00 capsule contains about 975 mg of the same substance. Only sizes 3 through 00 are available through the Federal Stock System.

PHARMACEUTICAL INSTRUMENTS

LEARNING OBJECTIVE: *Identify commonly used pharmaceutical instruments and describe the purpose of each.*

In the process of preparing some pharmaceutical preparations, you may need to use specialized instruments. To acquaint you with some of the more commonly used pharmaceutical instruments, the following sections will give you a description of each instrument and explain its purpose. See figure 6-2 for an illustration of each instrument discussed.

Pharmaceutical Balances

Two types of pharmaceutical balances are in common use in the Navy: torsion balances (shown in figure 6-2) and electronic balances (not shown). These balances are classified as either "Class A" or "Class B." Class A balances are used for weighing loads from 120 mg to 120 g. All dispensing pharmacies are required to have at least one Class A balance on hand at all times. Class B balances weigh loads of more than 648 mg, and they must be conspicuously marked

"Class B." Class B balances are optional equipment in the pharmacy.

Ribbed Funnel

Ribbed funnels are utensils used in the filtering process. They are most commonly made of glass, but other substances (tin, copper, rubber) are occasionally used. The funnel is shaped so that the inside surface tapers at a 60° angle, ending in a tapered delivery spout. The inside surface is "ribbed" to allow air to escape from between the glass and the filtering medium (improving the filtration process).

Erlenmeyer Flask

The Erlenmeyer flask is a glass container with metric measurements inscribed on it. It is used for mixing and measuring various medicinal ingredients.

Mortar and Pestle

These two items always go together, one being useless without the other. The mortar is basically a heavy bowl, with one distinct property: the inside concavity is geometrically hemispheric. The accompanying pestle is primarily a handtool that has a tip made of identical material as the mortar, and its convexity forms a perfect hemisphere. The reason for the two opposing hemispheres is to provide an even grinding surface. Mortars and pestles are made of glass, metal, or unglazed pottery called wedgewood. Glass is used when triturating (reducing substances to fine particles or powder by rubbing or grinding) very pure products (such as eye ointments), and when the preparations contain stains.

NOTE: Metal mortars and pestles should never be used when the drugs are likely to react with the metals.

Spatula

The spatula is a knifelike utensil with a rounded, flexible, smoothly ground blade, available in various sizes. The spatula is used to "work" powders, ointments, and creams in the process of levigation (the rubbing, grinding, or reduction to a fine powder with or without the addition of a liquid) and trituration. It is also used to transfer quantities of drugs from their containers to the prescription balance. Spatulas should not be used to pry open cans or as knives for opening boxes. Once the surface is scratched or the edges bent,

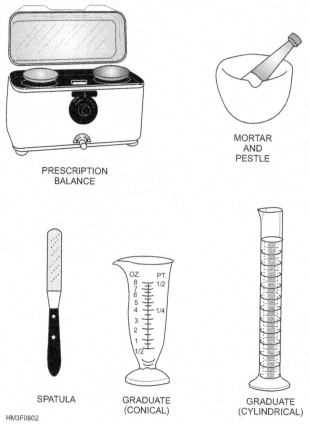

PRESCRIPTION
BALANCE

MORTAR
AND
PESTLE

SPATULA

GRADUATE
(CONICAL)

GRADUATE
(CYLINDRICAL)

HM3F0802

Figure 6-2.—Pharmaceutical instruments.

the spatula is ruined, and it becomes useless for pharmacy work.

Graduates

Graduates are conical or cylindrical clear glass containers, graduated in specified quantities and used to measure liquids volumetrically. Measuring should always be done at eye level.

DRUG INCOMPATIBILITIES, CONTRAINDICATIONS, AND ADVERSE EFFECTS

Occasionally, the drugs we use to improve a person's condition may not work in the manner intended. The outcome may be contrary to that which was expected, and, indeed, could even cause harm to the patient. It is important to be aware of symptoms that may indicate a drug is not doing its job properly.

Incompatibilities

LEARNING OBJECTIVE: *Identify the three classifications of drug incompatibility, and recall what causes these drug incompatibilities to occur.*

There are instances when a drug used simultaneously with another drug or substance does not perform as it was intended. These drugs or substances may be incompatible together and, therefore, should not be administered at the same time. A drug incompatibility can also occur when drugs are compounded together in the pharmacy. There are three classes of drug incompatibilities: therapeutic, physical, and chemical. In the following sections, each class of drug incompatibility is discussed.

THERAPEUTIC INCOMPATIBILITIES.— Therapeutic incompatibilities occur when agents antagonistic to one another are prescribed together. Such circumstances seldom occur, but when they do, the Hospital Corpsman should bring the perceived incompatibility to the attention of the physician. The pharmaceutical agents may have been used together for one agent to modify the activity of the other. The physician will verify the prescription as necessary.

PHYSICAL INCOMPATIBILITIES.—
Physical incompatibilities are often called pharmaceutical incompatibilities and are evidenced by the failure of the drugs to combine properly. It is virtually impossible for uniform dosages of medicine to be given from such solutions or mixtures. Ingredients such as oil and water (which are physically repellant to each other) and substances that are insoluble in the prescribed vehicle are primary examples of physical incompatibilities.

CHEMICAL INCOMPATIBILITIES.—
Chemical incompatibilities occur when prescribed agents react chemically upon combination to alter the composition of one or more of the ingredients (constituents).

MANIFESTATIONS OF INCOMPATIBI ITY.—
The following list outlines the various ways incompatibility between or among drug agents may be manifested. The respective type of incompatibility is also noted.

- Insolubility of prescribed agent in vehicle (physical)

- Immiscibility of two or more liquids (physical)

- Precipitation due to change in menstrum that results in decreased solubility (called **salting out**) (physical)

- Liquification of solids mixed in a dry state (called **eutexia**) (physical)

- Cementation of insoluble ingredients in liquid mixtures (physical)

- Evolution in color (chemical)

- Reduction or explosive reaction (called **oxidation**) (chemical)

- Precipitation due to chemical reaction (chemical)

- Inactivation of sulfa drugs by procaine HCl (therapeutic)

Although it is, of course, impossible to eliminate all drug-agent incompatibilities, some combinations

may respond to one of the following corrective measures.

- Addition of an ingredient that does no alter the therapeutic value (such as the addition of an ingredient to alter solubility of an agent)

- Omission of an agent that has no therapeutic value or that may be dispensed separately

- Change of an ingredient (e.g., substitution of a soluble form of an ingredient for an equivalent insoluble form)

- Change of a solvent

- Utilization of special techniques in compounding

Contraindications

LEARNING OBJECTIVE: *Recall drug contraindications, adverse drug reactions, and interactions.*

A contraindication is any condition the patient might display that makes a particular treatment or procedure inadvisable. These conditions include, but are not limited to, the disease process and other administered medications.

Adverse Drug Reactions

Adverse drug reactions may occur when a drug, administered in a dose appropriate for human prophylaxis, diagnosis, or therapy, has an unintended and noxious effect on the patient receiving it. As a Hospital Corpsman, you must be aware of the possibility of adverse effects of medications so that you can prevent an occurrence, or at least minimize the impact on the patient.

Drug Interactions

Patients may receive more than one medication at a time (as happens frequently in the case of hospitalized patients). Combining medications can cause the individual drugs to interact with each other—either positively or negatively—to produce an outcome that would not have occurred if each drug had been administered singly. Such interactions may affect the intensity of a drug's response, the duration of its effect, and side effects that may occur. As stated above, drug interactions can be positive as well as negative, and two or more medications are often administered to achieve a greater therapeutic effect.

Information Concerning Drug Contraindications, Adverse Reactions, and Interactions

Descriptions of drug contraindications, adverse reactions, and interactions may be found in several publications, most notably the *Physicians' Desk Reference*. However, the most important location for finding this information is the manufacturer's package insert and associated literature that accompanies each drug.

PRESCRIPTIONS

LEARNING OBJECTIVE: *Recall the parts of a prescription, authorized prescribers and how prescriptions are written, filled, verified, labeled, and filed.*

The most important tool used by the pharmacy is the prescription. A prescription is a written or computerized order from a healthcare provider (prescriber) directing the pharmacy to compound and dispense a drug or medication for a patient to use.

Of special importance is your understanding and conformance to the following protocols:

- All information pertaining to a prescription is confidential and should not be divulged to any persons not specifically involved in the treatment.

- No prescription or any of its parts may be applied or transferred to any person other than the patient specified.

To fill a prescription correctly, you must thoroughly understand the prescription writing and filling process. Because regulations and policies governing pharmacies sometimes change, it is important for you to be familiar with pharmacy policies in the *Manual of the Medical Department* (MANMED), NAVMED P-117. The MANMED is the basic guide to pharmacy operations.

PARTS OF THE PRESCRIPTION

Currently, there are two standardized forms used for prescriptions: the *DoD Prescription*, DD Form

1289 (fig. 6-3) and the *Polyprescription*, NAVMED 6710/6 (fig. 6-4). Information placed on these forms must be either typewritten or legibly handwritten in ink or indelible pencil. In addition to these two forms, many of today's fixed medical facilities (e.g., naval hospitals and medical clinics) now have automated pharmacy systems that allow healthcare providers to enter prescription requests into computers in their offices instead of handwriting prescriptions. Prescriptions, written or computerized, have, for the most part, the same information requirements. The only major difference is that automated prescriptions do not require the prescriber's signature.

DD 1289 is used extensively for outpatient prescriptions. For this reason, the key parts of DD 1289 will be discussed in the following sections. See figure 6-3 for examples of specific block entries.

Patient Information Block

In the patient information block, located at the top of the DD 1289, the patient's full name and date of birth are required. At most medical facilities, however, additional patient information is added to this block. This additional information usually includes the patient's duty station; social security number with family member prefix; rate; and branch of service.

Medical Facility and Date Block

The medical facility block, located below the patient information block, should contain the name of the medical facility or ship where the prescription was written. Completion of this block is important if the source of the prescription needs to be traced.

The date block, located to the right of the medical facility block, should contain the date in which the prescription was written.

Prescription Block

The large block in the center of the DD 1289 is the prescription block. It contains four parts: the superscription, the inscription, the subscription, and the signa.

SUPERSCRIPTION.—The superscription "Rx" means "take" or "take thou" or, in effect, "I want this patient to have the following medication."

INSCRIPTION.—The inscription is that part of the prescription that lists the names and quantities of the ingredients to be used. This part of the prescription is of utmost importance, since the spelling of many unrelated drugs is similar. **Whenever there is doubt as to the drug or the amount listed in the inscription, the individual filling the prescription should always verify the inscription with the prescriber.**

NOTE: The drug should be written generically, and the dosage size or strength written metrically.

SUBSCRIPTION.—The subscription follows the inscription and is that part of the prescription that gives directions to the compounder.

DD FORM **1289**

1 NOV 71

DOD PRESCRIPTION

FOR (Full name, address, & phone number) (If under 12, give age)

John R. Doe, HM3, USN

U.S.S. Neverforgotten (DD 178)

MEDICAL FACILITY *U.S.S. Neverforgotten (DD 178)*	DATE *23 Jan 99*

℞ (Superscription)   gm or ml.

(Inscription)

Tr Belladonna   *15* | *ml*

Amphogel qsad   *120* | *ml*

(Subscription)

M & ft Solution

(Signa)

Seg: 5ml tid a.c.

MFGR: *Wyeth*	EXP DATE: *12/02*
LOT NO: *P39K106*	FILLED BY: *KMT*

Jack R. Frost
LCDR. MD. USNR

℞ NUMBER   **10072**

SIGNATURE RANK AND DEGREE

EDITION OF 1 JAN 60 MAY BE USED FOR
S/N 0102-LF-012-6201

HM3F0603

Figure 6-3.—DOD Prescription form.

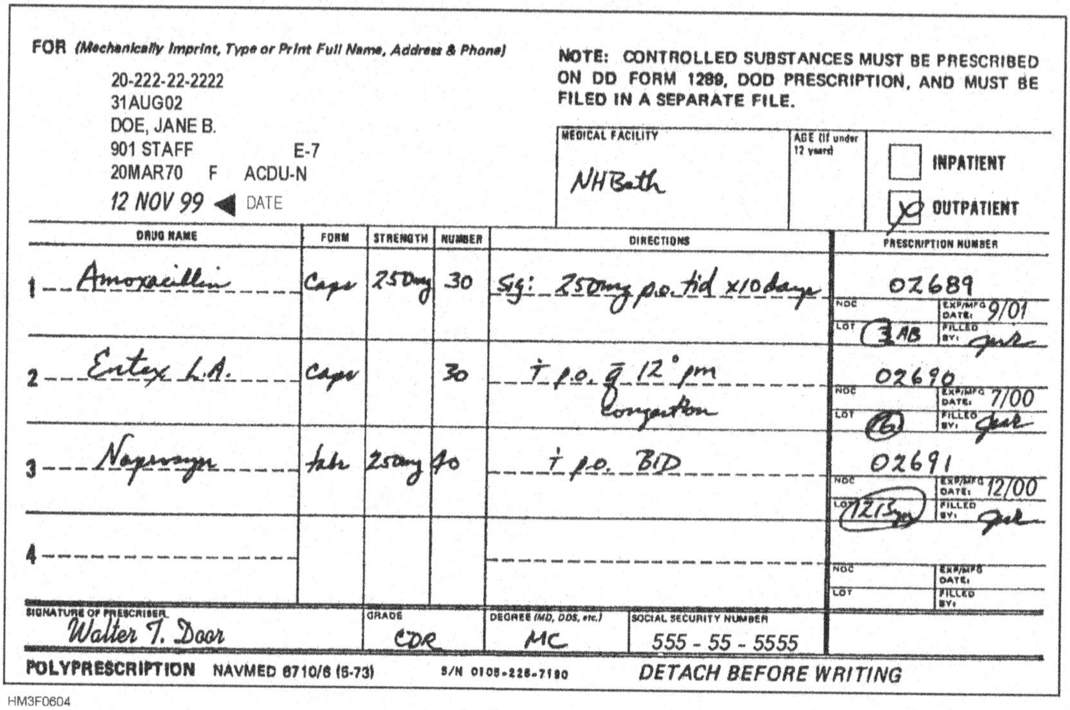
FOR (Mechanically Imprint, Type or Print Full Name, Address & Phone)
20-222-22-2222
31AUG02
DOE, JANE B.
901 STAFF E-7
20MAR70 F ACDU-N
12 NOV 99 ◀ DATE

NOTE: CONTROLLED SUBSTANCES MUST BE PRESCRIBED ON DD FORM 1289, DOD PRESCRIPTION, AND MUST BE FILED IN A SEPARATE FILE.

MEDICAL FACILITY: NHBeth
AGE (If under 12 years)
INPATIENT
☒ OUTPATIENT

	DRUG NAME	FORM	STRENGTH	NUMBER	DIRECTIONS	PRESCRIPTION NUMBER
1	Amoxacillin	Caps	250mg	30	Sig: 250mg p.o. tid x10days	02689; EXP/MFG DATE: 9/01; LOT: 3AB; FILLED BY: gsk
2	Entex L.A.	Caps		30	i p.o. q 12° pm congestion	02690; EXP/MFG DATE: 7/00; LOT: 6; FILLED BY: gsk
3	Naprosyn	tabs	250mg	40	i p.o. BID	02691; EXP/MFG DATE: 12/00; LOT: 1213; FILLED BY: gsk
4						NDC; LOT; EXP/MFG DATE; FILLED BY

SIGNATURE OF PRESCRIBER	GRADE	DEGREE (MD, DDS, etc.)	SOCIAL SECURITY NUMBER
Walter T. Door	CDR	MC	555 - 55 - 5555

POLYPRESCRIPTION NAVMED 6710/6 (6-73) S/N 0105-228-7190 DETACH BEFORE WRITING

HM3F0604

Figure 6-4.—Polyprescription form.

SIGNA.—The signa, not to be confused with the prescriber's signature, is the part of the prescription that gives the directions for the patient. This portion is preceded by the abbreviation "Sig."

Prescriber Signature Block

Finally, the prescriber signature block, located at the bottom of the form, **must** contain a legible signature of the prescriber, as well as the prescriber's full name, rank, corps, and service, stamped, typed, or handprinted. Mimeographed, preprinted, or rubber-stamped prescriptions may be used, but signatures must be original and in the handwriting of the prescriber. Facsimiles are not acceptable.

AUTHORIZED PRESCRIBERS

According to the MANMED, the following persons are authorized to write prescriptions:

- Medical and Dental Corps Officers
- Medical Service Corps optometrists, physician assistants, and podiatrists
- Civilian physicians employed by the Navy
- Independent duty Hospital Corpsmen
- Nurse practitioners (may prescribe when authorized in writing by the commanding officer)
- Nurse anesthetists and midwives (may prescribe within the scope of their practice when authorized in writing by the CO or delegated representative)

Prescriptions written by civilian prescribers, other than those employed by the Navy, may be filled for authorized beneficiaries, provided the prescribed item is on the medical facility's formulary (a published listing of medications) and the prescribed quantity is within limitations established by the command.

With the exception of the polyprescription, prescriptions are limited to one item per prescription. The quantity of the drug prescribed should be a reasonable amount needed by the patient. Excessive or unrealistic quantities should not be prescribed. Erasures on prescriptions are prohibited, and interlineations (information inserted between lines of writing) must be initialed.

Finally, persons authorized to prescribe cannot write prescriptions for themselves or members of their immediate families.

FILLING PRESCRIPTIONS

When you receive a prescription for filling, you should follow certain basic steps to make sure that the right patient gets the right medicine in the right amount in the right way. There are no shortcuts—in the pharmacy things are done right or not at all!

Prescription Verification

First of all, satisfy yourself that the prescription you have received is a bonafide one and that the person you have received it from is entitled to have it filled by your pharmacy. You don't need to be tedious about verification. The simplest and best way is to ask for an ID card and verify the expiration date on the ID card.

Study the prescription carefully and make sure that the drug prescribed is reasonable, that its amount or dosage is realistic in consideration of the patient's age, and that the quantity of the medication is practical. A prescription calling for 1,000 tetracycline tablets or a pint of paregoric, for example, warrants further inquiry.

If, in the process of verification, you feel that there is a discrepancy, an ambiguity, or an incompatibility, or for any reason you find it is necessary to consult the prescriber, never allow the patient to suspect that anything is amiss. You should never fill a prescription you do not completely understand or that you feel is incorrect. What appears to be an overdose may be the desired dose for a specific patient, but the prescriber will appreciate being called for verification.

When you are sure you understand the prescription and are satisfied that it is in all respects correct, you should give its filling your undivided attention. Most mistakes are made when the person filling the prescription is either interrupted while doing so or is trying to accomplish more than one task at a time.

During the process of filling a prescription, the label on the containers used in filling the prescription should be verified at least three times. Initially, the label should be read when the container is taken from the shelf. Then it should be read again when the contents are removed from the container. And finally, the container's label should be read before it is returned to the shelf. By following these three verification steps for each prescription you fill, you will reduce the possibility of making a prescription error.

Prescription Labeling

Proper labeling of a prescription is as important as filling it correctly. It is reasonable to assume that if a great deal of accuracy is necessary to properly compound a prescription, it is just as important that the patient take the correct amount of medication in the right manner to receive its maximum benefits. Improperly written or misunderstood directions on a prescription label can be disastrous. Make sure all labels are typed clearly and their directions translated into simple layman's language. Keep in mind that the prescription label serves two purposes. First and most important, it gives the patient directions pertaining to the medication; second, in case of misuse or error, it is the quickest means by which the contents of the prescription container, the person who wrote the prescription, and the person who filled it can be traced. Consequently, the following information, illustrated in figure 6-5, should always be on the label:

- The name and phone number of the dispensing facility

- A serialized number that corresponds with the number on the prescription form, (see figure 6-3)

- The date the prescription is filled

- The patient's name

- The directions to the patient, transcribed accurately from the prescription, in clear, concise layman's language

- The prescriber's name and rate or rank

- The initials of the compounder

- Authorized refills, if any

- The expiration date, if applicable

- Name, strength, and quantity of medication dispensed

    NOTE: Pharmaceutical preparations should be identified and labeled with the generic name. However, trade or brand names may be used if the trade or brand name is actually on the container.

Other information that may need to be attached to the prescription container are labels reading "Shake Well Before Using" or "For External Use Only." "Poison" labels should be omitted when a preparation

```
NAVAL HOSPITAL                         Phone
BETHESDA, MD      20814                295-2113
  (keep out of reach of children)      295-550

John R. Doe, HM2, USN                  4/28/99kk

Take one (1) tablet every 12 hours if needed
for cold symptoms.

Dimetapp #30          Dr. Johnson
No Refills
                                       117765
```

HM3F0605

Figure 6-5.—Prescription label.

is intended for external use, as many physicians prefer the "For External Use Only" labels.

After the prescription is labeled, check the ingredients again by some systematic method to ensure accuracy.

As an added precaution and to aid expeditious identification of drugs in case of undesirable effects, note the manufacturer and the lot number of the proprietary drug dispensed on the prescription form (fig. 6-3). This procedure, however, does not apply to medications consisting of a mixture of several ingredients. The initials or the code of the person filling the prescription must also be written on the prescription form (fig. 6-3).

FILING PRESCRIPTIONS

Prescriptions that have been filled must be maintained in one of several separate files:

- **Schedule II and III narcotics**—Prescriptions containing narcotics are numbered consecutively, preceded by the letter "N," and filed separately.

- **Alcohol**—These prescriptions are numbered consecutively, preceded by the letter "A," and filed separately.

- **Schedule III (nonnarcotic), IV, and V drugs**—These prescriptions are part of and are numbered in the same manner as the general files; however, they are maintained separately.

- **General files**—All other prescriptions are numbered consecutively and filed together.

Currently, prescriptions are required to be kept on file for at least 2 years after the date of issue.

REGULATIONS AND RESPONSIBILITIES PERTAINING TO CONTROLLED SUBSTANCES, ALCOHOL, AND DANGEROUS DRUGS

LEARNING OBJECTIVE: *Recall Hospital Corpsman responsibilities and accountability pertaining to controlled substances; identify controlled substance schedules; and recall controlled substance security, custody, inventory, and survey procedures.*

Hospital Corpsmen who handle controlled substances and other drugs are held responsible for the proper distribution and custody of those substances and drugs. Nowhere is the demand for strict integrity more important. Misuse, abuse, loss, and theft of these substances have always, sooner or later, ended in tragedy and severe consequences. No one has ever profited by their misappropriation.

It behooves every Hospital Corpsman to thoroughly understand the responsibility concerning the custody and handling of controlled substances and other drugs and to be familiar with the regulations and laws pertaining to them.

RESPONSIBILITY

Although the MANMED specifically assigns custodial responsibility for controlled substances, alcohol, and dangerous drugs to a commissioned officer (and more specific control to the Nursing Service), you, as a Hospital Corpsman, have the responsibilities of administering and securing them properly. All controlled substances and other drugs are to be kept under lock and key. Neither keys nor drugs should ever be entrusted to a patient.

ACCOUNTABILITY

Hospital Corps personnel are held accountable for drugs entrusted to them. Great care should be exercised to prevent the loss or unauthorized use of drugs. No drug should be administered without proper authority. In addition, U.S. Navy Regulations forbid the introduction, possession, use, sale, or other transfer of marijuana, narcotic substances, or other controlled substances.

CONTROLLED SUBSTANCE SCHEDULES

Controlled substances and drugs require special handling and security measures. The Controlled Substance Act of 1970 established five schedules (categories) related to a drug's potential for abuse, medical usefulness, and degree of dependency, if abused.

Controlled substances may migrate between schedules, and new products may be added. These changes will be promulgated by the Navy Materiel Support Command in the Medical and Dental Materiel Bulletin.

Schedule I

Schedule I substances have high abuse potential and no accepted medical use (e.g., heroin, marijuana, LSD).

Schedule II

Schedule II substances have high abuse potential and severe psychological and/or physical dependence liability. Examples of schedule II substances include narcotics, amphetamines, and barbiturates. Prescriptions for schedule II substances can never be ordered with refills and must be filled within 7 days of the date originally written.

Schedule III

Schedule III substances have less abuse potential than schedule II substances and moderate dependence liability. Examples of schedule III substances include nonbarbiturate sedatives, nonamphetamine stimulants, and medications that contain a limited quantity of certain narcotics. Prescriptions must be filled within 30 days of the date written and may be refilled up to five times within 6 months.

Schedule IV

Schedule IV substances have less abuse potential than schedule III substances and limited dependence liability. Prescriptions must be filled within 30 days of the date written and may be refilled up to five times within a 6-month period.

Schedule V

Schedule V substances have limited abuse potential. Schedule V substances are primarily antitussives or antidiarrheals that contain small amounts of narcotics (codeine). Prescriptions must be filled within 30 days of the date written and may be refilled up to five times within 6 months.

DANGEROUS DRUGS

Poisonous drugs, chemicals, and similar substances are classified as dangerous drugs. Because these substances are powerful, their containers should have a distinctive color, size, or shape, and the container should be placed in a special storage area so they are not mistaken for other drugs. In addition, the following safeguards should be enforced:

- Label all containers of dangerous substances appropriately.

- Store caustic acids (such as glacial acetic, sulfuric, nitric, concentrated hydrochloric, or oxalic acids) in appropriate containers, and do not issue to wards or outpatients.

- Account for and issue methyl alcohol (methanol) to be used by medical activities in the same manner as other controlled substances. Methanol should not be stored, used, or dispensed by the pharmacy, ward, or outpatient treatment facility.

SECURITY AND CUSTODY OF CONTROLLED SUBSTANCES

Schedule I and II controlled substances and ethyl alcohol require vault or safe storage and inventory by the Controlled Substance Inventory Board (discussed in more detail in the section entitled "Inventory of Controlled Substances"). Working stock may be kept in a locked area within the pharmacy. A copy of the safe combination must be kept in a sealed envelope deposited with the CO or representative.

Schedule III, IV, and V controlled substances require locked cabinet security for storage of bulk drugs. A minimum amount of working stock may be dispersed among other pharmacy stock, provided the pharmacy stock itself is secure. Otherwise, all stock in this category must be kept in locked cabinets.

Custodial responsibility for controlled substances, ethyl alcohol, and dangerous drugs at naval hospitals is entrusted to a commissioned officer or a civilian pharmacist who is appointed in writing by the CO. At remote branch clinics that do not have a commissioned officer or a civilian pharmacist, the CO will designate in writing a member of the branch clinic as custodian. On board large naval vessels, the CO will appoint an officer of the Medical Department or another officer in writing as the bulk custodian. This officer will be responsible for, and maintain custody of, all bulk controlled substances. On board smaller naval vessels, access to controlled substances is limited to the bulk custodian and the senior medical department representative (SMDR). Only individuals whose official duties require access to such spaces are provided the safe combinations.

INVENTORY OF CONTROLLED SUBSTANCES

Monthly (or more frequently, if necessary), the Controlled Substances Inventory Board takes an unannounced inventory of controlled substances.

NOTE: An exception to this frequency may be made for ships with an Independent Duty Corpsman. On these ships, the inventory may be conducted on a quarterly basis if there have been no transactions of controlled substances (including filled prescriptions or receipts of items requisitioned from supply).

The CO appoints the members of the board in writing. The board consists of three members, at least two of whom are commissioned officers. After the board conducts the inventory, it submits a report to the CO. The officer having custodial responsibility cannot be a member of the board. On small ships and installations, the SMDR may be a board member. For further guidance on controlled substance inventory procedures, refer to NAVMEDCOMINST 6710.9, *Guidelines for Controlled Substances Inventory*.

SURVEY OF CONTROLLED SUBSTANCES

Schedule I and II controlled substances, ethyl alcohol, and locally controlled drugs that have become outdated, deteriorated to the point of not being usable, are of questionable purity or potency, or have had their identity compromised, must be reported to the CO. If destruction is indicated and directed by the CO, destruction must be accomplished in the presence of a member of the Controlled Substance Inventory Board. A certification of destruction form contains the complete nomenclature and quantity of the substances to be destroyed together with the method of destruction to be used. After certification is completed, approved by the CO, and signed by the members witnessing the destruction, the certification of destruction is retained and filed as required by current instructions. The destroyed substances should then be removed from the stock records and the controlled substance log.

SUMMARY

Inpatients and the majority of outpatients will receive pharmaceutical products as part of their treatment. As a healthcare provider who may administer these products or fill prescriptions, it is crucial for you to have a good foundation of knowledge in pharmacology, toxicology, and the proper handling of prescriptions and controlled substances. This chapter touched on each of these topics to assist you in your duties. However, you should consult the recommended publications, such as the *Manual of the Medical Department*, *Drug Facts and Comparisons*, and the *Physicians' Desk Reference*, to provide you with the guidance and knowledge you will need to provide the best possible care for your patients.

CHAPTER 7

CLINICAL LABORATORY

A basic knowledge of clinical laboratory procedures is critical for all Hospital Corpsmen, particularly those working at small dispensaries and isolated duty stations without the supervision of a medical officer. A patient's complaint may be of little value by itself, but coupled with the findings of a few easily completed laboratory studies, a diagnosis can usually be surmised and treatment initiated.

Hospital Corpsmen who can perform blood and urine tests and interpret the results are better equipped to determine the cause of illness or request assistance. Since they can provide a more complete clinical picture to the medical officer, their patients can be treated sooner.

In this chapter, we will discuss laboratory administrative responsibilities, ethics in the laboratory, the microscope, blood collection techniques, and step-by-step procedures for a complete blood count and urinalysis. Also included are basic testing procedures for bacteriologic, serologic, and fungal identification.

THE HOSPITAL CORPSMAN AND THE CLINICAL LABORATORY

LEARNING OBJECTIVE: *Recall clinical laboratory administrative procedures and ethics policy.*

The Hospital Corpsman is not expected to make diagnoses from test findings or to institute definitive treatment based upon them. However, with the availability of modern communications facilities, having the results of these tests available will greatly assist the Corpsman in giving a clearer clinical picture to the supporting medical officer.

Needless to say, accuracy, neatness, and attention to detail are essential to obtain optimum test results. Remember also that these tests are only aids to diagnosis. Many other clinical factors must be taken into consideration before treatment may be started.

ADMINISTRATIVE PROCEDURES AND RESPONSIBILITIES

The ability to perform clinical laboratory tests is a commendable attribute of the Hospital Corpsman. However, the entire testing effort could be wasted if proper recording and filing practices are ignored and the test results go astray. As a member of the medical team, it is your responsibility to make sure that established administrative procedures are followed with regard to accurate patient and specimen identification. It is your further responsibility to ensure laboratory reports in your department are handled and filed properly.

Since the test results are a part of the patient's clinical picture, their precision and accuracy are vital. Test results have a vital bearing upon the patient's immediate and future medical history. They are, therefore, made part of the patient's health record (inpatient or outpatient). Laboratory reports of inpatients are placed in the inpatient health record, while laboratory reports of outpatients are placed in the outpatient health record.

Laboratory Request Forms

The armed forces have gone to great lengths to produce workable, effective laboratory forms that serve their purpose with a minimum of confusion and chance for error. These forms are standard forms (SF) in the 500 series. Their primary purpose is to request, report on, or record clinical laboratory tests. With the exception of SF-545 (*Laboratory Report Display*), SF laboratory forms are multicopied and precarbonized for convenience. The original copy of the laboratory report forms are attached to the SF-545 (located inside the patient's heath record), and the carbon copy becomes part of the laboratory's master file. For a complete listing of SF forms and their purposes, refer to the *Manual of the Medical Department* (MANMED), NAVMED P-117.

SF laboratory request forms are not the only means by which healthcare providers can order laboratory tests. Many of today's naval medical facilities have computerized laboratory systems. Computerized laboratory systems enable healthcare providers to enter laboratory test requests into computers located in their spaces. Once healthcare providers enter their test requests, patients may report immediately to the Laboratory Department, where specimens are obtained and tests are performed.

Use of Laboratory Request Forms

Write information on the SF laboratory request forms in black or blue-black ink. Use a separate SF laboratory request form for each patient and for each test. Document the patient's full name, family member prefix and social security number, rate/rank, dependency status, branch of service, and status in the "Patient Identification" block. Also identify the ward or department ordering the test in this block. See figure 7-1 for an illustration of the *Urinalysis* request form, SF-550. Computer-generated laboratory test requests require the same patient identification data as SF laboratory requests.

Since the results of the requested laboratory test are usually closely associated with the patient's health and treatment, the requesting healthcare provider's name should also be clearly stated in the "Requesting Physician's Signature" block on the request form (fig. 7-1). The doctor requesting the urinalysis should sign in this block. Alternatively, you may type/print the doctor's name in the block and initial the entry to authenticate it. This practice ensures that the report will get back to the provider as soon as possible.

Enter the requested test in the "Remarks" block (e.g., "Clean catch midstream to R/O urinary tract infection"). Because the data requested, the date reported, and the time of specimen collection are usually important in support of the clinical picture, these pieces of information should be clearly written on the request in the areas provided for them (fig. 7-1).

Patient and Specimen Identification

Before accepting laboratory request forms and specimens in the laboratory, check patient identification information on both the request form and the specimen container label for completeness and legibility. Proper documentation of patient identification information on these items can prevent a great number of errors. Also, make sure the specimen(s) submitted is in fact the specimen of the patient submitting it. You need not stand over the patient while the specimen is being collected; however, keep in mind that for certain tests (such as drug or alcohol screening tests) individuals may attempt to substitute specimens.

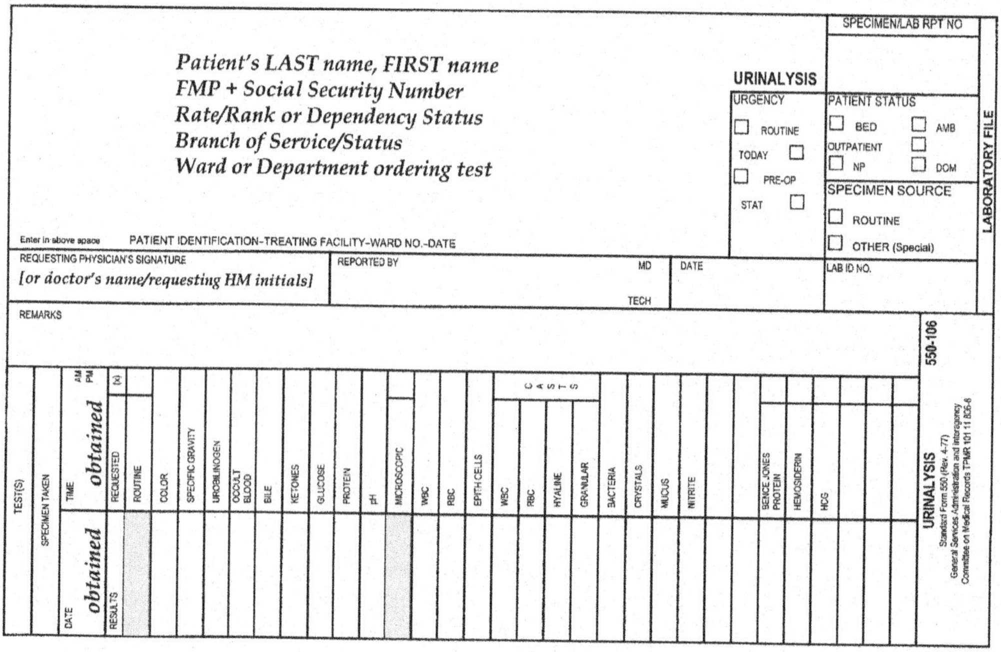
Patient's LAST name, FIRST name
FMP + Social Security Number
Rate/Rank or Dependency Status
Branch of Service/Status
Ward or Department ordering test

Enter in above space PATIENT IDENTIFICATION-TREATING FACILITY-WARD NO.-DATE

URINALYSIS

URGENCY: ROUTINE / TODAY / PRE-OP / STAT

SPECIMEN/LAB RPT NO

PATIENT STATUS: BED / AMB / OUTPATIENT / NP / DOM

SPECIMEN SOURCE: ROUTINE / OTHER (Special)

LABORATORY FILE

REQUESTING PHYSICIAN'S SIGNATURE *[or doctor's name/requesting HM initials]* | REPORTED BY | MD | TECH | DATE | LAB ID NO.

REMARKS

550-106

TEST(S) | SPECIMEN TAKEN: TIME *obtained* AM PM, DATE *obtained* | REQUESTED (x) | RESULTS | ROUTINE | COLOR | SPECIFIC GRAVITY | UROBILINOGEN | OCCULT BLOOD | BILE | KETONES | GLUCOSE | PROTEIN | pH | MICROSCOPIC | WBC | RBC | EPITH CELLS | CASTS: WBC | RBC | HYALINE | GRANULAR | BACTERIA | CRYSTALS | MUCUS | NITRITE | BENCE JONES PROTEIN | HEMOSIDERIN | HCG

URINALYSIS
Standard Form 550 (Rev. 4-77)
General Services Administration and Interagency
Committee on Medical Records FPMR 101 11.806-8

HM3f0701

Figure 7-1.—SF-550, Urinalysis Request Form.

Filing Laboratory Forms

After healthcare providers have reviewed laboratory test reports, they will initial the form. Initialing the form indicates the healthcare provider has reviewed the test results. After the healthcare provider releases the laboratory report, it should be filed in the patient's inpatient or outpatient health record, as appropriate. If a standard form is used to record test results, it should be attached **chronologically** to the SF-545, *Laboratory Report Display*, inside the patient's health record. The SF-545 functions as a display form for multiple laboratory reports. See figure 7-2. Use the preglued areas provided on the lab forms. However, since the glue is notorious for losing its grip after a while, you may use tape or staples to attach the form to the SF-545. Each SF-545 can accommodate a limited number of laboratory reports, so do not overcrowd the display form. When the SF-545 is full, add a new SF-545 to the health record and place it in front of the old SF-545. In this way, the most current lab reports will remain in chronological order.

Automated or computer-generated laboratory test reports, depending on the form's size, may be either mounted on the SF-545 or placed adjacent to the SF-545 in the health record. Keep in mind that these automated or computer-generated forms should also be filed chronologically.

ETHICS AND GOOD PRACTICES IN THE LABORATORY

The nature of laboratory tests and their results must be treated as a confidential matter between the patient, the healthcare provider, and the performing technician. Chapter 16 of the MANMED outlines the Navy's ethics policy with regard to disclosure of the contents of a patient's medical record, including lab reports. It is good practice to prevent unauthorized access to these reports, to leave interpretation of the test results to the attending provider, and to refrain from discussing the results with the patient.

BLOOD COLLECTION

LEARNING OBJECTIVE: *Identify the correct steps to perform blood collection by the finger puncture method and venipuncture method, and recall Standard Precautions and other safety precautions that apply to blood collection.*

There are two principal methods of obtaining blood specimens: the finger puncture method and the venipuncture method. For most clinical laboratory tests requiring a blood specimen, venous blood obtained by venipuncture is preferred. Blood collected by venipuncture is less likely to become contaminated, and the volume of blood collected is greater. Infection control practices, equipment requirements, and step-by-step instructions on performing both of these blood collection methods will be discussed in the following sections.

STANDARD PRECAUTIONS

Under the concept of "Standard Precautions" outlined by the Centers For Disease Control and Prevention (CDC), blood and other bodily fluids should be considered as potentially infectious. To protect medical personnel from direct contact with blood during phlebotomy (blood collection), gloves are required to be worn. Gloves should be disposed of after each patient.

Needles and sharps used in the blood collection process should be handled with extreme caution and disposed of in biohazard sharps containers. Sharps containers should be conveniently located near phlebotomy work sites.

Absorbent materials, such as cotton 2 x 2's used to cover blood extraction sites, normally contain only a small amount of blood and can be disposed of as general waste. However, if a large amount of blood is absorbed, the absorbent material should be placed in a biohazard waste container and treated as infectious waste.

Clean phlebotomy work site equipment and furniture daily with a disinfectant.

FINGER PUNCTURE

The finger puncture method is used when a patient is burned severely or is bandaged so that the veins are either covered or inaccessible. Finger puncture is also used when only a small amount of blood is needed.

Materials Required for Finger Puncture Procedure

To perform a finger puncture, the following materials are required:

- Sterile gauze pads (2" x 2")

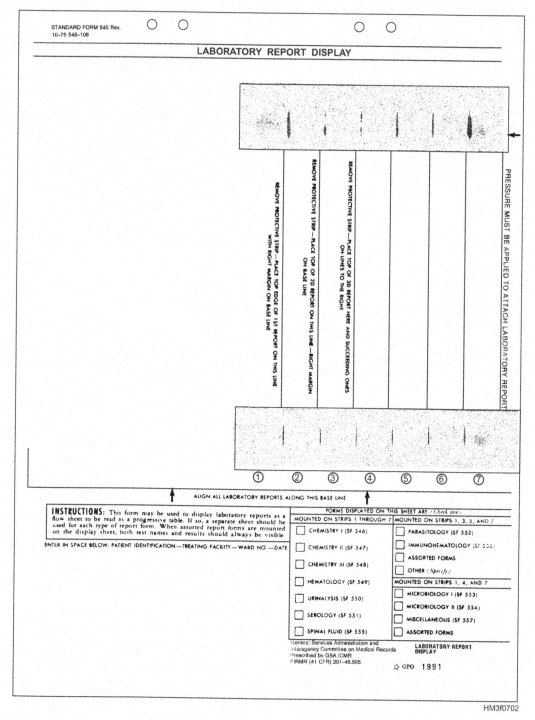

Figure 7-2.—SF-545, Laboratory Report Display.

- 70% isopropyl alcohol or povidone-iodine solution pads
- Blood lancets
- Capillary tubes
- Bandages

Arrange your equipment in an orderly manner and have it within easy reach. Also, wash your hands before and after each procedure.

Finger Puncture Procedure

To perform a finger puncture, follow the steps given below.

1. Explain the procedure to the patient.

2. Using the middle or ring finger, massage or "milk" the finger down toward the fingertip. Repeat this "milking" five or six times.

3. Cleanse the fingertip with an alcohol pad or povidone-iodine solution and let dry.

4. Take a lancet and make a quick deep stab on the side of the finger (off-center). To obtain a large rounded drop, the puncture should be across the striations of the fingertip. See figure 7-3.

5. Wipe away the first drop of blood to avoid dilution with tissue fluid. Avoid squeezing the fingertip to accelerate bleeding as this tends to dilute the blood with excess tissue fluid, but gentle pressure some distance above the puncture site may be applied to obtain a free flow of blood.

6. When the required blood has been obtained, apply a pad of sterile gauze and instruct the patient to apply pressure, then apply a bandage.

When dealing with infants and very small children, the heel or great toe puncture is the best method to obtain a blood specimen. This method is performed in much the same way.

VENIPUNCTURE (VACUTAINER METHOD)

The collection of blood from veins is called venipuncture. For the convenience of technician and patient, arm veins are best for obtaining a blood sample. If arm veins cannot be used due to interference from bandage or IV therapy, thrombosed or hardened veins, etc., consult your supervisor for instructions on the use of hand or foot veins.

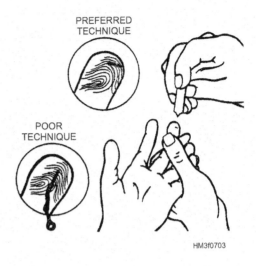

PREFERRED TECHNIQUE

POOR TECHNIQUE

HM3f0703

Figure 7-3.—Finger puncture.

NOTE: Do not draw blood from an arm with IV fluid running into it. Choose another site. The IV fluid will alter tests results.

Materials Required for Venipuncture Procedure

To perform a venipuncture, the following materials are required:

- Sterile gauze pads (2" x 2")
- 70% isopropyl alcohol or povidone-iodine solution pads
- Tourniquet
- Vacutainer needles and holder
- Vacutainer tube appropriate for the test to be performed

Arrange your equipment in an orderly manner and have it within easy reach. Also, wash your hands before the procedure.

Venipuncture Procedure

Position the patient so that the vein is easily accessible and you are able to perform the venipuncture in a comfortable position. Always have the patient either lying in bed or sitting in a chair with the arm propped up.

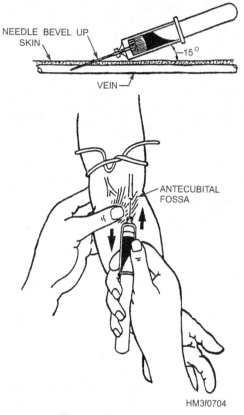

Figure 7-4.—Venipuncture.

To perform venipuncture, follow the steps given below.

1. Explain the procedure to the patient.

2. Apply tourniquet around the arm approximately 2 to 3 inches above the antecubital fossa (the depression in the anterior region of the elbow, see figure 7-4) with enough tension so that the VEIN is compressed, but not the ARTERY. A BP cuff (sphygmomanometer) may be used instead of a tourniquet if a patient is difficult to draw.

3. Position the patient's arm extended with little or no flexion at the elbow.

4. Locate a prominent vein by palpation (feeling). If the vein is difficult to find, it may be made more prominent by massaging the arm with an upward motion to force blood into the vein.

5. Cleanse the puncture site with a 70% alcohol pad or povidone-iodine solution and allow to dry.

6. "Fix" or hold the vein taut. This is best accomplished by placing the thumb under the puncture site and exerting a slight downward pressure on the skin or placing the thumb to the side of the site and pulling the skin taut laterally (fig. 7-4).

7. Using a smooth continuous motion, introduce the needle, bevel side up, into the side of the vein at about a 15-degree angle with the skin (fig. 7-4).

8. Holding the vacutainer barrel with one hand, push the tube into the holder with the other hand and watch for the flow of blood into the tube until filling is completed.

9. Once all the specimens have been collected, hold the vacutainer with one hand and release the tourniquet with the other.

10. Place a sterile gauze over the puncture site and remove the needle with a quick, smooth motion.

11. Apply pressure to the puncture site and instruct the patient to keep the arm in a straight position. Have the patient hold pressure for at least 3 minutes.

12. Take this time to invert any tubes that need to have anticoagulant mixed with the blood.

13. Label specimens.

14. Reinspect the puncture site to make sure bleeding has stopped, and apply a bandage.

THE MICROSCOPE

LEARNING OBJECTIVE: *Identify the parts of the microscope, and determine their functions.*

Before any attempts are made to view blood smears, urinary sediments, bacteria, parasites, etc., it is absolutely essential that beginners know the instrument with which they will be spending considerable time—the microscope. The microscope is a precision instrument used extensively in clinical laboratories to make visible objects too small to be seen by the unaided eye. Most laboratories are equipped with binocular (two-eyepiece) microscopes, but monocular microscopes are also commonly used. The type of microscope most often used in the laboratory is referred to as the **compound microscope**. See figure 7-5. A compound microscope contains a system of lenses of sufficient magnification and resolving power (ability to show, separate, and distinguish) so that small elements lying close together in a specimen appear larger and distinctly separated. In the following sections, the compound microscope's framework, illumination system, magnification system, and focusing system will be discussed.

FRAMEWORK

The framework of the compound microscope consists of four parts: the arm, the stage, the mechanical stage, and the base (fig. 7-5).

Arm

The arm is the structure that supports the magnification and focusing system. It is the handle by which the microscope is carried.

Stage

The stage is the platform on which a specimen is placed for examination. In the center of the stage is an aperture or hole that allows the passage of light from the condenser.

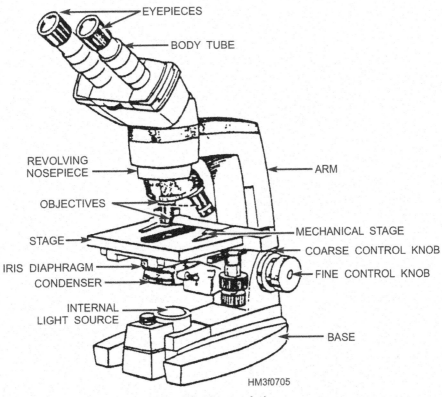

EYEPIECES

BODY TUBE

REVOLVING NOSEPIECE

OBJECTIVES

STAGE

IRIS DIAPHRAGM

CONDENSER

INTERNAL LIGHT SOURCE

ARM

MECHANICAL STAGE

COARSE CONTROL KNOB

FINE CONTROL KNOB

BASE

HM3f0705

Figure 7-5.—Compound microscope.

7-7

Mechanical Stage

The mechanical (movable) stage holds the specimen in place and is the means by which the specimen may be moved about on the stage.

Base

The base is the structure on which the microscope rests.

ILLUMINATION SYSTEM

Ideal illumination of a specimen viewed under the microscope requires even light distribution. The objectives must also be entirely filled with light from the condenser. To fulfill these requirements, the illumination system of the compound microscope consists of three parts: an internal light source, a condenser, and an iris diaphragm. See figure 7-5.

Internal Light Source

The internal light source is built into the base of the microscope. It provides a precise and steady source of light into the microscope.

Condenser

The condenser is composed of a compact lens system and is located between the light source and stage. The condenser concentrates and focuses light from the light source directly through the specimen.

Iris Diaphragm

An iris diaphragm located on the condenser controls the diameter of the light source's beam. To improve resolution, the operator should adjust the opening of the iris diaphragm to approximately the same size as the face of the objective lens. In addition to the diaphragm on the condenser, an iris diaphragm may be located on the internal light source. This iris diaphragm controls the amount of light sent to the condenser from the internal light source.

MAGNIFICATION SYSTEM

The magnification system of the compound microscope contains at least two lens systems. The two lens systems are mounted on either end of a tube called the body tube. The lens nearest the object is called the objective lens, and the lens nearest the eye is the ocular lens or eye piece. See figure 7-5.

Objective Lenses

On a compound microscope, there is usually a set of three objective lenses (or "objectives"). This set of objectives is the component most responsible for the magnification and resolution of detail in a specimen. Each objective lens has a different focus distance and magnification power. A set of objectives normally consists of a low-power lens (approximate focus 16 mm, magnification 10X), a high-power lens (approximate focus 4 mm, magnification 45X), and an oil-immersion lens (approximate focus 1.8 mm, magnification 100X). Objective lenses are color coded for easy recognition: 16 mm-10X (green), 4 mm-45X (yellow), and 1.8 mm-100X (red).

Revolving Nosepiece

The revolving nosepiece contains openings into which objective lenses are fitted, and revolves objectives into desired position.

Body Tube

The body tube is a tube that permits light to travel from the objective to the ocular lens.

Ocular Lenses

Ocular lenses, or eyepieces, are located on top of the body tube and usually have a magnification power of 10X. To calculate the total magnification of a specimen, you multiply the magnification power of the objective by the magnification power of the ocular lens. Examples of total magnifications are provided in table 7-1.

FOCUSING SYSTEM

Focusing is accomplished by moving the stage up or down with the coarse and fine control knob (fig. 7-5). Whether the stage needs to be raised or lowered depends on the focal length of the objective

Table 7-1.—Examples of Total Magnifications

Objective Lens	Color Code	10X Ocular	Total Magnification
16 mm-10X	Green	10X	100X
4 mm-45X	Yellow	10X	450X
1.8 mm-100X	Red	10X	1000X

being used. For example, the high-powered objective of short focal length (4 mm) will need the stage raised so the objective is very close to the specimen, while the low-powered objective of a longer focal length (16 mm) will need the stage lowered so the objective is farther from the specimen.

The coarse control knob is used initially to bring the specimen's image into approximate focus. Once this is accomplished, the fine control knob sharpens the image.

Coarse Control Knob

The coarse control knob is the larger and inner knob. Rotating the coarse control knob allows the image to appear in approximate focus.

Fine Control Knob

The fine control knob is the smaller and outer knob. Rotating this control knob renders the image clear and well-defined.

FOCUSING THE MICROSCOPE

The process of focusing consists of adjusting the relationship between the optical system of the microscope and the object to be examined so that a clear image of the object is obtained. The distance between the upper surface of the glass slide on the microscope stage and the faces of the objective lens varies depending upon which of the three objectives is in the focusing position. It is a good practice to obtain a focus with the low-power objective first, then change to the higher objective required to avoid accidentally damaging the objective lens, the specimen, or both. Most modern microscopes are equipped with parfocal objectives (meaning that if one objective is in focus, the others will be in approximate focus when the nosepiece is revolved). With the low-power objective in focusing position, observe the following steps in focusing.

1. Seat yourself behind the microscope, then lower your head to one side of the microscope until your eyes are approximately at the level of the stage.

2. Using the coarse adjustment knob, lower the body tube until the face of the objective is within 1/4 inch of the object. Most microscopes are constructed in such a way that the low-power (green) objective cannot be lowered and make contact with the object on the stage.

3. While you are looking through the ocular, you should use the coarse adjustment knob to elevate the body tube until the image becomes visible. Then use the fine adjustment knob to obtain a clear and distinct image. Do not move the focusing knob while changing lenses.

4. If the high-power objective (yellow) is to be used next, bring it into position by revolving the nosepiece (a distinct "click" indicates it is in proper alignment with the body tube). Use the fine adjustment knob only to bring the object into exact focus.

5. If specimen is too dark, you can increase lighting by opening the iris diaphragm of the condenser.

6. The oil-immersion objective (red) is used for detailed study of stained blood and bacterial smears. Remember that the distance between objective lens and object is very short, and great care must be employed so the specimen is not damaged. After focusing with the high-power objective and scanning for well-defined cells, raise the objective, place a small drop of immersion oil, free of bubbles, on the slide, centering the drop in the circle of light coming through the condenser. Next, revolve the nosepiece to bring the oil-immersion objective into place, and, by means of the coarse adjustment knob, slowly lower the body tube until the lens just makes contact with the drop of oil on the slide. The instant of contact is indicated by a flash of light illuminating the oil. The final step in focusing is done with the fine adjustment knob. It is with this lens in particular that lighting is important. The final focus, clear and well-defined, will be obtained only when proper light adjustment is made.

CARE OF THE MICROSCOPE

The microscope is an expensive and delicate instrument that should be given proper care.

Moving or transporting microscopes should be accomplished by grasping the arm of the scope in one hand and supporting the weight of the scope with the other hand. Avoid sudden jolts and jars.

Keep the microscope clean at all times; when not in use, microscopes should be enclosed in a dustproof cover or stored in their case. Remove dust with a camel hair brush. Lenses may be wiped carefully with lens tissue. When the oil-immersion lens is not being used, remove the oil with lens tissue. Use oil solvents (such as xylene) on lenses only when required to remove dried oil and only in the minimal amount necessary. **Never use alcohol or similar solvents to clean lenses**.

COMPLETE BLOOD COUNT

LEARNING OBJECTIVE: *Identify the five parts of a complete blood count, and recognize the testing procedures for the following: Unopette® Red Blood Cell Count, Microhematocrit, Unopette White Blood Cell Count, and Differential White Blood Cell Count.*

A complete blood count consists of the following five tests:

- Total red blood cell (RBC) count

- Hemoglobin determination

- Hematocrit reading

- Total white blood cell (WBC) count

- Differential white blood cell count

The complete blood count, commonly referred to as a CBC, is used in the diagnosis of many diseases. Blood collected for these tests are capillary or peripheral blood and venous blood. CBCs may be performed either manually or by using automated hematology analyzers. The manual method is used in isolated locations and on board some naval vessels where a hematology analyzer installation is not practical. For this reason, and because machines break down on occasion, the manual method will be covered in the following sections.

COUNTING BLOOD CELLS

To manually count red blood cells (erythrocytes) and white blood cells (leukocytes), you will need a microscope and an instrument called a **hemacytometer**. See figure 7-6. The hemacytometer is a thick glass slide with three raised parallel platforms on the middle third of the device. The central platform is subdivided by a transverse groove to form two halves, each wider than the two lateral platforms and separated from them and from each other by moats. The central platforms each contain a counting chamber and are exactly 0.1 mm lower than the lateral platforms.

Each counting chamber has precisely ruled lines etched into the glass, forming a grid. This grid or ruled area is so small that it can only be seen with the aid of a microscope. The grid used by most laboratories is the Improved Neubauer Ruling. See figure 7-7 for an example of the Improved Neubauer Ruling. The Improved Neubauer Ruling is 3 by 3 mm (9 mm^2) and subdivided into nine secondary squares, each 1 by 1 mm (1 mm^2).

A thick cover glass, ground to a perfect plane, accompanies the counting chamber (fig. 7-6). Ordinary cover glasses have uneven surfaces and should not be used. When the cover glass is in place on the platform of the counting chamber, there is a space exactly 0.1 mm thick between it and the ruled platform.

Counts of red blood cells and white blood cells are each expressed as concentration: cells per unit volume of blood. The unit of volume for cell counts is expressed as cubic millimeters (mm^3) because of the linear dimensions of the hemacytometer chamber.

TOTAL RED BLOOD CELL COUNT

The total red blood cell (erythrocyte) count is the number of red cells in one cubic millimeter of blood. The normal red blood cell count is as follows:

Adult male. . . . . .4.2 to 6.0 million per mm^3

Adult female . . . . .3.6 to 5.6 million per mm^3

Newborn. . . . . .5.0 to 6.5 million per mm^3

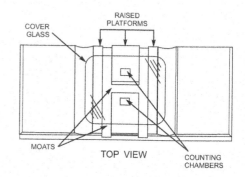

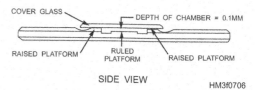

Figure 7-6.—Top and side views of a hemacytometer.

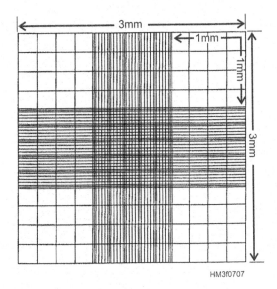

Figure 7-7.—Improved Neubauer Ruling.

As we said earlier, the red cell count is used in the diagnosis of many diseases. For example, a red cell count that drops below normal values may indicate anemia and leukemia. On the other hand, a red cell count that rises above the normal values may indicate dehydration.

The Unopette® Method is used to manually count red blood cells. Material requirements and the step-by-step procedures for performing this procedure are provided in the following sections.

Materials Required for Unopette Procedure

The Unopette procedure consists of a disposable diluting pipette system that provides a convenient, precise, and accurate method for obtaining a red blood cell count. To perform a red blood cell count using the Unopette method, you will need to obtain the following materials:

- A disposable Unopette (see fig. 7-8) for RBC counts. The Unopette consists of

  —a shielded capillary pipette (10 microliter (μl) capacity), and

  —a plastic reservoir containing a premeasured volume of diluent (1:200 dilution).

- Hemacytometer and coverglass

- Microscope with light source

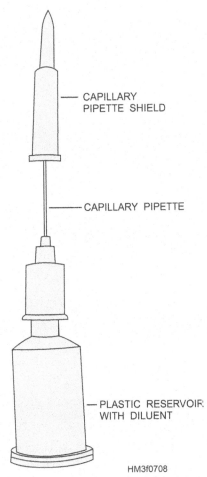

Figure 7-8.—Unopette® for RBC count.

- Hand-held counter

- Laboratory chit

Unopette Procedure

The Unopette procedure for counting red blood cells is as follows:

1. Puncture the diaphragm in the neck of the diluent reservoir with the tip of the capillary shield on the capillary pipette. See figure 7-9.

2. After obtaining free-flowing blood from a lancet puncture of the finger, remove the protective plastic shield from the capillary pipette. Holding the capillary pipette slightly above the horizontal, touch the tip to the blood source (see fig. 7-10, view A). The pipette will

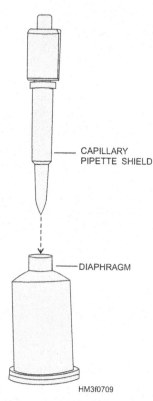

CAPILLARY
PIPETTE SHIELD

DIAPHRAGM

HM3f0709

Figure 7-9.—Puncturing the diaphragm of diluent with the capillary pipette shield.

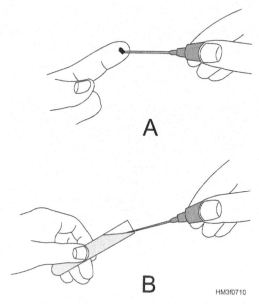

A

B

HM3f0710

Figure 7-10.—Drawing blood into the Unopette capillary tube: A. From a finger puncture; B. From a venous blood sample.

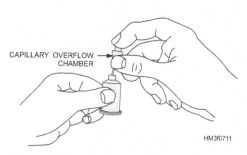

CAPILLARY OVERFLOW
CHAMBER

HM3f0711

Figure 7-11.—Preparing reservoir to receive blood from the capillary tube.

fill by capillary action. When blood reaches the end of the capillary bore in the neck of the pipette, filling is complete and will stop automatically. The amount of blood collected by the capillary tube is 10 μl. Wipe any blood off the outside of the capillary tube, making sure no blood is removed from inside the capillary pipette. (An alternative source of blood is a thoroughly mixed fresh venous blood sample obtained by venipuncture. See figure 7-10, view B.)

3. With one hand, gently squeeze the reservoir to force some air out, but do not expel any diluent (fig. 7-11). Maintain pressure on the reservoir. With the other hand, cover the upper opening of the capillary overflow chamber with your index finger and seat the capillary pipette holder in the reservoir neck (see fig. 7-11).

4. Release pressure on the reservoir and remove your finger from the overflow chamber opening.

Suction will draw the blood into the diluent in the reservoir.

5. Squeeze the reservoir gently two or three times to rinse the capillary tube, forcing diluent into but not out of the overflow chamber, releasing pressure each time to return diluent to the reservoir. Close the upper opening with your index finger and invert the unit several times to mix the blood sample and the diluent. See figure 7-12.

6. For specimen storage, cover the overflow chamber of the capillary tube with the capillary shield.

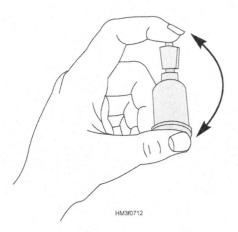

HM3f0712

Figure 7-12.—Mixing blood sample and diluent.

7. Immediately prior to cell counting, mix again by gentle inversion, taking care to cover the upper opening of the overflow chamber with your index finger.

8. Place the coverglass on the hemacytometer counting chamber, making sure coverglass is clean and free of grease. (Fingerprints must be completely removed.)

9. Remove the pipette from the reservoir. Squeeze the reservoir and reseat the pipette in the reverse position, releasing pressure to draw any fluid in the capillary tube into the reservoir. Invert and fill the capillary pipette by gentle pressure on the reservoir. After discarding the first 3 drops, load (charge) the counting chamber of the hemacytometer by gently squeezing the

reservoir while touching the tip of the pipette against the edge of the coverglass and the surface of the counting chamber (fig. 7-13). A properly loaded counting chamber should have a thin, even film of fluid under the coverglass (fig. 7-14, view A). Allow 3 minutes for cells to settle. If fluid flows into the grooves (moats) at the edges of the chamber or if air bubbles are seen in the field, the chamber is flooded and must be cleaned with distilled water, dried with lens tissue, and reloaded (fig. 7-14, view B). If the chamber is underloaded, carefully add additional fluid until properly loaded.

10. Place the loaded hemacytometer into a petri dish with a piece of dampened tissue to keep the hemacytometer from drying out (fig. 7-15). Allow 5 to 10 minutes for the cells to settle.

11. Once the cells have settled, place the hemocytometer on the microscope. Use the low-power lens to locate the five small fields (1, 2, 3, 4, and 5) in the large center square bounded by the double or triple lines. See figure 7-16. Each field measures $1/25 \text{ mm}^2$, $1/10$ mm in depth, and is divided into 16 smaller squares. These smaller squares form a grid that makes accurate counting possible.

12. Switch to the high-power lens and count the number of cells in field 1. Move the hemacytometer until field 2 is in focus and repeat the counting procedure. Continue until the cells in all five fields have been counted. Note the fields are numbered clockwise around the chamber, with field 5 being in the center.

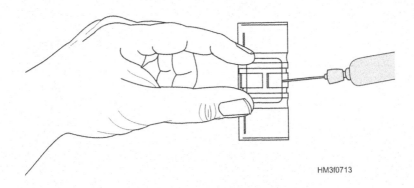

HM3f0713

Figure 7-13.—Loading the counting chamber.

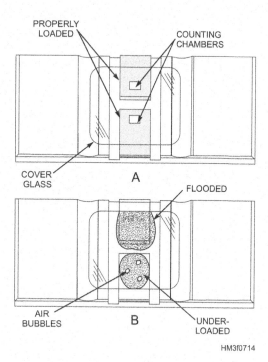

Figure 7-14.—Loading hemacytometer: A. Hemacytometer properly loaded; B. Hemacytometer improperly loaded.

Count the fields in this order. To count the cells in each field, start in the upper left small square and follow the pattern indicated by the arrow in field 1 of figure 7-16. Count all of the cells within each square, including cells touching the lines at the top and on the left. **Do not count any cells that touch the lines on the right or at the bottom**.

13. Total the number of cells counted in all five fields and multiply by 10,000 to arrive at the number of red cells per cubic millimeter of blood.

Example: Total number of cells counted = 423.

Multiply:

423 x 10,000 = 4,230,000

Total red cell count = **4,2300,000 cells/mm^3**

NOTE: The number of cells counted in each field should not vary by more than 20. A greater variation may indicate poor distribution of the cells in the fluid, resulting in

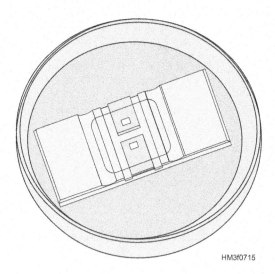

Figure 7-15—Loaded hemacytometer placed inside petri dish.

an inaccurate count. If this happens, the test must be repeated.

HEMOGLOBIN DETERMINATION

A routine test performed on practically every patient is the hemoglobin determination. Hemoglobin determination, or hemoglobinometry, is the measurement of the concentration of hemoglobin in the blood. Hemoglobin's main function in the body is to carry oxygen from the lungs to the tissues and to assist in transporting carbon dioxide from the tissues to the lungs. The formation of hemoglobin takes place in the developing red cells located in bone marrow.

Hemoglobin values are affected by age, sex, pregnancy, disease, and altitude. During pregnancy, gains in body fluids cause the red cells to become less concentrated, causing the red cell count to fall. Since hemoglobin is contained in red cells, the hemoglobin concentration also falls. Disease may also affect the values of hemoglobin. For example, iron deficiency anemia may drop hemoglobin values from a normal value of 14 grams per 100 milliliters to 7 grams per 100 milliliters. Above-normal hemoglobin values may occur when dehydration develops. Changes in altitude affect the oxygen content of the air and, therefore, also affect hemoglobin values. At higher altitudes there is less oxygen in the air, resulting in an increase in red cell counts and hemoglobin values. At lower altitudes there is more oxygen, resulting in a decrease in red cell counts and hemoglobin values.

HEMACYTOMETER (COUNTING CHAMBER)

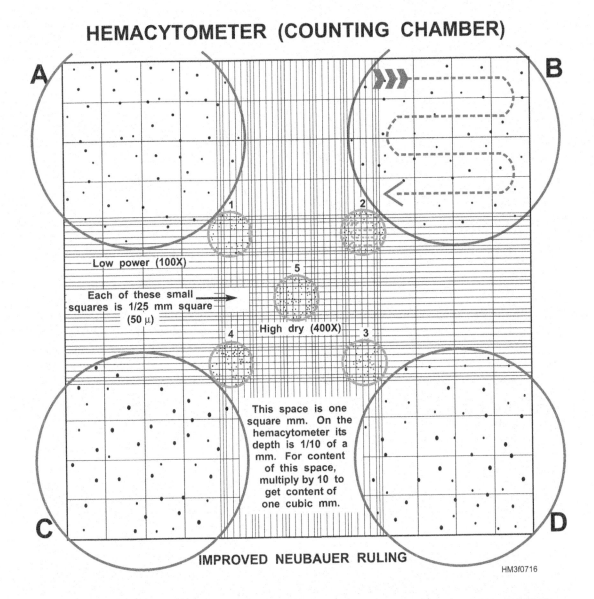

A

B

1

2

Low power (100X)

5

Each of these small squares is 1/25 mm square (50 μ)

High dry (400X)

4

3

This space is one square mm. On the hemacytometer its depth is 1/10 of a mm. For content of this space, multiply by 10 to get content of one cubic mm.

C

D

IMPROVED NEUBAUER RULING

HM3f0716

A - B - C - D ARE FIELDS USED IN DOING THE WHITE BLOOD CELL COUNT.

1 - 2 - 3 - 4 - 5 ARE FIELDS USED IN DOING THE RED BLOOD CELL COUNT.

(Letters, numbers, and arrows are not actually seen in the counting chamber. They are for illustration only. Circles depict areas seen through the microscope.)

Figure 7-16.—Hemacytometer counting chamber.

The normal values for hemoglobin determinations are as follows:

	Grams per 100 ml blood	Percent
Woman	12.5 to 15	83 to 110
Men	14 to 17	97 to 124
Newborn infants	17 to 23	97 to 138

Methods for hemoglobin determination are many and varied. The most widely used automated method is the **cyanmethemoglobin method**. To perform this method, blood is mixed with Drabkin's solution, a solution that contains ferricyanide and cyanide. The ferricyanide oxidizes the iron in the hemoglobin, thereby changing hemoglobin to methemoglobin. Methemoglobin then unites with the cyanide to form cyanmethemoglobin. Cyanmethemoglobin produces a color which is measured in a colorimeter, spectrophotometer, or automated instrument. The color relates to the concentration of hemoglobin in the blood.

Manual methods for determining blood hemoglobin include the **Haden-Hausse** and **Sahli-Hellige methods**. In both methods, blood is mixed with dilute hydrochloric acid. This process hemolyzes the red cells, disrupting the integrity of the red cells' membrane and causing the release of hemoglobin, which, in turn, is converted to a brownish-colored solution of acid hematin. The acid hematin solution is then compared with a color standard.

HEMATOCRIT (PACKED CELL VOLUME) DETERMINATION

The hematocrit or packed cell volume (PCV) determines the percentage of red blood cells (RBCs) in whole blood.

The normal hematocrit value for men is 42% to 52%; for women, 37% to 47%; and for newborns, 53% to 65%. When hematocrit determinations are below normal, medical conditions such as anemia and leukemia may be present. Above-normal hematocrit determinations indicate medical conditions like dehydration, such as occur in severe burn cases.

Currently, automated hematology analyzers supply most hematocrits. However, when hematology analyzers are not available, hematocrit determinations can be manually performed by the microhematocrit method or macrohematocrit method. Both methods call for the blood to be centrifuged, and the percentage of packed red cells is found by calculation.

The microhematocrit method is the most accurate manual method of determining blood volume and should be used whenever feasible. Material requirements and the step-by-step procedures for performing the microhematocrit method will be covered in the following sections.

Materials Required for Microhematocrit Procedure

To perform a hematocrit using the microhematocrit method, the following materials are required.

- Capillary tubes, plain or heparinized
- Modeling clay sealant
- Microhematocrit centrifuge
- Microhematocrit reader

Microhematocrit Procedure

To perform the microhematocrit method, you should follow the steps listed below:

1. Fill the capillary tube two-thirds to three-quarters full with well-mixed, oxalated venous blood or fingertip blood. (For fingertip blood use heparinized tubes, and invert several times to mix.)

2. Seal one end of the tube with clay.

3. Place the filled tube in the microhematocrit centrifuge, with the plugged end away from the center of the centrifuge.

4. Centrifuge at a preset speed of 10,000 to 12,000 rpm for 5 minutes. If the hematocrit exceeds 50 percent, centrifuge for an additional 3 minutes.

5. Place the tube in the microhematocrit reader. Read the hematocrit by following the manufacturer's instructions on the microhematocrit reading device.

TOTAL WHITE BLOOD CELL COUNT

The total white cell (leukocyte) count determines the number of white cells per cubic millimeter of blood. A great deal of information can be derived from white cell studies. The white blood cell count (WBC) and the differential count are common laboratory tests, and they are almost a necessity in determining the nature and severity of systemic infections. Normal WBC values in adults range from 4,500 to 11,000 cells per cubic millimeter; in children the range is from 5,000 to 15,000 cells per cubic millimeter; and in newborns the range is from 10,000 to 30,000 cells per cubic millimeter.

White blood cell counts are performed either manually or with automated hematology analyzers. Only the manual method will be covered in this chapter. After a brief discussion on abnormal white blood cell counts, we will cover the Unopette method for manually counting white blood cells.

Abnormal White Cell Counts

When white cell counts rise above normal values, the condition is referred to as **leukocytosis**. Leukocytosis frequently occurs when systemic or local infections (usually due to bacteria) are present. Counts for infections are highly variable. Examples of some infections and their representative white cell counts are as follows:

Pneumonia—20,000 to 30,000/mm^3

Meningitis—20,000 to 30,000/mm^3

Appendicitis—10,000 to 30,000/mm^3

Dyscrasia (the diseased condition) of blood-forming tissues, such as occurs in leukemia (due to a malfunctioning of lymph and marrow tissues) also results in leukocytosis, with extremely high white cell counts. These white cell counts sometimes exceed 1,000,000/mm^3.

Other physiological conditions that can cause leukocytosis and a white cell count as high as 15,000/mm^3 may occur as follows:

- Shortly after birth

- During late pregnancy

- During labor

- Accompanying severe pain

- After exercise or meals

- After cold baths

- During severe emotional upset

An abnormally low count, known as **leukopenia**, may be caused by the following conditions:

- Severe or advanced bacterial infections (such as typhoid, paratyphoid, and sometimes tularemia), or when the bacterial infection has been undetected for a period of time (as with chronic beta streptococcal infections of the throat).

- Infections caused by viruses and rickettsiae, such as measles, rubella, smallpox (until the 4th day), infectious hepatitis, psittacosis, dengue, tsutsugamushi fever, and influenza (when it may fall to 1,500/mm^3, or shift to leukocytosis if complications develop).

- Protozoal infections (such as malaria) and helminthic infections (such as trichinosis). (For example, with victims of malaria, slight leukocytosis may develop for a short time during paroxysm (the sudden intensification of symptoms). Shortly thereafter, however, leukopenia ensues.)

- Overwhelming infections when the body's defense mechanisms break down.

- Anaphylactic shock

- Radiation

Materials Required for Unopette Procedure

The Unopette method uses a disposable diluting pipette system that provides a convenient, precise, and accurate method for obtaining a white blood cell count. When the Unopette method is used, whole blood is added to a diluent. The diluent lyses (destroys) the red blood cells, but preserves the white blood cells. Once the red cells are completely lysed, the solution will be clear. The diluted blood is then added to a hemacytometer. Once the hemacytometer is loaded, the cells should be allowed to settle for 10 minutes before counting proceeds.

The following materials are required to perform a white blood cell count using the Unopette method:

- Disposable Unopette for WBC counts, which consists of

 —a shielded capillary pipette (20 microliter (μl) capacity), and

 —a plastic reservoir containing a premeasured volume of diluent (1:100 dilution).

- Hemacytometer and coverglass

- Microscope with light source

- Hand-held counter

- Laboratory chit

Unopette Procedure

The Unopette disposable diluting pipette system used to count WBCs is almost identical in shape and application to the Unopette system for RBC counts. The only major difference is that the reservoir contains a different diluent and the capillary pipette capacity differs (RBC 10 μl and WBC 20 μl). To assist you in performing the Unopette procedure for WBCs, we will refer to illustrations for the Unopette procedure for RBCs in this section.

The Unopette procedure for counting white blood cells is as follows:

1. Puncture the diaphragm in the neck of the reservoir with the tip of the capillary pipette shield. See figure 7-9.

2. After you obtain free-flowing blood from a lancet puncture of the finger, remove the protective plastic shield from the capillary pipette. Hold the capillary pipette slightly above the horizontal and touch the tip to the blood source (fig. 7-10, view A). The pipette will fill by capillary action. When blood reaches the end of the capillary bore in the neck of the pipette, filling is complete and will stop automatically. The amount of blood collected by the capillary tube is 20 μl. Wipe any blood off the outside of the capillary tube, making sure no blood is removed from inside the capillary pipette. (An alternative source of blood is a thoroughly mixed fresh venous blood sample obtained by venipuncture. See figure 7-10, view B.)

3. With one hand, gently squeeze the reservoir to force some air out, but do not expel any diluent (fig. 7-11). Maintain pressure on the reservoir. With the other hand, cover the upper opening of the capillary overflow chamber with your index finger and seat the capillary pipette holder in the reservoir neck (fig. 7-11).

4. Release pressure on the reservoir and remove your finger from the overflow chamber opening. Suction will draw the blood into the diluent in the reservoir.

5. Squeeze the reservoir gently two or three times to rinse the capillary tube, forcing diluent into but not out of the overflow chamber, releasing pressure each time to return diluent to the reservoir. Close the upper opening with your index finger and invert the unit several times to mix the blood sample and diluent. See figure 7-12.

6. For specimen storage, cover the overflow chamber of the capillary tube with the capillary shield.

7. Immediately prior to cell counting, mix again by gentle inversion, taking care to cover the hole with your index finger.

8. Place the coverglass on the hemacytometer counting chamber, making sure the coverglass is clean and grease-free. (Fingerprints must be completely removed.)

9. Remove the pipette from the reservoir. Squeeze the reservoir and reseat the pipette in the reverse position. Release pressure to draw any fluid in the capillary tube into the reservoir. Invert and fill the capillary pipette by gentle pressure on the reservoir. After discarding the first 3 drops, load (charge) the counting chamber of the hemacytometer by gently squeezing the reservoir while touching the tip of the pipette against the edge of the coverglass and the surface of the counting chamber (fig. 7-13). A properly loaded counting chamber should have a thin, even film of fluid under the coverglass (fig. 7-14, view A). Allow 3 minutes for the cells to settle. If fluid flows into the grooves (moats) at the edges of the chamber or if you see air bubbles in the field, the chamber is flooded and must be cleaned with distilled water, dried with lens tissue, and reloaded (fig. 7-14, view B). If the chamber is underloaded, carefully add additional fluid until properly loaded.

10. Place the loaded hemacytometer into a petri dish with a piece of dampened tissue to keep the hemacytometer from drying out (fig. 7-15). Allow 5 to 10 minutes for the cells to settle.

11. Once the cells have settled, place the hemacytometer on the microscope. Using the high-power objective, count the WBCs in the four corner fields of the hemacytometer chamber (fields A, B, C, and D of figure 7-16). Each field is composed of 16 small squares. To count the cells in each field, start in the upper left small square and follow the pattern indicated by the arrow in field B of figure 7-16. Count all of the cells within each square, including cells touching the lines at the top and on the left. **Do not count any cells that touch the lines on the right or at the bottom.**

12. When all the cells in the 4 fields have been counted, multiply the count by 50. This will give you the total number of white cells per cubic millimeter of blood.

Example:	25 cells in field #1
	23 cells in field #2
	26 cells in field #3
	<u>26 cells in field #4</u>
	100 total cells in all fields
Multiply:	
100 x 50	= 5,000
Total white cell count	**= 5,000 cells/mm³**

DIFFERENTIAL WHITE BLOOD CELL COUNT

A total white blood cell count is not necessarily indicative of the severity of a disease, since some serious ailments may show a low white cell count. For this reason, a differential white cell count is performed. A differential white cell count consists of an examination of blood to determine the presence and the number of different types of white blood cells. This study often provides helpful information in determining the severity and extent of an infection, more than any other single procedure used in the examination of the blood.

The role of white blood cells, or leukocytes, is to control various disease conditions. Although these cells do most of their work outside the circulatory system, they use the blood for transportation to sites of infection.

Five types of white cells are normally found in the circulating blood. They are

- eosinophils,
- basophils,
- neutrophils,
- lymphocytes, and
- monocytes.

Cell Identification

To perform a differential white cell count, you must be able to identify the different types of white cells. The ability to properly identify the different

types of white cells is not difficult to develop, but it does require a thorough knowledge of staining characteristics and morphology (the study of the form and structure of organisms). This knowledge can be gained only by extensive, supervised practice.

To acquaint you with the developmental stages of each type of leukocyte, a colorized illustration (fig. 7-17) has been provided. This illustration also displays the developmental stages of the red blood cell (erythrocyte) and the blood platelet cell (thrombocyte). To further assist you, identifying characteristics of each type of leukocyte as they appear on a stained blood smear will be covered in the following sections.

Laboratories use a **blood smear** to obtain a differential white cell count. To prepare a blood smear, a blood specimen is spread across a glass slide, stained to enhance leukocyte identification, and examined microscopically. Material requirements and the step-by-step procedure for performing a blood smear will be covered later in this chapter.

NEUTROPHILS.—Neutrophils account for the largest percentage of leukocytes found in a normal blood sample, and function by ingesting invading bacteria. On a stained blood smear, the cytoplasm of a neutrophil has numerous fine, barely visible lilac-colored granules and a dark purple or reddish purple nucleus (see figure 7-17). The nucleus may be oval, horseshoe, or "S"-shaped, or segmented (lobulated). Neutrophils are subclassified according to their age or maturity, which is indicated by changes in the nucleus. The subclassifications for neutrophilic cells are metamyelocyte, band, segmented, and hypersegmented.

Neutrophilic Metamyelocyte.—A neutrophilic metamyelocyte, also called a "juvenile" cell, is the youngest neutrophil generally reported. The nucleus is fat, indented, and is usually "bean"-shaped or "cashew nut"-shaped (fig. 7-17).

Neutrophilic Band.—A neutrophilic band, sometimes called a "stab" cell, is an older or intermediate neutrophil. The nucleus has started to elongate and has curved itself into a horseshoe or S-shape. As the band ages, it matures into a segmented neutrophil (fig. 7-17).

Segmented Neutrophil.—A segmented neutrophil is a mature neutrophil. The nucleus of a segmented neutrophil is separated into two, three, four, or five segments or lobes (fig. 7-17).

DEVELOPMENT OF BLOOD CELLS X 1500

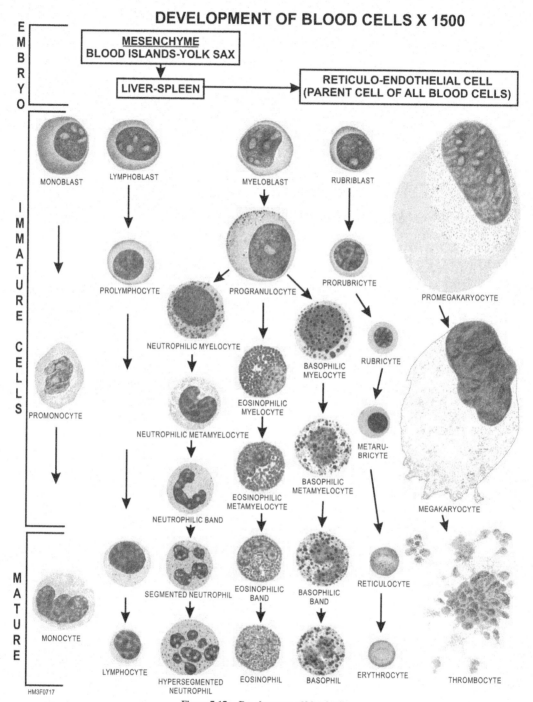

Figure 7-17.—Development of blood cells.

Hypersegmented Neutrophil.—A hypersegmented neutrophil is a mature neutrophil. The nucleus of a hypersegmented neutrophil is divided into six or more segments or lobes (fig. 7-17).

EOSINOPHIL.—Eosinophils aid in detoxification. They also break down and remove protein material. The cytoplasm of an eosinophil contains numerous coarse, reddish-orange granules, which are lighter colored than the nucleus (fig. 7-17).

BASOPHIL.—The function of basophilic cells is unknown. It is believed, however, that basophilic cells keep the blood from clotting in inflamed tissue. Scattered large, dark-blue granules that are darker than the nucleus, characterize the cell as a basophil (fig. 7-17). Granules may overlay the nucleus as well as the cytoplasm.

LYMPHOCYTE.—The function of lymphocytes is also unknown, but it is believed that they produce antibodies and destroy the toxic products of protein metabolism. The cytoplasm of a lymphocyte is clear sky blue, scanty, with few unevenly distributed, azurophilic granules with a halo around them (fig. 7-17). The nucleus is generally round, oval, or slightly indented, and the chromatin (a network of fibers within the nucleus) is lumpy and condensed at the periphery.

MONOCYTE.—The monocyte, the largest of the normal white blood cells, destroys bacteria, foreign particles, and protozoa. Its color resembles that of a lymphocyte, but its cytoplasm is a muddy gray-blue (fig. 7-17). The nucleus is lobulated, deeply indented or horseshoe-shaped, and has a relatively fine chromatin structure. Occasionally, the cytoplasm is more abundant than in the lymphocyte.

Materials Required for the Differential Count Procedure

To perform a differential count, the following materials are required:

- Four plain glass microscope slides, clean and dry

- Wright-Giemsa stain solution (follow manufacturer's directions for use and storage)

- Staining containers

- Deionized or distilled water

- Microscope with light source

- Immersion oil

- Blood cell counter

Differential Count Procedure

The procedure for the differential white cell count is done in 4 steps:

Step 1:	Making the blood smear
Step 2:	Staining the cells
Step 3:	Counting the cells
Step 4:	Reporting the count

Each step of this procedure will be discussed in the following sections.

MAKING THE BLOOD SMEAR.—The simplest way to count the different types of white cells is to spread them out on a glass slide. The preparation is called a blood smear. There are two methods of making a blood smear: the slide method (covered in this chapter) and the cover glass method.

It is very important to make a good blood smear. If it is made poorly, the cells may be so distorted that it will be impossible to recognize them. You should make at least two smears for each patient, as the additional smear should be examined to verify any abnormal findings.

To prepare a blood smear for a differential count, follow the steps below:

1. Using a capillary tube, collect anticoagulated blood from a venous blood sample.

2. Deposit a drop of blood from capillary tube onto a clean, grease-free slide. Then place the slide on a flat surface, blood side up.

3. Hold a second slide between your thumb and forefinger and place the edge at a 23-degree angle against the top of the slide that holds the drop of blood (see figure 7-18, view A). Back the second slide down until it touches the drop of blood. The blood will distribute itself along the edge of the slide in a formed angle (see figure 7-18, view B).

4. Push the second slide along the surface of the other slide, drawing the blood across the surface in a thin, even smear (see figure 7-18, view C). If this is done in a smooth, uniform manner, a gradual tapering effect (or "feathering") of the blood will occur on the slide. This "feathering" of the blood is essential to the counting process and is the principal characteristic of a good blood smear (see figure 7-18, view D). When

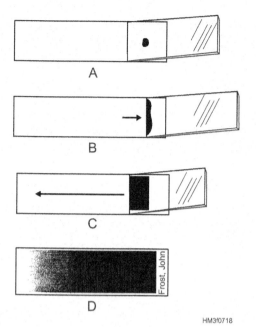

Figure 7-18.—Making a blood smear: A. Placing second slide at a 23°angle; B. Blood distributing itself along second slide's edge; C. Drawing blood across surface of slide; D. Example of a properly prepared blood smear.

(eosin) are called eosinophils. Other cells that prefer the basic dye are called basophils.

WARNING

Wright's staining solution contains methanol, which is considered a hazardous material. It is classified as flammable, a poison, and an irritant. Methanol must be kept away from heat, sparks, and open flames. Good ventilation in usage areas is paramount since exposure to vapors can irritate eyes, nose, throat, and mucous membranes of the upper respiratory tract. When not in use, methanol containers should be closed tightly and stored upright to prevent leakage. Gloves and protective clothing (e.g., lab coat or apron) and eyewear should be worn to avoid contact with the solution. Absorption through skin can cause permanent blindness. Death may result from ingestion or exposure to high vapor concentrations of methanol.

you are making the smear, prevent blood from reaching the extreme edges of the slides. Allowing the smear to reach the edges of the slide will aggravate the tendency of large cells to stack up on the perimeter of the smear. A smear with wavy lines or blanks spots should be discarded, and a new smear made.

5. Once the blood smear is made, let it dry (it will take a few minutes). Then write the patient's name in pencil on the bottom edge of the slide, as illustrated in figure 7-18, view D). Proceed to step 2, staining the cells.

STAINING THE CELLS.—Once a blood smear is made, it should be stained. Staining the blood smear highlights the differences among the different types of leukocytes for easier recognition during the counting process. The most popular stain used for this purpose is Wright's stain. Wright's stain is a methyl alcohol (methanol) solution of an acid dye and a basic dye. The acid dye in Wright's stain is known as eosin and is red in color. The basic dye in Wright's stain is known as methylene blue and is blue in color. Generally, white cells are identified by their affinity to the dye they prefer. For example, cells that prefer the acid dye

There are a variety of staining products on the market today. Some of these staining products have combined Wright's solution with other staining solutions, such as Giemsa stain. When using a new product, you should always review the manufacturer's usage and safety recommendations.

The staining process that we will cover in this chapter is known as a **quick stain**. A quick stain has very few equipment requirements and only a few procedural steps. An example of a quick stain is One Step II Wright-Giemsa Stain Solution® by Criterion Sciences. To stain a blood smear with this product, follow the steps below.

1. Prepare two staining containers by filling one with One Step II stain solution and the other with deionized or distilled water. The use of tap water instead of deionized or distilled water is not recommended since the pH of tap water varies. If tap water is used, its pH should between 5.8 and 7.03.

2. Immerse the slide (blood smear) in the stain for 15 to 30 seconds. (To prevent debris or precipitate from contaminating the slide, do not add new stain to old.)

3. Remove the slide and allow excess stain to drain from the edge of the slide.

4. Immerse the slide in the deionized or distilled water for 5 to 15 seconds. (Change the water

when it becomes dark blue or when film forms on the surface.) **NOTE:** Rinse time is critical and must be shorter than the stain time.

5. Drain excess water and wipe the back of the slide to reduce background color.

6. Place slide in horizontal position on table and allow to air dry. **NOTE:** Do not accelerate drying time by placing slide on a warmer or in front of a fan. The film of water on the slide is important for the color development.

7. Once the slide is dry, proceed to step 3, counting the cells.

COUNTING THE CELLS.—Once the blood smear has been stained, it is placed under a microscope, and the differential count is conducted.

To perform a differential white cell count, you should follow the steps listed below:

1. Place the slide under the microscope. Switch the oil immersion objective (red) (100X) into position above the stage. Turn the coarse adjustment to raise the oil immersion objective about 1 inch above the opening in the stage. Open the condenser and switch on the microscope light.

2. Place a large drop of immersion oil on the thin area of the blood smear. See figure 7-19.

3. Hold the slide so the thin area is on your left. Then fix the slide firmly in the jaws of the mechanical (movable) stage. Move the mechanical stage so the drop of oil on the slide is directly over the bright light coming up from the condenser.

4. Using the coarse control knob, you should now slowly lower oil immersion objective into the

drop of oil (on the slide). When the objective is in the drop of oil, continue turning the coarse adjustment until the objective is touching the glass slide.

5. Now, while continually looking through the eyepiece, VERY SLOWLY rotate the coarse adjustment toward you until you see some cells. After you have brought the cells into view with the coarse adjustment, bring the cells into perfect focus by rotating the fine adjustment. **NOTE:** Always rotate the fine adjustment back and forth when identifying cells. This step will help you see the various layers of the cell and thereby help you to identify the different types of white cells.

6. Count 100 consecutive white cells, pressing the correct key on the cell counter for each type of white cell identified. (If the cell counter is not available, record cell type and number of cells encountered on a piece of paper.) Follow path similar to one illustrated in figure 7-20 to count cells.

7. Total each type of white cell. If you count 20 lymphocytes among the 100 cells, the differential count for lymphocytes is 20%. Continue this process until your count totals 100%. This differential count is referred to as a **relative count**. Another differential count that may be requested is an **absolute count**. To perform an absolute count, multiply the total white cell count by the individual cell percentages. See the example below.

Example:

Patient has a total white cell count of 8,000. Differential count shows 20% leukocytes.

Multiply:

8,000 x 0.20 (20%) = 1,600

Patient has 1,600 lymphocytes/mm^3

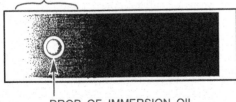

THIS THIN AREA OF THE
BLOOD SMEAR IS FOR
IDENTIFYING THE CELLS

DROP OF IMMERSION OIL

HM3f0719

Figure 7-19.—Placement of immersion oil on blood smear.

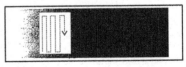

HM3f0720

Figure 7-20.—Counting path for differential count.

NOTE: When performing the white cell count, you may observe abnormal white cells such as distorted lymphocytes, smudge cells, and disintegrated cells. **Distorted lymphocytes**, which appear squashed or distorted, are caused by excessive pressure on the cell during the process of making the smear. Distorted cells should be recorded as normal lymphocytes. **Smudge cells** are white cells that have ruptured and only the nucleus remains. A few smudge cells may be found in a normal blood smear. Smudge cells should not be added to the count or recorded. **Disintegrated cells** are ruptured cells, but the nucleus and cytoplasm still remain. Disintegrated cells should not be counted as one of the 100 cells, but should be recorded on the report as "disintegrated cells."

8. Once the differential count is completed, proceed to step 4, reporting the count.

NOTE: If it is desirable to save a smear for reexamination, remove the immersion oil by placing a piece of lens tissue over the slide and moistening the tissue with xylene. Draw the damp tissue across the slide, and dry the smear with another piece of lens paper.

REPORTING THE COUNT.—When you have calculated the differential count, the report is given according to either the **Schilling classification** or **filament and nonfilament classification methods**. We will be covering the Schilling classification, since it is the simplest and most popular method.

The Schilling Classification.—The Schilling classification was established when Victor Schilling, a German hematologist, noticed that in many diseases there is an increase in the percentage of immature neutrophils. The blood chart he developed reported the percentages of the different neutrophilic cell types and (in part) was arranged in the following manner:

Normal %	Myelocytes	Meta-myelocytes	Band Cells	Segmented Cells
	0	0	2 to 6	55 to 75

Note that the immature cells are on the left side of the chart. If percentages of immature cell increased, Schilling referred it as a "shift to the left." When the shift to the left was accompanied by a low white cell count, Schilling called it a "degenerative shift to the left." A degenerative shift to the left is seen in such diseases as typhoid fever. This shift is caused by a depression of the cell factories in the bone marrow.

When the shift to the left is accompanied by a high white cell count, it is called a "regenerative shift to the left." A regenerative shift to the left is seen in such diseases as pneumonia. This shift is caused by a stimulus of the cell factories in the bone marrow.

A "shift to the right" implies an increase in hypersegmented neutrophils. It may be seen in pernicious anemia, an anemia caused by the malabsorption of vitamin B_{12}.

The Schilling classification for an adult differential white cell count is provided below in table 7-2.

NOTE: Normal values for differential counts vary with the age of the patient. For example, children's blood normally contains 0% to 2% basophils, 0% to 5% eosinophils, 25% to 75% neutrophils, 30% to 70% lymphocytes, and 0% to 8% monocytes. Normal values may also be adjusted by hospitals that have evaluated the normal differential value for their local population.

General Interpretations of Leukocyte Changes.—Together, the total white cell count and differential count aid physicians in interpreting the severity of infections. Some general interpretations of leukocyte changes are as follows:

• Leukocytosis with an increase in the percentage of neutrophils indicates a severe infection with a

Table 7-2.—Schilling Classification of the Differential White Cell Count

Cell	Normal %
Neutrophilic myelocytes	0
Neutrophilic metamyelocytes	0
Neutrophilic band cells	2 to 6
Neutrophilic segmented cells	55 to 75
Lymphocytes	20 to 35
Monocytes	2 to 6
Eosinophilic segmented cells	1 to 3
Basophilic segmented cells	0 to 1

good response of the bone marrow. The primary bacteria-destroying cells (known as phagocytes) are the neutrophils, and the bone marrow should supply large numbers of these to combat the infection. The greater the "shift to the left" (increase in immature neutrophils), the more severe the infection. The appearance of numerous juvenile cells (metamyelocytes) indicates irritation of the bone marrow with regeneration. If the infection continues and the patient's resistance declines, the shift advances further to the left. If improvement ensues, the shift declines and recedes to normal.

- A falling white cell count with the number and maturity of neutrophils progressing toward normal indicates recovery.

- A continued "shift to the left" with a falling total white cell count indicates a breakdown of the body's defense mechanism and is a poor prognosis.

- The percentage of eosinophils, lymphocytes, and monocytes generally decreases in acute infections.

- In tuberculosis, an increase in monocytes (monocytosis) indicates activity in the infected area. An increase in lymphocytes (lymphocytosis) indicates healing.

- Eosinophils increase in parasitic infections and allergic conditions.

BACTERIOLOGY

LEARNING OBJECTIVE: *Recall bacteria classifications, common bacteria, and procedural steps for making smears, Gram staining, and reading and reporting smears.*

Bacteriology is the study of bacteria. Of primary interest to Hospital Corpsman is medical bacteriology, which deals with the bacteria that cause disease in man.

Bacteria are prokaryotic microorganisms of the kingdom Protista. They reproduce asexually by transverse binary fission in which the cell divides into two new cells. Bacteria are found almost everywhere, and the human body harbors vast numbers. Many bacteria are beneficial and essential to human life; only a few are harmful to man.

BACTERIA CLASSIFICATION

Since there are thousands of types of bacteria, a method of classification is essential. Bacteria are classified according to their respective

- disease-producing ability,

- growth requirements,

- morphologic characteristics,

- colonial morphology,

- toxins produced, and

- Gram's stain reaction.

Disease-Producing Ability

The disease-producing ability of bacteria is referred to as either **pathogenic** or **nonpathogenic**. Pathogens are bacteria that cause diseases, and nonpathogens are harmless bacteria. Bacteria that are essential to our body are, in their proper environment, called common or normal flora. For example, alpha streptococcus in the throat is common flora, but when it is found elsewhere (such as in the blood stream, possibly as a result of tooth extraction), it may cause diseases such as septicemia and endocarditis.

Growth Requirements

The four growth requirements for bacteria are

- temperature,

- oxygen,

- nutrition, and

- moisture.

TEMPERATURE REQUIREMENTS.— Temperature requirements are divided into the following three categories.

- **Psychrophilic**—bacteria that reproduce best at 15°C to 20°C

- **Mesophilic**—bacteria that reproduce best at 20°C to 45°C

- **Thermophilic**—bacteria that reproduce best at 50°C to 55°C

OXYGEN REQUIREMENTS.—The amount of oxygen needed for an organism to grow or reproduce varies with the type of organism. **Aerobes** are organisms that reproduce in the presence of oxygen. **Obligate aerobes** are organisms that grow only in the presence of free oxygen. **Anaerobes** are organisms that do not reproduce in the presence of oxygen, and **obligate anaerobes** are organisms that grow only in the absence of free oxygen and are killed if exposed to free oxygen. **Facultative organisms** are organisms that grow in the presence of free oxygen and in an oxygen-free atmosphere. **Microaerophilic organisms** are organisms that grow only in low amounts of free oxygen.

NUTRITION REQUIREMENTS.—Nutrition requirements for the various types of bacteria depends on what their particular environment provides. **Autotrophic bacteria** are self-nourishing, and **heterotrophic bacteria** are not self-sustaining.

MOISTURE REQUIREMENTS.—Moisture is indispensable for bacterial growth.

Morphologic Characteristics

The structural (or morphologic) characteristics of bacteria are based on three distinct shapes or categories:

- **Coccus** (*pl.* cocci)—spherical, appears singly, in pairs, chains, clusters, or packets.

- **Bacillus** (*pl.* bacilli)—rod-shaped, appears singly, in chains, or in palisades.

- **Spirillum** (*pl.* spirilla)—spiral-, corkscrew-, or comma-shaped, appearing singly only.

Three special structures, present on some bacteria, aid in the classification process of bacteria. The special structures are the capsule, the spore, and the flagellum. The **capsule** is a gummy, gelatinous, or mucoid structure surrounding certain bacteria. The **spore** is an inactive, resting, and resistant form produced within the organism, usually as a result of unfavorable environmental conditions. The third and final special structure is the **flagellum**, a hairlike structure that provides motility.

Colonial Morphology

A colony is a cohesive mass composed of many millions of bacterial cells, growing on or in a medium (such as blood agar, a gel enriched with blood that is used in the preparation of solid culture media for microorganisms) as a result of the multiplication and division of a single cell. The size, color, shape, edge, topography, consistency, and odor of the colony vary with each organism.

Toxins Produced

Generally, toxins produced are waste products of metabolism in a bacterial cell. Some bacteria produce toxins that attack red blood cells in a culture medium such as blood agar. Examples of toxins produced by bacteria are listed below:

- **Alpha hemolysin**—produces partial hemolysis (the disruption of the integrity of the red cell membrane causing release of hemoglobin) and changes the medium to a green color.

- **Beta hemolysin**—completely lyses the RBC, leaving a clear zone of hemolysis.

- **Endotoxin** (low potency)—comprises part of the cell wall and is released as the bacterial cell spontaneously destroys itself with self-generated enzymes (a process known as autolysis).

- **Exotoxin** (high potency)—derives from the bacteria during its growth but is found outside the bacterial cell in the surrounding medium. Exotoxins are highly poisonous, soluble, and protein in nature.

Gram's Stain Reaction

To differentiate and identify bacteria, you must make them visible by staining. The staining procedure, devised by Dr. Hans Christian Joachim Gram, stains microorganisms such as bacteria with crystal violet, treats them with 1:15 dilution of strong iodine solution, decolorizes them with ethanol or ethanol-acetone, and counterstains them with a contrasting dye, usually safranin. Microorganisms that retain the crystal violet stain (a dark blue-black color) are said to be gram-positive, and those that lose the crystal violet stain by decolorization but stain with counterstain (a deep pink or reddish color) are said to be gram-negative.

COMMON BACTERIA

Bacteria are named by genus and species. The first word (capitalized) indicates the genus; the second word (not capitalized) indicates the species, a subdivision of the genus. For example:

GENUS	SPECIES
Neisseria	gonorrhoeae

Table 7-3 will familiarize you with commonly encountered bacteria. This table lists the bacteria's morphologic shape, Gram stain response, genus and species, and the type of infection it produces.

BACTERIOLOGIC METHODS

There are a variety of methods used in the laboratory to identify bacteria. However, only a few of these bacteriologic methods can be performed in isolated duty locations or on board naval vessels. One of these methods is the smear. The smear permits healthcare personnel to examine specimens microscopically. Material requirements and the step-by-step procedures for making smears is covered in the following sections.

Smear

A smear is the procedure in which a specimen–a body fluid or a discharge–is spread across a glass slide for microscopic examination. To enhance the visualization of microorganisms on the smear, Gram staining (introduced earlier in this chapter) is used. Once the smear is stained, it is ready to be examined under the microscope. Normally, smears are examined by laboratory technicians who prepare reports of their findings.

MATERIALS REQUIRED FOR SMEAR.—To perform a smear, the following materials are required:

- Glass slide

Table 7-3.—Common Bacteria

COMMON BACTERIA			
Morphologic Shape	Gram-Positive or -Negative	Genus & Species	Type of Infection
Cocci	Positive	Streptococcus pneumoniae	Pneumonia
		Streptococcus pyogenes (Beta Streptococci Group A)	Strep throat
		Staphylococcus aureus	Boils, furuncles, osteomyelitis, pneumonia, septicemia, endocarditis, and impetigo
	Negative	Neisseria gonorrhoeae	Gonorrhea
		Neisseria meningitidis (meningococcus)	Meningitis
Bacilli	Positive	Corynebacterium diphtheriae	Diphtheria
		Clostridium (all are anaerobic and spore producers) • perfringens (welchii) • tetani • botulinum	Gas gangrene Tetanus Botulism
	Negative	Yersinia (Pasteurella) pestis	Bubonic plague
		Brucella abortus	Brucellosis
		Bordetella pertussis	Whooping cough

- Microscope
- Wooden applicator stick
- Saline solution
- Forceps
- Bunsen burner

PROCEDURE FOR MAKING SMEARS.—To prepare smears for microscopic examination, follow these steps:

1. Spread the specimen with a wood applicator stick across a slide that has been cleaned with alcohol or acetone and polished with lens paper. The smear should be thin and uniformly spread. If the smear is opaque, it is too thick and should be emulsified with a drop or two of saline.

2. Label the smear and circle the material to be stained with a diamond point pen for easier identification and location of the material after staining.

3. Let the smear air dry. Do not use forced heat drying; forced drying will distort bacterial cells and other materials.

4. Hold the smear with forceps and fix the smear by passing it through a flame (smear side up) three or four times. Avoid overheating the smear; overheating will cause cellular wall destruction.

5. Let the slide cool. Once the slide is cooled, it is ready to be stained.

Gram's Stain

As previously explained, the most common staining procedure used in bacteriologic work is the Gram stain. This method yields valuable information and should be used on all smears that require staining. Gram's stain is also used for examining cultures to determine purity and for identification purposes.

PRINCIPLE OF GRAM STAINING.—As touched on previously, the crystal violet stain, the primary stain, stains everything in the smear blue. The Gram's iodine acts as a mordant, a substance that causes the crystal violet to penetrate and adhere to the gram-positive organisms. The acetone-alcohol mixture acts as the decolorizer that washes the stain away from everything in the smear except the gram-positive organisms. The safranin is the counter-stain that stains everything in the smear that has been decolorized: pus cells, mucus, and gram-negative organisms. The gram-negative organisms will stain a much deeper pink than the pus cells and mucus will stain even lighter pink than the pus cells.

MATERIALS REQUIRED FOR GRAM STAINING.—To Gram stain a smear, the following materials are required:

- Gram stain kit, which consists of:

  —Crystal violet stain

  —Iodine or stabilized iodine (mordant)

  —Acetone-alcohol decolorizer

  —Safranin stain

- Staining rack

- Blotting paper or paper towel

PROCEDURE FOR GRAM STAINING SMEARS.—After smears have been dried, heat-fixed, and cooled, proceed as follows:

1. Place the slide on a staining rack. Then flood slide with primary stain (crystal violet). Let stand 1 minute.

2. Remove the primary stain by gently washing with cold tap water.

3. Flood the slide with mordant (iodine or stabilized iodine) and retain on slide for 1 minute.

4. Remove mordant by gently washing with tap water.

5. Tilt slide at a 45-degree angle and decolorize with the acetone-alcohol solution until the solvent that runs from the slide is colorless (30 to 60 seconds).

6. Wash the slide gently in cold tap water.

7. Flood the slide with counter-stain (safranin) and let stand for 30 to 60 seconds.

8. Wash slide with cold tap water.

9. Blot with blotting paper or paper towel or allow to air dry.

10. Examine the smear under an oil immersion objective.

Reading and Reporting Smears

Place a drop of oil on the slide and, using the oil immersion objective of the microscope, read the smear. All body discharges contain extraneous materials, such as pus cells and mucus. Of interest, however, are the types of bacteria that may be present. The stained smear reveals only two features: the morphology and the staining characteristics of the bacteria present. Positive identification requires cultures and further studies.

Hospital Corpsmen should report only what they see. For example, "Smear shows numerous gram-negative bacilli." If two or more types of bacteria are seen in a smear, the rule is to report them in order of predominance. For example:

"1. Numerous gram-positive cocci in clusters

2. Few gram-negative bacilli"

Gram-positive organisms are easy to see because they stain a deep blue or blue-black. Gram-negative organisms stain a deep pink, but since the background material is also pink, minute and detailed inspection is necessary before reporting the results.

In the presence of gonorrhea, the smear will reveal large numbers of pus cells with varying numbers of intracellular and extracellular gram-negative, bean-shaped cocci in pairs. Such a finding could be considered diagnostic. It is important to point out that only a few of the thousands of pus cells on the slide may contain bacteria, and sometimes it requires considerable search to find one.

SEROLOGY

LEARNING OBJECTIVE: *Recall principles and procedures for the Rapid Plasma Reagin (RPR) Card Test and the Monosticon DRI-DOT® Slide Test.*

Serology consists of procedures by which antigens and reacting serum globulin antibodies may be measured qualitatively and quantitatively. Serologic tests have been devised to detect either antigens present or antibodies produced in a number of conditions. Most tests are based on agglutination reactions between an antigen and a specific antibody.

An **antigen** is a substance that, when introduced into an individual who does not already possess that substance, may stimulate the individual's cells to produce specific antibodies that react to this substance in a detectable way. The five basic characteristics of an antigen are that it must be foreign to the body, it must

possess a high molecular weight, it must be structurally stable, it must be complex, and it must have a high specificity to stimulate tissues to produce a defensive protein substance called an antibody.

Antibodies are the specific defensive proteins produced when an antigen stimulates individual cells. Antibodies are produced by the host in response to the presence of an antigen and are capable of reacting with antigens in some detectable way.

The **antigen-antibody reaction** takes place when a reaction occurs between specific antibodies in the plasma and the antigen present on cell surfaces.

Principles and procedures of two serologic tests, the rapid plasma reagin (RPR) card test and the Monosticon DRI-DOT® Slide Test are covered in the following sections.

RAPID PLASMA REAGIN (RPR) CARD TEST

The RPR Card test is a sensitive, easily performed screening test for syphilis. The test is performed on unheated plasma or serum. Everything needed for the test is in a kit that is available commercially. This test kit is very useful aboard ship and at small stations.

Principle of the RPR Card Test

In the RPR Card test method of syphilis detection, a specific antigen (carbon-particle cardiolipin) detects "reagin," a substance present in the serum of persons who are infected with syphilis. Specimens that contain reagin cause formation of particles (called flocculation) or coagulation of the carbon particles to occur on the RPR Card antigen. Reactive specimens appear as black clumps against a white background. Nonreactive specimens appear as an even, light-gray color.

Materials Required for RPR Test

To perform an RPR Card test, the following materials are required:

- Serum sample—venous blood collected in tubes without anticoagulant. **NOTE:** Use clear, unhemolyzed serum that has been separated from the blood cells as soon after collection as possible.

- RPR Card Test Kit, which consists of the following components:

  —RPR Card antigen suspension

—Plastic dispensing bottle

—20-gauge, galvanized needle, blunt cut

—Test cards

—Pipette/stirrers, 50 microliter (μl)

- One 1 ml tuberculin syringe

- Distilled water

- Mechanical rotator (adjusted to 100 rpm)

- RPR Card Test Control Cards (each consisting of three labeled test areas containing lyophilized (meaning a stabilized preparation of a biological substance, such as blood, that has been frozen rapidly and then dehydrated under a high vacuum) control specimens with designated patterns of reactivity: Reactive, Reactive-Minimal-to-Moderate, and Nonreactive.)

  NOTE: RPR Card Test Antigen and Control Cards must be stored at 4°C when not in use. Both items are stable until the expiration date. Store "in use" antigen suspension in the dispensing bottle at 4°C. The antigen suspension is stable for 3 months or until the expiration date, whichever occurs first.

Preliminary Preparations for RPR Test

The following preliminary preparations must be performed before RPR testing can begin:

1. Remove the antigen suspension vial and one control card envelope from the refrigerator. Allow the items to warm to room temperature.

2. Resuspend the contents of the vial by vigorously shaking the antigen vial.

3. Snap the neck of the vial.

4. Attach the needle (provided in the kit) to a 1 ml tuberculin syringe. Slowly draw up into the syringe from the vial approximately 1 ml of the antigen suspension.

5. Hold the syringe perpendicular to the surface and count the number of drops dispensed from a 0.5 ml volume. Allow the drops to fall into the antigen vial. **NOTE:** The needle is accurate if 30 drops, plus or minus 1 drop, are dispensed from the 0.5 ml volume.

6. Slowly expel the remainder of the antigen solution in the syringe back into the antigen vial.

7. Remove the needle from the syringe. Place the needle on the tapered fitting of the plastic dispensing bottle (provided in the kit).

8. Slowly withdraw all the contents of the antigen vial by collapsing the dispensing bottle and using it as a suction device.

9. Allow the rotator to warm up for 5 to 10 minutes; adjust to 100 rpm.

RPR Test Procedure

To detect syphilis using the RPR Card test, follow the steps below:

1. Open the foil package and remove the control card.

2. Use a pipette/stirrer to reconstitute each control card circle with 0.5 ml of distilled water.

3. Mix solution in control card circle with pipette/stirrer until the dehydrated control specimen is dissolved. Spread specimen over entire area of circle. Use a separate pipette/stirrer for each circle.

4. Draw the patient's sample by holding the pipette/stirrer between the thumb and forefinger near the stirring or sealed end and squeeze. Do not release pressure until the open end is below the surface of the specimen, then release pressure to draw up the sample.

5. Hold the pipette/stirrer in a vertical position, directly over the card test area where the specimen is to be delivered; squeeze pipette/stirrer, allowing 1 drop to fall onto the test area.

6. Invert the pipette/stirrer and, with the sealed end, spread specimen within the circle. Discard the pipette/stirrer when done.

7. Continue the steps above until one or two test cards are filled with patient's samples.

8. Gently shake the antigen dispensing bottle before use. Hold the bottle in the vertical position and dispense several drops into the dispensing bottle cap to ensure the needle passage is clear. Allow 1 "free-falling" drop to fall onto each test area. Do not stir; the mixing of antigen suspension and specimen is accomplished by rotation.

9. Put the card(s) on the rotator and cover with the humidifying cover. Rotate cards for 8 minutes

at 100 rpm. To help differentiate nonreactive from reactive results, you should briefly rotate and tilt the card by hand (3 or 4 back-and-forth motions).

10. Immediately read the card macroscopically (with the unaided eye) in the "wet" state under a high-intensity lamp.

11. Compare the patient's tests to the controls for correct interpretations. The reactive control should show small to large clumps. The nonreactive control should show no clumping or very slight roughness. The reactive-minimal-to-moderate control should show slight but definite clumping.

12. Report the test as

- **reactive**, if agglutination or flocculation is present, or

- **nonreactive**, if no agglutination is present.

NOTE: The RPR Card test is used as a screen for syphilis. If a patient's RPR is reactive, the patient should be sent to a laboratory to have a FTA-ABS (Fluorescent Treponemal Antibody Absorption Test) performed. The FTA-ABS, a more precise test, is used to confirm primary, secondary, and late syphilis.

MONOSTICON DRI-DOT SLIDE TEST

Mononucleosis imitates many diseases so well that diagnosis is confirmed only by selective serologic testing. The Monosticon DRI-DOT Slide Test is an accurate, 2-minute disposable test designed to detect the presence of infectious mononucleosis antibodies in serum, plasma, or whole blood.

Principle of the Monosticon DRI-DOT Slide Test

The Monosticon DRI-DOT Slide Test consists of specially prepared, stable sheep and/or horse erythrocyte antigen (dyed) and guinea pig antigen on a disposable slide. When serum, plasma, or whole blood is mixed with these antigens on the slide, the test result for infectious mononucleosis will be positive or negative. A positive result is indicated by agglutination and a negative result is indicated by no agglutination.

Materials Required for Monosticon DRI-DOT Slide Test

To perform the Monosticon DRI-DOT Slide Test, the following materials are required:

- Serum or plasma specimen

- Monosticon DRI-DOT Test kit, which consists of:

  —Monosticon DRI-DOT Test slides

  —Positive I.M. (infectious mononucleosis) serum control

  —Negative I.M. serum control

  —Dropper bottle

  —Dispenstirs® (designed to deliver a 0.03 ml drop)

- Distilled water

- Centrifuge

- DRI-DOT slide holder (available commercially, but not necessary to perform test)

Controls for Monosticon DRI-DOT Slide Test

Both a positive and negative control are included in each kit to check the effectiveness of the reagents. The positive I.M. serum control (human) is a dilution of human sera (*sing.* serum) containing the specific heterophile antibody of infectious mononucleosis. The negative I.M. serum control (human) is a dilution of human sera containing no detectable antibody to infectious mononucleosis. Both controls have been dried and placed in a vial with color-coded cap and label. Since both controls are of human origin, they are potentially infectious and must be handled with care.

Both controls (positive and negative) should be tested before performing test with serum, plasma, or whole blood. Controls are prepared in the same manner as serum and plasma test described in the next section, but instead of adding serum or plasma to the slide, the control is added. Before each control is used, it must be reconstituted with 0.5 ml of distilled water. If results of the control tests are not as expected, do not use the test kit.

Monosticon DRI-DOT Slide Test Procedure

To detect mononucleosis using the Monosticon DRI-DOT Slide Test, follow the steps below.

1. Centrifuge the blood specimen for 10 minutes to obtain the plasma or serum to be tested.

2. Fill the dropper bottle with distilled water.

3. Remove the disposable slide by tearing the envelope where indicated. (Remove only enough slides to perform the tests at hand.)

4. Set the slide in a holder or on a flat surface.

5. Place one drop of water from the dropper bottle **next to but not on** the blue dot within the circle on the slide.

6. Use a Dispenstir to squeeze the closed end between thumb and forefinger, and place the open end into the plasma or serum to be tested. Release pressure to draw up the specimen into the Dispenstir.

7. Hold the Dispenstir perpendicularly over the buff-colored dot (guinea pig antigen) within the circle of the slide. Place one drop of specimen onto the dot.

8. Use the flared end of the Dispenstir to mix the water, specimen, and the guinea pig antigen (bluff-colored dot) thoroughly.

9. Blend this mixture thoroughly with the blue dot (horse/sheep antigen).

10. Rock the slide (or slide holder) back and forth gently in a figure-8 motion for 2 minutes so that the liquid slowly flows over the entire area within the circle.

11. After 2 minutes, read the results under a strong, glaring light.

12. Report test as

   - **positive**, if agglutination is present, or

   - **negative**, if no agglutination is present.

See figure 7-21 for an illustration of positive and negative test results.

   NOTE: A positive test result usually occurs between the fourth day and the twenty-first day of illness, and may persist for several months.

FUNGUS TEST

LEARNING OBJECTIVE: *Recall how potassium hydroxide (KOH) preparation is used in the detection of fungi.*

Fungi (*sing.* fungus) are chlorophyll-free, heterotrophic (not self-sustaining) of the same family of plants (i.e., Thyllophyta) as algae and lichens. They reproduce by spores that germinate into long filaments called **hyphae**. As the hyphae continue to grow and branch, they develop into a mat of growth called the mycelium (*pl.* mycelia). From the mycelium, spores are produced in characteristic patterns. These spores, when dispersed to new substances, germinate and form new growths. Reproduction is often asexual, usually by budding (as in yeast), but certain fungi have sexual reproduction.

Common superficial infections of the skin caused by fungi are athlete's foot and ringworm of the scalp.

A simple and frequently used method of detecting fungi is the **potassium hydroxide (KOH) preparation**. Fungi are seen in clustered round buds with thick walls, accompanied by fragments of

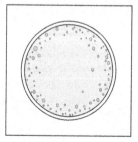

POSITIVE - AGGLUTINATION

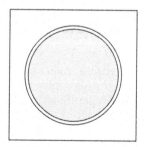

NEGATIVE - NO AGGLUTINATION

HM3f0721

Figure 7-21.—Illustration of positive and negative Monosticon DRI-DOT Slide Test Results.

mycelia. Scrapings from the affected area of the skin are mounted in 10% KOH for positive laboratory diagnosis.

To detect fungi in infected tissue using the KOH preparation, follow the steps below.

1. Place skin, hair, or nail scrapings from the affected area on a glass slide and add one drop of 10% KOH. (Dissolve 10 g of KOH in 100 ml of distilled water.)

2. Place a coverslip on the preparation.

3. Warm the preparation gently over a flame, being careful not to boil it, and allow it to stand until clear. Do not allow the preparation to dry out.

4. Examine the preparation by using the high-power objective on microscope with subdued light.

   • Fungi on the skin and nails appear as refractile fragments of hyphae.

   • Fungi in the hair appear as dense clouds around the hair stub or as linear rows inside the hair shaft.

URINALYSIS

LEARNING OBJECTIVE: *Recall the three types of urine specimens, the methods used to preserve urine specimens, and the procedure for performing a urinalysis.*

Since the physical and chemical properties of normal urine are constant, abnormalities are easily detected. The use of simple tests provides the physician with helpful information for the diagnosis and management of many diseases.

This section deals with the three types of urine specimens, methods used to preserve urine specimens, the procedure for performing a routine and microscopic examination of urine specimens, and some of the simpler interpretations of the findings.

URINE SPECIMENS

Urine specimens for routine examinations must be collected in aseptically clean containers. Unless circumstances warrant, avoid catheterization because it may cause a urinary tract infection. Specimens of female patients are likely to be contaminated with albumin and blood from menstrual discharge, or with albumin and pus from vaginal discharge. For bacteriologic studies, care must be taken to ensure that the external genitalia have been thoroughly cleansed with soap and water. The patient must void the initial stream of urine into the toilet or a suitable container and the remainder directly into a sterile container. All urine specimens should either be examined when freshly voided, or refrigerated to prevent decomposition of urinary constituents and to limit bacterial growth. In the following sections, we will cover three types of urine specimens: random, first morning, and 24-hour.

Random Urine Specimen

A random urine specimen is urine voided without regard to the time of day or fasting state. This sample is satisfactory for most routine urinalyses. It is the least valid specimen, since test results may reflect a particular meal or fluid intake.

First Morning Urine Specimen

The first morning urine specimen is the first urine voided upon rising. It is the best sample for routine urinalysis, because it is usually concentrated and more likely to reveal abnormalities. If positive results are obtained from the first morning specimen, the physician may order a 24-hour specimen for quantitative studies.

Twenty-Four Hour Urine Specimen

The 24-hour urine specimen measures the exact output of urine over a 24-hour period. Use the following steps to collect this specimen.

1. Have patient empty bladder early in the morning and record time. Discard this urine.

2. Collect all urine voided during next 24 hours.

3. Instruct patient to empty bladder at 0800 the following day (end of 24-hour period). Add this urine to pooled specimen.

Refrigerate specimen during collection, and, depending on the test being performed, add a preservative to the first specimen voided.

The normal daily urine volume for adults ranges from 800 to 2000 ml, averaging about 1,500 ml. The amount of urine excreted in 24 hours varies with fluid intake and the amount of water lost through perspiration, respiration, and bowel activity. Diarrhea or profuse sweating reduces urinary output; a high-protein diet tends to increase it. Daytime urine output is normally two to four times greater than nighttime output.

PRESERVATION OF URINE SPECIMENS

To delay decomposition of urine, use the following methods of preservation:

- Refrigeration
- Preservatives
  —Hydrochloric acid
  —Boric acid
  —Glacial acetic acid

Other preservatives used include formaldehyde, toluene, and thymol. The preservative used must be identified on the label of the container. If no preservative is used, this, too, should be noted.

> NOTE: Before adding a preservative to a urine specimen, contact the laboratory performing the test to find out what preservative to use and the quantity to add. Preservative requirements vary from laboratory to laboratory.

ROUTINE URINE EXAMINATION

A routine urinalysis includes the examination of physical characteristics, chemical characteristics, and microscopic structures in the sediment. A sample for urinalysis (routine and microscopic) should be at least 15 ml in volume (adult), and either a random or first morning specimen. Children may only be able to provide a small volume, but 10-15 ml is preferred.

Physical Characteristics

Physical characteristics evaluated during a routine urinalysis include color, appearance, and specific gravity.

COLOR.—The normal color of urine varies from straw to light amber. Diluted urine is generally pale; concentrated urine tends to be darker. The terms used to describe the color of urine follow.

- Colorless
- Light straw
- Straw
- Dark straw

- Light amber
- Amber
- Dark amber
- Red

The color of urine may be changed by the presence of blood, drugs, or diagnostic dyes. Examples are:

- **red or red-brown** (smokey appearance), caused by the presence of blood.
- **yellow or brown** (turning greenish with yellow foam when shaken), caused by the presence of bile.
- **olive green to brown-black**, caused by phenols (an extremely poisonous compound, used as an antimicrobial agent).
- **milky white**, caused by chyle. (Chyle, which consists of lymph and droplets of triglyceride, is a milky fluid taken up by lacteal vessels from the food in the intestine during digestion.)
- **dark orange**, caused by Pyridium® (a topical analgesic used in the treatment of urinary tract infections).
- **blue-green**, caused by methylene blue (used as a stain or dye for various diagnostic tests).

APPEARANCE.—Urine's appearance may be reported as clear, hazy, slightly cloudy, cloudy, or very cloudy. Some physicians prefer the term "turbidity" instead of "transparency," but both terms are acceptable.

Freshly passed urine is usually clear or transparent. However, urine can appear cloudy when substances such as blood, phosphates, crystals, pus, or bacteria are present. A report of transparency is of value only if the specimen is fresh. After standing, all urine becomes cloudy because of decomposition, salts, and the action of bacteria. Upon standing and cooling, all urine specimens will develop a faint cloud composed of mucus, leukocytes, and epithelial cells. This cloud settles to the bottom of the specimen container and is of no significance.

SPECIFIC GRAVITY.—The specific gravity of the specimen is the weight of the specimen compared to an equal volume of distilled water. The specific gravity varies directly with the amount of solids dissolved in the urine and normally ranges from 1.015 to 1.030 during a 24-hour period.

The first morning specimen of urine is more concentrated and will have a higher specific gravity than a specimen passed during the day. A high fluid intake may reduce the specific gravity to below 1.010. In the presence of disease, the specific gravity of a 24-hour specimen may vary from 1.001 to 1.060.

Specific gravity is measured with an index refractometer, available as standard equipment at most duty stations. See figure 7-22. The index refractometer may be held manually or mounted on a stand like a microscope. The specific gravity of urine is determined by the index of light refraction through solid material.

Measure the specific gravity with an index refractometer in the following manner:

1. Hold the index refractometer in one hand. Use the other hand and an applicator stick to place a drop of urine on the glass section beneath the coverglass.

2. Hold the refractometer so that the light reflects on the glass section, and look into the ocular end. Read the number that appears where the light and dark lines meet. This is the specific gravity.

Chemical Characteristics

Chemical characteristics evaluated during a routine urinalysis include pH, protein, glucose, ketones, and blood. Some laboratories also include tests for bilirubin, urobilinogen, and nitrite, depending on the test strip used. Currently, most medical facilities use the Multistix® and Color Chart, which detects pH, protein, glucose, ketones, blood, bilirubin, and urobilinogen. The Multistix is a specially prepared multitest strip. The strip is simply dipped into the urine specimen and compared to the color values for the various tests on the accompanying chart. The color chart also indicates numerical pH values, which should be reported.

Microscopic Examination of Urine Sediment

Microscopic examination of urine sediment is usually performed in addition to routine procedures.

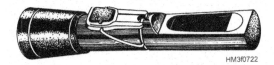

HM3f0722

Figure 7-22.—Index refractometer.

This examination requires a degree of skill acquired through practice under the immediate supervision of an experienced technician. The specimen used for microscopic examination should be as fresh as possible. Red cells and many formed solids tend to disintegrate upon standing, particularly if the specimen is warm or alkaline.

PREPARING SPECIMENS FOR MICROSCOPIC EXAMINATION.—To prepare urine specimens for microscopic examination, follow the steps below.

1. Stir the specimen well.

2. Pour 15 ml of urine into a conical centrifuge tube, and centrifuge at 1,500 rpm for 5 minutes.

3. Invert the centrifuge tube and allow all of the excess urine to drain out. **Do not shake the tube while it is inverted**. Enough urine will remain in the tube to resuspend the sediment. Too much urine will cause dilution of the sediment, making an accurate reading difficult.

4. Resuspend the sediment by tapping the bottom of the tube.

5. With a medicine dropper, mount one drop of the suspension on a slide and cover it with a coverslip.

6. Place the slide under the microscope, and scan with the low-power objective and subdued lighting.

7. Switch to the high-power objective for detailed examination of a minimum of 10 to 15 fields.

CLINICALLY SIGNIFICANT FINDINGS.—Leukocytes, erythrocytes, and casts may all be of clinical significance when found in urine sediment.

Leukocytes.—Normally, 0 to 3 leukocytes per high-power field will be seen on microscopic examination. More than 3 cells per high-power field probably indicates disease somewhere in the urinary tract. Estimate the number of leukocytes present per high-power field and report it as the "estimated number per high-power field."

Erythrocytes.—Red cells are not usually present in normal urine. If erythrocytes are found, estimate their number per high-power field and report it. Erythrocytes may be differentiated from white cells in several ways:

- White cells are larger than red cells.

- When focusing with the high-power lens, the red cells show a distinct circle; the white cells tend to appear granular with a visible nucleus.

- One drop of 5% acetic acid added to the urine sediment disintegrates any red cells, but it does not affect the white cells (except that the nuclei become more distinct).

Casts.—These urinary sediments are formed by coagulation of albuminous material in the kidney tubules. Casts are cylindrical and vary in diameter. The sides are parallel, and the ends are usually rounded. Casts in the urine always indicate some form of kidney disorder and should always be reported. If casts are present in large numbers, the urine is almost sure to be positive for albumin.

There are seven types of casts. They are as follows:

- **Hyaline casts** are the most frequently occurring casts in urine. Hyaline casts can be seen in even the mildest renal disease. They are colorless, homogeneous, transparent, and usually have rounded ends.

- **Red cell casts** indicate renal hematuria. Red cell casts may appear brown to almost colorless and are usually diagnostic of glomerular disease.

- **White cell casts** are present in renal infection and in noninfectious inflammation. The majority of white cells that appear in casts are hypersegmented neutrophils.

- **Granular casts** almost always indicate significant renal disease. However, granular casts may be present in the urine for a short time following strenuous exercise. Granular casts that contain fine granules may appear grey or pale yellow in color. Granular casts that contain larger coarse granules are darker. These casts often appear black because of the density of the granules.

- **Epithelial casts** are rarely seen in urine because renal disease that primarily affects the tubules is infrequent. Epithelial casts may be arranged in parallel rows or haphazardly.

- **Waxy casts** result from the degeneration of granular casts. Waxy casts have been found in patients with severe chronic renal failure, malignant hypertension, and diabetic disease of the kidney. Waxy casts appear yellow, grey, or colorless. They frequently occur as short, broad casts, with blunt or broken ends, and often have cracked or serrated edges.

- **Fatty casts** are seen when there is fatty degeneration of the tubular epithelium, as in degenerative tubular disease. Fatty casts also result from lupus and toxic renal poisoning. A typical fatty cast contains both large and small fat droplets. The small fat droplets are yellowish-brown in color.

SUMMARY

Clinical laboratory medicine is a very dynamic field of medicine, with new testing procedures and equipment being invented all the time. The goal of this chapter is to introduce you to some basic laboratory tests that do not require state-of-the-art equipment and that can be easily performed in isolated duty stations and aboard naval vessels. These tests will assist you in establishing diagnoses and will enable you to provide the best possible medical care for your patients.

CHAPTER 8

MEDICAL ASPECTS OF CHEMICAL, BIOLOGICAL, AND RADIOLOGICAL WARFARE

In this chapter we will discuss the history of chemical, biological, and radiological (CBR) warfare, and the recognition and treatment of CBR-produced conditions. We will also discuss the Medical Department's role in meeting the medical aspects of CBR defense, which includes protection from CBR hazards, mass casualty decontamination, decontamination stations, and supplies for decontamination. Table 8-1 provides a summary of CBR symptoms and treatments.

CHEMICAL WARFARE

LEARNING OBJECTIVE: *Select the appropriate treatment and decontamination procedure for chemical, biological, or radiological exposures.*

The use of chemical agents in warfare, frequently referred to as "gas warfare," is defined as the use of chemical agents in gaseous, solid, or liquid states to harass personnel, produce casualties, render areas impassable or untenable, or contaminate food and water. The chances of surviving a chemical attack are increased as knowledge of the nature of the agents and of the use of correct protective measures is increased.

HISTORY

The first large-scale use of chemical agents came in World War I when, in 1915, the Germans released chlorine gas against the Allied positions at Ypres, Belgium. Over 5,000 casualties resulted. There were other gas attacks by both combatant forces during World War I, and it is well documented that approximately one-third of all American casualties in this conflict were due to chemical agent attacks.

During the interval between World Wars I and II, each of the major powers continued to develop its capability for chemical warfare, in spite of a ban by the Geneva Treaty. In isolated cases in the late 1930s, toxic chemicals were used; however, they were not used during World War II. Nor were toxic chemicals authorized for use in Korea, Vietnam, or Desert Storm.

Defoliants and riot-control agents were used with some degree of effectiveness in the jungles of Vietnam, in tunnel and perimeter-clearing operations.

DISPERSAL

Chemical agents are dispersed by modern weapons for strategic as well as tactical purposes. However, the areas of their use are limited by the range of the weapons or aircraft used by the combatant force.

A naval unit afloat finds itself in a unique situation with respect to defending against toxic chemical agents. Agents can be released as clouds of vapor or aerosol. These can envelope the exterior of a vessel and penetrate the hull of the ship. Extensive contamination can result from such an attack, and the ship must be decontaminated while the personnel manning it continue to eat, sleep, live, and fight on board.

To properly meet the medical needs of the ship, the medical officer or Hospital Corpsman on independent duty must organize the Medical Department well in advance of the actual threat of a chemical agent attack. All hands must be indoctrinated in the use of protective equipment and self-aid procedures, and close liaison and planning must be maintained with damage control personnel responsible for area decontamination.

SELF-PROTECTION AND TREATMENT

In a chemical attack, the first priority is to ensure your own survival so that you may then treat casualties. There are several items available to help you survive a chemical attack, and you should know how to use them. Along with protective clothing, there is a protective mask, which should be put on at the first indication of a chemical attack. The mask will filter out all known chemical agents from the air and allow you to work in a chemically contaminated area. A chemical agent on the skin can be removed effectively by using the M291 skin decontamination kit (fig. 8-1). The M291 skin decontamination kit replaces the M258A1 (fig. 8-2). Upon receipt of the M291, discontinue use of the M258A1.

Table 8-1.—Summary of CBR Agents, Effects, and Treatment

TYPE OF AGENT	PHYSICAL CHARACTERISTICS	SYMPTOMS IN MAN	EFFECTS ON MAN	RATE OF ACTION	PERSONNEL DECONTAMINATION	TREATMENT
NERVE AGENT Tabun (GA) Sarin (GB) Soman (GD) VX	Colorless to light brown liquid Odorless to faint sweetish or fruity vapor Tasteless	Miosis, rhinorrhea, dimmed vision, salivation, nausea, abdominal cramping, increased bronchial secretions, dyspnea, pulmonary edema, headache, vertigo	Incapacitates; kills if high concentrations are inhaled or if contaminated skin is not decontaminated in time.	Very rapid with inhalation Slow through the skin.	None for aerosols or vapors. Flush eyes with water. Wash skin with soap and water, or use skin pad from M-13 kit; M-5 kit for VX.	Atropine IM or IV Artificial ventilation Oximes (2-PAM Cl) as adjunct to atropine
VESICANTS Mustard (HD) Nitrogen Mustard (HN) Lewisite (L) Phosgene Oxime (CX)	Odor of garlic or horseradish (HD) None to slightly fishy odor (HN) Fruity odor or odor or geranium (L) Disagreeable (CX) Colorless to dark brown liquid Vapors not usually visible	Lacrimation, eye pain, photophobia, cough, respiratory irritation, abdominal pain, nausea, vomiting, diarrhea Skin erythema and itching, headache	Generally nonlethal. Blisters skin, is destructive to upper respiratory tract; can cause temporary blindness. Some agents sting and form welts on skin, and others sear eyes.	Mustards: delayed effect. Arsenicals and CX: rapid and intense	Remove contaminated clothing, wash skin with soap and water, or use M-5 ointment or M-13 kit.	Analgesics, sterile dressings, antibiotics, and treat for shock. For arsenicals, BAL in oil IM. For CX, sodium bicarbonate dressings.
BLOOD AGENTS Hydrocyanic acid (AC) Cyanogen chloride (CK)	Colorless gas Faint bitter almond odor (AC) Irritating odor (CK)	Increased respiration followed by dyspnea, nausea, vertigo, headache, convulsions, and coma	Inhibits cytochrome oxidase. Incapacitates; lethal if high concentrations are inhaled.	Rapid	None needed.	Amyl nitrate ampules Artificial respiration Sodium thiosulfate/sodium nitrite IV
CHOKING AGENTS Phosgene (CG)	Colorless gas odor of corn, grass, or new mown hay	Coughing, choking, tightness in chest, nausea, and headache	Lethal. Floods lungs, causes pulmonary edema	Immediate to 3 hours	None needed.	Res, oxygen, antibiotics
VOMITING AGENTS Adamsite (DM)	Yellow or white to nonvisible gas Odor of burning fireworks	Pepperlike irritation of upper respiratory tract and eyes with lacrimation Uncontrolled sneezing and coughing and excessive salivation	Incapacitates. Local irritant.	Immediate	None needed.	Supportive Chloroform inhalation for symptomatic relief Physical exercise shortens duration and speeds recovery Recovery spontaneous
INCAPACITING AGENTS BZ	Odorless, colorless, tasteless	Unpredictable, irrational behavior; may be accompanied by coughing, nausea, vomiting, and headache. Dilation of pupils.	Temporarily incapacitates, mentally and physically. Anticholinergic. Psychotropic.	Delayed	Wash with soap and water.	Observation and physical restraint if indicated Physostigmine salicylate 2-3 mg IM every 1-2 hours for duration of symptoms
IRRITANTS Riot control agents CS, CN, CR, CA	Colorless to white vapor Pepperlike odor	Immediate lacrimation Coughing Skin irritation	Incapacitating. Local irritant.	Instantaneous	None needed.	Removal to fresh air
BIOLOGICAL AGENTS	Microscopic live organisms	Variable, depending on agent and resistance of victim	Lethal or incapacitating, depending on agent.	Delayed for days or longer	Wash with soap and water.	Variable, specific if agent is known Supportive
NUCLEAR BURST	Bright intense flash of light Heat, wind, shock wave Earth tremors	Temporary blindness Thermal burns Radiation burns Physical injuries	Blast destruction. Radiation sickness.	Immediate for blast Delayed for radiation	Wash with soap and water. Shower. Monitor.	Immediate decontamination Treatment of physical injuries Antibiotics for radiation exposure

HM3T0801

8-2

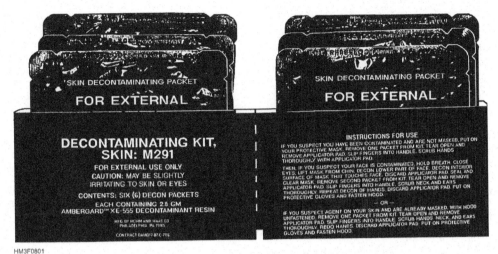

HM3F0801

Figure 8-1.—M291 skin decontamination kit.

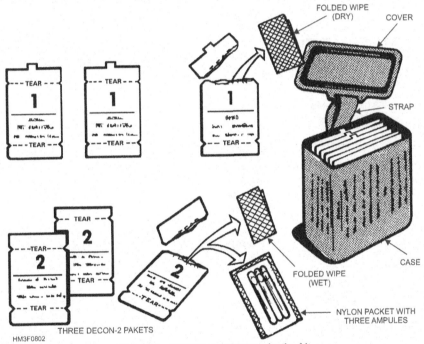

HM3F0802

Figure 8-2.—M258A1 skin decontamination kit.

Chemical agents penetrate ordinary clothing rapidly. However, significant absorption through the skin requires a period of minutes. The effects of clothing penetration may be reduced by quickly removing the contaminated clothing and neutralizing the chemical agent on the skin by washing, blotting, or wiping it away.

Prompt decontamination (decon) of the skin is imperative. Decon of chemical agents on the skin within 1 minute after contamination is perhaps 10 times more effective than if decontamination is delayed 5 minutes. Detailed instructions on the use of skin decontamination kits can be found in the NAVMED P-5041, *Treatment of Chemical Agent Casualties and Conventional Military Chemical Injuries*, and in the kits themselves.

Finally, there are two types of antidote autoinjectors—atropine and 2-PAM Cl—for your own use if you become a nerve-agent casualty. The autoinjectors will be discussed later in this chapter. Familiarize yourself with your equipment. Know how it works before you need it.

DECONTAMINATION

The guiding principle in personnel decontamination is to avoid spreading contamination to clean areas and to manage casualties without aggravating other injuries.

Casualty Priorities

It will often be necessary to decide whether to handle the surgical condition or the chemical hazard first. If the situation and the condition of the casualty permit, decontamination should be carried out first. The longer the chemical remains on the body, the more severe will be the danger of spreading the chemical to other personnel and equipment.

The following order of priority for first aid and decontaminating casualties is recommended:

1. Control of massive hemorrhage

2. First aid for life-threatening shock and wounds

3. Decontamination of exposed skin and eyes

4. Removal of contaminated clothing and decontamination of body surfaces (if not in a toxic environment)

5. Adjustment of patient's mask, if mask is necessary

6. First aid in less severe shock and wounds

The basic steps in sorting and handling casualties are indicated in figure 8-3. This plan should be modified to fit specific needs.

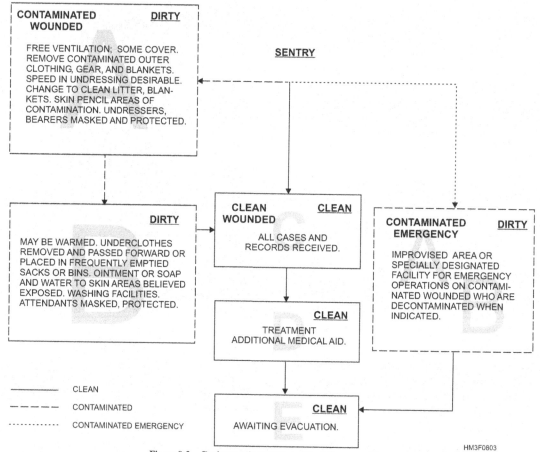

Figure 8-3.—Basic steps in sorting and handling casualties.

HM3F0803

Decontamination Station Organization

In general, the decontamination station, or "dirty" area, receives casualties contaminated with a chemical agent. The arrangement of this area will vary with the site of the medical unit and the facilities available for decontamination.

Each ship will have a minimum of at least two decontamination stations, insofar as the hull design permits. The "dirty" areas should be topside or in some well-ventilated space. Personnel manning these areas should be provided with protective equipment.

In the "dirty" area, casualties will be decontaminated, undressed, showered, and passed along to clean areas. Both areas should be clearly marked as either "clean" or "contaminated," as appropriate. Decontamination kits, protective ointment, and an abundant supply of soap and water must be provided. In addition, standard first-aid items should be on hand. When possible, improvise supports (e.g., small boxes, blocks of wood, etc.) for stretchers to keep them raised off the deck.

Handling of Contaminated Casualties

The spread of contamination to uncontaminated personnel or to spaces not set aside to receive contamination must be avoided. Contaminated personnel, clothing, or equipment must be kept out of uncontaminated areas since the subsequent decontamination of such spaces is quite difficult. Contaminated clothing and gear must be placed in designated dump areas and, whenever practically possible, kept in metal cans with tightly fitting covers.

Supplies

The Medical Officer or Senior Medical Department Representative (SMDR) is responsible for maintaining adequate supplies for decontamination and treatment of CBR casualties. Medical decontamination supplies are supplied to ships on a personnel-strength basis, as listed in current Authorized Medical Allowance List (AMAL).

The decontamination supply cabinets will be kept locked, and the keys will be in custody of the Damage Control Assistant (DCA). Cabinets and chests will be stenciled with a red cross and marked "DECONTAMINATION MEDICAL SUPPLIES."

CHEMICAL AGENTS

Chemical agents are grouped under several classifications. The broadest classification we will use is based on the general effect produced (i.e., severe casualty, harassment, or incapacitation). Within each general group, there are further breakdowns, the most convenient of which (from a medical point of view) is the classification by physiologic effect. Chemical agents may also be classified as lethal or nonlethal. Nonlethal agents will not kill you. Lethal agents are those that result in a 10 percent or greater death rate among casualties. They are further classified as persistent or nonpersistent, depending on the length of time they retain their effectiveness after dissemination.

In the following paragraphs, we discuss the agents that produce the greatest number of fatalities and casualties among personnel who have been exposed to them.

Nerve Agents

Nerve agents produce their effect by interfering with normal transmission of nerve impulses in the parasympathetic autonomic nervous system. Physically, nerve agents are odorless, almost colorless liquids, varying greatly in viscosity and volatility. They are moderately soluble in water and fairly stable unless strong alkali or chlorinating compounds are added. They are very effective solvents, readily penetrating cloth either as a liquid or vapor. Other materials, including leather and wood, are fairly well penetrated. Butyl rubber and synthetics, such as polyesters, are much more resistant.

Pharmacologically, the nerve agents are cholinesterase inhibitors (interfering with normal transmission of nerve impulses in the parasympathetic autonomic nervous system). Their reaction with cholinesterase tends to be irreversible, and reaction time varies with the agent.

SIGNS AND SYMPTOMS OF EXPOSURE.— Nerve-agent intoxication can be readily identified by its characteristic signs and symptoms. If a vapor exposure has occurred, the pupils will constrict, usually to a pinpoint. If the exposure has been through the skin, there will be local muscular twitching where the agent was absorbed. Other symptoms will include rhinorrhea, dyspnea, diarrhea and vomiting, convulsions, hypersalivation, drowsiness, coma, and unconsciousness.

TREATMENT.—Specific therapy for nerve agent casualties is atropine, an acetylcholine blocker. **When exposed**, each member of the Navy and Marine Corps is issued three 2 mg autoinjectors of atropine and three 600 mg autoinjectors of 2-PAM Cl. **DO**

NOT give nerve agent antidotes for preventive purposes **before** contemplated exposure to a nerve agent.

The atropine autoinjector consists of a hard plastic tube containing 2 mg (0.7 ml) of atropine in solution for intramuscular injection. It has a pressure-activated coiled-spring mechanism that triggers the needle for injection of the antidote solution. These injectors are designed to be used by individuals on themselves when symptoms appear. For medical personnel, the required therapy is to continue to administer atropine at 15-minute intervals until a mild atropinization occurs. This can be noted by tachycardia and a dry mouth. Atropine alone will not relieve any respiratory muscle failure. Prolonged artificial respiration may be necessary to sustain life.

A second autoinjector containing oxime therapy (using pralidoxime chloride, or 2-PAM Cl) can also be used for regeneration of the blocked cholinesterase. Since 2-PAM Cl is contained in the kit of autoinjectors, additional oxime therapy is not generally medically recommended for those who have already received treatment by autoinjection. The 2-PAM Cl autoinjector is a hard plastic tube that, when activated, dispenses 600 mg of 2-PAM Cl (300 mg/ml) solution. It also has a pressure-activated coiled-spring mechanism identical to that in the atropine autoinjector.

Self-Aid.—If you experience the **mild** symptoms of nerve-agent poisoning, you should **IMMEDIATELY** hold your breath and put on your protective mask. Then, administer **one set** of (atropine and 2-PAM Cl) injections into your lateral thigh muscle or buttocks, as illustrated in figures 8-4 and 8-5. Position the needle end of the **atropine** injector against the injection site and apply firm, even pressure (not jabbing motion) to the injector until it pushes the needle into your thigh (or buttocks). Make sure you **do not** hit any buttons or other objects. Using a jabbing motion may result in an improper injection or injury to the thigh or buttocks.

Hold the **atropine** injector firmly in place for **at least 10 seconds.** The seconds can be estimated by counting "one thousand one, one thousand two," and so forth. Firm pressure automatically triggers the coiled mechanism and plunges the needle through the clothing into the muscle and at the same time injects the atropine antidote into the muscle tissue.

Next, inject yourself in the same manner with the **2-PAM Cl** injector, using the same procedure as you

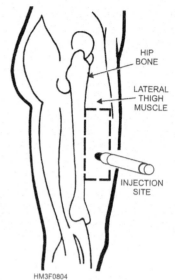

HM3F0804

Figure 8-4.—Thigh injection site.

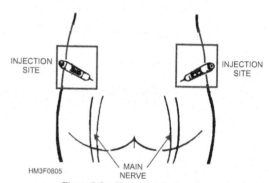

HM3F0805

Figure 8-5.—Buttocks injection site.

did for the atropine. This will now complete one set of nerve-agent antidotes. Attach the used injectors to your clothing (fig. 8-6) (to indicate the number of injections you have already received).

After administering the first set of injections, wait 10 to 15 minutes (since it takes that long for the antidote to take effect) before administering a second set, if needed. If the symptoms have not disappeared within 10 to 15 minutes, give yourself the second set of injections. If the symptoms still persist after an additional 15 minutes, a third set of injections may be given by nonmedical personnel.

After administering each set of injections, you should decontaminate your skin, if necessary, and put on any remaining protective clothing.

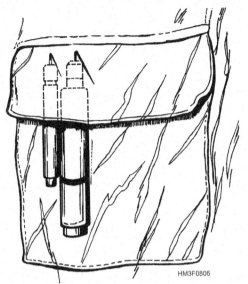

Figure 8-6.—One set of used autoinjectors attached to a pocket flap.

Buddy Aid.—If you encounter a service member suffering from severe signs of nerve-agent poisoning, you should provide the following aid:

- Mark the casualty, if necessary. Do not fasten the hood.

- Administer, in rapid succession, **three** sets of the nerve-agent antidotes. Follow the procedures for administration as described previously in the self-aid section.

  NOTE: Use the casualty's own autoinjectors when providing aid. Do not use your injectors on a casualty. If you do, you may not have any antidote available when needed for self-aid.

Blister Agents (Vesicants)

Blister agents, or vesicants, exert their primary action on the skin, producing large and painful blisters that are incapacitating. Although vesicants are classed as nonlethal, high doses can cause death.

Common blister agents include mustard (HD), nitrogen mustard (HN), and Lewisite (L). Each is chemically different and will cause significant specific symptoms. They are all similar in their physical characteristics and toxicology. Mustards are particularly insidious because they do not manifest their symptoms for several hours after exposure. They attack the eyes and respiratory tract as well as the skin.

There is no effective therapy for mustard once its effects become visible. Treatment is largely supportive: to relieve itching and pain, and to prevent infection.

MUSTARD (HD) AND NITROGEN MUSTARD (HN).—HD and HN are oily, colorless or pale yellow liquids, sparingly soluble in water. HN is less volatile and more persistent than HD but has the same blistering qualities.

Signs and Symptoms of Exposure.—The eyes are the most vulnerable part of the body to mustard gas. Contamination insufficient to cause injury elsewhere may produce eye inflammation. Because the eye is the most sensitive part of the body, the first noticeable symptoms of mustard exposure will be pain and a gritting feeling in the eyes, accompanied by spastic blinking of the eyelids and photophobia. Vapor or liquid may burn any area of the skin, but the burns will be most severe in the warm, sweaty areas of the body: the armpits, groin, and on the face and neck. Blistering begins in about 12 hours but may be delayed for up to 48 hours. Inhalation of the gas is followed in a few hours by irritation of the throat, hoarseness, and a cough. Fever, moist rales, and dyspnea may develop. Brochopneumonia is a frequent complication. The primary cause of death is massive edema or mechanical pulmonary obstruction.

Treatment.—There is no specific antidotal treatment for mustard poisoning. Physically removing as much of the mustard as possible, as soon as possible, is the only effective method for mitigating symptoms before they appear. All other treatment is symptomatic, that is, the relief of pain and itching, and control of infection.

LEWISITE (L).—Lewisite is an **arsenical** (an arsenic-based compound). This blistering compound is a light- to dark-brown liquid that vaporizes slowly.

Signs and Symptoms of Exposure.—The vapors of arsenicals are so irritating that conscious persons are immediately warned by discomfort to put on the mask. No severe respiratory injuries are likely to occur, except in the wounded who are incapable of donning a mask. The respiratory symptoms are similar to those produced by mustard gas. While distilled mustard and nitrogen mustard cause no pain on the skin during absorption, Lewisite causes intense pain upon contact.

Treatment.—Immediately decontaminate the eyes by flushing with copious amounts of water to remove liquid agents and to prevent severe burns. Sodium sulfacetamide, 30 percent solution, may be used to combat eye infection within the first 24 hours after exposure. In severe cases, morphine may be given to relieve pain.

In cases of systemic involvement, British Anti-Lewisite (BAL), dimercaprol, is available in a peanut oil suspension for injection. BAL is a specific antiarsenical that combines with the heavy metal to form a water-soluble, nontoxic complex that is excreted. However, BAL is somewhat toxic, and an injection of more than 3 mg/kg will cause severe symptoms.

Aside from the use of dimercaprol for the systemic effects of arsenic, treatment is the same as for mustard lesions.

Blood Agents

Blood agents interfere with enzyme functions in the body, i.e., block oxygen transfer. Hydrocyanic acid (AC) and cyanogen chloride (CK) are cyanide-containing compounds commonly referred to as blood agents. These blood agents are chemicals that are in a gaseous state at normal temperatures and pressures. They are systemic poisons and casualty-producing agents that interfere with vital enzyme systems of the body. They can cause death in a very short time after exposure by interfering with oxygen transfer in the blood. Although very deadly, they are nonpersistent agents.

SIGNS AND SYMPTOMS OF EXPOSURE.— These vary with concentration and duration of exposure. Typically, either death or recovery takes place rapidly. After exposure to high concentrations of the gas, there is a forceful increase in the depth of respiration for a few seconds, violent convulsions after 20 to 30 seconds, and respiratory failure with cessation of heart action within a few minutes.

TREATMENT.—There are two suggested antidotes in the treatment of cyanides: amyl nitrite in crush ampules (provided as first aid) and intravenous sodium thiosulfate solution.

In an attack, if you notice sudden stimulation of breathing or an almond-like odor, hold your breath and don your mask immediately. In treating a victim, upon notification by competent authority that there are no blood agents remaining in the atmosphere, crush two ampules of amyl nitrite in the hollow of your hand and hold it close to the victim's nose. You may repeat this procedure every few minutes until eight ampules have been used. If the atmosphere is contaminated and the victim must remain masked, insert the crushed ampules into the mask under the face plate.

Whether amyl nitrite is used or not, sodium thiosulfate therapy is required after the initial lifesaving measures. The required dose is 100 to 200 mg/kg, given intravenously over a 9-minute period.

The key to successful cyanide therapy is speed; cyanide acts rapidly on an essential enzyme system. The antidotes act rapidly to reverse this action. If the specific antidote and artificial respiration are given soon enough, the chance of survival is greatly enhanced.

Choking or Lung Agents

The toxicity of lung agents is due to their effect on lung tissues; they cause extensive damage to alveolar tissue, resulting in severe pulmonary edema. This group includes phosgene (CG) and chlorine (Cl), as well as chloropicrin and diphosgene. However, CG is most likely to be encountered, and its toxic action is representative of the group.

Phosgene is a colorless gas with a distinctive odor similar to that of new-mown hay or freshly cut grass. Unfortunately, even at minimal concentrations in the air (i.e., below the threshold of olfactory perception), CG can cause damage to the eyes and throat. Generally speaking, CG does not represent a hazard of long duration; therefore, an individual exposed to a casualty-producing amount should be able to smell it.

SIGNS AND SYMPTOMS OF EXPOSURE.— There may be watering of the eyes, coughing, and a feeling of tightness in the chest. More often, however, there will be no symptoms for 2 to 6 hours after exposure. Latent symptoms are rapid, shallow, and labored breathing; painful cough; cyanosis; frothy sputum; clammy skin; rapid, feeble pulse; and low blood pressure. Shock may develop, followed by death.

TREATMENT.—Once symptoms appear, complete bed rest is mandatory. Keep victims with lung edema only moderately warm, and treat the resulting anoxia with oxygen. Because no specific treatment for CG poisoning is known, treatment has to be symptomatic.

Incapacitating Agents

Incapacitating agents, which are mainly comprised of psychochemicals, produce mental confusion and an inability to function intelligently.

The psychochemicals temporarily prevent an individual from carrying out assigned actions. These agents may be administered by contaminating food or water, or they may be released as aerosols. The following are characteristics of the incapacitants:

- High potency (i.e., an extremely low dose is effective) and logistic feasibility

- Effects produced mainly by altering or disrupting the higher regulatory activity of the central nervous system

- Duration of action comprising hours or days, rather than momentary or transient action

- No permanent injury produced

SIGNS AND SYMPTOMS OF EXPOSURE.— The first symptoms appear in 30 minutes to several hours and may persist for several days. Abnormal, inappropriate behavior may be the only sign of intoxication. Those affected may make irrational statements and have delusions or hallucinations. In some instances, the victim may complain of dizziness, muscular incoordination, dry mouth, and difficulty in swallowing.

The standard incapacitant in the United States is 3-quinuclidinyl benzilate (BZ), a cholinergic blocking agent, which is effective in producing delirium that may last several days. In small doses it will cause an increase in heart rate, pupil size, and skin temperature, as well as drowsiness, dry skin, and a decrease in alertness. As the dose is increased to higher levels, there is a progressive deterioration of mental capability, ending in stupor.

TREATMENT.— The first aid is to prevent victims from injuring themselves and others during the toxic psychosis. Generally, there is no specific therapy for this type intoxication. However, with BZ and other agents in the class of compounds known as glycolates, physostigmine is the drug treatment of choice. It is not effective during the first 4 hours following exposure; after that, it is very effective as long as treatment is continued. However, treatment does not shorten the duration of BZ intoxication, and premature discontinuation of therapy will result in relapse.

Riot-Control/Harassment Agents

"Riot-control agents" is the collective term used to describe a collection of chemical compounds, all having similar characteristics which, though relatively nontoxic, produce an immediate but temporary effect in very low concentrations. These agents are used to harass enemy personnel or to discourage riot actions. Generally, patients require no therapy; removal from the environment is sufficient to effect recovery in a short time.

There are two classes of riot-control/harassment agents: lacrimators and vomiting agents.

LACRIMATORS.— Lacrimators (or tear gases) are essentially local irritants that act primarily on the eyes. In high concentrations, they also irritate the respiratory tract and the skin. The principal agents used are chloracetophenone (CN) and orthochlorobenzilidine malanonitrile (CS). Although CS is basically a lacrimator, it is considerably more potent than CN and causes more severe respiratory symptoms. CN is the standard training agent and is the tear gas most commonly encountered because it is not as potent. CS is more widely used by the military as a riot-control agent.

Protection against all tear agents is provided by protective masks and ordinary field clothing secured at the neck, wrists, and ankles. Personnel handling CS should wear rubber gloves for additional protection.

Signs and Symptoms of Exposure.— Lacrimators produce intense pain in the eyes with excessive tearing. The symptoms following the most severe exposure to vapors seldom last over 2 hours. After moderate exposure, they last only a few minutes.

Treatment.— First aid for lacrimators is generally not necessary. Exposure to fresh air and letting wind blow into wide open eyes, held open if necessary, is sufficient for recovery in a short time. Any chest discomfort after CS exposure can be relieved by talking.

An important point to remember is that this material adheres tenaciously to clothing, and a change of clothing may be necessary. Do not forget the hair (both head and facial) as a potential source of recontamination.

VOMITING AGENTS.— Vomiting agents comprise the second class of agents in the riot-control category. The principal agents of this group are diphenylaminochloroarsine (Adamsite (DM)), diphenylchloroarsine (DA), and diphenylcyanoarsine (DC). They are used as training and riot-control agents. They are dispersed as aerosols and produce their effects by inhalation or by direct action on the eyes. All of these agents have similar properties and pathology.

Signs and Symptoms of Exposure.—Vomiting agents produce a strong pepper-like irritation in the upper respiratory tract, with irritation of the eyes and lacrimation. They cause violent uncontrollable sneezing, coughing, nausea, vomiting, and a general feeling of malaise. Inhalation causes a burning sensation in the nose and throat, hypersalivation, and rhinorrhea. The sinuses fill rapidly and cause a violent frontal headache.

Treatment.—It is of the utmost importance that the mask be worn in spite of coughing, sneezing, salivation, and nausea. If the mask is put on following exposure, symptoms will increase for several minutes in spite of adequate protection. As a consequence, victims may believe the mask is ineffective and remove it, further exposing themselves. While the mask must be worn, it may be lifted from the face briefly, if necessary, to permit vomiting or to drain saliva from the face piece. Carry on duties as vigorously as possible. This will help to lessen and shorten the symptoms. Combat duties usually can be performed in spite of the effects of vomiting agents if an individual is motivated.

First aid consists of washing the skin and rinsing the eyes and mouth with water. A mild analgesic may be given to relieve headache. Recovery is usually spontaneous and complete within 1 to 3 hours.

SCREENING SMOKES.—Screening smokes fit in with riot-control agents. Their primary use is to obscure vision and to hide targets or areas. When used for this purpose outdoors, they are not generally considered toxic. However, exposure to heavy smoke concentration for extended periods, particularly near the source, may cause illness or death. Under no circumstances should smoke munitions be activated indoors or in closed compartments.

Symptomatic treatment of medical problems or discomfort resulting from exposure to screening smokes will generally suffice.

WHITE PHOSPHORUS.—White phosphorus (WP) is a pale, waxy solid that ignites spontaneously on contact with air to give a hot, dense, white smoke composed of phosphorus pentoxide particles. While field concentrations of the smoke may cause temporary irritation to the eyes, nose, and throat, casualties from the smoke have not occurred in combat operations. No treatment is necessary, and spontaneous recovery is rapid once the patient is removed from the WP source.

White phosphorus smoke not only creates an obscuring smoke, but it also has a secondary effect upon personnel if it contacts the skin. When burning particles of WP embed in the skin, they must be covered with water, a wet cloth, or mud. A freshly mixed 0.5 percent solution of copper sulfate (which produces an airproof black coating of copper phosphide) may be used as a rinse but must not be used as a dressing. The phosphorus particles must be removed surgically.

BIOLOGICAL WARFARE

Epidemics arising from natural causes have plagued military forces for centuries and in many instances have determined the outcome of campaigns. Recognition of this drain on personnel undoubtedly has led to attempts to produce illness in epidemic proportions, through pollution of water and food supplies as well as through other means. The dissemination of disease-producing organisms has never been employed on any significant scale as a weapon of war.

HISTORY

Biological warfare has become a very real possibility since World War II because of the advance of knowledge in the various biological science fields. Many countries have indulged in research on the use of microorganisms as a weapon of war, and in the hands of an unscrupulous enemy, antianimal and antiplant agents could be powerful instruments of war, reducing or destroying a nation's food supply. In this chapter, however, we are concerned only with agents that would be effective against populations. Although their effectiveness has never been established by actual use in war, they are considered to have grave military capabilities.

DISPERSAL

Biological warfare has certain aspects in common with chemical warfare in that biological agents can be dispersed in the air and travel downwind in the same manner as a gas cloud. These agents may be inhaled unless a protective mask is worn, and they may cause disability or death. They are capable of contaminating clothing, equipment, food, and water supplies. Some types of agents may persist in the target area for considerable periods of time.

Biological agents, unlike most war gases or vapors, cannot be detected by the physical senses or by chemical detectors. Their presence or identity can be determined only by laboratory examination of air samples or contaminated objects. The time between exposure and onset of disease symptoms will usually be a matter of days rather than hours, as is the case with most chemical agents. Though they may be exposed to the same dosage of biological agent, not all personnel will be affected the same way. Some may become seriously ill, while others may have a very mild attack. Still others may escape the disease entirely.

PROTECTION

In this section, we will discuss both individual and group protection, as well as the methods of protecting food and water supplies.

Individual Protection

The natural resistance of the body and its maintenance in the best possible physical condition constitute important lines of defense against biological agents. Immunity and good health alone, however, cannot be expected to triumph over massive onslaughts of biological agents. These agents may have been tailored to create varying degrees of incapacitation, including death. To reduce the effectiveness of such attacks, the military provides protective equipment and a series of protocols to its members. In general, these measures closely parallel those provided for defense against chemical attack.

PORTALS OF ENTRY.—Inhalation of airborne organisms is considered the greatest potential hazard in biological warfare. The protective mask is an important piece of defensive equipment. A mask that is in good condition and has been properly fitted will greatly reduce the possibility of your inhaling infectious material. Since you cannot detect the presence of biological agents, the use of the mask and other protective equipment will depend upon early warning.

To produce disease, biological agents must gain entrance into the body. A concentration of biological agents on the skin might, in time, be transferred to a portal of entry. Any type of clothing will provide some protection by reducing the quantity of agents coming in contact with the skin. The degree of protection afforded is dependent upon how well the fabric stops penetration and the number of layers of clothing being worn. Since this protective effect is due to the mechanical filtering or screening action of the cloth, it is important that shirt and jacket collars be fastened. Sleeves should be rolled down and cuffs buttoned, trouser cuffs stuffed inside tops of boots or socks, and all other garment openings tied or otherwise secured. Following this procedure will minimize the entry of airborne organisms and reduce the risk of bodily contact with biological agents that may be present on the surface of the ground or in the air.

EQUIPMENT AND ACTION.—Military headgear helps safeguard the hair from heavy contamination, and ordinary gloves or mittens provide protection for the hands. The type of clothing issued for protection against chemical agents is impregnated with an impermeable barrier and provides a higher degree of protection than the ordinary uniform. Whenever it is available, it should be used.

Upon notification of an attack with biological agents, or before entering an area known to be contaminated by them, the following steps should be taken:

1. Put on protective mask and check it for correct fit.

2. Button clothing. Tie clothing at wrists and ankles with string or extra shoelaces. Put on special protective clothing, if available.

3. Put on gloves, if available.

4. While in the contaminated area, maintain the provisions outlined above.

Upon leaving the area, proceed with decontamination measures to the extent the situation permits.

Group Protection

In biological as well as chemical and radiological warfare, a tightly constructed shelter offers great protection. The shelter must be pressurized to prevent entrance of the microorganisms. Pressurization is accomplished by introducing filtered air into the shelter. If the shelter is reasonably tight, this incoming air will force exhausted and/or contaminated air outward. Nonpressurized buildings, shelters, or field fortifications provide only limited protection from aerosols. Eventually, microorganisms will penetrate through cracks, creating a respiratory hazard requiring the use of a protective mask. As in the case of other protective equipment, the sooner a shelter is used following contamination, the more effective the shelter will be in arresting or staying in contact with biological agents.

Protection of Food and Water

Food and water supplies are especially susceptible to deliberate contamination. Civilian supplies— which all too frequently do not receive careful supervision and protection—must always be suspected of accidental or deliberate contamination. It should also be emphasized that water is not necessarily pure just because it comes from a faucet. In some countries pure water is the exception rather than the rule. The safest rule is to consume only food and drinks received from military sources. Procedures for protection of the water supply and routines for inspection and decontamination are well defined in the military and, if diligently observed, will protect from deliberate contamination.

FOOD.—In the event of a known or suspected biological attack, all exposed or unpackaged foods not in critical supply should be destroyed. In most instances, food can be rendered safe for consumption by application of moist-heat cooking procedures. In some instances, deep-fat cooking is adequate. Some foods, however, cannot be sterilized because the treatment would render them unacceptable for consumption.

WATER.—Chlorination is by far the almost universal method of purifying water, and it destroys most of the biological agents. Boiling may be required to ensure proper decontamination in exceptional cases.

The military establishes water points in the field whenever possible. The equipment location at these points provides for filtration as well as chlorination and, when properly operated, is effective in removing organisms that produce disease. Some biological agents cannot be destroyed by normal water-purification techniques. When biological agents are known to have been used, all drinking water must be boiled. In the preparation of water for large numbers, the boiling procedure should be supervised. Water boiling may, of necessity, become an individual responsibility and may be so directed.

For small groups of people, the Lyster bag is provided as a suitable container for the storage of water that has already been treated. Water that has not been made potable previously is purified in the Lyster bag by means of chemicals. Water purification procedures are discussed in detail in the *Preventive Medicine Manual*, NAVMED P-5010.

DECONTAMINATION

Personal decontamination following actual or suspected exposure to biological agents will depend upon the existing tactical situation and the facilities available. If the situation permits, contaminated clothing should be carefully removed and the body washed thoroughly with soap and water before donning fresh clothing. Specific attention should be given to decontamination and treatment of skin lesions.

Normally, each individual is responsible for his own decontamination. If a person is physically unable to decontaminate himself, this process has to be performed by other available personnel. Since illness resulting from exposure to biological warfare may be delayed because of the incubation period, decontamination may occur before the individual becomes ill. Decontamination of the wounded is the responsibility of Medical Department personnel. When the situation and the condition of the casualty permit, decontamination should come first. However, massive hemorrhage, asphyxia, or other life-endangering conditions naturally receive priority.

In general, all candidates for decontamination should first have all exposed areas thoroughly washed with soap and large amounts of water, the mask adjusted, and all contaminated clothing removed. The casualty may then be moved to a clean area where the wounds can be treated.

Decontamination procedures are the same as those used for casualties of chemical warfare.

RADIOLOGICAL WARFARE

Radiological—the "R" in CBR—warfare is more frequently referred to as nuclear warfare. The principles of treatment of casualties, as developed from previous experiences in conventional warfare, are applicable in the treatment of casualties produced by radiological warfare. With the exception of ionizing radiation effects, the type of injuries produced in nuclear warfare are similar to those of conventional warfare. Standardized techniques of treatment must be adopted for all types of casualties so the greatest number of patients can receive maximum medical care in the shortest period of time with the greatest economy of medical personnel and equipment.

HISTORY

The death and devastation evidenced by the first and only use of nuclear power in wartime (in Hiroshima and Nagasaki, Japan, at the end of World War II) has, to date, kept it from being used again. Although a nuclear nonproliferation treaty has been signed by most of the major powers, nuclear weaponry is still a part of the arsenal of many countries of the world, some of which, if given the opportunity and excuse, would not hesitate to employ it to achieve victory at any cost.

History has shown that nuclear warfare is capable of producing a large disparity between the available medical care and the number of casualties requiring care. The capabilities of medical facilities and personnel must be surveyed to determine how and where they can best be utilized. Both professional and nonprofessional personnel must be trained in additional skills related as far as possible to their primary duties. Within medical organizations, efficiency will depend upon controlled patient flow, adequate supplies, and continuing essential housekeeping and administrative functions. To meet the requirements, it is essential that all medical service personnel be trained to assume some additional responsibilities.

EXPOSURE FACTORS

Teams entering contaminated areas to either remove casualties or work in decontamination stations have two major concerns. The first concern is the prevention of their own contamination, and the second is the prevention or reduction of radioactive exposure. Contamination can be avoided by decontaminating patients and equipment before handling, wearing appropriate protective clothing and equipment, avoiding highly contaminated areas, and strictly observing personal decontamination procedures. Exposure to radiation should also be avoided or minimized. Alpha and beta particles and gamma rays are emitted from radioactive contaminants and present a direct risk to the health and safety of personnel in the contaminated area. This risk can be avoided (or at least minimized) by following some simple guidelines and using common sense. Time, distance, and shielding are the major elements that guide actions to avoid exposure.

Time

Radioactive decay and the decomposition of fallout products progress rapidly in the early hours after a nuclear blast, and the hazards to rescue workers can be reduced considerably if operations can be delayed until natural decay has reduced the level of radioactivity. Use teams trained in the use of survey instruments since they will determine the intensity of radiation and mark perimeters of danger zones.

Limiting the time of exposure is essential if total avoidance is not possible. Rotating personnel entering an exposure risk area, planning actions to minimize time in the area, and prompt decontamination reduce the total time the individual is exposed, thereby reducing the dose of radiation absorbed by the body.

Distance

Both radioactive particles and electromagnetic waves (gamma rays) lose energy and consequently lose their ability to harm tissue as they travel away from their source. Therefore, the farther one is from the source, the more the danger of an exposure is minimized.

Shielding

Shielding is an essential component in preventing radiation exposure. Alpha and beta particles have very little penetrating power, and the intact skin forms an adequate barrier in most cases. Gamma radiation has much greater penetrating power and presents the greatest risk of exposure and damage to tissue.

Lead is the most effective shielding material. Wood, concrete, other metals, and heavy clothing will somewhat reduce the amount of gamma radiation that reaches the body. Most particle exposure is the result of inhalation or ingestion, although radiation particles may enter the body through burned, abraded or lacerated skin. In avoiding particle exposure, full personnel-protective clothing and a protective mask with hood provides the best protection. The protective mask and foul-weather gear will provide lesser but adequate protection. In cases where no protective breathing devices are available, some protection is afforded by breathing through a folded towel, handkerchief, or several surgical masks. Avoid hand-to-mouth contact, eating, or smoking in contaminated areas.

EFFECTS ON PERSONNEL

The injuries to personnel resulting from a nuclear explosion are divided into three broad classes: blast and shock injuries, burns, and ionizing radiation effects.

Apart from the ionizing radiation effects, most of the injuries suffered in a nuclear weapon explosion will not differ greatly from those caused by ordinary high explosives and incendiary bombs. An important aspect of injuries in nuclear explosions is the "combined effect," that is, a combination of all three types of injuries. For example, a person within the effective range of a weapon may suffer blast injury, burns, and also from the effects of nuclear radiation. In this respect, radiation injury may be a complicating factor, since it is combined with injuries due to other sources.

Blast and Shock Wave Injuries

Injuries caused by blast can be divided into primary (direct) blast injuries and secondary (indirect) blast injuries.

Primary blast injuries are those that result from the direct action of the air shock wave on the human body. These injuries will be confined to a zone where fatal secondary blast and thermal damage may be anticipated. Therefore, most surviving casualties will not have the severe injuries that result from the direct compressive effects of the blast wave.

Secondary blast injuries are caused by collapsing buildings and by timber and other debris flung about by the blast. Persons may also be hurled against stationary objects or thrown to the ground by the high winds accompanying the explosions. The injuries sustained are thus similar to those due to a mechanical accident: bruises, concussions, cuts, fractures, and internal injuries.

At sea, the shock wave accompanying an underwater burst will produce various "mechanical" injuries. These injuries will resemble those caused aboard ship by more conventional underwater weapons, such as noncontact mines and depth charges. Instead of being localized, however, they will extend over the entire vessel.

Equipment, furniture, gas cylinders, boxes, and similar gear, when not well secured, can act as missiles and cause many injuries.

Burn Injuries

A weapon detonated as an air burst may produce more burn casualties than blast or ionizing radiation casualties. Burns due to a nuclear explosion can also be divided into two classes: direct and indirect burns. **Direct burns** (usually called **flash** burns) are the result of thermal (infrared) radiation emanating from a nuclear explosion, while **indirect burns** result from fires caused by the explosion. Biologically, they are similar to any other burn and are treated in the same manner.

Since all radiation travels in a straight line from its source, flash burns are sharply limited to those areas of the skin facing the center of the explosion. Furthermore, clothing will protect the skin to some degree unless the individual is so close to the center of the explosion that the cloth is ignited spontaneously by heat. Although light colors will absorb heat to a lesser degree than dark colors, the thickness, air layers, and types of clothing (wool is better than cotton) are far more important for protection than the color of the material.

Eye Burns

In addition to injuries to the skin, the eyes may also be affected by thermal radiation. If people are looking in the general direction of a nuclear detonation, they may be flash blinded. This blindness may persist for 20 to 30 minutes.

A second and very serious type of eye injury may also occur. If people are looking directly at the fireball of a nuclear explosion, they may receive a retinal flash burn similar to the burn that occurs on exposed skin. Unfortunately, when the burn heals, the destroyed retinal tissue is replaced by scar tissue that has no light-perception capability, and the victims will have scotomas, blind or partially blind areas in the visual field. In severe cases, the net result may be permanent blindness. The effective range for eye injuries from the flash may extend for many miles when a weapon is detonated as an air burst. This effective range is far greater at night when the pupils are dilated, permitting a greater amount of light to enter the eye.

Radiation Injuries

Radioactivity may be defined as the spontaneous and instantaneous decomposition of the nucleus of an unstable atom with the accompanying emission of a particle, a gamma ray, or both. The actual particles and rays involved in the production of radiation injuries are the alpha and beta particles, the neutron, and the gamma ray. These particles and rays produce their effect by ionizing the chemical compounds that make up the living cell. If enough of these particles or rays disrupt a sufficient number of molecules within the cell, the cell will not be able to carry on its normal functions and will die.

ALPHA.—Alpha particles are emitted from the nucleus of some radioactive elements. Alpha particles produce a high degree of ionization when passing through air or tissue. Also, due to their large size and electrical charge, they are rapidly stopped or absorbed by a few inches of air, a sheet of paper, or the superficial layers of skin. Therefore, alpha particles do not constitute a major external radiation hazard. However, because of their great ionization power, they constitute a serious hazard when taken into the body through ingestion, inhalation, or an open wound.

BETA.—Beta particles are electrons of nuclear origin. The penetration ability of a beta particle is greater than an alpha particle, but it will only penetrate a few millimeters of tissue and will most probably be shielded out by clothing. Therefore, beta particles, like alpha particles, do not constitute a serious external hazard; however, like alpha particles, they do constitute a serious internal hazard.

NEUTRONS.—Neutrons are emitted from the nucleus of the atom. Their travel is therefore unaffected by the electromagnetic fields of other atoms. The neutron is a penetrating radiation which interacts in billiard-ball fashion with the nucleus of small atoms like hydrogen. This interaction produces high-energy, heavy-ionizing particles that can cause significant biological damage similar to that produced by alpha particles.

GAMMA RAYS.—Gamma rays are electromagnetic waves. Biologically, gamma rays are identical to x-rays of the same energy and frequency. Because they possess no mass or electrical charge, they are the most penetrating form of radiation. Gamma rays produce their effects mainly by knocking orbital electrons out of their path—thereby ionizing the atom so affected—and imparting to the ejected electron. Neutrons and gamma rays are emitted at the time of the nuclear explosion, along with light. Gamma rays and beta particles are present in nuclear fallout along with alpha particles from unfissioned nuclear material. Neutrons and gamma rays are an important medical consideration in a nuclear explosion since their range

is great enough to produce biologic damage, either alone or in conjunction with blast and thermal injuries.

PROTECTION AND TREATMENT

Preparations for the protection and treatment of projected casualties of a nuclear attack must be made in advance of any such assault.

Action before Nuclear Explosion

If there is sufficient warning in advance of an attack, head as quickly as possible for the best shelter available. This is the same procedure as would be used during an attack by ordinary, high-explosive bombs. At the sound of the alarm, get your protective mask ready. Proceed to your station or to a shelter, as ordered. If you are ordered to a shelter, remain there until the "all clear" signal is given.

In the absence of specially constructed shelters during a nuclear explosion ashore, you can get some protection in a foxhole, a dugout, or on the lowest floor or basement of a reinforced concrete or steel-framed building. Generally, the safest place is in the basement near walls. The next best place is on the lowest floor in an interior room, passageway, or hall, away from the windows and, if possible, near a supporting column. Avoid wooden buildings when possible. If you have no choice, take shelter under a table or bed rather than going out into the open. If you have time, draw the shades and blinds to keep out most of the heat from the blast. Only those people in the direct line of sight of thermal emission will be burn casualties; that is, anything that casts a shadow will afford protection. Tunnels, storm drains, and subways can also provide effective shelter.

In the event of a surprise attack, no matter where you are—out in the open on the deck of a ship, in a ship compartment, out in the open ashore, or inside a building—drop to a prone position in a doorway or against a bulkhead or wall. If you have a protective mask with you, put it on. Otherwise, hold or tie a handkerchief over your mouth and nose. Cover yourself with anything at hand, being especially sure to cover the exposed portions of the skin, such as the face, neck, and hands. If this can be done within a second of seeing the bright light of a nuclear explosion, some of the heat radiation may be avoided. Ducking under a table, desk, or bench indoors, or into a trench, ditch, or vehicle outdoors, with the face away from the light, will provide added protection.

Treatment of Nuclear Casualties

Most injuries resulting from the detonation of a nuclear device are likely to be mechanical wounds resulting from collapsing buildings and flying debris, and burns caused by heat and light liberated at the time of detonation.

A burn is a burn, regardless of whether it is caused by a nuclear explosion or by napalm, and its management remains the same. This is also true of fractures, lacerations, mechanical injuries, and shock. In none of these is the treatment dictated by the cause. For most of the conventional injuries, standard first-aid procedures should be followed.

The following word of caution should be considered when you are treating wounds and burns: Dressings for wounds and burns should follow a closed-dressed principle, with application of an adequate sterile dressing using aseptic techniques. Make no attempt to close the wound, regardless of its size, unless authorized by a physician. If signs of infection and fever develop, give antibiotics. When a physician is not available to direct treatment, the Corpsman should select an antibiotic on the basis of availability and appropriateness, and administer **three times** the recommended amount. If the antibiotic does not control the fever, switch to another. If the fever recurs, switch to still another. Overwhelming infection can develop rapidly in the patients due to burns or damage from radiation. Whenever a broad-spectrum antibiotic is given, administer oral antifungal agents.

To date, there is no specific therapy for injuries produced by lethal or sublethal doses of ionizing radiation. This does not mean that all treatment is futile. Good nursing care and aseptic control of all procedures is a must. Casualties should get plenty of rest, light sedation if they are restless or anxious, and a bland, nonresidue diet.

DECONTAMINATION

If you suspect that you are contaminated, or if detection equipment indicates you are, report to a personnel decontamination facility as soon as possible.

Facilities

In a large-scale nuclear catastrophe, there may be numerous casualties suffering not only from mechanical injuries and thermal burns, but from radiation injuries and psychological reactions as well.

The medical facility should consist of a personnel monitoring station, both clean and contaminated emergency treatment stations, a decontamination station, a sorting station, and various treatment stations. It should be set up so that personnel must pass through a monitoring station prior to sorting for medical care. If there is a need for decontamination, the casualty should be routed through the decontamination station on the way to the sorting station. The physical layout should be arranged so that no casualty can bypass the monitoring station and go directly to a treatment station. Also, casualties who are contaminated should be unable to enter clean areas without first passing through a decontamination station. The medical facility flow chart shown in figure 8-3 illustrates an appropriate schema for handling those exposed to nuclear radiation.

TEAMS.—Patients brought in by the rescue teams or arriving on their own should first proceed through the monitoring station to determine whether or not they are contaminated with radioactive material. No medical treatment should be instituted in the monitoring station. Only personnel who have had training and experience as members of Radiological Safety/Decontamination teams or as members of Damage Control parties should be assigned to the monitoring station. Those operating the monitoring station should have a basic knowledge of and experience with radiac instruments. Of the personnel available to the treatment facility, several of those most experienced and knowledgeable in radiological safety and radiation protection should be assigned supervisory jobs in the decontamination station. Also, it is highly desirable to have some personnel with operating room experience to decontaminate patients with traumatic injuries. It is not necessary for the other personnel working in the decontamination station to have any appreciable training or experience other than that given when the medical facility is put into operation.

MONITORS.—After the patients are monitored, they are directed or taken down one of four avenues, depending upon their physical conditions. Those requiring immediate lifesaving measures should be considered contaminated and routed directly through the monitoring station to the contaminated emergency treatment station. Definitive monitoring for these individuals may be performed at the decontamination station. Both treatment stations are set up much the same and should have only those facilities necessary for immediate lifesaving forms of treatment. Personnel working in these stations should be better versed in emergency first-aid care than those used for monitoring and for rescue teams, but they need not be trained in radiation monitoring.

SORTING.—After emergency lifesaving procedures have been attended to, casualties from the clean emergency treatment station should be taken directly to the sorting station, and those from the contaminated treatment station should be taken to the decontamination station. Casualties not requiring immediate emergency treatment should be taken or sent from the monitoring station directly to the sorting station or to the decontamination station, whichever is appropriate. The decontamination station should be set up to take, hold, and dispose of all contaminated clothing and to supply clean replacement clothing after the casualty has been decontaminated. Monitoring equipment will also be required, as will showering and washing facilities, and some capability for surgical (e.g., wound) decontamination when necessary.

Cleaning

Early removal of radioactive "contamination" will reduce radiation burns, radiation dosage, and the chances of inhaling or ingesting radioactive material. There are two rules to be remembered in the removal of radioactive contamination:

- Contamination is easily spread, so "spot" cleaning must be attended to before general decontamination procedures are started.

- Removal of radioactive contamination is best accomplished with soap and water.

SPOT CLEANING.—Cotton swabs or gauze may be used to decontaminate moist areas. Use gummed tapes to decontaminate dry areas. If, after the first cleansing, decontamination is inadequate, the process should be repeated three to five times. If contamination persists, a preparation consisting of a mixture of 50 percent detergent and 50 percent cornmeal, with enough water added to make a paste, should be tried. The contaminated area should be scrubbed (preferably with a soft-bristle surgical brush) for 5 minutes, then rinsed.

GENERAL CLEANING.—After the hot spots have been removed, the second step is to shower with soap and water. Scrub the entire body, including the hair and nails. After the shower, monitor again; if any contamination remains, repeat spot cleaning and shower procedures. If the hair is contaminated, shampoo it several times. If it becomes apparent that shampooing has not removed the radioactive material, cut the hair as close to the scalp as necessary to remove the radioactive material.

If areas become tender from excessive washing, it may be necessary to restore some of the skin oils by gently rubbing in a small amount of lanolin or ordinary hand or face cream. This will soothe the skin and prepare it for further decontamination if additional steps are necessary. Decontamination should be continued until the radioactivity has been reduced to the "safe" level set by the responsible Medical Department representative. Wounds or body parts that resist decontamination may have to be covered and the patient referred to a higher-level medical treatment facility.

UNCONTAMINATED AREAS.—Protect any uncontaminated cut, scratch, or wound with an impermeable tape or other suitable material while decontaminating the rest of the body. If a wound is already contaminated, the simplest and least drastic decontamination method available should be tried first, always by trained medical personnel. First, the wound should be carefully bathed or flushed with sterile water, and a reasonable amount of bleeding should be encouraged. Following decontamination, standard triage procedures are used.

Additional information pertaining to the initial management of irradiated or radioactively contaminated individuals may be obtained from the current version of BUMEDINST 6470.10, *Initial Management of Irradiated or Radioactively Contaminated Personnel.*

Contaminated Material and Supplies

Radiological material may be removed but not destroyed. Water then becomes a special problem. Distillation frees water of radioactive material, providing emergency drinking water. Water coming from an underground source usually is free from radioactive materials and is therefore usable; however, water coming from a reservoir that has to depend upon a surface watershed for its source may not be usable. Fortunately, regular water-treatment processes that include coagulation, sedimentation, and filtration will remove most fallout material, and if the reservoir water can be properly treated, it will be usable again. But for safety's sake, never drink untested water.

SUPPLIES AND FOOD.—Supplies and food can be protected from residual radiation by storage in dust-proof containers. Although the outside of the containers may become contaminated, most of this radioactive material can be removed by washing. The container can then be opened and the contents removed and used without fear of causing significant contamination.

The outer wrappings on medical supplies and the peelings on fruit and vegetables also afford protection to their contents. After carefully removing the outer coverings and checking the contents, it may be found that these materials will be safe to use.

CLOTHING.—Contaminated clothing should be handled with care. Such clothing should never be casually placed on furniture, hung on walls, or dropped on floors, but, instead, should be stored in garbage cans or disposable containers. If these are not available, contaminated clothing should be placed on pieces of paper large enough to be rolled and secured. Grossly contaminated clothing should be properly disposed of by an authorized method, such as burial at sea or in deep pits or trenches, whichever is appropriate. If clothing is in short supply, lightly contaminated clothing may be salvaged by special laundering. Three washings in hot water with detergent should be sufficient. To be sure that this procedure has freed the clothing from radioactive material, each article should be monitored before it is released for reuse. Rubber and plastic materials are readily decontaminated in a warm detergent wash.

SUMMARY

In this chapter we discussed the recognition and treatment of chemical, biological, and radiological (CBR) hazards, and the Medical Department's role in meeting the medical aspects of CBR defense. These included protection from CBR hazards, mass-casualty decontamination, decontamination stations, and supplies for decontamination.

CHAPTER 9

DIET AND NUTRITION

This chapter is concerned with the nutritional requirements for the healthy person, and for the sick, wounded, and convalescing patient. Research has confirmed that good health depends in part upon the availability of essential nutrients the body requires throughout life. The well-nourished individual is usually mentally alert, is at a maximum of physical capability, and has a high resistance to disease. The daily basic minimum nutritional requirements must be met and often supplemented during periods of illness to meet the changing needs of the body and its ability to use foods. Therefore, the diet is an important factor in the therapeutic plan for each patient.

The important role of nutrition in overall health is widely recognized. As a member of the Navy, you must be healthy to perform your professional duties. Part of maintaining a healthy lifestyle starts with eating a well-balanced diet and maintaining a good fitness regimen. Many people in the Navy and Marine Corps do not maintain a proper daily diet. As a Hospital Corpsman, you may be responsible for providing nutritional counseling and, perhaps, even motivation. You have an added responsibility to observe for additional nutritional needs and omissions and to advise your shipmates when necessary. If you stay healthy and energetic, the knowledge and experience you share and the example you set may help your shipmates adopt and maintain a healthier lifestyle.

Balancing energy intake and expenditure can be difficult, both when activity levels are high as well as when they are very low. Typically, body weight remains constant when energy intake equals expenditure (fig. 9–1). The energy balance equation can be "unbalanced" by changing energy intake, energy expenditure, or both. To gain or lose 1 pound requires that approximately 3,500 extra calories be consumed or burned.

FOOD CLASSIFICATION

LEARNING OBJECTIVE: *Identify the components of good nutrition.*

Foods are substances from animal and plant sources that yield heat and energy when ingested and

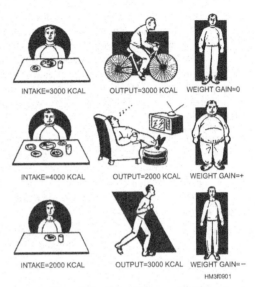

INTAKE=3000 KCAL   OUTPUT=3000 KCAL   WEIGHT GAIN=0

INTAKE=4000 KCAL   OUTPUT=2000 KCAL   WEIGHT GAIN=+

INTAKE=2000 KCAL   OUTPUT=3000 KCAL   WEIGHT GAIN=–

HM3f0901

Figure 9–1.—Balancing energy intake.

absorbed by the body. Food nutrients build and renew tissues and regulate the body processes. The unit commonly used for describing energy intake and energy expenditure is the calorie. Good food sources contain substantial amounts of nutrients in relation to caloric content and provide upwards of 10 percent of the U.S. Recommended Dietary Allowance for each specific nutrient. Most people can get enough of each required nutrient daily by eating a wide variety of foods.

PROTEINS

Proteins are the "building blocks" of the body and provide important required nutritive elements. Proteins are needed for growth, maintenance, and replacement of body cells, and they form hormones and enzymes used to regulate body processes. Extra protein is either used to supply energy or is changed into body fat. Found in both the animal and plant kingdoms, all proteins are composed of amino acids. Some amino acids are absolutely essential to maintain life and are necessary for repair, growth, and body development. Of the approximately 20 amino acids, our body can produce all but nine. These nine amino acids are termed "essential amino acids." We must get them from food, and we need all nine at one time so our body can use them effectively.

Proteins, which promote tissue growth and renewal, have long been recognized as the main structural unit of all living cells. Each gram (g) of protein yields 4 calories in the process of metabolism. Although proteins yield energy, they are an expensive source. If sufficient carbohydrates are not supplied, the body will use protein for energy requirements. This protein may be obtained from muscle tissue, producing the "wasting effect" of long-term starvation and some diseases.

A constant protein source is required in the daily diet. The normal daily protein intake for adults should be 0.8 gram per kilogram (g/kg) (2.2 lbs) of body weight, or 12 percent of the total caloric intake. Pregnant women require an additional 10 grams of protein a day over the normal daily intake.

Proteins play an important role in recovering from fractures, burns, and infections. They are also important in healing wounds and recovering from surgical procedures. In cases of recovery, protein intake should be increased in accordance with the severity of the condition, and carbohydrates and fats can be added liberally. While proteins can supply energy, they are not a main source of energy like carbohydrates and fat.

Ideally, the patient should receive protein by mouth; however, it is sometimes necessary to meet the minimum requirements parenterally. Glucose parenteral solution, given during an acute emergency period, will prevent some loss of protein. Protein deficiency may stunt growth, promote a secondary anemia, or induce nutritional edema. Dietary sources of protein and the nine essential amino acids are milk, yogurt, eggs, meats, fish, cheese, poultry, peanut butter, legumes, and nuts. Protein from plant sources is best when combined with animal protein, such as milk plus peanut butter, or when legumes are combined with grains, such as Navy beans plus rice.

FATS

The chief functions of fats are to supply energy and transport fat-soluble vitamins. Each gram of fat yields 9 calories. Fats provide the most concentrated source of calories (and, therefore, energy) of all the food nutrients. Fats are found in both the animal and vegetable kingdoms. Fatty acids and glycerol are the end products of the digestion of fats.

Many fats act as carriers for the fat-soluble vitamins A, D, E, and K. They also act both as a padding for vital organs, particularly the kidneys, and as subcutaneous tissue to help conserve body heat. Fat is stored as adipose (fatty) tissue to form a reserve supply in time of need. Dietary fats delay gastric emptying and promote a feeling of fullness. Excess calories from fats may produce obesity, the forerunner of arteriosclerosis, hypertension, gallbladder disease, and diabetes. A diet high in fat, especially saturated fat and cholesterol, contributes to elevated blood cholesterol levels in many people. Adults over the age of 30 should have a serum cholesterol level of less than 200 mg/dl. Health experts agree that less than 30 percent of our total calories per day should come from fat. Saturated fat intake should be no more than 10 percent of the total calories.

Reducing dietary fat is also a good way to limit calories. Decreased fat intake results in fewer calories without a reduction of most nutrients. Too little fat in the diet may lead to being underweight, having insufficient padding for the vital organs, and lowered energy. Butter, margarine, cream cheese, fatty meats, whole milk, olives, avocados, egg yolks, nuts, commercial bakery products, and vegetable oils are all sources of dietary fat.

CARBOHYDRATES

Carbohydrates (sugar and starches) are the most efficient sources of energy and are known as the "fuel of life." They are abundantly found in most plant food sources. Complex carbohydrates (starches) are in breads, cereals, pasta, rice, dry beans and peas, and other vegetables, such as potatoes and corn. Simple carbohydrates are found in sugars, honey, syrup, jam, and many desserts. The new nutritional guidelines established by the Food and Drug Administration (FDA) recommend that complex carbohydrates and naturally occurring sugars (found primarily in fruit) make up approximately 50 percent of one's total caloric intake. The FDA also recommends that refined and processed sugars make up no more than 10 percent of the calories in one's diet.

Each gram of carbohydrate yields 4 calories in the process of its metabolism. Carbohydrates must be reduced to glucose before the body can use them. Carbohydrates are stored in the muscles to fuel their movement, and in the liver as glycogen, which is then broken down and released as glucose at the exact rate needed by the body. This latter mechanism is controlled largely by insulin from the pancreas. During fasting, liver glycogen is rapidly depleted, leading the body to use its fat for energy. Carbohydrates that are not needed for energy are converted to and stored as adipose (fat) tissue.

The main functions of carbohydrates are to

- furnish the main source of energy for muscular work and nutritive processes,

- help maintain body temperature,

- form reserve fuel,

- assist in oxidation of fats, and

- spare protein for growth and repair.

MINERALS

Although mineral elements constitute only a small portion of the total body weight, they enter into the activities of the body to a much greater degree than their weight would indicate. Certain mineral elements are essential for specific body functions. While it is not yet known exactly how many of the mineral elements are indispensable to the body functions, seemingly small changes of mineral concentration can be fatal. These essential inorganic elements contribute overwhelmingly to the skeletal framework of the body and teeth, and they are an essential part of many organic compounds.

Minerals form an integral part of basic cell structure and circulate in body fluids. They also exercise specific physiologic influences on the function of body tissues. For mineral needs to be met satisfactorily, consumption of each element must be sufficient to cover body tissue requirements and to meet changing physiological needs. At one time, it was erroneously believed that any diet adequate in other respects would also provide an adequate intake of essential minerals. This is not so. Foods vary greatly in their mineral—as well as their overall nutritional—content, depending on growing conditions, storage, and preparation procedures. Among the major minerals are calcium, phosphorus, iron, potassium, zinc, and magnesium. Table 9–1 lists the essential elements, the foods that contain them, and their functions.

VITAMINS

Vitamins are essential compounds that are present in food in minute quantities. Although vitamins do not furnish energy or act as tissue-building materials, they do act as catalysts in many body chemical reactions and are necessary for normal metabolic functions, growth, and the health of the human body. Their absence results in malnutrition and specific deficiency diseases. Vitamin chemistry is complex and nutritional experimentation is difficult, so our knowledge of them is being continually supplemented and revised. It is quite possible that additional vitamins will be discovered or that some of those already recognized may prove to contain more than one factor.

Vitamins are so widely distributed in food that a properly prepared normal diet usually provides an adequate amount. Vitamins can be destroyed during the preparation or preservation of certain foods; however, manufacturers frequently add vitamins to their products to replace those destroyed or removed in processing. Since fat-soluble vitamins can be stored in the body, it is possible to develop hypervitaminosis by consuming excessive amounts of these nutrients, and death may result in extreme cases. Fat-soluble vitamins include A, D, E, and K.

- **Vitamin A** is involved in the formation and maintenance of healthy skin, hair, and mucous membranes. Vitamin A helps us to see in dim light and is necessary for proper bone growth, tooth development, and reproduction. Good sources of vitamin A include yellow, orange, and dark green vegetables; fruits; and liver, eggs, cheese, butter, and milk.

- **Vitamin D** promotes calcium and phosphorus absorption and is required for the formation of healthy bones and teeth. Good sources include fortified milk, egg yolk, liver, tuna, and cod liver oil. Vitamin D is produced in the body on exposure to sunlight.

- **Vitamin E** protects vitamin A and essential fatty acids from oxidation in the body cells and prevents breakdown of body tissues. Good sources include vegetable oils, fortified cereals, whole-grain cereals and bread, nuts, wheat germ, and green leafy vegetables.

- **Vitamin K** includes a group of vitamins that promote normal clotting of the blood and helps maintain normal liver functions. Good sources

Table 9–1.—Mineral Elements in Nutrition

Element	Rich Sources	Function in the Body
Iodine	Seafood, water, and plant life in nongoiterous regions, and iodized salt	Assists in normal functioning of the thyroid gland.
Sodium	Table salt, seafood, animal products, and foods processed with sodium	Regulates osmotic pressure, pH balance, and heartbeat.
Potassium	Avocados, bananas, oranges, potatoes, tomatoes, nuts, meat, coffee, tea, milk, and molasses	Regulates osmotic pressure and pH balance. A constituent of all cells.
Magnesium	Nuts, whole-grain cereals, legumes, and vegetables	Assists in maintaining mineral balance.
Calcium	Milk, yogurt, cheese, some green vegetables, molasses, sardines, and salmon	Assists in blood coagulation; regulates heartbeat, aids in regulating mineral metabolism and muscle and nerve response. A constituent of bones and teeth.
Phosphorus	Milk, yogurt, poultry, fish, meats, cheese, nuts, cereals, and legumes	Aids in metabolizing organic foodstuffs and maintains pH balance. A constituent of bones and teeth.
Iron	Liver, egg yolks, oyster, legumes, whole or fortified grains, dark and green vegetables, and dried fruit	Helps carry oxygen throughout the body. A constituent of hemoglobin, blood, and tissue.
Chlorine	Table salt, seafoods, and animal products	Regulates osmotic pressure. A constituent of gastric acid.
Sulphur	Protein foods	Promotes hair and nail formation and growth. A constituent of all body tissue.
Copper	Liver, kidney, nuts, dried legumes, some shellfish, and raisins	Aids in the use of iron in hemoglobin synthesis.
Zinc	Meat, liver, eggs, seafood (especially oysters), milk, and whole-grain products	Regulates growth, taste acuity, and appetite. A constituent of enzymes.

are green leafy vegetables, liver, soybean, and other vegetable products.

Water-soluble vitamins, such as vitamin C and the B-complex vitamins, are not stored in the body to any great extent. Rather, they are used as necessary by the body, and any amounts that remain are excreted in the urine. As a result, these vitamins must be replenished daily to ensure optimum health.

- **Vitamin C** (ascorbic acid) is necessary for normal growth and cell activity and is important for maintaining blood vessel strength. It helps the body resist upper respiratory infections and is necessary for the proper development of teeth and gums. Wounds and burns require vitamin C for healing. A deficiency of ascorbic acid causes an individual to bruise easily. A severe deficiency leads to a condition known as scurvy. Good sources include citrus fruits, raw leafy vegetables, and tomatoes.

- **Vitamin B (Complex)** includes more than 12 separate B vitamins. Some of the more common B vitamins are

—**Thiamin (B$_1$)** is necessary for normal growth, normal carbohydrate metabolism and normal functioning of the heart, nerves, and muscles. Thiamin deficiency results in retarded growth and nerve disorders, and a condition known as beriberi. Good sources include pork, fish, eggs, and whole-grain cereals.

—**Riboflavin (B$_2$)** is required for normal growth, vigor, healthy skin and mucosa, and normal eye function. Riboflavin is found in milk products, green leafy vegetables, and eggs. Other good sources of vitamin B$_2$ are the organ meats, heart, kidney, and liver.

—**Niacin (B$_3$)** is necessary for normal growth and skin health, normal functioning of the stomach and intestines, nervous and circulatory systems, and for carbohydrate, fat, and protein metabolism. The best sources are meat, liver, poultry, and peanuts.

—**Pyridoxine (B$_6$)** is necessary for fat, carbohydrate, and protein metabolism, and is sometimes used to treat nausea in pregnancy. Sources include liver, yeast, wheat germ, pork, potatoes, and milk. Vitamin B$_6$ is usually prescribed with Isonizid (INH) treatment since INH often causes a pyridoxine deficiency.

—**Cyanocobalamin (B$_{12}$)** is necessary for the health of nervous tissue and assists in iron metabolism and the maturation process of red blood cells. B$_{12}$ is used to prevent pernicious anemia. The best sources are liver and kidneys, milk, eggs, fish, and cheese.

See Appendix IV for more information on vitamins.

VITAMIN AND MINERAL SUPPLEMENTS

Vitamin supplements are usually not necessary if a diet includes a wide variety of foods. Exceptions may occur in prenatal diets in which iron is low, as well as in patients who are deficient in a specific vitamin. Vitamin supplements should be taken only on a physician or dietitian's recommendation.

Vitamin and mineral supplements are being widely used by physically active people because of all the performance-enhancing claims made by supplement manufacturers. It is estimated that 40–50 percent of athletes use some form of vitamin/mineral supplements. Some doses range from amounts similar to the Recommended Dietary Allowances (RDA) up to levels many times the RDA. Supplements are useful under a variety of conditions, such as if an individual

- has an existing vitamin or mineral deficiency;

- has poor nutrient intake and/or dietary habits; or

- is exposed to extreme environmental conditions, such as altitude.

Often, laxatives are prescribed in conjunction with some medical treatments and may cause decreased absorption of vitamins, loss of minerals and elec- trolytes, or inhibition of glucose uptake. Therefore, any patient on laxatives should be carefully monitored, and supplementary nutritives should be administered as necessary.

Taking a general multivitamin supplement appears to be without measurable performance enhancing effects in healthy, well-nourished, physically active personnel. Similarly, no improvements in muscle strength or endurance have been noted in strength athletes, such as body builders, who tend to use megadoses of vitamin and mineral supplements. The indiscriminate use of high-potency vitamins and minerals is of growing concern since excessive amounts of vitamins and/or minerals can be harmful and may result in nutrient imbalances. Excessive intake of some vitamin and mineral supplements can result in adverse—and possibly toxic–side effects.

WATER

Water is often called the "forgotten nutrient." Water is needed to replace body fluids lost primarily in urine and sweat. A person can survive weeks without food but only days without water. Water makes up 70 percent of body weight and is found in every cell in the body. It is the medium through which nutrients are transported from the digestive tract to the cells where they are needed. Water is also the medium through which the by-products of cell metabolism are removed.

Water also serves as the medium in which the chemical processes of life take place. It is normally taken into the body in beverages, soups, and in the form of solid foods. Fluid needs are increased with sweating, vomiting, diarrhea, high-protein diets, and in hot environments. An insufficient intake may cause dehydration, evidenced by loss of weight, increased body temperature, and dizziness.

GUIDE TO GOOD EATING

LEARNING OBJECTIVE: *Recall the elements of the USDA Food Guide Pyramid and recommended dietary guidelines.*

Calculating a therapeutic diet can be complicated and is best left to dietitians. It is now common practice for dietitians or dietary kitchens to select foods for diets using the food groups outlined in figure 9–2, the Food Guide Pyramid. These foods are classified according to their nutritional value and the number of servings that should be eaten each day.

THE FOOD GUIDE PYRAMID

The Food Guide Pyramid emphasizes foods from the five food groups shown in the sections of the pyramid. Each of these groups provides some, but not all, of the nutrients we require. For good health we need them all. For everyday living, the simplest and most practical plan is to follow those same guidelines, selecting from the various food groups the type and amount of food recommended.

DIETARY GUIDELINES

The food pyramid graphically communicates the message of the Dietary Guidelines for Americans. Diets should be built upon a base of complex carbohydrates and less fats. The placement of the food groups starting at the base of the pyramid conveys the current recommendations. These recommendations are as follows:

- Eat more grains, vegetables, and fruits

- Eat moderate amounts of lean meats and dairy foods

- Use sweets, fats, and oils sparingly

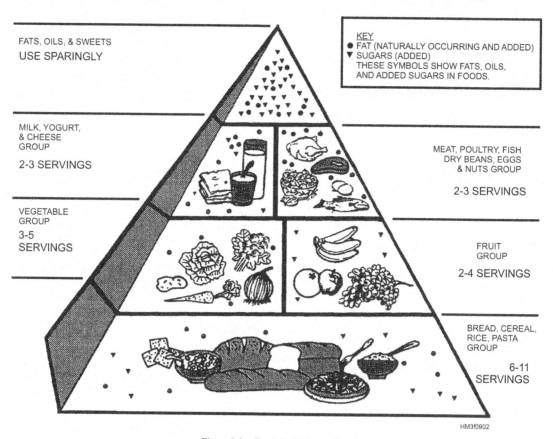

FATS, OILS, & SWEETS
USE SPARINGLY

KEY
● FAT (NATURALLY OCCURRING AND ADDED)
▼ SUGARS (ADDED)
THESE SYMBOLS SHOW FATS, OILS, AND ADDED SUGARS IN FOODS.

MILK, YOGURT, & CHEESE GROUP
2-3 SERVINGS

MEAT, POULTRY, FISH DRY BEANS, EGGS & NUTS GROUP
2-3 SERVINGS

VEGETABLE GROUP
3-5 SERVINGS

FRUIT GROUP
2-4 SERVINGS

BREAD, CEREAL, RICE, PASTA GROUP
6-11 SERVINGS

HM3f0902

Figure 9-2.—Food Guide Pyramid.

Generally accepted guidelines suggest that you eat a diet that is high in complex carbohydrates and low in protein and fat. Your diet should consist of at least five combined servings of fruits and vegetables each day. Avoid fat when possible. Eat at regular intervals when possible, and avoid snacking late at night. For detailed information on nutrition, consult *Navy Nutrition and Weight Control Guide,* NAVPERS 15602; and the *Fat, Cholesterol and Calorie List for General Messes,* NAVSUP 580.

DIET THERAPY

LEARNING OBJECTIVE: *Select the appropriate diet for various medical conditions.*

It is often necessary to cater to a patient's appetite, since many individuals become especially hard to please when sick. In some disease states, such as cancer, patients experience marked taste changes. Because of the importance of the nutritional elements in feeding the sick, try to carry out the patient's wishes whenever possible. A tactful and observant Hospital Corpsman can be of great benefit to the physician and dietitian in carrying out the dietary regimen. You must be aware of what comprises a well-balanced diet and should be able to recognize when dietary adjustments need to be made in special situations. This is important to meet the changing needs of the diseased body's ability to make use of foods.

The patient should be made to feel that the utmost cleanliness and care have been observed in the preparation and service of their food. The patient's face and hands should be cleaned before food is served, and the lips and teeth cleaned before and after the meal. If the mouth is dry, it should be moistened periodically.

When special or modified diets are ordered, check the contents of the tray with the written orders. An error in serving a special diet may cause discomfort, serious illness, or even death.

OBJECTIVES OF DIET THERAPY

The objectives of diet therapy are as follows:

- To increase or decrease body weight

- To rest a particular organ

- To adjust the diet to the body's ability to use certain foods

- To produce a specific effect as a remedy (e.g., regulation of blood sugar in diabetes)

- To overcome deficiencies by the addition of food rich in some necessary element (e.g., supplementing the diet with iron in treating macrocytic anemia)

- To provide ease of digestion by omitting irritating substances, such as fiber, spices, or high-fat foods

TYPES OF DIETS

Diets used in the treatment of disease are often spoken of by specific names that show a special composition and often indicate the purpose for which the diet is intended.

Regular Diet

The regular diet is composed of all types of foods and is well balanced and capable of maintaining a state of good nutrition. It is intended for convalescing patients who do not require a therapeutic diet.

Modified or Therapeutic Diets

Modified or therapeutic diets are modifications of the regular diet and are designed to meet specific patient needs. These include

- method of preparation (e.g., baking, boiling, or broiling),

- consistency (e.g., ground or chopped),

- total calories (e.g., high or low calorie),

- nutrients (e.g., altering carbohydrate, protein, fat, vitamins, and minerals), and

- allowing only specific foods (e.g., diabetic diet).

SOFT DIET.—The soft diet is soft in texture and consists of liquids and semi-solid foods. It is indicated in certain postoperative cases, for convalescents who cannot tolerate a regular diet, in acute illnesses, and in some gastrointestinal disorders. A soft diet is an intermediate step between a liquid and regular diet and is low in connective tissue and indigestible dietary fiber. Little or no spices are used in its preparation.

The soft diet includes all liquids other than alcohol, and foods that may be incorporated into a soft diet include well-cooked cereals, pastas, white bread and crackers, eggs, cottage cheese, tender meat, fish, poultry, and vegetables (including baked, mashed, and scalloped potatoes). Vegetables can be puréed and meats ground for dental patients. Permitted desserts are custards, gelatin puddings, soft fruits, and simple cakes and cookies. Foods prohibited in a soft diet include fried foods, raw vegetables, and nuts.

LIQUID DIET.—A liquid diet consists of foods that are in a liquid state at body temperature. This type of diet is indicated in some postoperative cases, in acute illnesses, and in inflammatory conditions of the gastrointestinal (GI) tract. It is important that feedings consisting of 6 to 8 ounces or more be given every 2 to 3 hours while the patient is awake.

Liquid diets are usually ordered as clear, full, or dental liquid. A **clear liquid diet** includes clear broth, black tea or coffee, plain gelatin, and clear fruit juices (apple, grape, and cranberry), popsicles, fruit drinks, and soft drinks. This diet is inadequate in all nutrients. A **full liquid diet** includes all the liquids served on a clear liquid diet, with the addition of strained cream soups, milk and milk drinks, ice cream, puddings, and custard. The full liquid diet is inadequate in iron, niacin, and possibly Vitamin A and thiamin. A **dental liquid diet** includes regular foods blended and strained in liquid form and all foods allowed on clear and full liquid diets. Vitamin and mineral supplements may be necessary with the dental liquid diet if the recommended amounts of food are not tolerated.

HIGH-CALORIE DIET.—The high-calorie diet is of a higher caloric value than the average patient normally requires. A high-calorie diet is indicated when an increase of total calories is required by malnourished, underweight, postsurgical, or convalescing patients, especially those recovering from acute illnesses such as infections, burns, and fevers. The increase in calories is obtained by supplementing or modifying the regular diet with high-calorie foods or commercial supplements, by giving larger portions, or by adding snacks. It is given to meet a need for energy caused by the more rapid metabolism that accompanies certain diseases (especially fever, hyperthyroidism, poliomyelitis, and tuberculosis). In the liquid or soft diet, adding fats and carbohydrates increases the caloric value. The high-calorie diet is often ordered along with high protein. Proteins are added to prevent depletion of proteins in the plasma (a condition known as hypoproteinemia). As the patient progresses, a more solid diet is given.

Good sources of high-calorie foods are whole milk, cream, sweets, butter, margarine, fried foods, gravy, sauces, and ice cream. Between-meal feedings consisting of milk, milkshakes, cheese, cookies, or sandwiches are recommended, but these feedings should not interfere with the patient's appetite at mealtime.

HIGH-PROTEIN DIET.—As previously stated, protein is essential for tissue growth and regeneration. A high-protein diet is indicated in almost all illnesses (e.g., nephrosis, cirrhosis of the liver, infectious hepatitis, burns, radiation injury, fractures, some GI disorders, conditions in which the protein blood level is low, and in preoperative and postoperative cases).

In some acute illnesses and disorders, such as infectious hepatitis, GI disorders, and postoperative conditions, patients may be unable to consume solid foods or the daily requirement of protein and calories because of pain or nausea. In these cases, intravenous fluids with nutrient additives are required for the patient to receive the required amount of protein.

Protein-calorie deficiency is a definite factor in postoperative wound disruption. This disruption can best be prevented by preemptive nutritional measures before surgery. Antibody production will be decreased if the patient receives inadequate protein. Remember, the daily recommended intake of proteins for adults is at least 0.8 g/kg of body weight (approximately 56 g). A high-protein diet should provide a minimum of 1.5 g of protein per kg of body weight (approximately 105 g). The seriously burned and radiation injury patients should receive at least 3.0 g/kg daily.

Supplement the regular diet with high-quality protein foods, such as meat, fish, cheese, milk, and eggs.

LOW-CALORIE DIET.—The low-calorie diet is useful in the treatment of obesity, but it may also be used to control weight in medical conditions such as arthritis, hypertension, diabetes, cardiac disease, or hypothyroidism. A loss of 1 to 2 pounds per week is the medically acceptable limit for weight reduction. A low-calorie diet consists of 1,000 to 1,800 calories per day. Calorie levels are determined by physicians and dietitians to help meet specific individual patient weight-loss goals. The daily intake of proteins should be at least 0.8 g/kg of standard body weight. Supplemental vitamins may be ordered if the prescribed diet is less than 1,200 calories.

Patients on low-calorie diets should be instructed by the dietitian (if available) or other medical personnel knowledgeable in proper eating habits. The dietitian conducts patient interviews to learn the patient's eating behaviors, usual portions, preparation of foods, meal patterns, nutritional adequacy, exercise, and so forth. Individual programs should then be recommended to assist patients to attain and maintain their ideal weight.

The *Handbook of Clinical Dietetics,* published by the American Dietetic Association, lists the following formula for determining ideal body weight. For females, the basic weight for 5 feet is 100 pounds. Add 5 pounds for every inch over 5 feet. For males, the basic weight for 5 feet is 106 pounds, with 6 pounds added for every inch over 5 feet. Adjustments must be made for body build. Reduce desired weight by 10 percent for a small frame; increase it by 10 percent for a large frame. Total caloric requirements are based on ideal body weight plus activity.

Many patients on low-calorie diets experience hunger. To satisfy this hunger or appetite, low-calorie foods such as raw vegetables, broth, black coffee or tea, and other unsweetened or diet beverages should be provided. Water and sodium need not be restricted unless there are cardiac complications or edema, and the restrictions are ordered by the physician.

LOW-PROTEIN DIET.—As the name implies, the low-protein diet is made up of foods that furnish only small amounts of protein and consist largely of carbohydrates and fats (e.g., foods such as marshmallows, hard candy, and butter). This diet is used in renal diseases associated with nitrogen retention or liver disorders. Limited amounts of protein are sometimes advocated in certain kidney diseases (such as chronic nephrotic edema). Low-protein diets for renal failure are usually restricted in sodium and potassium, because these two elements are not excreted properly during this condition. In some cases of chronic renal insufficiency, the protein content of the diet is varied, usually between 40 and 60 g per day, so that there will be sufficient complete protein to maintain nitrogen equilibrium.

In some metabolic disturbances, such as amino acids in the urine, protein restriction may be of therapeutic value.

HIGH-RESIDUE DIET.—The high-residue (high-bulk, high-fiber, high-roughage) diet is indicated in atonic constipation, spastic colon, irritable bowel syndrome, and diverticulosis. This diet encourages regular elimination by stimulating muscle tone, creating softer and larger stools that are more easily propelled through the colon, thereby reducing the pain and cramping that accompany spastic colon or irritable bowel syndrome.

The patient is given a regular diet, with the inclusion of high-residue foods. The main sources of fiber are whole-grain breads and cereals, bran cereals, fresh fruits, and vegetables that are raw or cooked until tender. Whole grain breads and cereals that contain wheat bran have a greater laxative effect than fruits and vegetables, because the bran acts to absorb water within the colon, creating a bulk effect. Fiber intake should be increased gradually to minimize potential side effects of bloating, cramps, and diarrhea. At least one serving of 100 percent wheat bran cereal is recommended daily. Cereals such as raisin bran, Bran Flakes®, Shredded Wheat®, and oatmeal may be used occasionally, but they contain less than half the amount of fiber found in All-Bran® or Bran Buds®. Fresh fruits and vegetables with edible skins, such as apples and grapes, are higher in fiber content than canned fruits or vegetables and their juices.

Dietary intake of refined sugars and starches should be decreased because they are poor sources of fiber. Also, limit white flour products, refined cereals, pies, cakes, and cookies.

Too little fluid in the high-residue diet may cause dehydration and lead to constipation. The patient must drink at least eight 8-ounce glasses of water or other fluids daily, particularly when consuming the recommended amount of bran. Drinking too much alcohol, beverages containing caffeine (such as coffee, cola, tea, and soft drinks), however, can irritate a sensitive colon and can cause dehydration. When possible, use decaffeinated coffee. One or two glasses of water in the morning help to stimulate peristalsis. Excessive intake of foods like dried beans, fruits with seeds and skins, nuts, popcorn, and strong spices may cause irritability, especially during the inflammation period of colon disease states. These foods should be individualized to the patient.

When one is progressing from a low-residue diet after an acute infection or diverticulitis, increase fiber in the diet gradually. Start by adding one serving of 100 percent bran cereal and three servings of whole-grain bread to the low-residue menu pattern. Gradually increase the amount of raw vegetables and fresh fruits to at least four servings per day.

LOW-RESIDUE DIET.—The low-residue diet is indicated in ulceration, inflammation, and other gastric disorders (such as partial intestinal obstruction or diverticulitis). It is also used in certain postoperative states that affect any part of the GI tract, e.g., a hemorrhoidectomy. Low-residue diets are also used in treating dysenteries of long duration.

The purpose of this diet is to provide non-stimulating, non-irritating, and easily digested material that leaves little residue, thus avoiding mechanical irritation of the GI tract. Various commercially prepared low-residue elemental diet supplements may be given to provide complete nutrition.

LOW-SODIUM DIET.—A low-sodium diet consists of foods containing a very small percentage of sodium, with no salt added in preparation or by the patient. It is impossible to prepare an absolutely sodium-free diet.

The low-sodium diet is indicated when edema is present, in renal diseases, hypertension, and certain cardiac conditions.

The nephrotic patient is often unable to excrete sodium in a normal manner because the kidneys' retention of sodium leads to edema. A low-sodium diet is thus indicated, with no restriction on salt-free liquids. Such patients should be encouraged to drink 2,000 to 3,000 milliliters (ml) of low-sodium fluids daily.

The allowance of sodium in a strict low-sodium diet is 250 to 1,000 mg daily. The allowance of sodium in a moderate low-sodium diet is 2,000 mg or 2 g. Regular diets with no salt added contain 2.4 to 4.5 g of sodium.

Any diet in which the amount of sodium is drastically reduced has possible side effects. The patient who is on this diet regimen must be constantly observed—particularly in warm climates—for lassitude, complaints of weakness, anorexia, nausea and vomiting, mental confusion, abdominal cramps, and aching skeletal muscles. Electrolyte imbalances can have serious consequences. If you observe symptoms such as those described above, notify a medical officer.

BLAND DIET.—A bland diet may be helpful for gastritis, hyperacidity, hemorrhoids, peptic ulcers, and other GI disorders. Dietary management of patients with chronic ulcer disease has been the subject of much controversy. Bland diets have traditionally been used for these patients. However, experiments show that there is no significant difference in the response of patients with an active duodenal ulcer to a bland diet. Known irritants to the gastric mucosa include alcohol, black pepper, caffeine, chili powder, cocoa, coffee, certain drugs, and tea.

Emphasizing *how* to eat is as important as indicating *what* foods to eat, since there are individual responses to bland diets. Offer the following suggestions to the patient:

- Avoid worry and emotional upsets at mealtime
- Chew food well and eat slowly
- Rest before and after meals
- Avoid foods of extreme temperatures

If fruits and juices between meals cause distress, try including them with meals. Meals must be kept small to reduce gastric acidity and distention. Among foods to avoid in the bland diet are

- fatty meats,
- fried foods,
- whole-grain breads and cereals,
- dried beans and peas,
- cabbage-family vegetables,
- chocolate,
- nuts and seeds, and
- carbonated beverages, caffeine, coffee, and tea.

Patients on a bland diet may use spices and condiments such as allspice, cinnamon, mace, paprika, sage, thyme, catsup, cranberry or mint jelly, and extract and flavorings without chocolate or vinegar.

The bland diet allows a more liberal food selection than other restrictive diets. This diet reduces the number of meals to three, and increases the quantity of foods given. Individualize the diet to the patient.

The "Regular-No Stimulants Diet" (also called "liberal bland"), a type of bland diet, eliminates **only** those items that have been shown scientifically to irritate the gastric mucosa (i.e., alcohol, black pepper, caffeine, chili powder, cocoa, coffee, certain drugs, and tea).

Decaffeinated coffee may be restricted in most types of bland diets. Recent studies show that it causes increased gastric acid secretion and esophageal pressure causing gastric acid reflux in the esophagus. Decaffeinated coffee is only offered on the bland diet and the regular-no stimulants diet if it is tolerated by the patient.

Chronic and excessive use of antacids to treat hyperacidity and related conditions may result in thiamin deficiency, presumably because of alkaline destruction of thiamin within the bowel lumen. Excessive intake of milk with antacids may cause systemic alkalosis and hypercalcemia. Milk may be contraindicated in patients with allergic reactions or lactose intolerance.

LOW-CARBOHYDRATE, HIGH-PROTEIN DIET.—A low-carbohydrate, high-protein diet is used in the treatment of hypoglycemia. This diet limits simple carbohydrates that are quickly absorbed into the blood. A marked rise in blood sugar stimulates the pancreas to overproduce insulin, which leads to a hypoglycemic state as too much sugar is transported out of the blood.

Individualize the diet to the patient, since hypoglycemic reactions may occur at any time for various reasons. For example, meal skipping, inadequate calorie intake with excessive energy expenditure, and drinking alcohol may precipitate a low-blood-sugar reaction.

The foods may be divided into three to six or more small meals. Liberal amounts of protein and fat are used, as they are more slowly digested and absorbed. The diet includes meats, fish, poultry, cheese, eggs, fats, low-starch vegetables, and limited amounts of unsweetened fruit and juices, breads, cereals, and high-starch-content vegetables (like corn, peas, and potatoes). Because milk contains the sugar lactose, limit it to 2 cups a day for an adult.

Sweets such as candy, sugar, jams, jellies, soft drinks, and pastries should be avoided to help prevent hypoglycemic reactions. They should be consumed only when necessary to quickly increase blood-sugar levels during a hypoglycemic reaction. If reactions are frequent, it is helpful to carry hard candy for quick and easy use. Handy high-protein snacks to help prevent hypoglycemic reactions may include cheese, peanut butter, milk, and hard-boiled eggs.

SUMMARY

Fulfilling the daily requirement of eating a wide variety of foods, in the correct amounts, will contribute directly to a healthy lifestyle. Well-nourished crewmembers with good health are much more able to resist infections, are able to sleep soundly and awake with a pleasant demeanor. By using your knowledge of diet therapy and nutrition to train and treat your crew, your job will be made significantly easier.

EMERGENCY DENTAL CARE AND PREVENTIVE MEDICINE

TERMINAL OBJECTIVE: *Be familiar with the subject matter and technical publications relating to emergency dental care and preventive medicine.*

Because of the nature of our rating and the many responsibilities placed upon us, Hospital Corpsmen must have a general understanding of many areas of medicine. Emergency dental care and preventive medicine practices are two of those areas. Both of these subjects are extremely important, but because they are both already discussed in great detail in other Navy publications, this chapter will present only a brief overview of them. Emergency Dental Care is covered in Section I, and Preventive Medicine is addressed in Section II. For in-depth information, refer to the publications outlined respectively in table 10-1.

SECTION I

EMERGENCY DENTAL CARE

In the absence of a dental officer you, as the medical department representative (MDR), will be required to perform basic emergency dental first aid associated with the most common oral conditions and injuries. While this section will introduce you to the basics of dental anatomy and histology, dental terminology, oral diseases and injuries, and the dental record, you will find in-depth discussion of these areas in the DT and HM Advancement Handbooks; chapter 6 of *Dental Technician Training Manual, Volume 1,* NAVEDTRA 12572; and in chapter 6 of the *Manual of the Medical Department,* NAVMED P-117.

The primary function of this emergency dental care is to alleviate pain, arrest hemorrhage, or prevent further or complicating injury to dental structures. Ensuring that the entire crew is in good dental health before deployment will prevent most dental-related

Table 10-1.—Publication List

Dental	*DT Advancement Handbook*
	HM Advancement Handbook
	Dental Technician Training Manual, Vol. 1, NAVEDTRA 12572
	Dental Technician Training Manual, Vol. 2, NAVEDTRA 12573
	Manual of the Medical Department, NAVMED P-117, chapter 6
	Various BUMED notes and instructions
	Various SECNAV and OPNAV notes and instructions
Preventive Medicine	*HM Advancement Handbook*
	Manual of Naval Preventive Medicine, NAVMED P-5010
	Control of Communicable Diseases Manual, NAVMED P-5038
	Naval Supply Publication 486
	Various BUMED notes and instructions
	Various SECNAV and OPNAV notes and instructions

problems. Therefore, predeployment examinations are very important.

You must administer only **emergency** dental care. Refer routine cases to a dental treatment facility, and refer any cases treated by nondental personnel for follow-up at the earliest opportunity.

DENTAL ANATOMY AND HISTOLOGY

To provide emergency dental care, you will need to be familiar with dental anatomy and histology. The following sections will provide you with basic information; however, if you require more detailed information on dental anatomy and histology, consult the *Dental Technician Training Manual, Volume 1,* NAVEDTRA 12572, or contact your local dental treatment facility for references.

Dental Anatomy

The adult mouth normally has 32 permanent teeth. On board ship, you will usually be able to refer a patient to a dentist for a dental problem. When you do have to make such a referral, you must be able to correctly describe the problem and its location (e.g., which tooth, which surface of the tooth, etc.) in appropriate dental terminology. Because referrals are infrequent, this required information will not be covered here. However, the information is available in detail in the *Dental Technician Training Manual, Volume 2,* NAVEDTRA 12573.

Dental Histology

Dental anatomy deals with the external form and appearance of the teeth. Dental histology studies the tissues and internal structure of the teeth, along with the tissues that surround and support them. It will be helpful to have a knowledge of dental histology in case you need to provide emergency dental treatment.

Dental Terminology

Knowledge of dental terminology is important to interpret emergency treatment plans prepared by dentists and to prepare consultation sheets for referral to dental treatment facilities. Make sure you use standard dental abbreviations when recording entries in a patient's dental record. You will find some important basic dental-related words and definitions in the next section, "Oral Diseases and Injuries." Both the *Dental Technician Training Manual Volume 2,* NAVEDTRA 12573, and the *Manual of the Medical Department,* NAVMED P-117, will provide you with a more in-depth listing of dental terminology.

ORAL EXAMINATION

Before performing an oral examination, you should review the patient's medical and dental histories. Note the medications the patient is currently taking. The dental health questionnaire should be updated if any significant changes in the patient's health status have occurred since the form was last updated by the patient.

When you examine the oral cavity, use a thorough and systematic approach. You must have a knowledge

of the normal dental anatomy and histology to recognize oral diseases and injuries. The chief complaint that brought the patient to seek treatment will fall into the category of either an oral disease or condition or an oral injury.

The following are brief descriptions of the major oral diseases or conditions and oral injuries that may be seen during an oral examination.

- **Dental caries** are the result of localized decay of the calcified tissues of teeth. Bacterial plaque is the most common cause of dental caries. Bacteria release acids and other toxins that attack tooth enamel and produce carious lesions called **cavities**.

- **Acute pulpitis** is a severe inflammation of the tooth pulp. Usually, it is the result of dental caries.

- A **periapical abscess** usually results from an infection of the tooth pulp, often developing as a result of unchecked pulpitis.

- **Gingivitis** is an inflammation of the gingival tissue. The most frequent cause of marginal gingivitis is poor oral hygiene.

- **Necrotizing ulcerative gingivitis (NUG)** is a severe inflammation of the gingival tissue. NUG may be also referred to as **trench mouth**. NUG is not contagious.

- **Periodontitis** is an inflammatory condition that involves the gingivae, the crest of the alveolar bone, and the periodontal membrane above the alveolar crest.

- A **periodontal abscess** is caused by an infection in the periodontal tissues.

- **Pericoronitis** is an inflammation of the gingiva around a partially erupted tooth. It may also result from constant contact between the tissue flap and a tooth in the opposing arch.

- **Stomatitis** is an inflammation of the oral mucosa.

- **Recurrent labial herpes** is an infection that produces a fever blister or cold sore. Such a lesion is usually found on the lip.

- **Postoperative hemorrhage** may occur any time from a few hours to several days after a tooth extraction. The bleeding from the extraction site may be light or heavy. Treat all abnormal postextraction bleeding as serious.

- **Alveolar osteitis**, also known as **dry socket**, results when a normal clot fails to form in the socket of a recently extracted tooth. Since this condition is usually very painful, always consider it a serious emergency.

- Pain in **fractured teeth** usually results from the irritation of the pulp tissue. Additional information concerning the types of fractures is contained in chapter 6 of the *Dental Technician Training Manual, Volume 1*, NAVEDTRA 12572.

DENTAL RECORD

Each service member's military dental treatment record consists of a *Dental Record Jacket*, NAVMED 6150/21-30, containing dental treatment forms. The form used to record dental treatment is EZ603A. It is imperative that all forms documenting patient care contain adequate treatment information. Additional information concerning dental forms is contained in chapter 2 of the *Dental Technician Training Manual, Volume 2*, NAVEDTRA 12573; and chapter 6 of the *Manual of the Medical Department*, NAVMED P-117.

SECTION SUMMARY

When dental emergencies occur and dental facilities are not readily available, medical personnel are expected to perform basic emergency dental care. This section has provided basic information on fundamental dental histology and a variety of dental conditions. We also discussed the importance of dental record maintenance and dental forms used by medical personnel.

SECTION II

PREVENTIVE MEDICINE

Prevention and control of disease are considered the most desirable means of maintaining good health. Information included in this overview should provide you with a general knowledge of the principles and practices of the Navy's Preventive Medicine afloat and ashore. This information is discussed in detail in the *Manual of Naval Preventive Medicine*, NAVMED P-5010.

SANITATION

Sanitation is defined as the formulation and application of measures designed to protect (military) public health, and the disposal of waste. The goal of the Navy's sanitation program is to provide personnel with a clean and healthy work and living environment.

Personal Hygiene

Because of the close living quarters in the Navy, particularly aboard ships, personal hygiene is of utmost importance: Uncleanliness or disagreeable ordor will surely affect the morale of your shipmates. Disease and other health problems can spread and rapidly affect an entire compartment or division. Good personal hygiene promotes health and prevents disease. You are responsible for presenting health education training programs to the personnel in your unit, including information on the basics of personal hygiene, and proper exercise, sleep, and nutritional requirements.

Sanitation of Living Spaces

You, as the MDR, perform sanitation inspections and provide recommendations to the commanding officer. The living spaces, their inspection, and living space cleaning and maintenance practices are discussed in detail in the *Manual of Preventive Medicine, NAVMED P-5010*.

HABITABILITY

Factors that can effect habitability of working and berthing spaces are air ventilation, heating, and air conditioning.

Measurements of thermal stress are used to monitor environmental conditions in which personnel work, live, and exercise. Monitoring environmental conditions is crucial to maintaining a safe environment for personnel. For more detailed information on the items discussed in this section, you should refer to *Manual of Naval Preventive Medicine*, NAVMED P-5010.

VECTOR AND PEST CONTROL

A **vector** is any animal capable of transmitting pathogens or producing human or animal discomfort or injury. Some of the commonly encountered vectors are insects, arthropods (insects with hard, jointed exoskeleton and paired, jointed legs), and rodents. **Pests**, on the other hand, are organisms (insects, rodents, fungi, bacteria, snakes, etc.) that adversely affect military operations and the well-being of man and animal; attack real property, supplies, and equipment; or are otherwise undesirable. For more detailed information on the items discussed in this section, you should refer to *Manual of Naval Preventive Medicine,* NAVMED P-5010.

FOOD-SERVICE SANITATION

Food-borne illnesses represent an ever-present threat to the health and morale of our military personnel. To prevent food-borne illnesses, you will need to ensure that all foods are procured from approved sources and processed, prepared, and served with careful adherence to recommended sanitary practices. When assigned as a medical department representative for a command or station, you may be given the responsibility of inspecting food, food-service facilities, and investigating food-borne illness outbreaks.

For guidance on safe time limits for keeping food, proper storage temperatures, and storage life of perishable and semi-perishable items, refer to tables in Naval Supply Publication 486.

Training and Hygiene of Food-Service Personnel

Food-service personnel should be thoroughly indoctrinated in personal hygiene and food sanitation procedures and in the methods and importance of preventing food-borne illness. Requirements for food service training are addressed in *Food Service Training Program,* SECNAVINST 4061.1.

Food-Service Inspection Report

Navy and Marine Corps food-service facilities are required to be inspected by a medical department representative, together with the food-service manager or officer or designated representative. The findings of the inspection are reported on a NAVMED Form 6240/1, *Food Service Sanitation Inspection.* A system has been established in which maximum defect points are awarded for each stated requirement. The inspector assigns an appropriate number of defect points up to the maximum possible and computes a sanitary compliance score (SCS). Complete step-by-step procedures for filing the report and computing the SCS are provided in the *Manual of Naval Preventive Medicine,* NAVMED P-5010.

IMMUNIZATIONS AND COMMUNICABLE DISEASES

Navy and Marine Corps personnel are exposed to a wide variety of environmental conditions, including climatic extremes, stressful situations, and close living quarters. Many of these personnel travel to foreign lands where conditions may not only be unsanitary, but where a high level of disease may also exist. Preventive medicine's major role is to minimize disability by emphasizing immunization programs.

Immunizations

Vaccines used to protect Navy and Marine Corps personnel against certain diseases before exposure to infection are called **prophylactic immunizations**. Prophylactic immunizations are limited to very serious diseases for which effective and reliable immunizing agents have been developed.

Immunizations procured for the Armed Forces are required to meet the minimum standards set by the Department of Health and Human Services (DHHS).

Immunizations for Military Personnel

Navy and Marine Corps personnel are required to be ready to deploy on a moment's notice. To make sure personnel are prepared for deployment, you should review their immunization records on a routine basis, and, before deployments, also review BUMEDINST 6230.15, *Immunizations and Chemoprophylaxis.* Initial and booster dosages and routes of administration are dictated by the vaccine manufacture, the U.S. Public Health Service Immunization Practices Advisory Committee (ACIP), or both.

Communicable Diseases

Communicable diseases, as the name implies, are diseases that may be transmitted from a carrier to a susceptible host. They may be transmitted from an infected person or animal or indirectly through an intermediate host, vector, or inanimate object. The illness produced is the result of infectious agents invading and multiplying in the host, or from the release of their toxins (poisons).

An important step in the control of communicable disease is the expedious preparation and submission of the **Medical Event Report**. Instructions and requirements for reporting to local, state, national, and international health authorities can be found in the preface of the *Control of Communicable Diseases Manual,* NAVMED P-5038. In addition, you should follow instructions for the *Medical Event Report* (MER), BUMEDINST 6220.12, when reporting communicable diseases affecting Navy and Marine Corps personnel.

WATER SUPPLY

A hygienically safe and continuously dependable water supply is a necessity of life. Drinking water should be free of disease-producing organisms, poisonous chemicals, as well as from objectionable color, odor, and taste. For more detailed instruction on these topics, you should review the *Manual of Naval Preventive Medicine,* NAVMED P-5010.

Water Supply Ashore

With rare exceptions, Navy and Marine Corps activities ashore within the continental limits of the United States are situated where a municipal water supply is available. BUMEDINST 6240.1, *Standards for Potable Water*, sets drinking water standards for U.S. naval establishments worldwide, both ashore and afloat.

Water Supply in the Field

Hospital Corpsmen are frequently called upon to approve field water sources and to recommend disinfection methods before water is considered safe to drink. Consider water acquired in the field as unsafe until it has been disinfected and tested. Approval of water sources should be based on a thorough surveillance of available water sources.

WATER QUANTITY REQUIREMENTS.— The daily water requirements for personnel in the field vary with a number of factors, including the season of the year, geographical location, and the tactical situation. Personnel who do not drink enough water can quickly become dehydrated both in extremely hot or extremely cold climates.

WATER TREATMENT.—Water treatment is the process of purifying water to make it potable (safe to drink). Various processes can be used to purify water. These processes include **aeration, coagulation, flocculation, filtration, reverse osmosis,** and **disinfection,** all of which are discussed in depth in NAVMED P-5010.

Water Supply Afloat

Potable water for shipboard use comes from one of several sources: the ship's distillation plant, shore-to-ship delivery, or ship-to-ship transfer. The ship's medical department is responsible for determining the quality of the water. The ships engineering section determines the quantity stored or produced, and performs the actual chlorination or bromination.

Water Testing

Naval vessels follow water testing requirements and procedures outlined in the latest edition of *Standard Methods for the Examination of Water and Wastewater,* published by the American Public Health Association (APHA), American Water Works Association (AWWA), and the Water Pollution Control Federation (WPCF).

Manufacture and Handling of Ice

Most ships and shore activities use ice machines to make ice. To reduce bacterial growth, ice used around food or in food or drink must be made from potable water. All ice must be prepared in a sanitary manner and afforded the same protection as potable water. The medical departments aboard ships are required to include ice samples in any bacteriological analyses they perform on water.

WASTEWATER TREATMENT AND DISPOSAL

Wastewater is the spent water of a ship, base, industrial plant, or other activity. This spent water contains wastes, such as soil, detergent, and sewage. The proper disposal of these waste materials is one of the most important measures for controlling water-borne diseases, such as cholera and typhoid fever.

Wastewater Treatment and Disposal Systems Ashore

The use of approved municipal or regional wastewater collection and disposal systems is the preferred method for disposing of wastes from shore activities. Accordingly, municipal or regional wastewater disposal systems are used by Navy shore activities whenever feasible.

Wastewater Treatment and Disposal Systems Afloat

The overboard discharge of untreated sewage from DoD ships within the navigable waters of the United

States and the territorial seas (within three nautical miles of shore) is prohibited by federal law. To comply with the law, naval vessels are being equipped with marine sanitation devices (MSDs) that either treat sewage before discharge or collect and hold it until it can be properly disposed of through dockside sewer connections or pumped overboard in unrestricted waters. For more detailed instruction on these topics, you should review *Manual of Naval Preventive Medicine*, NAVMED P-5010.

SECTION SUMMARY

This section discussed basic information pertaining to sanitation, habitability management, pest and vector control, food-borne illness, food-service sanitation, food-service inspections, and food-borne illness outbreak investigations.

We also discussed communicable diseases, water supply, and wastewater treatment and disposal procedures. This section discussed information on the safe and proper handling of potable water, bacteriological tests, treatment, and disinfection. A general review of wastewater treatment and disposal procedures for shore and afloat activities was also included in this section.

SUMMARY

This chapter has provided a general overview on a variety of fundamental dental conditions and preventive medicine situations. Because of the nature of our rating and the many responsibilities placed upon us, Hospital Corpsmen must have a general understanding of many areas of medicine. Dentistry and preventive medicine practices are two of those areas. For additional detailed information on these subjects, you should refer to the references listed at the beginning of this chapter.

CHAPTER 11

PHYSICAL EXAMINATIONS

The Department of Defense has established uniform physical standards for all members of the military service. Physical examinations are conducted to interpret each individual's physical qualification for initial entry, mobilization, retention, assignment to special duties, and training programs that lead to enlistment and commissioning. The purpose of the examination is to identify physical defects and psychological problems that would compromise a member's ability to perform duties normally assigned. Physical standards are intended to preclude acceptance of those individuals who present contagious or infectious hazards to other personnel, would be unable to perform assigned duties, or who have conditions likely to be aggravated by naval service.

The purpose of this chapter is to review the various types of physical examinations and their requirements, provide a general understanding of how physical examination forms and reports are completed, and cover some of the testing procedures and equipment for which you may be responsible. In your capacity as a Hospital Corpsman, you will function as both clerical and medical assistant to the medical examiner. To do this properly, you should be familiar with administrative regulations that apply to physical examinations. You should also ensure the patient's health record is correct and complete, all tests and laboratory results are recorded, and the completed report of medical examination and history are properly filed in the member's health record.

TYPES OF PHYSICAL EXAMINATIONS

LEARNING OBJECTIVE: *Differentiate between the types of physical examinations.*

Physical examinations, whether routine or special duty, are mandatory for members at certain times during their military careers. The first of these examinations is the entrance (enlistment, appointment, or commissioning) physical examination, and the last is the physical examination that occurs upon separation from the service. In addition to these two,

there may be several others, depending on the length of the member's service or special duty requirements.

Physical examinations of Marine Corps and Navy personnel, active and reserve, are performed by Navy medical officers or other credentialed providers. If a Navy medical officer or credentialed provider is not available, the medical examination may be performed by a Department of Defense (DoD) physician or credentialed civilian contracted physician. Dental examinations are normally performed by Navy dental officers. For further information on dental examinations for naval reserve personnel, refer to the *Manual of the Medical Department* (MANMED), NAVMED P-117.

Most physical examinations will require special studies (tests). Some of these special studies (which will be performed in advance of the physical examination by the medical examiner) may include laboratory tests to detect syphilis (RPR), HIV, and cholesterol levels; optometric evaluation to determine visual acuity; audiometric testing for hearing capabilities; and dental examination to determine dental fitness. For more information on special study requirements for each type of physical examination, refer to the MANMED and directives that address specific physical examinations.

ROUTINE PHYSICAL EXAMINATIONS

Essentially, there are four types of routine physical examinations you should know about. They are the **entrance**, **periodic**, **reenlistment**, and **separation** physicals. The MANMED provides specific instructions on how and when each type of physical is to be conducted.

Entrance (Enlistment, Appointment, and Commissioning) Physical Examination

The Department of Defense (DoD) establishes the standards for entry into military service (DoD Directive 6130.3). Entry physical standards for training programs leading to officer appointment are more stringent than the basic physical qualifications for enlistment or commissioning. This policy ensures qualification of the member at the time of his appointment.

Entrance physical examinations are normally performed at Military Entrance Processing Stations (MEPS). Entrance physical examination results are documented on the *Report of Medical Examination* (SF-88) and *Report of Medical History* (SF-93). The original completed physical examination forms are permanently filed in the member's health record. Copies of the completed examination forms are filed by the examining facility for a specified period of time. (See MANMED for current physical examination disposition requirements.) This policy applies to all of the physical examinations service members may have throughout their career. The forms used for the entrance physical (SF-88 and SF-93) are also used for many of the routine and special duty physical examinations that will be discussed in more detail later in this chapter.

Periodic Physical Examination

The purpose of the periodic examination is to determine physical qualification for retention on active duty and to maintain current medical data regarding physical qualification of personnel. Retention standards are not the same as entrance standards; the prime consideration for retention is the ability to continue active service. The periodic physical examination evaluates the member's current state of health. The examination also includes documentation of chronic or unresolved medical complaints from injuries or illnesses incurred during military service or complaints or injuries that may have existed before induction. The periodic physical examination is conducted at the intervals prescribed in the MANMED.

If the examining medical officer determines a defect exists that he cannot adequately evaluate, a consultation or referral for further evaluation may be initiated. If the defect is severe enough, the member may be referred to a medical board. A medical board is convened to evaluate and report on the diagnosis; prognosis for return to full duty; plan for further treatment, rehabilitation, or convalescence; estimate the length of further disability; and provide medical recommendations for disposition of the service member being evaluated.

A member may be considered physically qualified (PQ) despite the presence of certain medical conditions. However, if it is clearly determined that the condition interferes with the member's capability of functioning in the naval service effectively, the member may be processed for an administrative or medical discharge. Additional guidance is provided in the *Military Personnel Manual* (MILPERSMAN) and applicable Navy and Marine Corps directives.

Reenlistment Physical Examination

The purpose of the reenlistment physical examination is to determine if service members are physically qualified to be retained on active duty. A complete medical examination is not required if there is a valid examination (i.e., entrance, periodic, or special duty physical) in the service member's service record. The reenlistment physical consists of a medical record review and documentation of medical conditions that may need consideration or further inquiry by healthcare providers. The service member will also be interviewed by a healthcare provider. Reenlistment criteria specified in the MANMED should be followed during the health record review and the interview of patient.

The results of the reenlistment physical examination are recorded on form SF-600, *Chronological Record of Medical Care*. The healthcare provider will indicate on the SF-600 if the service member is physically qualified for reenlistment. After the physical examination is completed, the SF-600 will be filed in the member's health record.

Separation Physical Examination

Before being released from active duty, members receive a thorough physical examination. If the separation is the result of an evaluation by a medical board, the medical board report serves as the document for the physical examination.

Members who separate from the service—for any reason (i.e., retirement, end-of-enlistment, or administrative discharge)—are required to read the following statement at the time of their physical examination:

You are being examined because of your separation from active duty. If you feel you have a serious defect or condition that interferes, or has interfered, with the performance of your military duties, advise the examiner. If you are considered by the examiner to be not physically qualified for separation, you will be referred for further evaluation, and, if indicated, appearance before a medical board. If, however, you are found physically qualified for separation, any defects will be recorded in item 74 of the

SF-88 or on an SF-600. Such defects, while not considered disqualifying for military service, may entitle you to certain benefits from the Department of Veterans Affairs (DVA). If you desire further information in this regard, contact the DVA office nearest your home after your separation.

In the case of a service member separating from the Navy or Marine Corps before completion of 90 days of service, a similar statement as above must be read by the separating member. Refer to article 15-29 of the MANMED for this statement. In either case the separating member will be requested to sign the following entry in item 73 on the SF-88 or the SF-600.

I have been informed of and understand the provisions of article XX-XX of the *Manual of the Medical Department*.

Refusal of the member to sign this statement will not delay separation. Rather, the examiner will note in item 73 of the SF-88 or on the SF-600 that the provisions of MANMED article XX-XX have been fully explained to the member, who declined to sign a statement to that effect. Give each member released from active duty a signed, legible copy of the SF 88 or SF-600.

SPECIAL DUTY PHYSICAL EXAMINATIONS

Military personnel who are assigned to or applying for special duty such as aviation duty, diving duty, submarine duty, etc., are required to meet physical requirements above the basic entrance examination requirements. In addition, personnel are required to have a special duty physical if they have psychosocial considerations, are exposed to extreme physical hazards, or if they are to be assigned to sites with inadequate medical facilities. Other special duties requiring preplacement examinations include handling explosives, operating explosives vehicles, and duty as a fire fighting instructor. Specific details for each type of special duty physical examination is delineated in the MANMED.

As with routine physicals, special duty physical examinations are performed by medical officers or DoD civilian physicians. For operational units (squadrons or groups), the medical officer assigned will normally perform special duty examinations. If there is not a unit medical officer, a medical officer assigned to a supporting clinic, hospital, or related operational unit should perform the examination.

Physician assistants (PAs) and nurse practitioners may perform special duty examinations if a medical officer or DoD physician is not available or if the examination workload is too great. When a PA or nurse practitioner performs special duty examinations, the examination **MUST** be countersigned in block 80 of the SF 88 by a physician.

Physical examinations for special duty applicants must be completed before reporting for their special duty assignment. If a service member is determined by the medical examiner to be "not qualified for special duty," the member can usually remain in the service but will not be given special duty assignments. To maintain special duty status, service members may have more frequent physical examinations than service members not on special duty status. Validity periods for special duty physicals are discussed in the MANMED. Also, refer to Navy directives that apply to specific special duty examinations for current information on physical qualifications.

OVERSEAS/OPERATIONAL SUITABILITY SCREENING EXAMINATIONS

Upon receipt of accompanied orders overseas or to a remote assignment, the member and, as applicable, his family members will be screened to determine their physical and psychological suitability for transfer. Service members and families who are not screened—or who are improperly screened—can arrive at a duty station with requirements beyond the capability of the local medical, dental, educational, or community facilities. This may result in decreased quality of life, early return from assignment, billet gaps, etc. Proper screening helps ensure a positive and productive tour for the service member. All screening should be completed within 30 days of receipt of orders.

OCCUPATIONAL HEALTH MEDICAL SURVEILLANCE EXAMINATIONS

The Navy uses many materials in its work places, some of which are potentially hazardous to personnel. To minimize the risk associated with these hazardous substances, the Navy developed the *Navy Occupational Safety and Health (NAVOSH) Program*, OPNAVINST 5100.23. Within the NAVOSH Program is the *Medical Surveillance Program*. The Medical Surveillance Program provides physical examination and medical monitoring guidelines for personnel who are exposed to or work with hazardous materials.

Medical surveillance examinations assess the health status of individuals as it relates to their work. Although these exams are not physical examinations as described in this chapter, they are actually surveillance examinations that produce specific information with regard to an individual's health during actual or potential exposure to hazardous materials (i.e., the Asbestos Medical Surveillance Program [AMSP]). Specific guidance on the *Asbestos Medical Surveillance Program* is provided in OPNAVINST 5100.23. Another example of a medical surveillance program is the *Occupational Noise Control and Hearing Conservation Program*. Personnel who work in areas of high sound generation (e.g., flight deck of carrier) must be evaluated periodically for hearing loss. Specific guidance on the Occupational Noise Control and Hearing Conservation Program is provided in NAVMEDCOMINST 6260.5 and OPNAVINST 5100.23.

MEDICAL BOARD EXAMINATIONS AND REPORTS

Medical review boards are the single most important factor in determining fitness for duty in today's Navy. Medical boards are convened and reviews are conducted to determine the various degrees of fitness for military service. Local (re)evaluations are scheduled to assess patient progress and length of limited duty, or need for a formal evaluation at NAVPERSCOM or the Physical Evaluation Board (PEB). The following examples illustrate the legal guidelines, requirements, and job descriptions for the different types of medical boards and describe the duties of the personnel responsible.

Abbreviated Temporary Limited Duty (TLD) Medical Board Report

The abbreviated board report is used only when a member is expected to return to full duty after an adequate period of treatment. Processing time should not exceed 6 working days, and under most circumstances, the report should be completed in 3 working days. The board report is a local action taken by an appropriate medical or dental officer and does not require external departmental review by NAVPERSCOM. The form (NAVMED 6100/5) used for this report is a multi-copy form. It is a vehicle for recording basic medical findings, plans, and expectations in terms of prognosis and length of medical restriction of activity. It also provides for

parent command acknowledgment and comment. This form serves as excellent input for the "putting performance into practice" form in the member's health record; however, it is not a substitute for detailed documentation of conditions in the member's health record. The *Abbreviated TLD Medical Board Report* (NAVMED 6100/5) is to be used when **all** of the following criteria are met:

- The member is enlisted in the U.S. Navy or Marine Corps.

- The member suffers from an uncomplicated illness or injury which makes them temporarily unable to fully perform duties to which they are assigned or expected to be assigned, but will most likely be fit for full duty after an adequate period of treatment not exceeding 8 months.

- The member's health or clinical record contains adequate documentation on the nature and circumstances of the illness or injury, its course, prognosis, and treatment.

Patient (Re)evaluation/TLD Duration

Once a member has been placed on TLD, the physician, dental officer, or Independent Duty Corpsman (IDC) (when in an independent operational duty environment), will

- conduct a detailed treatment/rehabilitation assessment and develop a treatment/ rehabilitation plan;

- ensure follow-up evaluations every 2 months, documenting at each evaluation objective findings of continued unsuitability, progress toward recovery, findings and recommendations of specialty evaluations, modifications to the treatment/ rehabilitation plan, and prognosis for return to worldwide assignability; and

- obtain approval from NAVPERSCOM (NPC-821) or CMC (MMSR-4), via the patient administration Limited Duty (LIMDU) Coordinator for periods of TLD less than 8 months, or via a formal board (NPC-821 or MMSR-4) for periods longer than 8 months.

Approval must be obtained via formal board if the initial recommended period of TLD exceeds 8 months, and the total period a member can be on LIMDU must not exceed 16 months.

Uncorrected Condition

If the servicemember's condition cannot be corrected during the initial or subsequent period of TLD and treatment, or if it is clear that the condition will continually interfere with or preclude his ability to function effectively in an operational arena or to deploy worldwide, notify the transferring or parent command and NAVPERSCOM. Subsequent to the second period of TLD, if appropriate, a Physical Evaluation Board (PEB) will adjudicate the case. If the PEB (in Washington, DC) finds the member "fit to continue Naval Service," NAVPERSCOM will direct the command to initiate appropriate administrative action, which may include a recommendation of administrative separation (per MILPERSMAN 1910-120).

Formal Board Report

If conditions warrant (i.e., when the period of recovery is expected to exceed 8 months), the physician or dental officer will dictate a formal board report in accordance with SECNAVINST 1850.4 and MANMED, chapter 18, for submission to NAV-PERSCOM (NPC-821). The LIMDU Coordinator is responsible for reviewing the medical board, verifying the content and that the processing time is consistent with current policy. However, a command endorsement is not required on a formal board.

COMPLETING REQUIRED FORMS

LEARNING OBJECTIVE: *Select the appropriate form(s) used for physical examinations and recall how each form should be completed.*

While there are several forms used to record physicals, the scope and purpose of the physical dictates which form or forms should be used. For example, the preplacement and annual physical evaluation of food service personnel or personnel exposed to hazardous materials can, in most cases, be adequately documented on an SF 600. This section discusses the most commonly used physical examination forms.

REPORT OF MEDICAL EXAMINATION, SF 88

The SF 88, Report of Medical Examination, is the principal document for recording a complete physical examination (figs. 11-1 and 11-2). The SF 88 is, like most medical documentation, a legal document. Entries on the form must be legible. If you make a typographical or clerical error, correct the entry by drawing a single line through the erroneous entry, initialing above the error, and making the corrected entry in the same block. If space is not available in that block, make the corrected entry in block 42 (identifying the erroneous entry by number). Chapter 16 of the MANMED provides specific details on information for each block to complete this form properly.

Stamps are used routinely by many naval medical facilities to incorporate routine information or data onto medical documents, as illustrated in blocks 50 and 73 of figures 11-1 and 11-2. The use of stamps must, however, be in accordance with physical examination directives and the MANMED.

REPORT OF MEDICAL HISTORY, SF 93

The purpose of Standard Form (SF) 93, Report of Medical History, is to provide a complete personal medical history and to serve as a source of information that supplements information reported on the SF 88. The SF 93 provides a current, concise, and comprehensive record of a service member's personal medical history before entering the service and any subsequent changes in the member's medical status.

After the military entrance examination, any subsequent medical examinations that require the use of the SF 88 will also require an SF 93 to be completed. Any medical information entered by patients on the SF 93 is made only to document changes in medical history since their last physical examination. If no changes have occurred since the previous SF 93 was generated, the examiner should enter "no significant interval history" in block 25.

When you prepare the SF 93, complete items 1 through 7 in the same manner as you did the SF 88 (fig. 11-3). This information can be handwritten or typed. Inform examinees that they are responsible for completing items 8 through 25 (figs. 11-3 and 11-4). Item 8 should contain a handwritten statement from examinees regarding their present state of health and any medications they may be taking. Items 9 through 24 are checked either "yes," "no," or "don't know" by the examinees. Assist examinees by explaining unfamiliar medical terminology that appears on these items. Helping them complete the form will ensure an accurate accounting of the member's medical history. Keep in mind that the SF 93 is information of

REPORT OF MEDICAL EXAMINATION

1. LAST NAME—FIRST NAME—MIDDLE NAME: Frost, Jack Ronald, JR.	2. GRADE AND COMPONENT OR POSITION: PR1	3. IDENTIFICATION NO.: 777-77-7777
4. HOME ADDRESS (Number, street or RFD, city or town, State and ZIP Code): 212 Sandy Lake Drive Pensacola, FL 31189	5. PURPOSE OF EXAMINATION: Periodic	6. DATE OF EXAMINATION: 07 Mar 96

7. SEX: Male	8. RACE: Negroid	9. TOTAL YEARS GOVERNMENT SERVICE: MILITARY 10y3m CIVILIAN	10. AGENCY	11. ORGANIZATION UNIT: Naval Air Station Pensacola, FL

12. DATE OF BIRTH: 27 Feb 65

13. PLACE OF BIRTH: Aurora, PA

14. NAME, RELATIONSHIP, AND ADDRESS OF NEXT OF KIN: JACK R. FROST, SR. (FATHER), 1616 ABALONE LANE, Venice, FL 36521

15. EXAMINING FACILITY OR EXAMINER, AND ADDRESS: Branch Medical Clinic, NAS Pensacola, FL 32508-7601

16. OTHER INFORMATION: Religion - Roman Catholic

17. RATING OR SPECIALTY

TIME IN THIS CAPACITY (Total) | LAST SIX MONTHS

CLINICAL EVALUATION

NORMAL	(Check each item in appropriate column, enter "NE" if not evaluated.)	ABNORMAL
X	18. HEAD, FACE, NECK AND SCALP	
X	19. NOSE	
X	20. SINUSES	
X	21. MOUTH AND THROAT	
X	22. EARS—GENERAL (INTERNAL CANALS) (Auditory acuity under items 70 and 71)	
X	23. DRUMS (Perforation)	
X	24. EYES—GENERAL (Visual acuity and refraction under items 59, 60 and 67)	
X	25. OPHTHALMOSCOPIC	
X	26. PUPILS (Equality and reaction)	
X	27. OCULAR MOTILITY (Associated parallel movements nystagmus)	
X	28. LUNGS AND CHEST (Include breasts)	
X	29. HEART (Thrust, size, rhythm, sounds)	
X	30. VASCULAR SYSTEM (Varicosities, etc.)	
X	31. ABDOMEN AND VISCERA (Include hernia)	
X	32. ANUS AND RECTUM (Hemorrhoids, Fistulae) (Prostate, if indicated)	
X	33. ENDOCRINE SYSTEM	
	34. G-U SYSTEM	X
X	35. UPPER EXTREMITIES (Strength, range of motion)	
X	36. FEET	
X	37. LOWER EXTREMITIES (Except feet) (Strength, range of motion)	
X	38. SPINE, OTHER MUSCULOSKELETAL	
	39. IDENTIFYING BODY MARKS, SCARS, TATTOOS	X
X	40. SKIN, LYMPHATICS	
X	41. NEUROLOGIC (Equilibrium tests under item 72)	
X	42. PSYCHIATRIC (Specify any personality deviation)	
	43. PELVIC (Females only) (Check how done) ☐ VAGINAL ☐ RECTAL	

NOTES: (Describe every abnormality in detail. Enter pertinent item number before each comment. Continue in item 73 and use additional sheets if necessary)

#34 Urinary Tract Infection resolved

#39 Scar right elbow & tattoo left arm.

(Continue in item 73)

44. DENTAL (Place appropriate symbols, shown in examples, above or below number of upper and lower teeth.)

Restorable Teeth — Non-restorable teeth — Missing Teeth — Replaced by Dentures — Fixed Partial dentures

RIGHT: X 1 2 3 4 5 6 7 8 9 10 11 12 13 14 15 16 X LEFT

X 32 31 30 29 28 27 26 25 24 23 22 21 20 19 18 17 X

REMARKS AND ADDITIONAL DENTAL DEFECTS AND DISEASES: Type 2 Class 2 Qualified: Yes

LABORATORY FINDINGS

45. URINALYSIS: A. SPECIFIC GRAVITY

B. ALBUMIN

C. SUGAR

D. MICROSCOPIC

46. CHEST X-RAY (Place, date, film number and result)

47. SEROLOGY (Specify test used and result): RPR: NONREACTIVE DATE: 05 Mar 96

48. EKG

49. BLOOD TYPE AND RH FACTOR: B+

50. OTHER TESTS: FAST GLU 105 CHOL 220 TRIG 110 LDL 140 HDL 58 HCT ____ HIV Neg.

NSN 7540-00-753-4570
88-125

Standard Form 88 (Rev. 3-89)
General Services Administration
Interagency Comm. on Medical Records
FIRMR (41CFR) 201-45.505

HM3f1101

Figure 11-1.—Example of completed front side of SF 88.

MEASUREMENTS AND OTHER FINDINGS

51. HEIGHT	52. WEIGHT	53. COLOR HAIR	54. COLOR EYES	55. BUILD:		56. TEMPERATURE
75" (190.5)	200 (90.00)	Brown	Brown	☐ SLENDER ☒ MEDIUM ☐ HEAVY ☐ OBESE		98.7° F

57.	BLOOD PRESSURE (Arm at heart level)				58.	PULSE (Arm at heart level)				
A. SITTING	SYS. 110 DIAS. 80	B. RECUMBENT	SYS. DIAS.	C. STANDING	SYS. DIAS.	A. SITTING 72	B. AFTER EXERCISE	C. 2 MIN. AFTER	D. RECUMBENT	E. AFTER STANDING 3 MIN.

59.	DISTANT VISION		60.		REFRACTION			61.	NEAR VISION		
RIGHT 20/ 200+	CORR. TO 20/ 20		BY	S.		CX			CORR. TO	BY	
LEFT 20/ 200+	CORR. TO 20/ 20		BY	S		CX			CORR. TO	BY	

62. HETEROPHORIA (Specify distance)								
ES°	EX°	R.H.	L.H.	PRISM DIV.	PRISM CONV. CT		PC	PD

63.	ACCOMMODATION	64. COLOR VISION (Test used and result)	65. DEPTH PERCEPTION (Test used and score)	UNCORRECTED
RIGHT	LEFT	Falant Pass 9/9		CORRECTED
		66. RED LENS TEST	69. INTRAOCULAR TENSION	

66. FIELD OF VISION	67. NIGHT VISION (Test used and score)	
Full OU		

70. HEARING — 71. AUDIOMETER ANSI 69 — 72. PSYCHOLOGICAL AND PSYCHOMOTOR (Tests used and score)

				250 256	500 512	1000 1024	2000 2048	3000 2096	4000 4096	6000 6144	8000 8192
RIGHT WV	/15 SV	/15	RIGHT	XX	10	05	00	10	05	25	XX
LEFT WV	/15 SV	/15	LEFT	XX	10	10	00	05	10	15	XX

73. NOTES (Continued) AND SIGNIFICANT OR INTERVAL HISTORY

Neck: 16
Waist: 36
Body Fat %: 20%

THIS PHYSICAL EXAMINATION HAS BEEN
ADMINISTRATIVELY REVIEWED FOR
COMPLETENESS AND ACCURACY.

Floss A. Brush

(Floss A. Brush)   HM2   08 Mar 96

SIGNATURE	RATE	DATE

(Use additional sheets if necessary)

74. SUMMARY OF DEFECTS AND DIAGNOSES (List diagnoses with item numbers)

#59 Refraction errors corrected to 20/20 O.D. & 20/20 O.S.

75. RECOMMENDATIONS—FURTHER SPECIALIST EXAMINATIONS INDICATED (Specify)	76.	A. PHYSICAL PROFILE					
		P	U	L	H	E	S

77. EXAMINEE (Check)	B. PHYSICAL CATEGORY			
A. ☒ IS QUALIFIED FOR Full Duty	A	B	C	E
B. ☐ IS NOT QUALIFIED FOR				

78. IF NOT QUALIFIED, LIST DISQUALIFYING DEFECTS BY ITEM NUMBER

79. TYPED OR PRINTED NAME OF PHYSICIAN	SIGNATURE
Mary A. Christmas, LCDR, MC, USN 111-11-1111	*Mary A. Christmas*
80. TYPED OR PRINTED NAME OF PHYSICIAN	SIGNATURE
81. TYPED OR PRINTED NAME OF DENTIST OR PHYSICIAN (Indicate which)	SIGNATURE
Doe, John P., LT, DC, USNR 333-33-3333	*John P. Doe*
82. TYPED OR PRINTED NAME OF REVIEWING OFFICER OR APPROVING AUTHORITY	NUMBER OF ATTACHED SHEETS

SF 88 (Rev. 3-89) PAGE 2

☆ U.S. GPO:1993-342-197/81292

HM3f1102

Figure 11-2.—Example of completed back side of SF 88.

STANDARD FORM 93
REV. OCTOBER 1974
PRESCRIBED BY GSA/ICMR
FIRMR (41 CFR) 201-45.505

APPROVED
OFFICE OF MANAGEMENT AND BUDGET No. 29-R0191

REPORT OF MEDICAL HISTORY

(THIS INFORMATION IS FOR OFFICIAL AND MEDICALLY-CONFIDENTIAL USE ONLY AND WILL NOT BE RELEASED TO UNAUTHORIZED PERSONS)

1. LAST NAME—FIRST NAME—MIDDLE NAME	2. SOCIAL SECURITY OR IDENTIFICATION NO.
Frost, Jack Ronald	777-77-7777

3. HOME ADDRESS (No. street or RFD, city or town, State, and ZIP CODE)	4. POSITION (title, grade, component)
212 Sandy Lake Drive Pensacola, FL 31189	PR1

5. PURPOSE OF EXAMINATION	6. DATE OF EXAMINATION	7. EXAMINING FACILITY OR EXAMINER, AND ADDRESS (Include ZIP Code)
Periodic	07 Mar 96	Branch Medical Clinic NAS Pensacola, FL 32508-7601

8. STATEMENT OF EXAMINEE'S PRESENT HEALTH AND MEDICATIONS CURRENTLY USED (Follow by description of past history, if complaint exists)

I AM IN _____Excellent_____ HEALTH

I AM TAKING _____No_____ MEDICATIONS

I HAVE _____No_____ DRUG ALLERGIES

9. HAVE YOU EVER (Please check each item)

YES	NO	(Check each item)
	X	Lived with anyone who had tuberculosis
	X	Coughed up blood
	X	Bled excessively after injury or tooth extraction
	X	Attempted suicide
	X	Been a sleepwalker

10. DO YOU (Please check each item)

YES	NO	(Check each item)
X		Wear glasses or contact lenses
X		Have vision in both eyes
	X	Wear a hearing aid
	X	Stutter or stammer habitually
	X	Wear a brace or back support

11. HAVE YOU EVER HAD OR HAVE YOU NOW (Please check at left of each item)

YES	NO	DON'T KNOW	(Check each item)	YES	NO	DON'T KNOW	(Check each item)	YES	NO	DON'T KNOW	(Check each item)
	X		Scarlet fever, erysipelas		X		Cramps in your legs		X		"Trick" or locked knee
	X		Rheumatic fever		X		Frequent indigestion		X		Foot trouble
	X		Swollen or painful joints		X		Stomach, liver, or intestinal trouble		X		Neuritis
	X		Frequent or severe headache		X		Gall bladder trouble or gallstones		X		Paralysis (include infantile)
	X		Dizziness or fainting spells		X		Jaundice or hepatitis		X		Epilepsy or fits
	X		Eye trouble		X		Adverse reaction to serum, drug, or medicine		X		Car, train, sea or air sickness
	X		Ear, nose, or throat trouble						X		Frequent trouble sleeping
	X		Hearing loss		X		Broken bones		X		Depression or excessive worry
	X		Chronic or frequent colds		X		Tumor, growth, cyst, cancer		X		Loss of memory or amnesia
	X		Severe tooth or gum trouble		X		Rupture/hernia		X		Nervous trouble of any sort
X			Sinusitis		X		Piles or rectal disease		X		Periods of unconsciousness
	X		Hay Fever		X		Frequent or painful urination				
	X		Head Injury		X		Bed wetting since age 12				
	X		Skin diseases		X		Kidney stone or blood in urine				
	X		Thyroid trouble		X		Sugar or albumin in urine				
	X		Tuberculosis		X		VD—Syphilis, gonorrhea, etc.				
	X		Asthma		X		Recent gain or loss of weight				
	X		Shortness of breath		X		Arthritis, Rheumatism, or Bursitis				
	X		Pain or pressure in chest		X		Bone, joint or other deformity				
	X		Chronic cough		X		Lameness				
	X		Palpitation or pounding heart		X		Loss of finger or toe	12. FEMALES ONLY: HAVE YOU EVER			
	X		Heart trouble		X		Painful or "trick" shoulder or elbow				Been treated for a female disorder
	X		High or low blood pressure		X		Recurrent back pain				Had a change in menstrual pattern

13. WHAT IS YOUR USUAL OCCUPATION?	14. ARE YOU (Check one)
Parachute Rigger	[X] Right handed [ ] Left handed

HM3f1103

93 103

Figure 11-3.—Example of front side of SF 93.

YES	NO	CHECK EACH ITEM YES OR NO. EVERY ITEM CHECKED YES MUST BE FULLY EXPLAINED IN BLANK SPACE ON RIGHT	
	X	15. Have you been refused employment or been unable to hold a job or stay in school because of: A. Sensitivity to chemicals, dust, sunlight, etc.	
	X	B. Inability to perform certain motions.	
	X	C. Inability to assume certain positions.	
	X	D. Other medical reasons (If yes, give reasons.)	
	X	16. Have you ever been treated for a mental condition? (If yes, specify when, where, and give details).	
	X	17. Have you ever been denied life insurance? (If yes, state reason and give details.)	
	X	18. Have you had, or have you been advised to have, any operations? (If yes, describe and give age at which occurred.)	
	X	19. Have you ever been a patient in any type of hospitals? (If yes, specify when, where, why, and name of doctor and complete address of hospital.)	
X		20. Have you ever had any illness or injury other than those already noted? (If yes, specify when, where, and give details.)	Had Urinary tract infection April '95.
	X	21. Have you consulted or been treated by clinics, physicians, healers, or other practitioners within the past 5 years for other than minor illnesses? (If yes, give complete address of doctor, hospital, clinic, and details.)	
	X	22. Have you ever been rejected for military service because of physical, mental, or other reasons? (If yes, give date and reason for rejection.)	
	X	23. Have you ever been discharged from military service because of physical, mental, or other reasons? (If yes, give date, reason, and type of discharge: whether honorable, other than honorable, for unfitness or unsuitability.)	
	X	24. Have you ever received, is there pending, or have you applied for pension or compensation for existing disability? (If yes, specify what kind, granted by whom, and what amount, when, why.)	

I certify that I have reviewed the foregoing information supplied by me and that it is true and complete to the best of my knowledge. I authorize any of the doctors, hospitals, or clinics mentioned above to furnish the Government a complete transcript of my medical record for purposes of processing my application for this employment or service.

TYPED OR PRINTED NAME OF EXAMINEE	SIGNATURE
PR1 Jack R. Frost	PR1 Jack R. Frost

NOTE: HAND TO THE DOCTOR OR NURSE, OR IF MAILED MARK ENVELOPE "TO BE OPENED BY MEDICAL OFFICER ONLY."
25. Physician's summary and elaboration of all pertinent data (Physician shall comment on all positive answers in items 9 through 24. Physician may develop by interview any additional medical history he deems important, and record any significant findings here.)

#10 Wears eye glasses for correction of refraction errors - NCD

#20 UTI resolved with treatment. - NCD

TYPED OR PRINTED NAME OF PHYSICIAN OR EXAMINER	DATE	SIGNATURE	NUMBER OF ATTACHED SHEETS
Mary A. Christmas, LCDR, MC, USN	07 Mar 96	Ldr. Mary A. Christmas	

REVERSE OF STANDARD FORM 93

*U.S. GPO: 1994-300-892/60197

HM3f1104

Figure 11-4.—Example of back side of SF 93.

significant or chronic disorders instead of one-time events of minor illnesses or disorders.

An essential part of a complete physical examination is the review of patient's medical history. The medical examiner is responsible for reviewing items 9 through 24 of the SF 93. After reviewing these items, the medical examiner uses item 25 to elaborate on all "yes" responses (fig. 11-4). Examiners document conditions considered disqualifying as "CD" and those considered not disqualifying as "NCD." Examiner's signature and identification information should be documented at the bottom of the back side of the SF 93.

SPECIAL DUTY MEDICAL ABSTRACT, NAVMED 6150/2

The NAVMED 6150/2, Special Duty Medical Abstract, is a record of physical qualifications, special training, and periodic examinations of members designated to perform special duty, such as aviation, submarine, and diving. When members complete special duty physical examinations and special training, they should have entries made on their NAVMED 6150/2. NAVMED 6150/2 entries require the approval of a medical officer or designated specialty medical service corps officer (i.e., aerospace physiologist for aerospace physiology training).

If a special-duty-qualified service member is found to be physically or mentally unfit, the service member's special duty status will be suspended either temporarily or permanently. The reason(s) for the member's suspension and period of suspension are recorded on the NAVMED 6150/2. Special pay disbursements are often based on a member's physical and mental qualifications or continued requalification for performance in a special duty.

PHYSICAL EXAM TESTING PROCEDURES AND EQUIPMENT

LEARNING OBJECTIVE: *Recall visual acuity, color vision, audiometric, and EKG test equipment and procedures.*

Some of the basic procedures used to gather information for a physical examination are taught in Hospital Corpsman "A" School (e.g., vital signs, venipuncture, and height and weight measurements). However, other tests require advanced technical expertise, such as serological testing, and pressure and oxygen-tolerance testing. Some testing procedures may be learned by on-the-job training (OJT) or by short courses of instruction. These testing procedures and the equipment used will be discussed in this section.

VISUAL ACUITY

Visual acuity testing determines the ability of the eye to discriminate fine detail. It is the most important test of eye function. Throughout the Navy, there are two accepted methods for testing visual acuity: the Snellen chart and Jaeger cards, and the Armed Forces Vision Tester. The Snellen chart and Jaeger cards are used together to test visual acuity. The Snellen charts test distant visual acuity; the Jaeger cards are used to evaluate near visual acuity. The Armed Forces Vision Tester checks both distant and near visual acuity, and assists in evaluating other optical conditions.

The first step in testing for visual acuity is to find out if the patient wears corrective eyewear. On the day of their visual acuity testing, patients should bring in their glasses. Contact lenses are not recommended for use during visual acuity testing. Contact lenses cause an increase in time needed for testing purposes, and they tend to be an inconvenience for both the patient and healthcare provider. Acuity testing is performed with and without the glasses on, and the results are documented in blocks 59 and 61 on the SF 88. Visual acuity requirements are discussed in the MANMED.

Snellen Charts

Probably the most familiar of the visual testing equipment, Snellen charts, are the preferred method for testing distant visual acuity. Snellen charts can test both monocular and binocular visual acuity. Operational guidelines for Snellen charts are provided by the chart's manufacturer. Your local military optometrist or eye clinic can also provide you operational guidelines for Snellen charts. Specific details and current conditions for testing with Snellen charts are as follows:

- If the examinee wears corrective lenses, have them remove the lenses before the examination. Test the examinee first without corrective lenses, and then with the corrective lenses in place.

- Hang the chart on the wall so the 20/20 line is 64 inches from the floor. Direct the examinees to stand 20 feet from the chart. Test each eye individually, then both eyes together. Do not allow the examinee to squint or tilt his head.

- With the graduation of the size of the letters advocated by Snellen, the visual acuity is expressed according to his classical formula $V = d/D$, where "d" is the distance at which the letters are read, is divided by "D" the distance at which the letters should be read. Then record the smallest line read on the chart from the 20-foot distance as the vision; e.g., 20/20, 20/200.

Jaeger Cards

When the Armed Forces Vision Tester is not available, Jaeger cards are used to test near vision. There are six paragraphs on each card. Each paragraph is printed in a different size type and labeled as J-1 (the smallest print size), J-2,..., up to J-6.

When testing with these cards, you should hold the card at a distance of 14 to 16 inches from the examinee and tell the examinee to read the paragraphs. Record the visual acuity as the smallest type he can comfortably read and record the distance (e.g., J-2 at 14 inches).

NOTE: The **distance** of the card from the examinee may be converted to centimeters, but ensure the **results** of the test are also recorded in centimeters. Consistency is the key.

Armed Forces Vision Tester

The Armed Forces Vision Tester (AFVT) is a semiportable machine that has the capability to test near and distant visual acuity, horizontal and vertical phorias, and stereopsis (depth perception). It consists of two rotating drums that hold illuminated slides. The handles on the side of the machine rotate the drums to change the slides. A scoring key and instruction manual are provided with the machine.

COLOR VISION TESTING

The *Manual of the Medical Department* requires that all applicants for the naval service receive a color vision test. The Navy has two methods of testing color discrimination: the Farnsworth Lantern Test (FALANT) and the pseudoisochromatic plates (PIP). The FALANT is the preferred test, and in many cases it is the test prescribed by the MANMED as the only acceptable method for testing color vision.

Farnsworth Lantern Test

The purpose of the Farnsworth Lantern Test is to evaluate color perception. The Farnsworth Lantern is a machine with a light source directed at the examinee. What the examinee sees is two lights in a vertical plane. These lights appear in two of three possible colors, either red, green, or white, shown in varying combinations. The examinee is asked to identify the color combinations from top to bottom at a distance of 8 feet; the examiner rotates the drum to provide the different combinations. The examinee must identify a total of nine different combinations.

On the first run of nine lights, if the examinee correctly identifies all nine, the FALANT is passed. If the examinee incorrectly identifies any of the lights, two additional runs of nine lights are performed without interruption. The score is the average number of incorrectly identified lights of the second two runs. If the average score is 1 or less, the FALANT is passed. If the score is 2 or more, the FALANT is failed. If the score is 1.5, the test should be repeated after a 5-minute break. Do not retest scores of 2 or more since this will invalidate the test procedure.

NOTE: If examinees wear corrective lenses for distant vision, they should wear them during this test.

Pseudoisochromatic Plates

If the FALANT is not available, pseudoisochromatic plates (PIP) are used to determine color vision. Personnel so tested must be retested with the FALANT at the first activity they report to that has a Farnsworth Lantern. Two tests are available, the 18-plate test and the 15-plate test, each of which includes one demonstration plate not used for scoring.

When administering the PIP examination, you should hold the plates 30 inches from the examinee. Allow 2 seconds for each plate identification, and do not allow the examinee to touch the plates. To pass the 18-plate test, the examinee must identify a minimum of 14 of the 17 test plates; for the 15-plate test, a minimum of 10 of the 14 test plates. Record the score in block 64 of the SF 88 as PASSED PIP or FAILED PIP. Include the number of correct responses (e.g., PASSED PIP 17 of 17 or FAILED PIP 10 of 17).

AUDIOGRAM

An **audiogram** is a record of hearing thresholds an individual has for various sound frequencies. By evaluating an individual's frequency thresholds, hearing deficiencies can be detected. To test an individual's frequency thresholds, the technician will use an instrument called an **audiometer** (manual or computerized). Audiometers used by the Navy are calibrated to American National Standards Institute (ANSI) specifications.

Upon entry into the service, a baseline audiogram is performed and recorded on a DD 2215. Subsequent audiometric test results are recorded on a DD 2216 and performed as directed by OPNAVINST 5100.19 and the MANMED. Audiometric testing shall be performed only by personnel who have attended an audiometric training course and have been certified. All audiometric tracings or readings recorded on the SF 88 or other medical documentation should contain the certification number of the person performing the audiometric test.

ELECTROCARDIOGRAM

An **electrocardiogram** is a record of electrical impulses made by the heart. Electrocardiograms are produced by an instrument called an **electrocardiograph**. The electrocardiograph is used to examine and record electrical impulses produced by the contraction of the heart muscle. Abbreviated either EKG or ECG, the electrocardiogram is interpreted by a physician or cardiologist to determine the heart rate and rhythm, and evidence of any heart damage, especially damage associated with a heart attack.

EKGs are currently performed as part of the physical examination once the member reaches the age of 40, and routinely thereafter. Otherwise, EKGs are performed only as clinically indicated or required for special duty. Refer to BUMED instructions for current periodicity information on EKG testing. The Naval Medical Department routinely uses EKGs with 12 leads for physical examinations performed on Navy and Marine Corps personnel.

SUMMARY

A general review has been provided to you on various types of physical examinations, their requirements, and the documentation procedures of commonly used physical examination forms. We have also discussed physical examination testing equipment and procedures that evaluate vision, hearing, and cardiac function.

The physical examination is a key component of the Navy Medical Department's efforts to maintain the health of Sailors and Marines during times of war and peace. The importance of the physical examination cannot be overstated. The combination of medical history, medical testing, and medical examination furnishes the healthcare provider with a complete picture of the individual's health. Any indications of medical problems can be evaluated and managed more expediently and effectively through the use of the physical examination. Your assistance with medical testing and your detailed document management will ensure the patient receives the best possible medical evaluation by the medical examiner. More in-depth information is contained in the *Manual of the Medical Department*, NAVMED P-117.

CHAPTER 12

HEALTH RECORDS

Just as the Personnelman is responsible for the preparation and maintenance of the service record, so you, the Hospital Corpsman, are responsible in the same way for health records. A health record is the official medical history of Navy and Marine Corps personnel and eligible beneficiaries.

The military health record is an individual's chronological record of medical, dental, occupational health evaluations, and treatments. The health record is used by healthcare providers to plan and document patient care treatment. The medical history provided by the health record assists medical personnel who perform physical examinations, physical fitness evaluations, diagnosis decisions, and render care incident to injury or disease.

The health record has significant medicolegal value to the patient, the medical treatment facility (MTF) and dental treatment facility (DTF), the practitioner responsible for the patient, and the U. S. Government. For example, if a military member or eligible beneficiary is injured by a nonmilitary individual (e.g., car accident) and the naval hospital provides medical care, the naval hospital would, in turn, bill the nonmilitary individual or his insurance company (third-party payer) for the medical services it provided the injured military member or beneficiary. To justify the naval hospital's billing, send copies of medical documents from the injured individual's health record pertaining to the injury and subsequent treatment(s) to the third-party payer. Third-party payers depend substantially upon the information recorded in the medical record. Also, various officials and boards (i.e., special duty boards and medical boards) refer to information furnished by the health record in determining physical fitness or physical disability.

The health record provides statistical data for medical research, utilization management, risk management, and quality assurance. For all the reasons mentioned here, accurate and complete record entries and proper medical record maintenance are of the utmost importance.

This chapter will discuss the requirements for opening, maintaining, verifying, and closing active

duty and reserve personnel health records. Use of medical forms and form filing procedures will also be covered. For further details and up-to-date guidelines on health record management, as well as differences between medical records established by deployable units or under combat conditions, refer to chapter 16 of the *Manual of the Medical Department* (MANMED) and pertinent instructions or notices.

PRIMARY AND SECONDARY MEDICAL RECORDS

LEARNING OBJECTIVE: *Identify the various types of primary and secondary medical records, and recall the usage of each type.*

Primary medical records are the original records established to document the continuation of care to service members (active and retired) and their beneficiaries. Secondary medical records are established by a patient's healthcare provider and contain specific medical information needed by that healthcare provider. Secondary medical records are maintained separate from the primary medical record.

PRIMARY MEDICAL RECORDS

Three major categories of primary medical records are health records (HRECs), outpatient records (ORECs), and inpatient records (IRECs). Dental records (DRECs) are part of HRECs and ORECs.

Health Record

The HREC is a file of continuous care given to **active duty members** and documents all their outpatient care. While the HREC primarily documents ambulatory (outpatient) care, copies of inpatient narrative summaries and operative reports are also placed in the HREC to provide continuity of healthcare documentation.

Outpatient Record

The OREC is a file of continuous care that documents ambulatory treatment received by a person other than an active duty person.

Inpatient Record

The IREC is a medical file that documents care provided to a patient (inpatient) assigned to a designated inpatient bed in an MTF or ship.

SECONDARY MEDICAL RECORDS

Secondary medical records are separate from the primary medical record and must follow the guidelines established by the MANMED and the local medical records committee. These records are kept in a separate file secured in a specialty clinic or department of fixed MTFs (e.g., naval hospitals and branch medical clinics). The secondary medical records include convenience records, temporary records, and ancillary records.

Because primary healthcare providers of active duty personnel must be aware of their crew's medical status at all times, temporary and ancillary records will not be opened or maintained for active duty personnel. The exceptions to this policy are records for obstetrics/gynecology (OB/GYN), family advocacy, and psychology and psychiatry clinical records.

The healthcare provider creating a secondary medical record should write a note stating the nature of the secondary record, the patient's diagnosis, and the clinic or department name, address, and telephone number on the NAVMED 6150/20, *Summary of Care*, of the patient's primary medical record. The healthcare provider should make a second note entry on the NAVMED 6150/20 when the secondary record is closed.

Convenience Record

A convenience record contains excerpts from a patient's primary record and is kept within the MTF by a treating clinic, service, department, or individual provider for increased access to the information. When the convenience record's purpose has been served, the establishing clinic, service, department, or provider purges the record from its file, compares it to the primary medical record, and adds any medical documents that are not already in the primary medical record.

Temporary Record

A temporary record is an original medical record established and retained in a specialty clinic, service, or department in addition to the patient's primary

medical record. Its purpose is to document a current course of treatment. The temporary medical record becomes a part of the primary medical record when the course of treatment is concluded. This record is most commonly established in OB/GYN for a prenatal patient.

Ancillary Record

Ancillary records consist of original healthcare documentation withheld from a patient's primary HREC or OREC. In certain cases it may be advisable to not file original treatment information in the primary treatment record, but instead place this information into a secondary medical record, to which the patient, parent, or guardian has limited access. Examples of such instances include information that is potentially injurious to the patient, or information that requires extraordinary degrees of protection (such as psychiatric treatment or instances of real or suspected child or spouse abuse, etc).

THE MEDICAL RECORD

LEARNING OBJECTIVE: *Recall custody guidelines for medical records.*

All medical records are the property of the U.S. Government and must be maintained by MTFs (naval hospitals, medical clinics, and medical departments of ships, submarines, aviation squadrons, and isolated duty locations) that have primary cognizance over the care of the patient. Medical records are of continuing long-term interest to the government and the patient and must be maintained within an MTF. Patients may not retain original HRECs, ORECs, or dental records. Hand-carrying medical records by unauthorized individuals (e.g., spouses or siblings of the patient) without written permission is prohibited.

HEALTH RECORD CUSTODY

The HREC is retained in the custody of the medical officer on the ship, submarine, or aviation squadron to which the member is assigned. For those ships, submarines, and aviation squadrons that do not have medical officers, the health record may be placed in the custody of the medical department representative (MDR) at the discretion of the commanding officer (CO). Examples of MDRs are Independent Duty Corpsman or Squadron Corpsman. When Medical

Department personnel are not assigned, the CO may assign custody of the health records to the local representatives of the Medical Department who generally furnish medical support. The custody of health record by an individual is not permitted.

Health records are subject to inspection at any time by the commanding officer, superiors in the chain of command, the fleet medical officer, or other authorized inspectors. The health record is for official use only, and adequate security and custodial care are required.

There are many methods of providing adequate security and custodial control of health records. In general, health records should be stored in such a manner as to be inaccessible to the crew or general public. No records or record pages should be left unattended. This precaution also helps to prevent loss or misplacement of records.

Medical Department personnel will maintain a *Health Records Receipt, File Chargeout, and Disposition Record*, NAVMED 6150/7, for each health record in their custody. The completed charge out form should be retained in the file until the record is returned.

Medical officers or MDRs are responsible for the completeness of required health record entries while the record remains in their custody.

CROSS-SERVICING HEALTH RECORDS

The HREC of a Navy or Marine Corps member is normally serviced by personnel of the Medical Department of the Navy. However, if a Navy or Marine Corps member is performing an assignment with the Army or the Air Force, the health record may be serviced by Army or Air Force Medical Department personnel. This management of the health record may be done if the attendant service interposes no objection and considers the procedure feasible. Reciprocal procedures for servicing the health records of Army or Air Force personnel by personnel of the Medical Department of the Navy will be maintained whenever feasible, and if requested by authorized representatives of those services.

DEALING WITH LOST, DESTROYED, OR ILLEGIBLE HEALTH RECORDS

When a HREC is lost or destroyed, the HREC custodian will open a replacement health record. The designation "REPLACEMENT" will be prominently entered on the jacket and all forms replaced. A brief explanation of the circumstances requiring the replacement and the date accomplished should be entered on SF 600, *Chronological Record of Medical Care*. If the missing record is subsequently recovered, the information or entries in the replacement record will be inserted in the original record.

The HREC or any part of it should be duplicated whenever it becomes illegible or deteriorates to the point that it may endanger its future use or value as a permanent record. The duplicate record or duplicate portion must reproduce as closely to the original as possible. Pay particular attention to detail when you transcribe this information. When you duplicate an entire health record, place the designation "DUPLICATE RECORD" prominently on the front of the jacket above the wording OUTPATIENT MEDICAL RECORD.

When you duplicate only part of the record, identify the individual forms by printing "DUPLICATE" at the bottom of each form. Enter the circumstances necessitating the duplication and the date accomplished on an SF 600. Microfiche all forms replaced for protection and preservation, and make the envelope a permanent part of the medical record. On front of the envelope, record the member's full name, FMP (family member prefix) and SSN, date of birth, and list the original forms contained in the envelope.

If microfilming is not available to the MTF, place the original health forms (except forms contaminated with mold or mildew) inside a plain envelope for preservation and make them part of the permanent record. On the front of the envelope, record the member's identifying data (same as microfiche envelope) and list the contents of the envelope. Mark the envelope "ORIGINAL MEDICAL RECORDS —PERMANENT" and file as the bottommost item in part 2 of the 4-part health record jacket.

DISPOSING OF HEALTH RECORDS DURING HOSPITALIZATION

When a patient is transferred to an MTF, the HREC should accompany the patient. If members are admitted to a military hospital while away from their command, their HRECs should be forwarded as soon as possible to the hospital. If a discharged member is directed to proceed home and await final action on the recommended findings of a physical evaluation board, an entry to this effect should be recorded in the HREC.

If a member is admitted to a civilian hospital for treatment involving brief periods of hospitalization, the HREC should be retained by the activity until disposition is completed. The HREC will then be forwarded to the cognizant office of medical affairs or to the activity designated by the Commandant of the Marine Corps (CMC) for Marine Corps members. In instances where the parent activity retains the HREC, a summary of the hospitalization will be entered on an SF 600 when the member returns to duty.

When a member is hospitalized at a medical facility of a foreign nation, an entry of this fact should be made in the HREC. The HREC should be retained on board and continued until the patient either returns to duty or is transferred to another U.S. Navy vessel or U.S. military activity. Upon departure of the vessel from the port, the HREC should be delivered to the commanding officer for inclusion in the member's service record for forwarding to the nearest U.S. embassy or consulate.

SECURITY AND SAFEKEEPING OF MEDICAL RECORDS

LEARNING OBJECTIVE: *Recall security and safekeeping procedures for medical records.*

Each MTF or medical department develops policies to ensure that medical records are secure and a patient's privacy is protected. Security and safekeeping are major concerns and responsibilities of staff handling medical records. The medical record contains information that is personal to patients, treated as privileged information, and protected by the **Privacy Act of 1974**. The Privacy Act of 1974 protects a patient's right to privacy in respect to personal medical information. The Privacy Act permits only the patients and their legal representatives to obtain this information.

Medical facilities or departments should take precautions to avoid compromise of medical information during the movement and storage of medical records. Medical records should be handled by only authorized medical service personnel. Records should be stored in a locked area, room, or file to ensure safekeeping, unless there is a 24-hour watch in the records room. Refer to the MANMED for more detailed guidelines on medical record security and safekeeping.

RELEASING MEDICAL INFORMATION

LEARNING OBJECTIVE: *Recognize guidelines for releasing medical information.*

The Surgeon General (also titled Director, Naval Medicine) is the official responsible for administering and supervising the execution of SECNAVINST 5211.5, Department of the Navy Privacy Act Program (PAP), as it pertains to the Health Care Treatment Record System. Additionally, the Office of the Surgeon General authorizes requests for access and amendment to naval members' medical and dental records.

Commanding officers of Navy MTFs are designated as local systems managers for medical records maintained and serviced within their activities. Local systems managers are authorized to release information from health records located within the command if proper credentials have been established. The requesting office or individual will be advised that such information is private and must be treated with confidentiality. In all cases where information is disclosed, an entry must be made on OPNAV Form 5211/9, *Record of Disclosure-Privacy Act of 1974*, and should include the date, nature and purpose of the disclosure, and the name and address of the person or agency receiving the information. Maintain a copy of any such disclosure requests.

GUIDELINES FOR RELEASING MEDICAL INFORMATION

In the following paragraphs, we cover the policy for release of record transcripts. As will be noted, the appropriate rule for release to be implemented depends upon the intended recipient of the record transcript.

1. **Release to the Public**. Information contained in medical records of individuals who have undergone medical or dental examination or treatment is personal to the individual and considered private and privileged in nature. Consequently, disclosure of such information to the public would constitute an unwarranted invasion of personal privacy. Such information is exempt from release under the **Freedom of Information Act**.

However, MTF commanding officers may release some information to the public or the press without the patient's or patient's next of kin's (NOK) consent. This information is the patient's name; grade or rate; date of admission or disposition; age; sex; component, base, station, or organization; and general condition.

2. **Release to the Individual Concerned**. Release of healthcare information to the individual concerned (patient) falls within the purview of the Privacy Act and not the Freedom of Information Act. When individuals request information from their medical record, it will be released to them unless, in the opinion of the releasing authority, it might prove injurious to their physical or mental health. In such an event, the releasing authority will request authorization from the patients to send their medical information to their personal physician.

3. **Release to Representatives of the Individual Concerned.** Upon the written request from patients, healthcare information will be released to their authorized representatives. If an individual is mentally incompetent, insane, or deceased, the NOK or legal representative must authorize the release in writing. NOK or legal representatives must submit adequate proof that the member or former member has been declared mentally incompetent or insane, or furnish adequate proof of death if such information is not on file. Legal representatives must also provide proof of appointment, such as a certified copy of a court order.

4. **Release to Other Government Departments and Agencies.** When requested, healthcare information will be released to other government departments. These government departments and agencies must have a legitimate need for the information as listed in the "Routine Uses" section of the Medical Treatment Records System, which is annually set forth in SECNAVNOTE 5211, *Systems of Personal Records Authorized for Maintenance Under the Privacy Act of 1974*, 5 USC 552a (PL 93-579).

If the releasing authority is in doubt whether the requesting department has a legitimate need for the information, it will ask the requesting department to specify the purpose for which the information will be used. In some cases, the requesting department should be advised that the information will be withheld until the written consent of the individual concerned is obtained.

RELEASING MEDICAL INFORMATION TO FEDERAL AND STATE AGENCIES

In honoring proper requests, the releasing authority should disclose only information relative to the request. In the following three instances, for example, departments and agencies, both federal and state, may have a legitimate need for the information:

1. Health care information is required to process a governmental action involving an individual. (The Veterans Administration and the Bureau of Employees' Compensation process claims in which the claimant's medical or dental history is relevant). If an agency requests health care information solely for employment purposes, a written authorization is required from the individual concerned.

2. Health care information is required to treat an individual in the department's custody. (Federal and state hospitals and prisons may need the medical or dental history of their patients and inmates.)

3. Release to federal or state courts or other administrative bodies. The preceding limitations are not intended to prevent compliance with lawful court orders for health records in connection with civil litigation or criminal proceedings, or to prevent release of information from health records when required by law. If you have doubts about the validity of record requests, ask the Judge Advocate General (JAG) for guidance.

RELEASING MEDICAL INFORMATION FOR RESEARCH

Commanding officers of MTFs are authorized to release information from medical records located within the command to members of their staff who are conducting research projects. Where possible, the names of parties should be deleted. Other requests from research groups should be forwarded to Bureau of Medicine and Surgery (BUMED) for guidance.

FILING HEALTH RECORDS

LEARNING OBJECTIVE: *Recall filing procedures for health records.*

The Navy Medical Department uses the Terminal Digit Filing System (TDFS) to file health records. In this system, health records are filed according to the terminal digits (last two numbers) of the service member's social security number (SSN), color coding of the health record jacket, and use of a block filing system.

To understand the TDFS filing system, you will need to view the SSN in a different way. As you know, the nine digits of the SSN are divided into three number groups for ease in reading. This practice reduces the chance of transposing numbers. For example, in the TDFS system the SSN 123-45-6789 is visually grouped and read from right to left (instead of left to right), as follows:

Primary Group	Secondary Group	Third Group
89	67	123-45

On the health record, the family member prefix (FMP) is added to the patient's social security number. The FMP is a system used by the Navy to show a beneficiary's relationship to the sponsor. For instance, the FMP for active duty personnel is 20, while the FMP for a spouse is 30 (fig. 12-1).

Under the Terminal Digit Filing System, the central files are divided into 100 approximately equal sections. Each section is identified by a maximum of 100 file guides bearing the 100 primary numbers, **00** consecutively through **99**. Each of these 100 sections contain records whose terminal digits correspond to the section's **primary number** (fig. 12-1). For example, every record with the SSN ending in 56 is filed in section 56.

Within each of these 100 sections, health records are filed in numerical sequence according to their secondary numbers. The **secondary number** is the pair of digits immediately left of the primary number (fig. 12-1).

To make filing of health records easier, health record jackets are color-coded. The second to the last digit of the SSN is preprinted on the jacket. The color of the health record jacket corresponds to the preprinted digit as follows:

Preprinted Digit	Jacket Color
0	Orange
1	Green
2	Yellow
3	Gray
4	Tan
5	Blue
6	White
7	Almond
8	Pink
9	Red

Centralized files having records based upon more than 200 SSNs, or a file of more than 200 records, may

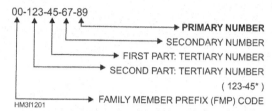

Figure 12-1.—Example of social security number grouping and family member prefix.

need to use the TERTIARY (third) NUMBER in filing. In a properly developed and maintained terminal-digit, color-coded and block-filing system, it is almost impossible to misfile a record. A record misfiled with respect to the left digit of its primary number (for example, a **45** that has been inserted among the **55**s) will attract attention because of its different record jacket color. A record jacket misfiled in respect to the right primary number (for example, a **45** that has been inserted among the **42**s) causes a break in the diagonal pattern formed by the blocking within a color group.

Authorized exemptions from the requirements of the TDFS are discussed in detail in the MANMED.

OPENING HEALTH RECORDS

LEARNING OBJECTIVE: *Determine when a health record should be opened, and select the appropriate record jacket and sequence of medical forms to be placed within a new record.*

This section will discuss the opening of active duty HRECs. HRECs are opened when an individual becomes a member of the Navy and Marine Corps, when a member on the retired list is returned to active duty, or when the original record has been lost or destroyed.

When establishing the four-part health record, the appropriate military health record jacket and required forms must be current and assembled in accordance with current directives.

OPENING HEALTH RECORDS FOR ACTIVE DUTY OFFICERS

Recruiting offices open HRECs for civilian applicants who are accepted for an officer appointment. The health record is then forwarded to the new officer's first duty station.

Midshipmen or former enlisted members appointed to commissioned officer or warrant officer grade continue to use their existing HREC. The MTF having custody of the record at the time of acceptance of appointment will make necessary entries to indicate the new grade and the designator or MOS. Also, the record custodian should prepare summary information entries on SF 600 and NAVMED 6150/4 to include date, place, and grade to which the member was appointed.

Health records of civilian candidates selected for appointment to the Naval Academy should be prepared at the Naval Academy at the time of appointment. Health records for civilian applicants selected for officer candidate programs should be opened upon enrollment in the program.

OPENING HEALTH RECORDS FOR ACTIVE DUTY ENLISTED PERSONNEL

The HREC is opened by the activity executing the enlistment contract upon original enlistment in the Navy or Marine Corps. An exception to this rule involves service members who are enlisted or inducted and ordered to immediate active duty at a recruit training facility. In this instance, the HREC will be opened by either the Naval Training Center (NTC) or Marine Corps Recruit Depot, as appropriate. Copies of the service member's SF 88, *Report of Medical Examination*, and SF 93, *Report of Medical History,* are sent to the appropriate NTC or recruit depot, and added to other applicable HREC forms in the member's HREC.

OPENING HEALTH RECORDS FOR RESERVISTS

The Naval Reserve Personnel Center (NRPC), New Orleans, is the HREC custodian for inactive reserve personnel. In addition, NRPC is responsible for the records' preparation and maintenance. When inactive reservists are called to active duty and their HRECs have not been received by their duty station, a request for their records should be initiated. Requests for Navy personnel are sent to NRPC. Marine Corps personnel requests are sent to the **Marine Corps Reserve Support Center**. For Navy and Marine Corps service members who were discharged before 31 January 1994, requests should be sent to the **National Personnel Records Center** (NPRC) for

record retrieval. For service members who were discharged after 31 January 1994, requests for record retrieval are sent to the **Department of Veterans Affairs** (DVA). Addresses of each of these activities are listed in the MANMED.

PREPARING THE HEALTH RECORD JACKET

A new **military health record jacket**, NAVMED 6150/20-29, should be prepared when an HREC is opened or when the existing jacket has been damaged or is deteriorating to the point of illegibility. The old jacket should be destroyed following replacement.

Preparing the Outside Front Cover and Inside Back Cover

A **felt-tip or indelible black-ink pen** should be used to record all identifying data, except in the "Pencil Entries" block on the upper left of the outer front cover of the HREC. As indicated, information in this block should be written in pencil, so it can be updated or changed. Figure 12-2 illustrates the completed outside front cover and inside back cover of a military health record jacket.

RECORD NUMBERING.—Each health record jacket has the second to the last digit of the SSN preprinted on it. The preprinted digit also matches the last digit of the form number (e.g., the preprinted digit on NAVMED 6150/26 is 6). The color of the treatment record jacket corresponds to the preprinted digit. In preparing a member's treatment record jacket, select a prenumbered NAVMED 6150/20-29 jacket by matching the second to the last number of the member's SSN.

SOCIAL SECURITY NUMBER.—Enter the rest of the member's SSN on the top of the inside back cover. For members who do not have an SSN (e.g., foreign military personnel), use NAVMED 6150/29 as the treatment record jacket. A "substitute" SSN should be created for these members by assigning the numbers "9999" as the last four digits of the SSN and assigning the first five digits in number sequence (e.g., first SSN 000-01-9999, the second SSN 000-02-9999). Place a piece of **black** cellophane tape over the number that corresponds to the last digit of the SSN in each of the two number scales on the inside back cover of the HREC (fig. 12-2).

FAMILY MEMBER PREFIX.—Enter the member's family member prefix (FMP) code in the two diamonds preceding the SSN on the top of the

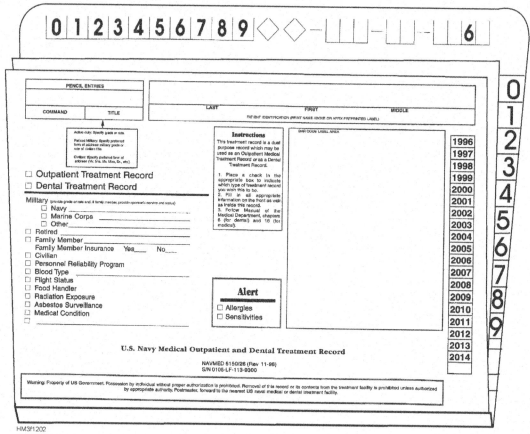

PENCIL ENTRIES

COMMAND TITLE

LAST FIRST MIDDLE
PATIENT IDENTIFICATION (PRINT NAME ABOVE OR AFFIX PREPRINTED LABEL)

Active duty: Specify grade or rate.

Retired Military: Specify preferred form of address: military grade or rate of civilian title.

Civilian: Specify preferred form of address (Mr, Mrs, Ms, Miss, Dr., etc.).

☐ Outpatient Treatment Record
☐ Dental Treatment Record

Military (provide grade or rate and, if family member, provide sponsor's service and status)
☐ Navy _____
☐ Marine Corps _____
☐ Other _____
☐ Retired _____
☐ Family Member _____
Family Member Insurance Yes___ No___
☐ Civilian
☐ Personnel Reliability Program
☐ Blood Type _____
☐ Flight Status _____
☐ Food Handler
☐ Radiation Exposure
☐ Asbestos Surveillance
☐ Medical Condition
☐ _____

Instructions

This treatment record is a dual purpose record which may be used as an Outpatient Medical Treatment Record or as a Dental Treatment Record.

1. Place a check in the appropriate box to indicate which type of treatment record you wish this to be.
2. Fill in all appropriate information on the front as well as inside this record.
3. Follow Manual of the Medical Department, chapters 6 (for dental) and 16 (for medical).

BAR CODE LABEL AREA

Alert

☐ Allergies
☐ Sensitivities

U.S. Navy Medical Outpatient and Dental Treatment Record

NAVMED 6150/26 (Rev 11-96)
S/N 0105-LF-113-9300

Warning: Property of US Government. Possession by individual without proper authorization is prohibited. Removal of this record or its contents from the treatment facility is prohibited unless authorized by appropriate authority. Postmaster, forward to the nearest US naval medical or dental treatment facility.

0 1 2 3 4 5 6 7 8 9

1996 1997 1998 1999 2000 2001 2002 2003 2004 2005 2006 2007 2008 2009 2010 2011 2012 2013 2014

HM3f1202

Figure 12-2.—Sample of completed outside front cover and inside back cover of a health record jacket (NAVMED 6150/26.)

inside back cover. Enter the FMP code of 20 for all Navy and Marine Corps members. Enter an FMP code of 00 for all foreign military personnel.

PATIENT'S NAME.—Enter the member's full name (last, first, middle initial, in that order) in the upper-right corner. Indicate no middle name by the abbreviation "NMN." If the member uses initials instead of first or middle names, show this by enclosing the initials in quotation marks (e.g., "J" "C"). Indicate titles, such as JR, SR, and III, at the end of the name. The name may be handwritten on the line provided or imprinted on a self-adhesive label and attached to the jacket in the patient identification box.

ALERT BOX—In the lower center area of the outside front cover, indicate in the alert box whether the member has drug sensitivities or allergies by entering an "X" in the appropriate box. If there are no allergies or sensitivities, leave it blank.

RECORD CATEGORY.—Indicate the appropriate record category by entering an "X" in the box marked "Health Record" on the outside front cover, just below the "Pencil Entries" block. Then attach ½-inch **red** tape to the record category block on the right edge of the inside back cover of the jacket; this indicates it's an active duty record.

PATIENT SERVICE AND STATUS.—Below the record category box is the patient service and status box. Mark an "X" in the appropriate service block.

SPECIAL CATEGORIES OF RECORDS.— Identify the records of personnel assigned to special duty or medical surveillance programs (e.g., personnel reliability program, flight status, or the Asbestos Medical Surveillance Program) by marking an "X" at the appropriate special category entry listed below the record category type.

Identify flag officers and general officers by stamping or printing "FLAG OFFICER" or

"GENERAL OFFICER," as appropriate, on the lower portion of the patient identification box. If a patient identification label is used, print or stamp the appropriate identification below the label.

PENCIL ENTRIES.—Following the instructions on the front cover, pencil in the appropriate title (i.e., grade or rate, if on active duty; preferred form of address, if retired or civilian), and include the current command (if active duty).

RECORD RETIREMENT TAPE BOX.— Leave the record retirement tape box on the inside back cover blank.

BAR CODE.—Some Navy medical facilities have bar coding capabilities. The bar code label indicates the patient's FMP, SSN, record type, and record volume number. Affix the label to the front of the record jacket in the box right of the alert box. If the bar code is part of the patient identification label (such as the patient identification label produced by the Composite Health Care System (CHCS) computers), place this label in the patient identification box.

LABELS.—Use of a self-adhesive label with the name of the MTF, ship, or other units having custodial responsibility for the record is optional. Ship or MTF logos are permitted as long as the necessary patient identifying information is not obscured. For further details see the appropriate MANMED article covering this subject.

Preparing the Inside Front Cover

Enter the following information in pencil on the inside front cover of the HREC jacket. Record the information in the inside of the front cover in pencil to permit changes and updating.

- Date of arrival

- Projected departure date

- Home address and telephone number

- Duty station and telephone number

Preparing the Middle Section

The middle section of the HREC contains a preprinted DD 2005, *Privacy Act Statement—Health Care Records*, on the front side. When opening an HREC, the service members are asked to read the Privacy Act Statement. After the members have read the statement, they will need to sign, date, and include their SSN at the bottom of the form. Signing this statement indicates the service members understand their right to confidentiality in regard to the medical documentation placed in their HREC.

On the reverse of the middle section is a Disclosure Accounting Record. This form should be annotated whenever the HREC is released to any individual or agency outside the MTF.

SEQUENCE OF HEALTH RECORD FORMS

When assembling an HREC, you should arrange the forms in chronological order by date. The most current document should be placed on top, and the least current documents below it. The HREC contains dividers that partition the record into four parts. A sequential listing of medical forms to be filed in each section is provided in table 12-1. The titles for each part of the HREC are as follows:

Part 1. Record of Preventive Medicine and Occupational Health

Part 2. Record of Medical Care and Treatment

Part 3. Physical Qualifications

Part 4. Record of Ancillary Studies, Inpatient Care, and Miscellaneous Forms

HEALTH RECORD FORMS

LEARNING OBJECTIVE: *Recall the purpose and completion procedures for the health record forms discussed in this section.*

In the last section, you learned there are many medical forms placed in the health record. Also, you learned each form has a specific location within the record. The methods for the management of major areas of health care, both ashore and afloat, are rapidly changing. The Composite Health Care System (CHCS), a secure, computer-based system, is now the primary means that healthcare practitioners use to schedule and process patient visits, track medical results, order labs and x-rays, and process orders for medications. CHCS is especially valuable for pier-side healthcare providers and furnishes a much higher standard for patient care.

Computerized medical documentation (e.g., laboratory test results, emergency room reports, etc.)

Table 12-1.—Sequential List of Health Record Forms

LEFT SIDE OF HREC FOLDER	RIGHT SIDE OF HREC FOLDER
(Top to bottom with most current entry on top within group of forms)	(Top to bottom with most current entry on top within group of forms)

Left Side - Part 1: Record of Preventive Medicine & Occupational Health

NAVMED 6150/20, Summary of Care Form *[Always on top.]*

SF 601, Immunization Record

NAVMED 6000/2, Chronological Record of HIV Testing

DD 771, Eyewear Prescription

NAVMED 6490/1, Visual Record

NAVMED 6470/10, Record of Occupational Exposure to Ionizing Radiation

NAVMED 6470/11, Record of Exposure to Ionizing Radiation from Internally Deposited Radionuclides *[Interfile behind 6470/10 with corresponding dosimetry issue period.]*

DD 2215, Reference Audiogram

DD 2216, Hearing Conservation Data

NAVMED 6224/1, TB Contact/Converter Follow-up

NAVMED 6260/5, Asbestos Medical Surveillance Program

DD 2493-1, Abestos Exposure-Part 1, Initial Medical Questionnaire *[Attach to correspondence NAVMED 6260/5.]*

DD 2493-2, Abestos Exposure-Part II, Periodic Medical Questionnaire

OPNAV 5100/15, Medical Surveillance Questionnaire

Other 5100 Forms-Occupational Health Series Forms

Right Side - Part 2, Section A: Record of Medical Care and Treatment

NAVPERS 5510/1, Record Identifier for personnel Reliability Program (PRP) *[Always top form, except for deaths.]* *[File all forms below in chronological order with most current form on top, regardless of form number. Be sure to group episodes of care together.]*

SF 558, Medical Record Emergency Care and Treatment Record of Ambulance Care

SF 600 HREC-Chronological Record of Medical Care *[If for outpatient surgery, dictate or document immediately after surgery and file with corresponding SF 516. Otherwise file as exhibited here.]*

SF 513, Medical Record Consultation Sheet

DD 2161, Referral For Civilian Medical Care

Top Forms in Part 2, Section A When a Patient is Deceased

Attestation Sheet

DD 2064, Certificate of Death

SF 503, Autopsy Protocol

SF 523, Authorization for Autopsy

SF 523A, Disposition of Body

SF 523B, Authorization For Tissue Donation

Right Side - Part 2, Section B: Inpatient Care, Ambulatory Surgeries, etc.

NAVMED 6300/5, Inpatient Admission/Disposition Record (Copy)

SF 502, Medical Record, Narrative Summary (Copy)

SF 539, Medical Record-Abbreviated Medical Record (Copy)

SF 509, Progress Notes

SF 516 Medical Record-Operation Report (Original for Outpatient Surgery) *[Dictate/document immediately after surgery.]*

SF 600 HREC-Chronolgocial Record of Medical Care *[Outpatient Surgery: To be dictated immediately after surgery] [File with corresponding SF 516.]*

SF 517, Anesthesia

SF 522, Request for Administration of Anesthesia *[File with corresponding SF 517.]*

SF 533 Medical Record-Prenatal and Pregnancy (Only for patients not admitted for delivery)

Civilian Medical Care Notes

DD 602, Patient Evacuation Tag *[Staple to current SF 600.]*

Left Side - Part 3: Physical Qualifications, Administrative Forms

NAVMED 1300/1, Medical & Dental Overseas Screening Review for Active Duty & Dependents

NAVPERS 1300/16, Report of Suitability for Overseas Assignment - Parts I, II, and III

NAVMED 6100/1, Medical Board Report Cover Sheet

NAVMED 6100/2, Medical Board Statement of Patient

NAVMED 6100/3, Medical Board Certificate

NAVMED 6100/5, Abbreviated Temporary Limited Duty

DD 2569, Third Party Collection Program *[See BUMEDINST 7000.7 series for additional guidance.]*

SF 2824C, Physicians Statement for Employee Disability Retirement

SF 47, Physical Fitness Inquiry For Motor Vehicle Operators

SF 78, Certificate of Medical Examination

DD 2005, Privacy Act Statement

Right Side, Part 4, Record of Ancillary Studies, Therapies, etc.

SF 217, Medical Report-Epilepsy

SF 88, Report of Medical Examination

SF 93, Report of Medical History *[File behind corresponding SF 88 or SF 78.]*

BUMED Waiver Letters with BUPERS Endorsement

NAVMED 6120/1, Competence for Duty Examination

NAVMED 6120/2, Officer Physical Examination Special Questionnaire *[File in place of SF 93 when used.]*

NAVMED 6120/3, Annual Certificate of Physical Condition

NAVMED 6150/2, Special Duty Medical Abstract

NAVMED 6150/4, Abstract of Service and Medical History

NAVJAG 5800/10, Injury Report

NAVJAG Report - Investigation to inquire into the circumstances surrounding the injury of (servicemember).

NAVPERS 1754/1, Exceptional Family Member (EFM) Program Application

Living Will or Medical Power of Attorney

OPNAV 5211/9, Record of Disclosure, Privacy Act of 1974

DD 877, Request for Medical/Dental Records

SF 515, Medical Record Tissue Examination

SF 519A, Radiographic Consultation Request/Report

SF 519B, Medical Record-Radiologic Consultation Request/Report

SF 519, Medical Record-Radiographic

SF 518, Medical Record-Blood or Blood Component Transfusion

SF 520, Medical Record-Electrocardiogram Request

SF 524, Radiation Therapy

SF 525, Radiation Therapy Summary

SF 526, Medical Record-Interstitial/Intercavity Therapy

SF 527, Group Muscle Strength, Join ROM, Girth and Length Measurements

SF 528, Medical Record-Muscle Function By Nerve Distribution: Face, Neck and Upper Extremity

SF 529, Medical Record-Muscle Function by Nerve Distribution: Trunk and Lower Extremity

SF 530, Neurological Examination

SF 531, Anatomical Figure *[May also be filed under a corresponding SF 600, SF 513, etc.]*

SF 541, Medical Record Gynecologic Cytology

SF 545, Laboratory Report Display

SF 546 - 557, Laboratory Reports. *[Attach through to SF 545 in chronological order.]*

SF 559, Medical Record-Allergen Extract Prescription New and Refill

SF 560, Medical Record-Electroencephalogram Request and History

SF 511, Vital Signs Record

SF 512, Plotting Chart

SF 512A, Plotting Chart Blood Pressure

HM3t1201

has become commonplace. However, the Navy Medical Department continues to use many government printed forms (e.g., NAVMED, DD, and SF). This section will cover selected (government-printed) medical forms, their purpose, and procedures for completing them.

Healthcare providers should enter their signature and identification data in the HREC in black or blue-black ink. Type, print, or stamp provider's name, grade or rating, and social security number below their signature. Stamped facsimile signatures are NOT to be used on any medical form in the HREC. The signing individual assumes responsibility for the correctness of the entry for which they sign.

All medical forms require an accurate and complete documentation of patient identification data. Patient identification data on medical documentation is critical. Complete and accurate documentation of patient identification data helps to ensure the documents are placed in the correct patient's record. Three methods are currently used to place patient identification on medical documents:

- embossed medical card,

- automated forms, and

- handwritten entries.

Embossed medical cards are used to imprint patient identification data on medical forms. Printouts of automated (computerized) forms should provide the information listed in table 12-1. Handwritten patient identification data should be entered in spaces at the bottom of the form. Each method should contain, at a minimum, the patient identification data listed in table 12-2.

SUMMARY OF CARE (NAVMED 6150/20)

The Summary of Care (fig. 12-3) contains a summation of relevant problems and medications that significantly affect the patient's health status. Properly maintained, the Summary of Care form aids healthcare providers by allowing them quick access to pertinent medical factors that may affect how they manage a patient's medical care. This form is a permanent part of the HREC.

Entries on the NAVMED 6150/20 should include significant medical and surgical conditions, allergies, untoward reactions to medication, and medications currently using or recently used. The Summary of Care form should be reviewed, and, if necessary,

Table 12-2.—Patient Identification Data

Item #	Patient Identification Data
1	Full name (last, first, middle)
2	FMP + SSN
3	Date of birth (YY-MM-DD)
4	Sex of patient (M or F)
5	Sponsor (self)
6	Sponsor's Agency or military service (USN, USMC, USCG,...)
7	Patient's paygrade (e.g., E7, O2)
8	MTF maintaining record (e.g., NH Pensacola, etc.)

revised during the patient's visit. The NAVMED 6150/20 should also be reviewed during yearly verification and before HREC transfers.

The Summary of Care form is divided into five sections: significant health problems, hospitalization/surgery, medical alert, medications, and health maintenance.

- **Significant health problems section:** Enter only significant medical conditions in this section. Significant medical conditions include chronic diseases (such as hypertension, diabetes, arthritis, etc.) and acute recurrent illnesses (such as recurrent urinary tract infections, recurrent otitis media, recurrent bronchitis, etc.)

- **Hospitalization/surgery section:** Enter significant surgical conditions. Include all procedures requiring general or regional anesthesia and any procedures likely to have a long-term effect on the patient's health status.

- **Medical alert section:** Note any allergies and significant reactions to drugs in the medical alert section. Record also in this section relevant alcohol and tobacco use.

- **Medications section:** Record all currently or recently used medications.

- **Medical maintenance section:** This section of the NAVMED 6150/20 contains a variety of medical information. It contains health maintenance functions, such as mammograms, chest X-rays, EKGs, and pap smears. Enter the date of the health maintenance functions in pencil, so it can be updated. Include in this section occupational health surveillance activities, such

Summary of Care
(This form is subject to the Privacy Act of 1974)

No.	Significant Health Problem	Date	Medical Alert	(SBE Prophylaxis, allergies, other)
1.	Right Thyroid Nodule	19Aug95	Aspirin	
2.	Influenza	30Jan97		
3.	Urinary Tract Infecton	16Nov99		
4.				
5.			Alcohol:	
6.			Tobacco:	

No.		Date	Medications	Start	Stop
7.				Start	Stop
8.			Tylenol (PRN)	30Jan97	
9.			Ciprofloxacin 250mg BID	16Nov99	25Nov99
10.			Pyridium 200mg TID	16Nov99	18Nov99
11.					
	Exceptional Family Member Program				

	Hospitalization/Surgery	Date	Health Maintenance	Date of Last Test (Pencil entry)
1.	Tonsillectomy	1974	Prostate Exam	N/A
2.	Wisdom Teeth extracted X 4	23Mar96	RPR	06 Feb 98
3.			G6PD / GPAB	06 Feb 98
4.			Stool GUAIAC	06 Feb 98
5.			Mammogram	
6.			Chest X-Ray	
7.			ECG	06 Feb 98
8.			Birth Control Method	
9.			PAP Smear	06 Feb 98
10.	Advance Directive Provided:		Sickle Cell Trait	06 Feb 98
11.	Advance Directive Returned:		HIV Screen	06 Feb 98
12.			Other	

(Continue significant health problems, medications, hospitalization/surgery on reverse)

Space for Mechanical Imprint			
	Patient's Name: Frost, Jane O.	Rank/Grade: HMCS	Sex: Female
	SSN/Identification Number: 20-123-45-6789	Status: Active Duty	Date of Birth: 02Dec69
	Branch of Service:	Organization: USS Reliable	
	Sponsor's Name: SSA	Relationship to Sponsor: Self	Records maintained at: USS Reliable

NAVMED 6150/20 (Rev. 1-94)
S/N 0105-LF-017-9000

HM3f1203

Figure 12-3.—Summary of Care, NAVMED 6150/20.

as involvement in the Asbestos Program, the Hearing Conservation Program, or exposure to lead. Include also the following laboratory tests: blood type, G6PD, and sickle trait.

CHRONOLOGICAL RECORD OF MEDICAL CARE (SF 600)

The *Chronological Record of Medical Care*, SF 600, provides a current, concise, and comprehensive record of a member's military medical history (fig. 12-4, view A and B). Use the SF 600 for all outpatient care and file in the HREC. Record all visits, including those that result in referrals to other MTFs, on the SF 600. Each person making an entry on the form must sign the entry and include his identification information (full name, grade or rate, profession [e.g., MC, NC, etc.], and SSN), either hand printed, typed, or stamped.

Properly maintained, the SF 600 facilitates the evaluation of a patient's physical condition and reduces correspondence necessary to obtain medical records. Appropriate use of the form also eliminates unnecessary repetition of expensive diagnostic procedures and serves as an invaluable permanent record of medical evaluations and treatments.

Completing the SF 600

Entries made on the SF 600 can be typewritten when practical. However, entries normally are handwritten with black or blue-black ink pens. When initiating an SF 600, patient identification data should be completed. Also, type or stamp the date (DD-MMM-YY) and the name and address of the activity responsible for the entry.

Use both sides of each SF 600. Preparation of a new SF 600 is not necessary each time the person is seen in a different MTF. If only a few entries are recorded on the SF 600 at the time of a move, stamp the designation and location of the receiving MTF below the last entry and use the rest of the page to record subsequent visits. If the back of the SF 600 is not used, then the back needs to be crossed out and the words "This side not used," printed in the middle of the form.

SF 600s are continuous and include the following information: complaints, duration of illness or injury, physical findings, clinical course, results of laboratory or other special examinations, treatment (including operations), physical fitness at the time of disposition, and disposition. The subjective complaint, observation, assessment, and plan (SOAP) format may be used for entries so long as the required information in table 12-3 is included.

Table 12-3.—Required Information on an SF 600

ITEM	REMARKS
Date	A complete date must be included with every entry in the HREC. When an undated page is misfiled, it is difficult to replace in proper sequence. Use the three-letter abbreviation for the month on all dates (e.g., 27 Apr 96).
MTF name	Name of hospital, clinic, or ship
Clinical department or service	(e.g., Military Sick Call, Orthopedic Department., etc.)
Chief complaint or purpose of visit	(e.g., headache, PRT screening, etc.)
Objective findings	
Diagnosis or medical impression	
Studies ordered and results	(e.g., laboratory, X-ray, etc.)
Therapies administered	
Patient disposition, recommendations, and patient instructions	(e.g., SIQ for 24 hours, referral to specialty clinic, etc.)
Healthcare provider's name and signature	Include the provider's grade or rate, profession (e.g., MC, NC), and SSN

Enter the following information indicated on table 12-3 on the patient's SF 600.

Record each visit and the complaint described, even if a member is returned to duty without treatment. Also, document if a patient leaves before being seen.

Other SF 600 Entries

Other SF 600 entries include the following:

- Imminent hospitalization

- Special procedures and therapy

- Sick call visit

NSN 7540-00-634-4176

HEALTH RECORD	CHRONOLOGICAL RECORD OF MEDICAL CARE
DATE	SYMPTOMS, DIAGNOSIS, TREATMENT TREATING ORGANIZATION *(Sign each entry)*

1 DEC 97 — NAVAL HOSPITAL, BLANK, VA

Member cut forehead when he slipped in shower and struck head on edge of shower stall. 1" (2.54 cm) laceration over left eyebrow. Wound cleaned and sutured with six 6-0 nylon sutures. Tetanus Toxoid booster given. To duty. To return to sick call on 6 Dec 97.

W. T. Door
W. T. DOOR
111-11-1111
LCDR, MC, USNR

6 Dec 97 — NAVAL HOSPITAL, BLANK, VA

Forehead laceration healing well. Sutures removed. No other complaints. To duty.

W. T. Door
W. T. DOOR
111-11-1111
LCDR, MC, USNR

10 Jan 98 — NAVAL HOSPITAL, BLANK, VA

Health and Dental records screened. Physically qualified for transfer.

Jack R. Frost
HM1 J. R. FROST, USN
222-22-2222

23 Feb 98 — USS CARRIER (CV-00)

Transcribed from DD 689 - NAS Dispensary, Blank, VA, dated 21 Feb 98

PATIENT'S IDENTIFICATION *(Use this space for Mechanical Imprint)*

RECORDS MAINTAINED AT: ► Naval Hospital, Blank, VA

PATIENT'S NAME *(Last, First, Middle initial)*			SEX
DOE, John R.			M
RELATIONSHIP TO SPONSOR	STATUS		RANK/GRADE
N/A	AD		HM3
SPONSOR'S NAME		ORGANIZATION	
N/A		Fighter Sq.-VF 143	
DEPART./SERVICE	SSN/IDENTIFICATION		DATE OF BIRTH
USN	20-123-45-6789		9 May 75

CHRONOLOGICAL RECORD OF MEDICAL CARE

STANDARD FORM 600 (REV. 5-84)
Prescribed by GSA and ICMR
FIRMR (41 CFR) 201-45-45.505

HM3F1204A

Figure 12-4.—Chronological Record of Medical Care, SF 600: A. Front view.

DATE	SYMPTOMS, DIAGNOSIS, TREATMENT TREATING ORGANIZATION *(Sign each entry)*
5 Mar 98	"Member injured right hand when he struck hand on backboard during COMNAVAIRLANT basketball game at 2030 this date. X-ray of right hand negative for fracture or dislocation. Impression: Contusion rt. hand. Treatment: Hot soaks for next several days and ASA 10 gr q4h prn for pain. To duty. /s/CDR P. T. BOATE, MC,USNR"
	A. B. Seaman HM2 A. B. SEAMAN, USN 333-33-3333
19 Mar 98	USS CARRIER (CV-00) DIAGNOSIS: Contusion, left thoracic region. ICDA Code No. 9220 Line of duty. Not due to own misconduct. While descending hatchway, slipped and fell, striking left chest against hatch combing. Patient complains of shortness of breath with pain and discomfort in left thoracic region. Examination indicates possibility of internal injuries, and as this ship is leaving port tomorrow on extended operation, it is deemed medically advisable to transfer this patient to a hospital.
19 Mar 98	Transferred to Naval Hospital, Blank, VA
	A. B. Smith A. B. SMITH, LT, MC, USN 444-44-4444
	APPROVED: Jack R. Frost J. R. Frost CAPT, MC, USN 555-55-5555
19 Mar 98	NAVAL HOSPITAL, BLANK, VA DIAGNOSIS: Contusion, left thoracic region. ICDA Code No. 9220 Line of duty. Not due to own misconduct. Admitted from USS CARRIER (CV-00) where while descending hatchway, patient slipped and fell, striking left chest against hatch combing. Complains of shortness of breath and severe pain in area of 4th thoracic rib. X-RAY: Examination of entire right and left thoracic regions reveals no evidence of fracture or bone pathology. TREATMENT: Heat application and bed rest. Slight pain with motion. Discomfort subsiding. On 24 Mar 98, patient developed acute sore throat. Temp. 101.2 (38.7); pharynx injected, tonsils inflamed. Exudate cultured.
	DIAGNOSIS CHANGED on 26 Mar 98 by reason of intercurrent diagnosis. Tonsillitis, Acute, Streptococcal, ICDA Code No. 4630 Line of duty. Not due to own misconduct. Placed on antibiotic therapy. (Penicillin) On 1 May 98, Temp. 98.6 (37.3); all medication discontinued. Slight discomfort and tenderness remain in left thoracic region. Ward privileges authorized.
4 May 98	No complaints. To duty. Well.
	V.C.Pistol V. C. PISTOL, LT, MC, USN 666-66-6666
	APPROVED: M. N. Chairman M. N. CHAIRMAN Chief Service CAPT, MC, USN 777-77-7777

*U.S.GPO: 1997-426-840/69077

STANDARD FORM 600 BACK (REV. 5-84)

HM3f1204B

Figure 12-4.—Chronological Record of Medical Care, SF 600: B. Back view.

- Injuries or poisonings

- Line-of-duty inquiries

- Binnacle list and sick list

- Reservist check-in and check-out statements

IMMINENT HOSPITALIZATION.—When an admission of a patient is imminent, admission notes can be made on an SF 600. However, the use of the SF 509, *Medical Record-Progress Report*, is preferred. The SF 509 form is routinely used for inpatient admission notes and are filed in the patient's IREC. Record referred or postponed inpatient admissions on the SF 600.

SPECIAL PROCEDURES AND THERAPY.—When patients are seen repeatedly for special procedures or therapy, such as physical and occupational therapy, renal dialysis, or radiation, note the therapy on the SF 600 and record interim progress statements. Initial notes, interim progress notes, and any summaries may be recorded on any appropriate authorized form, but should be referenced on SF 600. Write a final summary when special procedures or therapy are ended. This summary should include the result of evaluative procedures, the treatment given, the reaction to treatment, the progress noted, condition on discharge (when applicable), and any other pertinent observations.

SICK CALL VISITS.—Whenever a member is evaluated at sick call, an entry will be made on an SF 600 reflecting the complaints or conditions presented, pertinent history, treatment rendered, and disposition.

INJURY OR POISONING.—In the event of injury or poisoning, record the duty status of the member at the time of occurrence and the circumstances of occurrence per the guidelines in BUMEDINST 6300.3, *Inpatient Data System*.

LINE-OF-DUTY INQUIRIES.—When a member of the naval service incurs an injury that might result in permanent disability or results in his physical inability to perform duty for a period exceeding 24 hours, an entry should be made concerning line-of-duty misconduct. Such entries should include facts, such as time of injury, date, place, names of persons involved, and the circumstances surrounding the injury.

A line-of-duty inquiry is conducted to establish whether the injuries the patient sustained are the result of misconduct on the part of the member or others. For more details on line-of-duty inquiries, see the *Manual of the Judge Advocate General* (JAGMAN).

BINNACLE LIST AND SICK LIST.—When a member's name is placed on the Binnacle List for treatment, make an entry on the SF 600 showing date, diagnosis, and a summary of treatment.

When an active duty member is placed on the Sick List, the medical department representative (MDR) should enter information on the SF 600 about the nature of the disease, illness, or injury; pertinent history or circumstances of occurrence; treatment rendered; and disposition.

SERIOUSLY ILL/VERY SERIOUSLY ILL (SI/VSI) LIST.—Place personnel whose illness or injuries are severe on the SI/VSI List (as defined in MILPERSMAN 4210100) and make appropriate notification.

RESERVIST CHECK-IN AND CHECK-OUT STATEMENTS.—Naval Reserve personnel who are checking in, or out on orders for annual training (AT), active duty for training (ADT), or inactive duty training travel (IDTT)) should sign the following statements. The statements should be entered on an SF 600 and signed by the reserve member and the MDR.

For personnel checking in:

I certify that there have been no significant changes in my physical condition since my last physical examination or annual certification. Furthermore, I certify that I have no illness or injury that would preclude me from performing this period of (circle one) AT, ADT, IDTT.

(Member's and MDR's signature and date)

For personnel checking out:

I certify that I have/have not incurred or aggravated any injuries or illnesses during the period of Naval Reserve service.

(Member's and MDR's signature and date)

Special SF 600s

Two special SF 600s will be covered in the section. Both forms perform specific functions.

SPECIAL-HYPERSENSITIVITY SF 600.—Indicate any hypersensitivity to drugs or chemicals on a separate SF 600 (fig. 12-5). The SF 600 will be marked "SPECIAL-HYPERSENSITIVITY" at the

HEALTH RECORD	CHRONOLOGICAL RECORD OF MEDICAL CARE		
DATE	SYMPTOMS, DIAGNOSIS, TREATMENT TREATING ORGANIZATION *(Sign each entry)*		
	RETAIN IN PERMANENT HEALTH RECORD		
6 Jun 97	Determined to be hypersensitive to ASPIRIN		
8 Nov 97	Determined to be hypersensitive to INFLUENZA, POLY VALENT VACCINE		
21 Nov 97	Determined to be hypersensitive to EGGS		

"SPECIAL HYPERSENSITIVITY"

PATIENT'S IDENTIFICATION *(Use this space for Mechanical Imprint)*	RECORDS MAINTAINED AT: ► Naval Hospital, Blank, VA		
	PATIENT'S NAME *(Last, First, Middle initial)* SEAMAN, Able B.		SEX Male
	RELATIONSHIP TO SPONSOR Self	STATUS AD	RANK/GRADE BM3
	SPONSOR'S NAME N/A		ORGANIZATION USS CARRIER
	DEPART./SERVICE USN	SSN/IDENTIFICATION 20-123-45-6789	DATE OF BIRTH 15 May 75

CHRONOLOGICAL RECORD OF MEDICAL CARE   STANDARD FORM 600 (REV. 5-84)
Prescribed by GSA and ICMR
FIRMR (41 CFR) 201-45-45.505

HM3f1205

Figure 12-5.—Standard Form 600, Special-Hypersensitivity.

bottom of the page. Appropriate entries regarding the hypersensitivity should be made on the SF 601 (Immunization Record), SF 603 (Dental Report), NAVMED 6150/10-19 (HREC jacket), and the NAVMED 6150/20 (Summary of Care).

BLOOD GROUPING AND TYPING RECORD.—The Blood Grouping and Typing Record, which is generated at the member's initial entry processing point, is an SF 600 overprint. Information on the Blood Grouping and Typing Record identifies the individual by the appropriate ABO group and Rh type (positive or negative). Testing results are documented on the form and the original laboratory request filed with the SF 545, *Laboratory Result Display*, in the member's HREC. The Blood Grouping and Typing Record may also contain a syphilis screening test and other screening test for the presence of certain diseases.

IMMUNIZATION RECORD (SF 601)

The purpose of the SF 601 form (fig. 12-6) is to record prophylactic (disease preventive) immunizations; sensitivity tests; reactions to transfusions, drugs, sera (*sing.* serum), and food; known allergies; and blood-typing. The SF 601 contains specified blocks for various immunizations, such as yellow fever vaccine, typhoid vaccine, and influenza vaccine.

Preparing and Maintaining SF 601

An immunization record is prepared and maintained for each person with an HREC. Information on the SF 601 is recorded in designated blocks. When space is exhausted in any single category, prepare a new SF 601 and file in the HREC in chronological order. Verify previous entries and bring the most current immunizations forward. Retain the old SF 601 beneath the new SF 601. Replacement of the SF 601 is not required because of a change in grade, rating, name, or status of member. Never maintain the SF 601 separate from the HREC. Information recorded on the SF 601 is normally needed for government international travel, such as unit deployments or directed governmental travel.

Immunization Entries

The name of the medical officer or MDR administering the immunization or test or determining

HEALTH RECORD   IMMUNIZATION RECORD

All entries in ink to be made in block letters

VACCINATION AGAINST SMALLPOX *(Number of previous vaccination scars)*

	DATE	ORIGIN	BATCH NUMBER	REACTION	STATION	PHYSICIAN'S NAME
1						
2						
3						
4						
5						
6						

YELLOW FEVER VACCINE

	DATE	ORIGIN	BATCH NUMBER	STATION	PHYSICIAN'S NAME
1	05Jan98	Nat'l Drug Company	Y101	Naval Base, Norfolk, VA	J. B. Doe
2					
3					

TYPHOID VACCINE

	DATE	DOSE	PHYSICIAN'S NAME		DATE	DOSE	PHYSICIAN'S NAME
1	07Jun95	Vi 0.5/ Q 2 yrs	A. B. Smith	4			
2	23Jul97	4 caps/ Q 5 yrs	W. T. Door	5			
3				6			

TETANUS-DIPHTHERIA TOXOIDS

	DATE	DOSE	PHYSICIAN'S NAME		DATE	DOSE	PHYSICIAN'S NAME
1	05Jan98	0.5 cc	J. B. Doe	4			
2				5			
3				6			

CHOLERA VACCINE

	DATE	PHYSICIAN'S NAME		DATE	PHYSICIAN'S NAME		DATE	PHYSICIAN'S NAME
1	12Jan98	J. B. Doe	4			7		
2			5			8		
3			6			9		

PATIENT'S IDENTIFICATION *(Mechanically Imprint, Type of Print):*

```
SEAMAN, Able B.
Male 09May75
YN2   N/AD
20-123-45-6789
```

◄ Patient's Name— last, first, middle initial; Sex; Age or Year of Birth; Relationship to Sponsor; Component/Status; Department/Serevice.

◄ Sponsor's Name— last, first, middle initial; Rank/Grade; SSN or Identification Number; Organization.

601-105

IMMUNIZATION RECORD

Standard Form 601 October 1975 (Rev)
General Services Administration & Interagency
Committee on Medical Records
FIRMR (41 CFR) 201-45 505

HM3f1206A

Figure 12-6.—Immunization Record, SF 601: A. Front view.

ORAL POLIOVIRUS VACCINE

	DATE	DOSE	PHYSICIAN'S NAME		DATE	DOSE	PHYSICIAN'S NAME
1	05Jun00	0.5cc	J. R. Frost	3			
2				4			

INFLUENZA VACCINE

	DATE	DOSE	PHYSICIAN'S NAME		DATE	DOSE	PHYSICIAN'S NAME
3	15Nov96	0.5cc	A. B. Smith	3	01Nov98	0.5cc	J. B. Doe
4	15Oct97	0.5cc	W. T. Door	4	20Oct99	0.5cc	J. R. Frost

OTHER IMMUNIZATIONS

	DATE	TYPE	DOSE	PHYSICIAN'S NAME		DATE	TYPE	DOSE	PHYSICIAN'S NAME
1	27Aug99	MMR		J. R. Frost	5	06Jun00	HepatitisA#2	1.0cc	J. R. Frost
2	16Nov99	Varicella #1	0.5cc	J. R. Frost	6				
3	16Dec99	Varicella #2	0.5cc	J. R. Frost	7				
4	23Dec99	HepatitisA#1	0.1cc	J. R. Frost	8				

SENSITIVITY TEST (Tuberculin, etc.)

	DATE	TYPE	DOSE	ROUTE	RESULT	PHYSICIAN'S NAME
1	16Nov98	TB (Mantoux)	0.1cc	Intradermal	zero mm	J. B. Doe
2						
3						
4						
5						

REMARKS:

(1) HYPERSENSITIVITY TO ASPIRIN

(2) HISTORY MODERATELY SEVERE REACTION TO PARENTERAL PENICILLIN IN 1995

THIS RECORD IS ISSUED IN ACCORDANCE WITH ARTICLE 99, WHO SANITARY REGULATION NO. 2.

HM3f1206B

Figure 12-6.—Immunization Record, SF 601: B. Back view.

the nature of the sensitivity reaction should be typed or stamped on the SF 601 form. Signatures are not required; however, when signatures are used, make sure you can read them.

The medical officer or Medical Department representative administering the immunization is responsible for completing entries in the appropriate sections of SF 601. For smallpox (if administered), cholera, yellow fever and anthrax immunizations, record the manufacturer's name and batch or lot number.

NOTE: The specific protocol for recording anthrax immunizations is outlined in SECNAVINST 6230.4.

Type any hypersensitivity to drugs or chemicals under "Remarks and Recommendations" in capital letters (e.g., "HYPERSENSITIVITY TO ASPIRIN," "HYPERSENSITIVE TO LIDOCAINE"). This entry is in addition to a similar entry required on the SF 603, the SF 600 Special-Hypersensitivity form, and the NAVMED 6150/20 retained permanently in the HREC.

When recording positive results (10 mm or more induration) of the tuberculin skin test (PPD), refer to the *Tuberculosis Control Program* instruction, BUMEDINST 6224.8, for guidance.

Disposing of SF 601

When a service member is released from active duty or separated from the service, the SF 601 is to remain with the HREC.

INTERNATIONAL CERTIFICATES OF VACCINATION (PHS-731)

All personnel performing international travel should be immunized in accordance with NAVMEDCOMINST 6230.15, *Immunizations and Chemoprophylaxis*, and the current edition of FM 8-33/NAVMED P-5038, *Control of Communicable Diseases of Man*. Service members should have a properly completed and authenticated PHS-731 form (International Certificates of Vaccination) in their possession. The PHS-731 form is issued to service members for independent international travel. This form, kept by the individual, is a personal record of immunizations. The PHS-731 is not to be filed in the HREC at any time. Any immunizations recorded on the PHS-731 should be transcribed onto the SF 601.

According to international rules, entries on the PHS-731 require authentication for immunizations against smallpox (if administered), yellow fever, cholera, and anthrax. Authentication (proof the immunization has been given) is accomplished by stamping each entry with the Department of Defense (DoD) immunization stamp and by the healthcare provider's signature. The signature block may be stamped or typewritten and authenticated with the healthcare provider's signature.

ABSTRACT OF SERVICE AND MEDICAL HISTORY (NAVMED 6150/4)

This form provides a chronological history of the ships and stations to which a member has been assigned for duty and treatment, and an abstract of medical history for each admission to the Sick List.

A NAVMED 6150/4 (fig. 12-7) is prepared upon opening the health record, and it remains with the health record regardless of any change in the member's status. Continuation sheets are incorporated whenever a current abstract is completely filled. Complete columns of the NAVMED 6150/4 as follows:

- **Ship or Station column.** Enter the name of the ship or command to which the member is attached for duty or treatment.

- **Diagnosis, Diagnosis Number, and Remarks column.** Enter the diagnosis title and International Classification of Diseases (ICDA) number each time final disposition from the Sick List is made. When there is more than one diagnosis for a single admission, record each diagnosis.

- **Date column.** Indicate in the "From" and "To" subcolumns all dates of reporting and detachment for duty or dates of admission and discharge from the Sick List. Upon transfer for temporary duty (TDY), make an entry only if the HREC accompanies the individual to the place of TDY.

NAVMED 6150/4 is retained as a permanent part of the HREC. When the record is closed, make an entry indicating the date, title of servicing activity, and explanatory circumstances.

Upon discharge and immediate reenlistment, or change in status, an appropriate entry to this effect should be made on the current NAVMED 6150/4. Subsequent chronological entries are continued on the same form.

ABSTRACT OF SERVICE AND MEDICAL HISTORY
NAVMED 6150/4 (Rev. 12-87)   S I N. 0105 - 209 -5040
(Formerly NAVMED 1406)

| SHIP OR STATION | DIAGNOSIS, DIAGNOSIS NUMBER AND REMARKS | DATE | |
		FROM	TO
NAVAL TRAINING CENTER GREAT LAKES, IL	Duty	1 MAY 96	30 JUL 96
NAVSTA NORVA	Duty	1 AUG 96	15 NOV 97
USS CARRIER (CV 00)	Duty	16 NOV 97	19 MAR 98
	Contusion, left thoracic region ICDA Code No. 9220	19 MAR 98	19 MAR 98
NAVHOSP Blank, VA	Treatment	19 MAR 98	4 MAY 98
	Contusion, left thoracic region ICDA Code No. 9220	19 MAR 98	4 MAY 98
	Tonsillitis, acute #4630	26 MAR 98	4 MAY 98
USS CARRIER (CV 00)	Duty	4 MAY 98	3 MAY 99
USS UNDERWAY (LHD 00)	Duty	14 MAY 99	

| NAME (Last, first and middle) DOE, John James | BIRTH DATE 9 MAY 75 | BRANCH OF SERVICE USN | SERVICE/SOCIAL SECURITY NO. 20-123-45-6789 |

C-27849

HM3f1207

Figure 12-7.—Abstract of Service and Medical History, NAVMED 6150/4.

RECORD OF OCCUPATIONAL EXPOSURE TO IONIZING RADIATION (DD FORM 1141)

This form is initiated when military personnel are first exposed to ionizing radiation (with the exception of patients incurring such radiation while undergoing diagnostic treatment). This form becomes a permanent part of the member's health record.

Instructions for preparing DD Form 1141 are on the back of the form. Further instruction concerning the applicability and use of the form are contained in the *Radiation Health Protection Manual*, NAVMED P-5055.

ADJUNCT HEALTH RECORD FORMS AND REPORTS

This section provides instruction for using certain forms in the health record instead of transcribing their data to the SF 600, *Chronological Record of Medical Care*.

Narrative Summary (SF 502)

The purpose of the SF 502 is to summarize clinical data relative to treatment received during periods of hospitalization. The narrative summary should include all procedures and diagnoses, and must agree with information listed on the *Inpatient Admission/Disposition Report* (NAVMED 6300/5) and any information listed in the operation report.

The SF 502 should include the following information:

- Reason for hospitalization, including a brief clinical statement of the chief complaint and history of the present illness.

- All significant findings.

- All procedures performed and treatment given, including patient's response, complications, and consultations.

- The condition and relevant diagnosis at the time of patient's transfer or discharge.

- Discharge instructions given to patients or their families (i.e., physical activity permitted, medication, diet, and follow-up care).

- List of principal providers or attending physicians and their signatures.

A completed copy of the SF 502 should accompany patients who are transferred to another medical facility. Upon discharge from the hospital, a copy of the SF 502 should be taken to the member's parent command. The SF 502 informs the command of any limitations, medications, and follow-up care the service member may need. After command use, the SF 502 should be placed into the member's HREC. For more detailed instruction on the use of the SF 502, refer to the MANMED.

Abbreviated Clinical Record (SF 539)

The SF 539 may be used as a substitute for the narrative summary for those admissions of a minor nature that require less than 48 hours of hospitalization. A copy of SF 539 should be filed in the HREC.

Consultation Sheet (SF 513)

The SF 513 is used for outpatients who need to be referred to other healthcare providers or specialists, such as gynecologists, internists, optometrists, etc. The primary patient assessment should be entered onto the form. Include as well the results of examinations and tests on the SF 513. The patient remains the responsibility of the referring provider until the specialist takes over the care. In some cases, the specialist will perform an examination or procedure and refer the patient back to the original provider for continued care. The original consultation form stays in the HREC.

Medical Board Report (NAVMED 6100/1)

Whenever a member of the naval service is reported on by a medical board, place a legible copy of the report in the health record instead of transcribing the clinical data to the SF 600. Make a notation on the current SF 600 to indicate the clinical data is contained in the copy of the Medical Board Report incorporated in the health record, when the Medical Board Report is forwarded to the Navy Department for review and appropriate disposition. Enter a report of the departmental action on the current SF 600.

Eyewear Prescription (DD Form 771)

The purpose of DD form 771, *Eyewear Prescription* (fig. 12-8), is to order corrective prescription eyewear. Depending on its edition date (any of which is authorized), the DD form 771 may consist of a 3-copy carbon form (for use with pen), a 2-part carbonless form (printed on a tractor-feed printer) (fig. 12-8A), or a computer-generated form using virtual copies (fig. 12-8B). The original of the form will be sent to the optical laboratory, and a copy of the form will be placed in the patient's HREC. As with other standard forms, the DD 771 is frequently submitted via computer modem or fax, depending on availability.

Three major areas covered by the DD Form 771 are patient information, prescription information, and

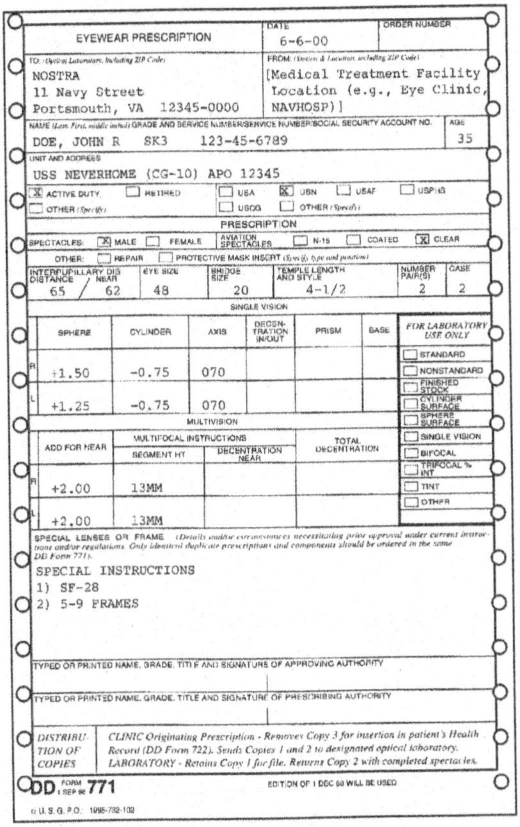
EYEWEAR PRESCRIPTION
DATE 6-6-00
ORDER NUMBER
TO: (Optical Laboratory, Including ZIP Code) NOSTRA 11 Navy Street Portsmouth, VA 12345-0000
FROM: (Station & Location, including ZIP Code) [Medical Treatment Facility Location (e.g., Eye Clinic, NAVHOSP)]
NAME (Last, First, middle initial) GRADE AND SERVICE NUMBER/SERVICE NUMBER/SOCIAL SECURITY ACCOUNT NO. AGE
DOE, JOHN R SK3 123-45-6789 35
UNIT AND ADDRESS
USS NEVERHOME (CG-10) APO 12345
[X] ACTIVE DUTY [ ] RETIRED [ ] USA [X] USN [ ] USAF [ ] USPHS
[ ] OTHER (Specify) [ ] USCG [ ] OTHER (Specify)
PRESCRIPTION
SPECTACLES: [X] MALE [ ] FEMALE AVIATION SPECTACLES [ ] N-15 [ ] COATED [X] CLEAR
OTHER: [ ] REPAIR [ ] PROTECTIVE MASK INSERT (Specify type and position)
INTERPUPILLARY DISTANCE / NEAR 65 / 62
EYE SIZE 48
BRIDGE SIZE 20
TEMPLE LENGTH AND STYLE 4-1/2
NUMBER PAIR(S) 2
CASE 2
SINGLE VISION
SPHERE CYLINDER AXIS DECENTRATION IN/OUT PRISM BASE
R +1.50 -0.75 070
L +1.25 -0.75 070
MULTIVISION
ADD FOR NEAR / MULTIFOCAL INSTRUCTIONS SEGMENT HT / DECENTRATION NEAR / TOTAL DECENTRATION
R +2.00 13MM
L +2.00 13MM
FOR LABORATORY USE ONLY
STANDARD
NONSTANDARD
FINISHED STOCK
CYLINDER SURFACE
SPHERE SURFACE
SINGLE VISION
BIFOCAL
TRIFOCAL % INT
TINT
OTHER
SPECIAL LENSES OR FRAME (Details and/or circumstances necessitating prior approval under current instructions and/or regulations. Only identical duplicate prescriptions and components should be ordered in the same DD Form 771.)
SPECIAL INSTRUCTIONS
1) SF-28
2) 5-9 FRAMES
TYPED OR PRINTED NAME, GRADE, TITLE AND SIGNATURE OF APPROVING AUTHORITY
TYPED OR PRINTED NAME, GRADE, TITLE AND SIGNATURE OF PRESCRIBING AUTHORITY
DISTRIBUTION OF COPIES
CLINIC Originating Prescription - Removes Copy 3 for insertion in patient's Health Record (DD Form 722). Sends Copies 1 and 2 to designated optical laboratory.
LABORATORY - Retains Copy 1 for file. Returns Copy 2 with completed spectacles.
DD FORM 1 SEP 86 771
EDITION OF 1 DEC 68 WILL BE USED
U.S.G.P.O. 1995-782-102

A

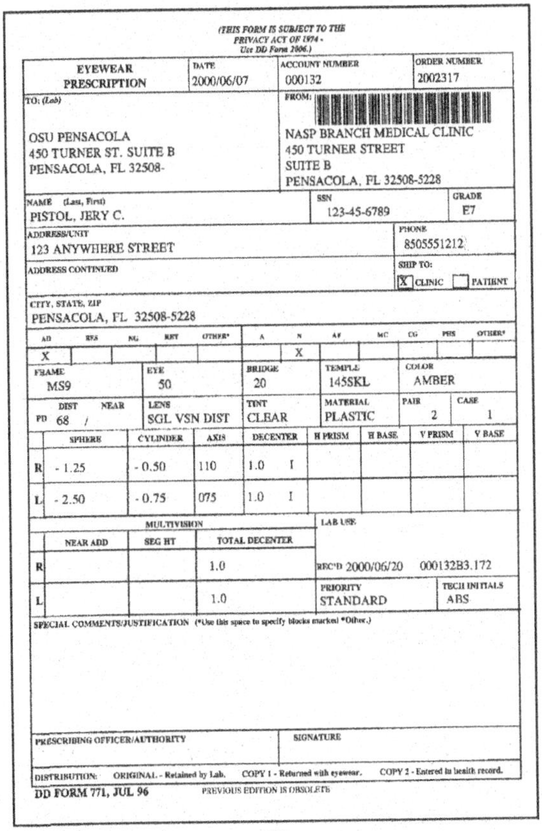
(THIS FORM IS SUBJECT TO THE PRIVACY ACT OF 1974 - Use DD Form 2005.)
EYEWEAR PRESCRIPTION
DATE 2000/06/07
ACCOUNT NUMBER 000132
ORDER NUMBER 2002317
TO: (Lab) OSU PENSACOLA 450 TURNER ST. SUITE B PENSACOLA, FL 32508-
FROM: NASP BRANCH MEDICAL CLINIC 450 TURNER STREET SUITE B PENSACOLA, FL 32508-5228
NAME (Last, First) PISTOL, JERY C.
SSN 123-45-6789
GRADE E7
ADDRESS/UNIT 123 ANYWHERE STREET
PHONE 8505551212
ADDRESS CONTINUED
SHIP TO: [X] CLINIC [ ] PATIENT
CITY, STATE, ZIP PENSACOLA, FL 32508-5228
AD RES NG RET OTHER* A N AF MC CG PHS OTHER*
X X
FRAME MS9
EYE 50
BRIDGE 20
TEMPLE 145SKL
COLOR AMBER
DIST NEAR PD 68 /
LENS SGL VSN DIST
TINT CLEAR
MATERIAL PLASTIC
PAIR 2
CASE 1
SPHERE CYLINDER AXIS DECENTER H PRISM H BASE V PRISM V BASE
R - 1.25 - 0.50 110 1.0 I
L - 2.50 - 0.75 075 1.0 I
MULTIVISION
NEAR ADD SEG HT TOTAL DECENTER
R 1.0
L 1.0
LAB USE
REC'D 2000/06/20 000132B3.172
PRIORITY STANDARD
TECH INITIALS ABS
SPECIAL COMMENTS/JUSTIFICATION (*Use this space to specify blocks marked *Other.)
PRESCRIBING OFFICER/AUTHORITY
SIGNATURE
DISTRIBUTION: ORIGINAL - Retained by Lab. COPY 1 - Returned with eyewear. COPY 2 - Entered in health record.
DD FORM 771, JUL 96
PREVIOUS EDITION IS OBSOLETE

B

HM3f1208

Figure 12-8.—Eyewear Prescription, DD Form 771: A. Computer-printed edition; B. Computer-generated edition.

miscellaneous information. These three areas are discussed as follows:

1. **Patient Information:** The specific information required is the patient's name, rank, SSN, duty station, mailing address, and military status. This information is required to establish eligibility and provide the requesting activity with an address for the patient upon receipt of the completed eyeglasses.

2. **Prescription Information:** Since the spectacle prescription is the technical portion of the order form, you should complete it with great care, ensuring that the prescription is transferred in its entirety. The essential elements of the prescription are interpupillary distance, frame size, temple length, plus and minus designators for both sphere and cylinder powers, segment powers and heights, prism, and prism base. It is not necessary to calculate decentration in the single vision or multifocal portions of the order. It is also unnecessary to try to transpose any prescription into plus or minus cylinder form. Leave the prescription as is, copy it onto the DD Form 771, and note in the remarks section that the prescription has been copied and is in the HREC.

3. **Miscellaneous Information:** This area is reserved for any information you feel the Navy Optical Laboratory may need. Information the laboratory may need includes special fabrication requirements, such as multifocal lenses, or proof of eligibility for specialized eyewear, such as aviator sunglasses. Standard issue items can be determined from NAVMEDCOMINST 6810.1, *Ophthalmic Services.*

DD Forms 771 should be typewritten or computer printed whenever possible. This practice eliminates any errors by misreading an individual's handwriting. It is critical you take the time to correctly order spectacles. Omission of any information or entering erroneous information will result in a delay at the fabricating facility or a patient's receiving an incorrect pair of eyeglasses, or both.

If you cannot read what has been written on an eyewear prescription, you should contact the optometrist for clarification. In the case where the optometrist cannot be contacted, as a last effort you can send a photostatic copy of the prescription to the optical laboratory, rather than transcribing information of which you are unsure. Make sure that the copy of the prescription is accompanied by a completed DD Form 771.

VERIFYING HEALTH RECORDS

LEARNING OBJECTIVE: *Identify health record items that should be reviewed during an annual verification.*

Health records are verified annually by medical personnel having custody of the record. Health records should also be reviewed when service members report and detach from their command, and at the time of their physical examinations.

Each record should be carefully reviewed, and any errors or discrepancies should be corrected. Items to be reviewed during an annual verification include: form placement, forms order (chronological), and completeness and accuracy of patient identification data on the record jacket and on each piece of medical documentation. In addition, verify that the Privacy Act Statement has been signed, the Summary of Care form is updated (as necessary), blood group and Rh factor are documented, and currency of immunizations and accuracy of allergy documentation are complete.

Upon completion of an annual HREC verification, you should make an SF 600 entry and black-out the corresponding year block on the front leaf of the jacket with a black felt-tip pen. With this procedure, records that have not been verified during the calendar year can be identified readily and the annual verification accomplished.

CLOSING HEALTH RECORDS

LEARNING OBJECTIVE: *Recall closing procedures for health records.*

A member's health record is to be closed under the following circumstances:

- Death or declared death
- Discharge
- Resignation
- Release from active duty
- Retirement
- Transfer to the Fleet Reserve or release to inactive duty
- Missing or missing in action (MIA)(when officially declared as such)
- Desertion (when officially declared as such)
- Disenrollment as an officer candidate or midshipman

When closing an HREC, make sure the record is in order, that there are no loose papers, and all identification data is consistent. Record closing entry on the NAVMED 6150/4, *Abstract of Service and Medical History.* Include the date of separation, title of servicing activity, and any explanatory circumstances.

Upon final discharge or death, send the entire HREC and dental record to the command maintaining the member's service record (no later than the day following separation) for inclusion in and transmittal with the member's service record. Make sure the original of the separation physical examination documents are included in the HREC before delivery to the command maintaining the member's service record, such as the PSD, PSA, etc. In case of death, send a copy of the death certificate along with the transmitted records.

A copy of the HREC is provided free of charge to members who requests one upon their release, discharge, or retirement.

MISSING OR MISSING-IN-ACTION MEMBERS

Whenever a member disappears and the available information is insufficient to warrant an administrative determination of death, enter a summary of the relevant circumstances on the SF 600. Include circumstances about the presumed disappearance of the individual, then status (missing or missing in action), and supporting documentation. Close the record and handle it as you would records for members being discharged from the service.

DESERTION

When a member is officially declared a deserter, explain this fact on the SF 600 and the NAVMED 6150/4. Deliver member's HREC and dental treatment record to the member's commanding officer (CO) for inclusion in and transmittal with the member's service record for both Navy and Marine Corps personnel.

When a deserter is apprehended or surrenders, the CO of the activity having jurisdiction is required to submit a request for the member's records to Bureau of Naval Personnel (BUPERS) or Commandant of the Marine Corps (CMC), as appropriate.

RETIREMENT

When a member of the naval service is placed on the retired list or Fleet Reserve List, close the HREC as you would on a discharge. However, upon request of the retiring member, a new medical record (OREC) is established. A **copy** of the retiring member's active duty HREC may be incorporated into a new NAVMED 6150/20-29 folder. Make an entry on an SF 600 in the HREC and in the new OREC, stating the date the HREC was closed.

DISABILITY SEPARATION OR RETIREMENT

The MTF should send a copy of the HREC of a member being separated for disability to the DVA (Department of Veteran Affairs) regional officer nearest to where the member will be residing. Send the medical record directly from the MTF to the DVA, so the record can be considered as a primary source of evidence in processing a claim for veteran's benefits. A record carried by the member is considered secondary evidence and is not used to process a claim. Send the record with the VA 526, *Claim of Benefits*, so the regional office can initiate the claim.

Members separating from the service and eligible for veteran's benefits should be provided a copy of their HREC on request. Members should be counseled to request a copy in the event they may make a claim for veteran's benefits in the future. Always offer to send a copy of their HREC to the regional DVA office for them.

SUMMARY

As a Hospital Corpsman, you will be responsible for managing health records. Health records are a vital tool in the healthcare delivery process. It is of the utmost importance that you learn and follow guidelines for establishing, handling, maintaining, and closing health records. Keep in mind, your handling of the health record can affect others. A well-maintained health record furnishes healthcare providers with current medical data, enabling the provider to give each patient timely and comprehensive medical care. Confidential treatment of a patient's medical information honors the patient's privacy and is in keeping with legal regulations. Following the guidelines in this chapter will assist you in properly managing health records under your care.

CHAPTER 13

SUPPLY

The responsibility of accounting for assets within the Department of the Navy comes down from the Secretary of the Navy (SECNAV) to the commanding officers of field activities throughout the Navy. Commanding officers must ensure proper fiscal administration by the directives, principles, and policies prescribed by the Comptroller of the Navy.

The Naval Supply Systems Command (NAVSUP) is responsible for administering supply management policies, to include cataloging, standardization, inventory control, storage, issue, and disposal of naval material. You, as a Hospital Corpsman, must be familiar with the methods of procuring and accounting for naval materials.

In this chapter we will discuss the proper procedures to use in estimating supply needs, procuring supplies and material, and accounting for supplies and operating funds. The last section of the chapter deals with contingency supply blocks and their maintenance.

NAVSUP MANUALS, PUBLICATIONS, AND DIRECTIVES

LEARNING OBJECTIVE: *Recognize the purpose and content of key supply manuals and instructions.*

To function well in the Navy supply system, you must be familiar with the NAVSUP manuals, publications, and directives that outline policy and procedures for different areas of supply. These manuals, publications, and directives are available in the Naval Logistics Library located on the NAVSUP homepage, www.navsup.navy.mil.

ALTERNATIVE TITLES FOR NAVSUP PUBLICATIONS

NAVSUP publications may be referred to in four different ways. For example, the *Operating Procedures Manual Military Standard Requisitioning and Issue Procedure*, and *Military Standard Transaction Reporting and Accounting Procedure* *(MILSTRIP/MILSTRAP)*, NAVSUP P437, may be referred to in various publications and directives as **NAVSUP Publication 437**, **NAVSUP P-437**, **NAVSUP Pub 437**, or **NAVSUP 437**. However, when referencing this publication (or other NAVSUP publications), cite it as "**NAVSUP P-437**" (and the applicable paragraph number).

CHANGES TO PUBLICATIONS

Regardless of how well you have learned to use the various supply publications, if they aren't kept up to date, you may encounter problems when you attempt to order an item. Also, you may be unaware of an item that has been recalled. Enter changes promptly when they are received to ensure that the latest information is being used. Always read accompanying instructions before making changes.

NAVAL SUPPLY SYSTEMS COMMAND (NAVSUP) MANUAL

The NAVSUP manual is designed to institute standardized supply procedures and consists of the following four volumes:

Volume I — *Introduction to Supply*

Volume II — *Supply Ashore*

Volume III — *Retail Clothing Stores and Commissary Stores*

Volume IV — *Transportation of Property*

OPERATING PROCEDURES MANUAL FOR MILITARY STANDARD REQUISITIONING AND PROCEDURES (NAVSUP P-437) AND MILITARY STANDARD TRANSACTION REPORTING AND ACCOUNTING PROCEDURES (MILSTRIP/MILSTRAP)

The MILSTRIP/MILSTRAP manual issues policy on the MILSTRIP/MILSTRAP system. This publication takes precedence over conflicting provisions contained in other supply system manuals or directives. The manual covers system management, requisitioning procedures for ashore activities, inventory control, financial matters, and other topics. The publication provides forms, formats, and codes, and serves as a comprehensive reference for persons involved in preparing or processing MILSTRIP documents. Since NAVSUP P-437 is not distributed afloat, afloat MILSTRIP/MILSTRAP operations are incorporated into NAVSUP P-485.

MILSTRIP/MILSTRAP DESK GUIDE, NAVSUP P-409

The NAVSUP P-409 was published as a handy reference for personnel responsible for originating and processing MILSTRIP/MILSTRAP documents, since NAVSUP P-437 is a large, comprehensive, three-volume publication. This small booklet contains common definitions, coding structures, and abbreviated code definitions used on a day-to-day basis. Blank space is provided for entering commonly used routing identifiers, funding codes, project codes, and locally assigned codes.

AFLOAT SUPPLY PROCEDURES, NAVSUP P-485

The *Afloat Supply Procedures*, NAVSUP P-485, establishes policies for operating and managing afloat supply departments and activities. It helps supply personnel understand and perform their individual tasks. Although this publication is designed primarily for nonautomated supply procedures, a significant amount of the information it contains also applies to automated systems.

The procedures contained in this publication are the minimum essential for acceptable supply management and are mandatory unless specifically stated as optional. The publication encompasses the procedures outlined in the NAVSUP Manual, volumes I, II, and V, and NAVSUP P-437 as they apply to afloat situations. It covers organization and administration, material identification, material procurement, material receipt, custody and stowage, material expenditure and shipment, inventory management, transportation, and special material.

NAVY MEDICAL AND DENTAL MATERIAL BULLETIN, NAVMEDLOGCOM NOTICE 6700

The *Navy Medical and Dental Material Bulletin*, NAVMEDLOGCOM NOTICE 6700, is issued monthly via the NAVMEDLOGCOM homepage, www-nmlc. med.navy.mil, by the Commander, Naval Medical Logistics Command. It contains information of importance and interest to medical supply departments, such as changes in stock numbers, addition and deletions, availability of excess equipment, and notification of material unfit for use and disposal instruction. Revisions to this publication should be read carefully for any changes to your files or references.

APPROPRIATIONS AND OPERATING BUDGETS

LEARNING OBJECTIVE: *Recognize how appropriations and operating budgets are conducted.*

An appropriation is referred to in the NAVCOMPT Manual as "... [an authorization] by an act of Congress to incur obligations for specified purposes and to make payments therefor out of the Treasury." The Navy uses appropriations received to pay for the construction of new ships, to fund the cost of operations and maintenance for the existing fleet, and to pay for training, personnel pay, and to operate shore establishments that support the fleet.

TYPES OF APPROPRIATIONS

Three types of appropriations are used by the Navy, depending upon the purpose for which the appropriation is issued. Most appropriations are for one fiscal year (FY). The FY runs from 01 October of a year to 30 September of the following year. The federal government uses this time period for budgeting normal operating costs of the armed services, including the Navy. Other types of appropriations may be granted without a time limitation or for a specific time that may exceed 1 year.

Annual Appropriations

Annual appropriations are provided for active and reserve military personnel expenses, as well as for operation and maintenance expenses. The appropriations become available for obligation and expenditure at the beginning of the fiscal year designated in the Appropriations Act. Obligations may be incurred only during this designated fiscal year; however, the obligated funds remain available for the payment of such obligations for an additional 5 years. At the end of the additional 5-year period, fund distribution differs, depending on the purpose of the appropriation.

Continuing Appropriations

A continuing appropriation, also referred to as a **no-year appropriation**, is one that is available for incurring obligations until the funding is exhausted or until the purpose for which it was made is accomplished without a fixed-period restriction. Examples of continuing appropriations are Military Construction Navy (construction projects that are planned up to 5 years ahead) and revolving funds such as the Defense Business Operating Funds (DBOF) (a projection of the predicted cost to operate the Navy).

Continuing appropriations become available for obligation and expenditure at the beginning of the FY following the passage of the Appropriations Act or may become immediately available when so specified in the Act. When the purpose of a continuing appropriation has been accomplished administratively or by Congress, DoD transfers an amount equal to the total of unliquidated obligations, less the total of reimbursements to be collected, to the surplus of the Treasury.

Multiple-Year Appropriations

Generally, multiple-year appropriations are made for appropriations that require a long lead time for planning and execution, such as procurement of aircraft, missiles, and ships. Multiple-year appropriations become available for obligation and expenditure at the beginning of the fiscal year (1 October) designated in the appropriation, unless otherwise stated in the Act. They are available for incurring obligations only during the FYs specified in the Act. However, they are available for paying such obligations for an additional 5 years.

At the end of the last FY included in the appropriation, when the appropriation expires for obligation purposes, the balance is transferred to the Treasury.

OPERATING BUDGETS

The operating budget is the annual budget of an activity and is assigned by the Chief of Naval Operations (CNO), Fiscal Management Division, to major claimants. A major claimant is an office, command, or Headquarters Marine Corps. The claimant is designated as the administering office under the operation and maintenance appropriation. Holders of operating budgets have the option of granting a degree of financial responsibility to subordinates by issuing operating targets (OPTARs). OPTARs are generally apportioned in four equal quarterly divisions that represent the maximum amount that can be spent for each quarter of the FY. By using this system, facilities are able to manage and effectively control the expenditure of funds. This system prevents overexpenditure of funds early in the fiscal year and helps prevent financial problems at the end of the year. Unused quarterly funds may be carried over to the next quarter simply by adding them to the new quarterly apportionment. At the end of the fourth quarter, all accounts are balanced and closed; new expenditures are not authorized until appropriated funds are made available for the new fiscal year.

Funds allotted to the medical department to purchase needed items are called the operating target (OPTAR). Medical OPTAR funds are the funds used to fulfill the following five major requirements:

- **Authorized Medical Allowance List (AMAL)**. The AMAL is the minimum amount of medical material to be maintained on board a ship or on order at any given time. The amount of material as noted in an AMAL is designated by BUMED for each class of ship and is based on past experience. Recommendations for changes to the AMAL should be forwarded through the chain of command to BUMED.

- **Authorized Dental Allowance List (ADAL)**. The ADAL is the minimum amount of dental material to be maintained on board a ship or on order at any given time. The amount of material as noted in an ADAL is designated by BUMED for each class of ship and is based on past experience. Recommendations for changes to the ADAL should be forwarded through the chain of command to BUMED.

- **Type Commander's (TYCOM) Requirements**. To supplement the AMAL, TYCOMs may have additional requirements to maintain units in a high state of readiness and allow units to be self-supporting in an emergency, such as a natural disaster or humanitarian mission. TYCOM requirements for medical considerations relate to such items as gun bags, airways, litters, and battle dressing supplies.

- **Special Mission Usage**. These missions include but are not limited to humanitarian, civilian rescue, and drug interdiction operations.

- **Administrative Requirements**. The purchase of consumable or medical OPTAR restricted items may be made from the medical OPTAR with the approval of the executive officer. Medical books and publications listed in NAVMEDCOMINST 6820.1 may also be purchased with this OPTAR.

FEDERAL SUPPLY CATALOG SYSTEM

LEARNING OBJECTIVE: *Recall the terms associated with the Federal Supply System and how to use the Federal Supply Catalog.*

The Department of Defense Supply System contains more than 4 million items; of this total the Navy stocks more than 1 million items. To order supplies effectively from this system, you must have a basic understanding of the DoD supply system terminology and structure. This includes the naming, description, classification, and numbering of all items carried under centralized control of the United States Government. Only one identification number is used for each item, from purchase to final disposal.

TERMINOLOGY

To effectively procure and account for naval materials, you will need to be familiar with terminology commonly used in the supply system. Some of the terms with which you should be familiar are discussed below:

BULK STOCK	Material in full, unbroken containers available for future use.
CONSUMABLE	Supplies that are consumed or disposed of after use.
EQUIPAGE	Items that require management control afloat because of high unit cost, vulnerability to pilferage, or indispensability to the ship's mission.
CONTROLLED EQUIPAGE	Items of equipage that require special management control because the material is essential for the mission or the protection of life, is relatively valuable, or easily converted to personal use.
EQUIPMENT	Any functional unit of hull, mechanical, electrical, ordnance, or electronic material, operated singly or as a component of a system or subsystem. Equipment is considered nonconsumable.
MATERIAL	All supplies, repair parts, equipment, and equipage used in the Navy/Marine Corps.
NON-CONSUMABLE	Supplies and materials that are not consumed or disposed of after their use. Buildings and equipment are nonconsumable items.
REPAIR PART	Any item that has an application and appears in an allowance parts list (APL), stock number sequence list (SNSL), integrated stock list (ISL), Naval Ship Systems Command drawings, or a manufacturer's handbook.
RESERVE STOCK	Items on hand and available for issue for a specific purpose, but not for general use (for example, decontamination supplies).
STANDARD STOCK	Material under the control of an inventory manager and identified by a National Item Identification Number (NIIN). The NIIN is the last nine-digits of the Federal Stock Number.
STOCK NUMBER	The smallest quantity of a supply item.

FEDERAL SUPPLY CLASSIFICATION SYSTEM

The Federal Supply Classification System is designed to permit the classification of all items of supply used by the federal government. Each item of supply will be included in one—AND ONLY ONE—FSC. The FSC is made up of 2 two-digit numeric codes: the federal supply group and the federal supply class. The federal supply group identifies, by title, the commodity area covered by the classes within each group.

An example of a Federal Supply Group and its classes is as follows:

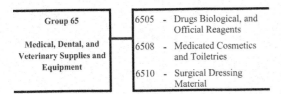

Group 65	6505	-	Drugs Biological, and Official Reagents
Medical, Dental, and Veterinary Supplies and Equipment	6508	-	Medicated Cosmetics and Toiletries
	6510	-	Surgical Dressing Material

NATIONAL STOCK NUMBERS

Every item in the Federal Supply Catalog is identified by a 13-digit stock number referred to as **National Stock Number** (NSN). The national stock number (NSN) for an item of supply consists of a four-digit federal supply classification (FSC group and class) and a nine-digit national item identification number (NIIN). The NIIN consists of a two-digit national codification bureau (NCB) code and seven digits that, in conjunction with the NCB code, identify each NSN item in the Federal Supply Distribution System.

The National Item Identification Number is a nine-digit number that identifies each item of supply used by the Department of Defense. Although the NIIN is part of the NSN, it is used independently to identify an item within a classification. Unlike the FSC, the NIIN is assigned serially, without regard for the name, description, or classification of the item.

An example NSN is: 3110-00-123-4567

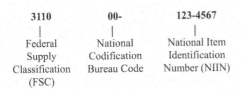

| 3110 | 00- | 123-4567 |
| Federal Supply Classification (FSC) | National Codification Bureau Code | National Item Identification Number (NIIN) |

NAVY ITEM CONTROL NUMBERS

Navy Item Control Numbers (NICN) identify items of material (such as pencils, staplers, sutures, and medications) that are not included in the FSC but are stocked in the Navy supply system. These numbers are 13-digits and are assigned by inventory control managers.

LOCAL ITEM CONTROL NUMBERS

Technically, any item identification number assigned by an activity for its own use is a Navy Item Control Number. To distinguish between NICNs that are authorized in supply transaction documents and those that are not, the term Local Item Control Number (LICN) is often used. A full explanation of the composition of NIINs, NICNs, and LICNs is contained in *Afloat Supply Procedures*, NAVSUP P-485.

COGNIZANCE SYMBOLS

Although cognizance symbols are not part of the NSN, they are used as supply management codes that identify the Navy inventory manager for the specific category of material requisitioned. This symbol consists of two parts, one numeric and one alphabetic. For example, the symbol for all Navy-owned bulk medical material is "9L."

FEDERAL SUPPLY CATALOG, MEDICAL MATERIAL SECTION

The Federal Supply Catalog contains all standard stock items available to agencies of the United States Government. It furnishes identification and management data for single-manager supply items. The sections of the catalog that are of special interest to the Hospital Corpsman are those dealing with medical items, as listed in the NAVSUP P-485, volume I, chapter 2. Each subsection deals with specific categories of material.

The following is a description of the subsections of Federal Supply Catalog, Medical Material, 6500 section:

- **Introduction**—provides a general overview of the contents and use of the catalog.

- **Alphabetical Index**—contains a list of item names, colloquial names, synonyms, common names, and trade names, referenced to index numbers, that help locate an item within the subsection.

- **Glossary of Colloquial Names and Therapeutic Index** (6505/6508 subsection only)—contains colloquial names, synonyms, and trade names arranged in alphabetical order and cross-referenced to appropriate National Item Names. Items are also classified by therapeutic use.

- **Identification List** (IL)—contains the following four sections:

1. **Preface**—Each subsection contains a preface that includes special instructions pertaining to that individual subsection.

2. **Alphabetical Index**—This list of National Item Names is cross-referenced to index numbers to help locate an item when the NSN is not known.

3. **National Stock Number Index**—This list of NSNs is arranged in numerical order and referenced to index numbers to help locate an item within a subsection.

4. **List of Items index number**—Some items are illustrated for clarity. Each item listed includes action codes; handling and/or storage codes, if any; NSN; and a brief description of the item.

- **Action Codes**—Additions, deletions, or revisions of published data are identified as follows:

  N-new — indicates items not previously included in the basic publica-tion, change bulletin, or change notice; or reinstaten-ment of a previously deleted item.

  C-change — indicates a change in data since the previous publication.

  D-deletion — indicates an item that is no longer available.

- **Index Numbers**—Items are presented in alphabetical order; index numbers are assigned in ascending sequence within each pamphlet. They are used solely as a locator device and not in place of NSNs.

- **National Stock Number Index**—NIINs are listed in numerical order.

- **Descriptive Data**—Important distinguishing characteristics are stated in this section.

- **Description**—Information which appears below the item name and above the box in which the index number, NSN, and data are arranged. Operational data may appear as a footnote such as "cold weather use only."

- **Notes**—Information regarding item special storage and handling procedures are as follows:

  B — corrosive or poisonous material

  C — contains one or more component items of the nature described under "R" below; used in connection with assemblies only

  F — subject to damage by freezing

  G — requires refrigeration between 2° to 8°C (35° to 46°F)

  I — flammable or oxidizing materials

  M — an item containing potentially recoverable precious metals

  P — an item with potency period or expiration date

  Q — drugs or other item requiring security storage and Schedule III, IV, and V

  R — alcohol, alcoholic beverages, precious metals, or other substances requiring vault storage and Schedule II

  W — item must be kept frozen for preservation

- **Navy Management Data List**—This list contains all items in the subsection and shows unit of issue, price, and authorized substitutions. A separate Navy Management Data List is published for each Identification List.

PROCUREMENT

LEARNING OBJECTIVE: *Recognize the various supply levels, and recall requisition form completion and processing procedures.*

Procurement is the act of obtaining materials or services. Material may be procured by requisition (items with federal stock numbers) or open purchase (items without federal stock numbers, procured from nonfederal sources). Requisitions are most frequently used, but open purchase is used for procuring nonstandard material and emergency items. In this section, we will cover supply levels, supply level terminology, requisition, requisition documents, purchase procedures, and the Uniform Material Movement and Issue Priority System (UMMIPS).

LEVELS OF SUPPLY

There must be some control over the level or quantity of supplies kept by medical departments. Without controls, policy changes or poor ordering procedures may result in some items being in short supply, while other items are stockpiled in quantities that would not be consumed for several years. To avoid such occurrences, it is necessary to develop rules governing stock levels.

Supply Level Terminology

Supply levels may be expressed in one of two ways: in numerical terms and in terms of months of usage. **Numerical** is expressed as the total amount of supplies on hand. **Months of usage** is the most commonly used measurement of supply levels. It is the best method to use in accounting for the amount of items that are used on a monthly basis. In expressing the supply level of any stock item, four measurements may be used: operating level, safety level, storage objective, and requisitioning objective.

OPERATING LEVEL.—This measurement indicates the quantity of an item that is required to sustain operations during the interval between requisitions or the receipt of scheduled successive shipments of supplies. The operating level should be based upon the length of the replenishment cycle. For example, if requisitions are submitted every 2 months, the operating level would be the quantity of the item that is consumed every 2 months. This level will vary for different items.

SAFETY LEVEL.—This measurement indicates the quantity of an item, over and above the operating level, that should be maintained to ensure that operations will continue if replenishment supplies are not received on time, or if there is an unpredictably heavy demand for supplies. This measurement simply provides a margin of safety.

STOCKAGE OBJECTIVE.—This measurement indicates the minimum quantity of a stock item that is required to support current operations. It is the sum of the operating level and the safety level. For example, if the operating level of an item is 80 units and the safety level is 20 units, the stockage objective

would be to maintain 100 units of that item in stock at all times.

REQUISITIONING OBJECTIVE.—This measurement indicates the maximum quantity of a stock item that should be kept on hand and on order to support operations. It is the sum of the operating and safety levels and the quantity of an item that will be consumed in the interval between the submission of a requisition and the arrival of the supplies. Figure 13-1 illustrates the relationship between the various levels of supply.

Usage Data

The most accurate guide in determining supply requirements is past experience, as reflected in accurate stock records. Stock record cards (which will be discussed in detail later in the chapter) should be kept current to assist in the material usage notes. Stock records should tell you how much of each item has been used in the past. From this past usage data, you can make a reasonable projection of future usage rates. SAMS (SNAP Automated Medical System) is an additional management tool. SAMS is the current approved shipboard computer program used to track all aspects of medical supply.

REQUISITIONS

A requisition is an order from an activity that is requesting material or services from another activity. Except for certain classes of material listed in NAVSUP P-485 and P-437, all items ordered from the Navy Supply System, other military installations, the Defense Logistics Agency (DLA), and the Government Services Administration (GSA) will be procured using the MILSTRIP system. MILSTRIP requisitioning is based upon the use of a coded, single-line-item document for each supply transaction discussed in the paragraphs that follow.

DoD Single-Line Item Requisition System Document (Manual), DD Form 1348

DD Form 1348 (fig. 13-2) is used as a requisition; requisition follow-up, modification, or cancellation; and tracer request on overdue shipments sent by insured, registered, or certified mail. This form is available in two-, four-, and six-part sets as follows:

- The two-part set is used by nonautomated ships for requisition follow-up, modification, or cancellation, and tracer requests;

- the four-part set is used for requisitioning from shore activities; and

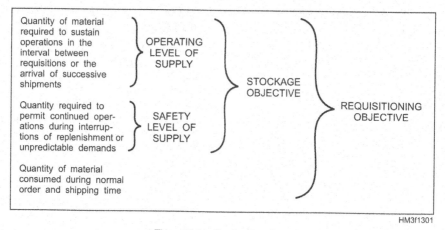

Figure 13-1.—Levels of supply.

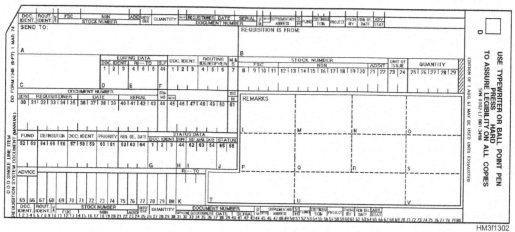

Figure 13-2.—MILSTRIP requisition document: DD Form 1348.

- the six-part set is used for requisitioning from other nonautomated ships (and from automated ships, when required).

Non-NSN Requisition (Manual), DD Form 1348-6

DD Form 1348-6 (fig. 13-3) is a six-part form used to requisition material that cannot be identified by an NSN, NATO stock number, or NICN other than permanent "LL"-coded NICNs. The form consists of two sections. The upper section includes essentially the same data elements as DD Form 1348. The lower section includes 10 data blocks for additional identification data.

Single-Line Item Consumption/Requisition Document (Manual), NAVSUP Form 1250-1

NAVSUP Form 1250-1 (fig. 13-4) is a seven-part multipurpose form used as a consumption document. It is also used as a MILSTRIP requisitioning document by nonautomated ships for procuring material or services from another ship, naval supply centers, naval supply depots, and Navy Inventory Control Point (NAVICP) Philadelphia.

Requisition and Invoice/Shipping Document, DD Form 1149

DD Form 1149 (fig. 13-5) is prepared for certain items that are excluded from MILSTRIP. These items are listed in NAVSUP P-485 and P-437. DD Form

ITEM IDENTIFICATION* (NSN, FSCM / Part No., Other)

DOCUMENT IDENTIFIER	ROUTING IDENTIFIER	M & S	FSCM	PART NUMBER	UNIT OF ISSUE	QUANTITY	S E N	REQUISITIONER
1 2 3	4 5 6	7	8 9 10 11 12 13 14 15 16	17 18 19 20 21 22	23 24	25 26 27 28 29	30	31 32 33 34 35
A Ø E	N D Z	6			E A	Ø Ø Ø Ø 1	R	5 2 1 9 2

DOCUMENT NUMBER

DOCUMENT NO. (Cont.) DATE	SERIAL	D E M A N D	S E R V	SUPPLEMENTARY ADDRESS	S I G N A L	FUND CODE	DISTRI- BUTION CODE	PROJECT CODE	PRIORITY	REQUIRED DELIVERY DAY OF YEAR	ADVICE CODE	BLANK
36 37 38 39 40 41 42	43	44 45 46 47	48 49 50 51	52 53	54 55 56	57	58 59	60 61	62 63 64	65 66	67 68 69
8 Ø 3 3 3 Ø 1 4	R	Y N E B	1 3 A N R					Ø 6			

IDENTIFICATION DATA

	REJECT CODE (FOR USE BY SUPPLY SOURCE ONLY)	*1. MANUFACTURE'S CODE AND PART NO. (When they exceed card columns 9 thru 22)
70 71 72 73 74 75 76 77 78 79 80	65 66	Ø5Ø73 N3 - 12291 - P1Ø4
1 5 Ø Ø Ø		

2. MANUFACTURE'S NAME
BABCOCK & WILCOX CO., NEW YORK, NY

3. MANUFACTURE'S CATALOG IDENTIFICATION

4. DATE (YY/MM/DD)

5. TECHNICAL ORDER NUMBER

6. TECHNICAL MANUAL NUMBER
NAVY TECH MANUAL 351 - 0048

7. NAME ITEM REQUESTED
ELEMENT, SOOT BLOWER, UNIT A

8. DESCRIPTION OF ITEM REQUESTED

8a. COLOR

8b. SIZE

9. END ITEM APPLICATION
BOILER, STEAM, MN, 634 PSI, 4617 CU FT, 1393 TB

9a. SOURCE OF SUPPLY
BABCOCK & WILCOX CO.

9b. MAKE

9c. MODEL NUMBER

9c. SERIES

9e. SERIAL NUMBER
Ø

10. REQUISITIONER (Clear text name and address)
USS JOHN PAUL JONES (DDG - 32)
FPO SAN FRANCISCO, CA 966Ø1

17818Ø84.7Ø2D/53824/Ø/Ø6Ø957/2D/R52192/ØØ8Ø333Ø/4NR

11 REMARKS
ADDL EQUIP DATA: APL # Ø212ØØØØ7,
MFR DW # MX 253ØØ1, EQUIP PATTERN # 12
ADDL ITEM DATA: NICN 441Ø - LL-CAO - ØØØ1:
$15Ø.ØØ

A.B. SMITH, LT, SC, USN

DD Form 1348 - 6, Feb.85 Edition of Apr. 77 may be used until exhausted. S/N 0102-LF-019-2273

DOD SINGLE LINE ITEM REQUISITION SYSTEM DOCUMENT (MANUAL - LONG FORM)

HM3f1303

Figure 13-3.—Example of a Non-NSN Requisition (DD Form 1348-6).

1149 may be used as a requisitioning document or a receipt document. As a requisitioning document, use this form to procure GSA contract items such as medical books, journals, and standard and nonstandard BUMED-controlled items requiring local purchase action.

BUMED-CONTROLLED ITEMS

BUMED-controlled items are essential to preserve life (medications), are easily pilferable (hemostats, etc.), and/or have a high acquisition or replacement cost (CAT scan, X-Ray equipment). Requisition standard stocked BUMED-controlled items on DD Form 1348, and forward the request through the chain of command to the Naval Medical Logistics Command (NAVMEDLOGCOM) for technical review.

PROFESSIONAL BOOKS AND PUBLICATIONS

The listing of all books and publications that are required to be maintained at an activity can be found in NAVMEDCOMINST 5600.1 and NAVMEDCOM-INST 6820.1. GSA periodically makes open-end contracts that cover the procurement of books. All professional books and publications are procured under the provisions of these contracts.

PURCHASES

Ships' supply officers and commanding officers of ships without Supply Corps officers may obtain supplies or services by purchase on the open market.

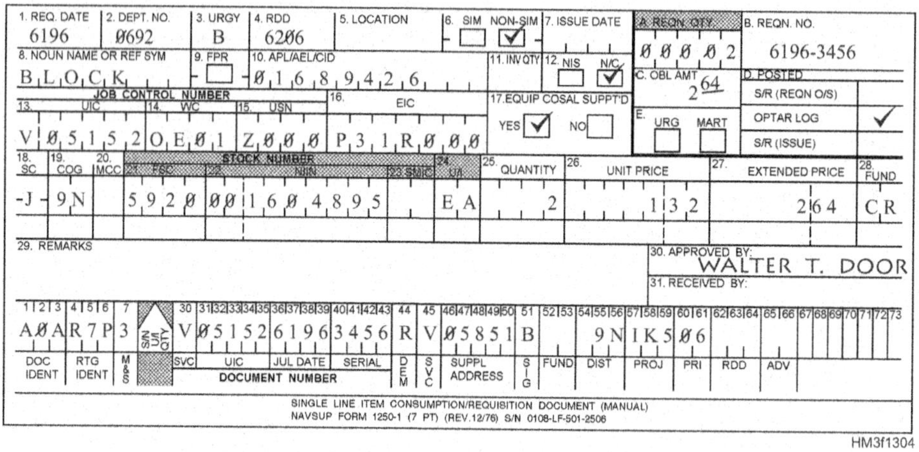

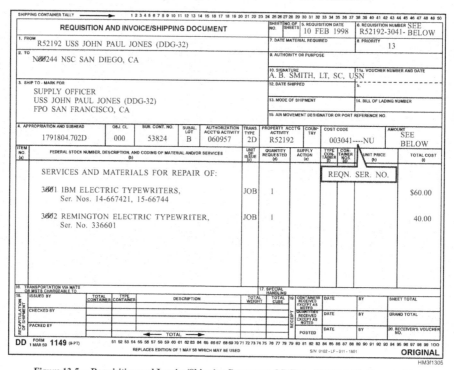

Figure 13-4.—MILSTRIP requisition document: NAVSUP Form 1250-1.

Figure 13-5.—Requisition and Invoice/Shipping Document, DD Form 1149 (multiple requests).

Purchases are made by one of the following three methods:

1. Purchase order for purchases not in excess of $25,000 CONUS or $50,000 outside CONUS.

2. Imprest fund (funds authorized by TYPE commander for immediate purchases) for cash purchases of $500 or less.

3. Orders under indefinite delivery-type contracts and blanket purchase agreements (BPAs) that have been negotiated by shore activities.

A single requirement may NOT be divided with more than one purchase action for the purpose of avoiding monetary limitations. Procedures for purchases by ashore activities are provided in NAVSUPINST 4200.85.

UNIFORM MATERIAL MOVEMENT AND ISSUE PRIORITY SYSTEM (UMMIPS)

The UMMIPS system assigns priorities to material movement. Issuing these priorities is a integral and vital part of MILSTRIP. In the movement and issue of material, it is necessary to establish a common basis to determine the relative importance of competing demands for resources of logistics systems. The method for determining the relative importance and urgency of logistics requirements is provided by the priority designator (PD), a two-digit code that ranges from 01 (highest) to 15 (lowest). The priority designator is determined from the urgency of need designator (UND) and the Force/Activity Designator (F/AD), as shown in table 13-1.

Force/Activity Designator (F/AD)

F/AD is a Roman numeral (I-V) that identifies and categorizes a force or activity on the basis of its military importance as shown below:

I   In Combat

II   Positioned for Combat

III Positioned to Deploy/Combat

IV   Other Active and Selected Reserve Forces

V   All Other

Table 13-1.—Listing of Priority Designators

| | URGENCY OF NEED DESIGNATORS* | | |
| | Unable to Perform Mission | Impaired Operational Capability | Routine |
Force/Activity Designators*	A	B	C
I In Combat	1	4	11
II Positioned for Combat	2	5	12
III Positioned to Deploy/Combat	3	6	13
IV Other Active & Selected Reserve Forces	7	9	14
V All Other	8	10	15

Numeric Priorities

*For additional detailed guidance concerning Force/Activity Designators and Urgency of Need Designators, see OPNAVINST 4614.1.

Urgency of Need Designator (UND)

The Urgency of Need Designator (UND) consists of an uppercase letter "A," "B," or "C." It is selected to indicate the relative urgency of a force's or activity's need for a required item of material. Assignment of UND is the responsibility of the force or activity making the requisition and is derived according to NAVSUP P-485. UNDs and their associated definitions are as follows:

UND		Definition
A	(1)	Requirement is immediate.
	(2)	Without material, the activity is unable to perform one or more of its primary missions.
	(3)	The condition noted in (2) above has been reported by established, not operationally ready supply/ casualty report (NORS/CAS-REPT) procedures.
B	(1)	Requirement is immediate or it is known that such a requirement will occur in the immediate future.
	(2)	The activity's ability to perform one or more of its primary missions will be impaired until the material is received.
	(3)	Deals with Q-COSAL Reactor Plant components.
C	(1)	Requirement is routine.
	(2)	Combat Logistics force.

Priority Designator (PD)

PD is a two-digit number (01-highest to 15-lowest) determined by using the table of priority designator shown in table 13-1. For example, if your ship is assigned an F/AD of III and your requirement is of a routine nature, assign priority 13.

In addition to providing standardized criteria for assigning priorities, UMMIPS provides acceptable maximum processing times for use by supply activities in furnishing material. Processing time standards and additional codes used in MILSTRIP and UMMIPS are included in NAVSUP P-485. For additional detailed guidance concerning Force/Activity Designator and Urgency of Need Designator, see OPNAVINST 4614.1.

PREPARING A MILSTRIP REQUISITION

LEARNING OBJECTIVE: *Recognize MILSTRIP requisition procedures and how they are used for material receipt, custody, and stowage.*

MILSTRIP uses coded data for processing requisitions with automatic data processing equipment. No matter what type of requisitioning document you use, use extreme care in selecting and entering the coded data elements. These codes apply to all levels of supply. Although they are too numerous for all to be included in this chapter, the codes can be found in the appendices of NAVSUP P-485. The following general rules apply to MILSTRIP requisition:

- Enter data by ball-point pen or typewriter. Do not use pencil; pencil marks can cause errors when the requisition is processed through mark sensing equipment.

- Data should be entered between the "tic" marks on the form. However, it is mandatory that entries be included within the data fields to which they pertain.

- To eliminate confusion between the numeral zero and the letter "O," use the communications zero (ϕ) on MILSTRIP requisitions when zeros are applicable.

Specific details for completing DD Form 1348 and NAVSUP Form 1250-1 can be found in NAVSUP P-485.

MATERIAL RECEIPT, CUSTODY, AND STOWAGE

For every procurement action taken, there is a receipt action that follows. Once the supplies are received, they must be identified, checked, and distributed to the appropriate storeroom or department, and documentation as to their receipt, custody and stowage must be accomplished.

Material Receipt

As in every situation, responsibility for actions taken must be assigned to key personnel. In the receipt of government-owned materials, responsibility for receipts takes on an added importance because of the many types of material receipts and the required accountability.

Receipt Documentation

There are several types of receipt papers, and which type is used depends upon the manner in which the material was requested, the issuing activity, and the modes of transportation used in delivery. The most commonly encountered receipt is the DoD Single Line Item Release/Receipt Document, DD Form 1348-1, (fig. 13-6). Regardless of the type of receipt document, the end-use receiver must

1. date the document upon receipt,

2. circle the quantity accepted, and

3. sign the document to indicate receipt.

Receiving Procedures

Small quantities of stores received on a daily basis require no special preparations for receipt. Stock large quantities of stores in a central area out of the traffic flow and hold there until preliminary identification and package count are completed. Then sort them according to the department or storeroom to which they will be distributed.

Report of Discrepancy

Item or packaging discrepancies attributable to the shipper (including contractors, manufacturers, or vendors) should be reported on the Report of

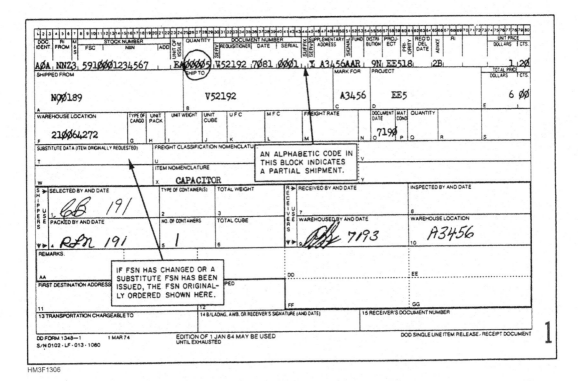

Figure 13-6.—DoD Single Item Release/Receipt Document, DD Form 1348-1.

Discrepancy (ROD), SF 364, by the receiving activity. The purpose of the ROD is to determine the cause of the discrepancy, effect corrective action, and prevent recurrence. When both item discrepancies and packaging discrepancies are noted on the same shipment, both blocks on the top of SF 364 should be checked and the types of discrepancies noted. The types of discrepancies required to be reported are described in chapter 4 of NAVSUP P-485. Detailed instructions for preparing and distributing of RODs are contained in the current version of SECNAVINST 4355.18.

Custody

The term **custody** refers to the responsibility for proper care, stowage, and use of Navy material and records pertaining to such. Stored material is required to be kept under lock and key, except when the material is too numerous or too large to make such stowage impractical. Lock storeroom spaces securely when not in use.

Stowage

Material in storerooms and other designated stowage areas should be arranged to

- ensure maximum use of available space,

- provide orderly stowage and ready accessibility,

- prevent damage to spaces or injury to personnel,

- reduce the possibility of material loss or damage,

- make it easy to issue the oldest stock first, and

- make it easy to inventory.

The preceding criteria and a "common-sense" approach will enable storeroom personnel to achieve stowage efficiency. To the maximum extent that available space permits, you should adhere to the following guidelines when stowing material:

- Locate heavy bulk material and materials handling equipment near hatches or doors to minimize the physical effort required for loading, stowage, and breakout.

- Locate light bulky materials in storerooms with high overhead clearances for maximum use of available space.

- Segregate materials that are dissimilar in type or classification.

- Locate frequently requested materials as close as possible to the point of issue.

- Locate shelf-life items in a readily accessible area to facilitate periodic screening.

- Install appropriate stowage aids (flashlight, paper, and pencil) in spaces where they are readily accessible.

- Make aisles at least 30 inches wide, if possible.

- Arrange material with identification labels facing outward to make issue and inventory easy.

- Avoid multiple locations for the same item.

If you follow the preceding criteria and guidelines, you should have no problems in maintaining your spaces and issuing and inventorying materials.

SPECIAL STOWAGE OF ITEMS

At times, you will have items that require special stowage. The *Naval Ships' Technical Manual (NSTM)* and the *Hazardous Materials Information System (HMIS)*, DoD 6050.5, outline the requirements for shipboard stowage of dangerous materials and lists the materials under each classification. We will now cover the classifications of material and discuss storage requirements for special types of material.

Hazardous Material

Hazardous material includes all types of compressed gases and materials that present a fire hazard or are otherwise dangerous. Paint and oil constitute the bulk of material in this category. Paint and flammable liquid storerooms are normally provided with alarm and CO_2 smothering systems that can be activated by automatic temperature-sensitive devices inside storerooms and by manual controls outside storerooms. A flooding system operated manually outside storerooms is an additional safety factor. These storerooms are located, when practical, below the full-load water line, near either end of the vessel, but not adjacent to a magazine. They are equipped with watertight doors that must be locked and dogged when not in use.

Compressed Gases

Stow compressed gases on the weather deck, and securely fasten them in a vertical position. Protect the cylinder valves from accumulations of ice and snow, and screen the cylinders from direct rays of the sun. NAVSUP P-485 contains more specific information concerning handling compressed gas cylinders.

Acid

Liquid acid, unless classified as safe material, is stowed in an acid locker. Acid lockers are leak-proof and lead-lined boxes, chests, or lockers specifically designed for stowing bottles or carboys of acid. Medical acids may be stored in a medical storeroom.

Alcohol

Alcohol should be stowed in a locked container in the paint and flammable liquid storeroom, to which only the supply officer (or other officer designated in writing by the commanding officer) has the key or combination.

SHELF-LIFE MATERIAL

Shelf-life material is subject to deterioration. These items are assigned a **shelf-life code** listed in the NMDL. The code denotes the shelf-life span of material from the date of manufacture to the date of disposal, or date of testing according to the inventory manager's instructions to extend the shelf life. Type I codes (alpha) apply to items for which shelf life cannot be extended. Type II codes (numeric) apply to items for which shelf life may be extended.

OTHER REPAIR PARTS

Repair parts should be stored in their original containers. With today's improving techniques and the material used in packaging, repair parts may be stored for a considerable time without damage from dust, shock, or humidity.

STOREROOMS

When you are in charge of a storeroom, you are also responsible for maintaining cleanliness of the space. Before you secure each night, sweep the storeroom and remove all trash. Periodically clean bins, shelves, ventilation ducts, and fans.

The overall condition of your space is also your responsibility. Rust is an ever-present enemy, and constant vigilance is required to keep it under control. Rust spots should be chipped, wire brushed or sanded, primed, and spot painted. Tighten loose bolts promptly to prevent possible damage to the storeroom or its contents. Examine pipes, valves, electrical systems, watertight fittings, and fire-fighting equipment daily, and report any defect to the supply officer.

Before getting underway into open seas, thoroughly inspect and secure storerooms to prevent stores from shifting due to the ship's motion. Lash bulk stores to bulkheads, stanchions, or battens, and secure the fronts of open bins and shelves to prevent stores from falling out on the deck. Unless approval is obtained from the commanding officer, do not stow personal gear in storerooms designated for supplies.

INVENTORY

LEARNING OBJECTIVE: *Recognize specific characteristics of each type of supply inventory, how inventories are to be conducted, and procedures for inventory reconciliation.*

Throughout this section, we will use various terms to refer to inventory control procedures. Some of these terms are defined here to help you understand them and apply them correctly. NAVSUP P-485 provides definitions for all the terms used in inventory control.

DEFINITIONS

In the following paragraphs, we will discuss definitions that are used in the supply system.

Inventory

Inventory is the quantity of stocks on hand for which stock records are maintained, or the function whereby the material on hand is physically inspected and counted and stock records reconciled accordingly.

Order and Shipping Time

Order and shipping time refers to the time elapsing between submitting a requisition and receiving the material requisitioned (also called **procurement lead time**).

Average Endurance Level

Average endurance level refers to the quantity of material normally required to be on hand to sustain operations for a stated period without resupply.

High Limit (Requisitioning Objective)

High limit is the maximum quantity of material to be maintained on hand and on order to sustain current operations normally for 9 months.

Low Limit (Reorder Point)

Low limit (reorder point) is the least amount of the stock required to be left on hand before the need to reorder is indicated.

Not Carried (NC) Items

Not carried (NC) items are items not stocked in storerooms or for which stock records are not maintained.

Not in Stock (NIS)

Not in stock (NIS) are items carried in stock but not on board when demand occurs.

Demand

Demand refers to the request for an NC item that will be procured or an issue of a stock item.

Frequency of Demand

Frequency of demand refers to the number of requests for an item within a given time frame, regardless of the quantity requested or issued.

Integrated Logistics Overhaul (ILO)

The ILO is an overhaul procedure divided into several phases, designed to weed out obsolete and unused items.

TYPES OF INVENTORIES

There are several types of inventories, each with a specific purpose. These types of inventory are bulkhead-to-bulkhead, specific commodity, special material, spot, velocity, and random sampling.

Bulkhead-to-Bulkhead

A bulkhead-to-bulkhead inventory is a physical count of all the material aboard a ship or within a specific storeroom. A bulkhead-to-bulkhead inventory of a specific storeroom is conducted when a random sampling of that storeroom fails to meet the inventory accuracy rate of 90 percent.

Specific Commodity Inventory

The specific commodity inventory is a physical count of all items under the same cognizance symbol or federal supply class (such as 6515/6505), or that support the same operational function (e.g., bandages, IV fluids, needles, etc.).

Special Material Inventory

A special material inventory requires the physical count of all items that, because of their physical characteristics, costs, or other reasons, are specifically designated for separate identification and inventory control. Special material inventories include but are not limited to stocked items designated as classified or hazardous. Physical inventory of such material is required on a scheduled basis, as prescribed in the NAVSUP P-485.

Medical supplies are examples of both the specific commodity and special material inventories.

Spot Inventory

A spot inventory is an unscheduled type of physical inventory to verify the existence of a specific item. It is usually conducted when a requisition is returned showing the item is not in stock but the stock records indicate the item is on hand. A spot inventory is also conducted when directed by higher authority or when a specific item has been found to be defective.

Velocity Inventory

A velocity inventory is based on the premise that the faster an item moves, the greater the room for error. This type of inventory is required on items with a relatively high turnover rate.

Random Sampling Inventory

A random sampling inventory is considered to be part of the annual scheduled inventory program. It is done to measure the stock record accuracy for a segment of material on hand.

INVENTORY PROCEDURES

Proper inventory procedures mandate a complete and correct item count. You must ensure that the total quantity of each item is determined as accurately as possible. Keeping in mind that inventories are conducted to bring stock and stock records into agreement, you can see the importance of a complete, accurate, and legible inventory. Documents authorized for conducting inventory counts of stock material include NAVSUP 1075 (whether or not maintained as locator records) and machine or manually prepared listings. Copies of *Stock Record Card, Afloat,* NAVSUP 1114, even when maintained in storerooms, are not to be used as inventory count documents.

Promptly upon completion of the physical inventory and before matching inventoried quantities against stock record balances, review the inventory documents to ensure that

- all items scheduled for inventory have been counted or verified as nonexistent,

- quantities counted are legibly recorded and compatible with related units of issue,

- all locations applicable to the inventory segment have been checked,

- "added" items are adequately identified and legibly recorded,

- items are documented in National Item Identification Number sequence, and

- documents are dated and initialed.

RECONCILIATION OF COUNT DOCUMENTS AND STOCK RECORDS

Upon completion of the physical count and review of the count documents (documents with the actual numerical count of the items), the next step in the inventory process is to reconcile count documents with the stock records. This is done to determine if a difference exists between the physical count and the amount recorded on stock records.

When the count documents are correct and complete, compare them, item by item, with the applicable stock records to determine whether differences exist. If no differences exist, post the matched count cards or items in the inventory listing to the applicable stock record. Enter the Julian date (numerical day of the year) of the inventory and the notation "INV" in the **DATE & SER/WCC** column, and enter the inventory quantity in the **ON-HAND** column. The inventory quantity and the on-hand number should match. See figure 13-7. If differences exist in the on-hand quantity, locations, or other stock record data, reconcile such differences using the procedures outlined in NAVSUP P-485.

STOCK RECORD CARDS

LEARNING OBJECTIVE: *Recall how to prepare and post stock record cards.*

Without stock record cards, it would be impossible to know if there were adequate stocks of material necessary for the operation of the medical department of a ship. Procurement of stock must be based on the information contained on the stock record cards. Use of approved computer programs are encouraged. Manual stock record cards are discussed in the paragraphs that follow.

The two stock record cards most commonly used in recording usage data are the *Stock Record Card, Afloat*, NAVSUP 1114, and the *Stock Record Card*.

These cards are maintained stock records for all items of stocked material.

DESCRIPTION OF NAVSUP 1114

The pre-printed captions appearing on the top line and at the bottom of the NAVSUP 1114 are identical to each other, and most of the captions are familiar and self-explanatory. Additional information on some of the top- and second-line data elements may help you understand the captions, as well as the source and use of the data shown.

Material Control Code (MCC)

The material control code (MCC) is a single alphabetical character assigned by the inventory control manager to segregate items into more manageable grouping of fast-, medium-, or slow-moving items, or to relate to field activities special reporting and control requirements. This is a first-line entry and is mandatory for repairable items.

Allowance Parts List/Allowance Equipage List (APL/AEL)

The APL/AEL is a system for numbering the repair parts and equipment-related consumable items. If the

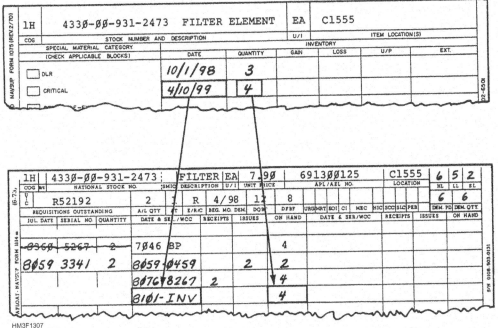

Figure 13-7.—Posting inventory to stock records

Integrated Stock List (ISL) indicated that more than one AEL or APL applies to the same item, enter the letter "M" instead of the AEL/APL number. Enter "General Use" or "GUCL" for non-equipment-related consumables.

Location

Location tells each area in which the item is stored.

High Limit, Low Limit, Safety Level (HL, LL, SL)

High limit, low limit, and safety level quantities are computed in accordance with NAVSUP P-485 and recorded on the NAVSUP 1114.

Allowance List Quantity (A/L QTY)

Allowance list quantity (A/L QTY) is filled in for items on the AMAL/ADAL and left blank for non-allowance items.

Allowance Type Code (AT)

The AT code is assigned by the Integrated Logistics Overhaul (ILO). It is a single-character numeric code based on the item use, requirement to be carried, or usage rates. When an item is added between ILOs, assign the appropriate AT code.

E/R/C Codes

The E/R/C codes are used for equipage items (E), repair parts and equipment-related consumables (R), or for general-use consumables (C). Equipage items (E) are for special accounting class 207 ships only.

BEG.MO.DE.

The BEG.MO.DE. codes are the beginning date of the demand period, generally the date of the last ILO. When the original (ILO-prepared) card is filled and a new card is prepared, bring this date forward to the new card with the demand and frequency of demand recorded on the original card. When a card is prepared between ILOs, the demand date is the date of the initial requisition.

Demand Frequency Brought Forward (DFBF)

The demand frequency brought forward (DFBF) code is the total brought forward from a filled stock record onto a new stock record.

URG

The URG code is a checkmark or "X" if the item is listed in the Consolidated Afloat Requisitioning Guide Overseas (CARGO).

MRT

The MRT code is a checkmark or "X" if the item is listed in the SERVMART shopping list of the local supply support activity.

Economic Order Item (EOI)

The economic order item (EOI) is a checkmark or "X" if the item is listed as an economic order item (low-cost item that may be ordered in a 90-day quantity if cost does not exceed $40).

Critical Item (CI)

The critical item (CI) is a checkmark or "X" if the item is listed as a critical item.

Military Essentiality Code (MEC)

The military essentiality code (MEC) is indicated in the Coordinated Shipboard Allowance List (COSAL) stock number sequence list (SNSL) for repair parts and equipment-related consumables.

Security Classification Code (SCC)

The security classification code (SCC) is used when applicable.

Shelf-Life Code (SLC)

The shelf-life code (SLC) is used when applicable.

Pre-Expended Bin (PEB) Item

The PEB code is a checkmark or "X" used on the NAVSUP 1114 when the item is designated as a pre-expended bin item (e.g., nuts, bolts), or when the unit of issue is large.

Requisition Outstanding

The requisition outstanding code is the Julian date, serial number, and quantity applicable to each procurement document.

PREPARING NEW CARDS

When the original card is filled, prepare a new card, duplicating the stock item information (except for usage data). Enter the beginning date on the new card. Bring forward the demand quantity and frequency demand totals from the old card to the new card. Also bring forward any requisitions still outstanding. Retain the old card, and file it according to local policy.

POSTING PROCEDURES

Post stock record cards daily as receipt and issue documents are received. Proper posting procedures include comparing the following data elements on receipt documents with those on the stock record cards:

- Cognizance symbols
- NSN
- Unit of issue
- Unit price
- Storage location
- Quantity received with quantity requisitioned

If the data elements on the receipt documents and the stock record card are in agreement, enter the Julian date of the receipt and the serial number of the related requisition in the DATE & SER/WCC column. Enter the quantity received in the RECEIPTS column, and increase the balance in the ON-HAND column by the quantity received. Draw a single line through the applicable requisition data for a full receipt (see fig. 13-8). For a partial receipt, if there is a suffix code in block 44 of DD Form 1348-1, draw a single line through the quantity and write the outstanding quantity next to it (fig. 13-8). If there is no suffix code in block 44, consider the requisition as complete. For supplies received in excess of the requisitioned amount, refer to NAVSUP P-485.

CONTROLLED SUBSTANCES

LEARNING OBJECTIVE: *Recall security and inventory procedures for controlled substances.*

Naval medical facilities dispensing pharmaceuticals range from large medical centers ashore to small sickbays aboard ships of the fleet. The custodial responsibility of controlled substances is vested in the commanding officer. An officer of the Medical Department or, in such an officer's absence, a commissioned officer designated by the commanding officer, keeps all unissued controlled substances in a separate, locked compartment. Controlled substances include tranquilizers, alcoholic beverages, alcohol, hypnotics, stimulants, and narcotics that require special custodial care. Medicinals are designated controlled substances by the symbol "Q" or "R" in the notes column of the Federal Supply Catalog. The Force

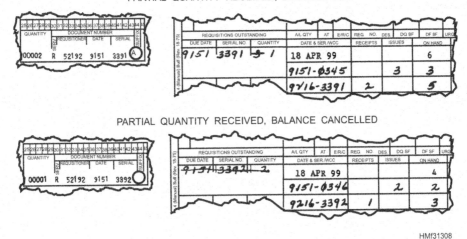

Figure 13-8.—Posting partial quantities to stock records.

Medical Officer also has authority to designate a medicinal as "controlled."

BULK CUSTODIAN

The commanding officer appoints in writing a commissioned officer to serve as the bulk custodian. This officer is responsible for and maintains custody of all bulk controlled substances.

SECURITY

Security of controlled substances is of utmost importance. Therefore, access to controlled medicinals is limited to the bulk custodian and the senior medical department representative (SMDR). Only individuals whose official duties require access to such spaces will be provided the safe combinations.

ACCOUNTABILITY

The bulk custodian and the SMDR are responsible for the receipt and custody of controlled substances. Each unit must maintain a detailed record of the receipt, transfer, survey, dispensing, and expenditure of controlled substances in accordance with MANMED, chapter 21.

INVENTORY BOARD

Monthly, or more frequently if necessary, the Controlled Substances Inventory Board will conduct an unannounced inventory of controlled substances. The commanding officer appoints three members to this board, at least two of whom are commissioned officers. The third member is an E-7 or above. The officer having custodial responsibility is not appointed to the board. After the board conducts the monthly inventory, it will submit a report to the commanding officer.

SURVEY OF CONTROLLED SUBSTANCES

The survey or inspection of the controlled substance inventory will be much easier if you adhere to proper documentation procedures. Destroy controlled substances in the presence of at least one member of the inventory board. Make appropriate entries to the stock records and the Controlled Substances Log. Items are destroyed in a manner that ensures total destruction and prevents subsequent use. The method of destruction must meet federal, state, and local environmental pollution control standards.

PROPERTY SURVEYS

A property survey is the procedure that is used when Navy property or Defense Logistics Agency material is lost, damaged, or destroyed. The purpose of a survey is to determine who or what is responsible for the loss, and to determine the actual loss to the United States Government. To make a true determination, the facts surrounding the loss or damage must be thoroughly investigated in a timely manner. The forms discussed in the following paragraphs are used in connection with survey procedures.

FINANCIAL LIABILITY INVESTIGATION OF PROPERTY LOSS, DD FORM 200

The *Financial Liability Investigation of Property Loss,* DD Form 200, is used if personal responsibility is evident, and if the commanding officer or higher authority so directs.

For more detailed information about the survey procedures, refer to the NAVSUP Manual, volumes I and II.

CONTINGENCY SUPPLY BLOCKS

LEARNING OBJECTIVE: *Recall assemblage and management procedures for medical contingency supply blocks.*

At some point in your career, you may be assigned to one of the six types (surgical, medical regulating, preventive medicine, specialist support, special psychiatric rapid intervention (SPRINT), or humanitarian support) of Mobile Medical Augmentation Readiness Teams (MMART), to a fleet hospital, or to some other contingency-related unit. MMARTs are specialty units that can be deployed anywhere in the world on short notice. The *Medical Augmentation Program (MAP),* BUMEDINST 6440.5, gives detailed information on policies, procedures, and responsibilities on the various types of teams. These specialty units require supplies and equipment that may not be available or are in limited supply in the area to which deployed. To circumvent this problem, contingency supply blocks have been established.

Contingency supply blocks consist of functionally packaged medical and dental equipment and supplies. Each block is assembled to meet the needs of a specific unit. For example, a surgical supply block contains enough equipment to establish one operating room and sufficient supplies for 100 major surgical cases. BUMEDINST 6440.6, *Mobile Medical Augmentation Readiness Team (MMART) Manual,* contains information about several other blocks and their support capabilities.

ASSEMBLING THE BLOCK

The contents of each contingency supply block are outlined in an Authorized Medical Allowance List (AMAL) specific to that block. The Naval Medical Logistics Command (NAVMEDLOGCOM) is responsible for developing, publishing, maintaining, and coordinating a comprehensive review of all AMALs on at least an annual basis. The AMAL is the basic source document used to sustain supply block management. The preface of the AMAL contains instructions for maintaining, packing, and marking the block.

MANAGING THE BLOCK

Contingency supply blocks contain dated, shelf-life, or deteriorative items such as pharmaceuticals, intravenous solutions, and prepackaged items. Proper management of the block ensures operational readiness. Dated items in the block must have an expiration date sufficiently far in the future to allow for a lengthy deployment (up to 6 months). The requirement for monthly status and quarterly readiness reports ensures the designated supply blocks are ready for rapid deployment. This reporting process also allows the team members to become familiar with the contents of the block and the operability of all equipment.

Navy medicine's primary mission—and most important responsibility—is to provide combat-ready professional medical personnel to support the Navy and Marine Corps team. A highly effective logistic management program is the cornerstone for any deployed mission.

SUMMARY

In this chapter we identified Naval Supply manuals and publications. We introduced the Federal Supply Catalog System, and we discussed the proper procedures used to estimate supply needs, procure supplies and material, and account for supplies and operating funds. We also discussed the several types of inventory used in the Navy and the proper procedures for conducting each inventory, as well as the importance of stock record cards and the information required to be recorded on them. Finally, we identified the importance of and specific procedures for safeguarding controlled substances.

CHAPTER 14

ADMINISTRATION

Although most of the their duties are performed in a clinical environment, Hospital Corpsmen may be assigned to clerical positions aboard ship, assigned to duty with the Fleet Marine Force, or detailed to staff duty where a knowledge of administrative procedures and reports is a must. Handling, correcting, and using official directives and publications are important administrative duties. The efficiency of your office depends upon the currency of its publications and directives and how well you know them.

As you progress in rate and assume greater responsibilities, you will be required to maintain the activity's Medical Department Journal, and various logs, records, and directives. Additionally, you may be required to draft, type, and file correspondence. You will use Navy directives and publications more and more as you learn your job. You may also be required to maintain computer data for command use.

In this chapter we will cover medical reports, logs, and records commonly used by the Navy Medical Department. We will also discuss the maintenance and disposal of instructions and notices, preparation of correspondence, and filing procedures. Additionally, we will discuss the organization of the Fleet Marine Force and Fleet Hospitals. Finally, we will discuss the steps required for the development of both a command medical readiness plan (to include Mobile Medical Augmentation Readiness Team (MMART) and unit augmentation) and a joint medical operation plan.

REPORTING REQUIREMENTS

LEARNING OBJECTIVE: *Recognize Medical Department reporting requirements.*

As a member of the Medical Department, whether in a clinic, on a ship, or working sick call, your duties may include the maintenance of various logs and the preparation of reports required by higher authority. These reports are in the *Manual of the Medical Department* (NAVMED P-117) and in the current version of BUMEDINST 5210.9. BUMED has distributed numerous forms to facilitate reporting, recordkeeping, and administrative efficiency throughout the Medical Department. Specific instructions for management of reports and forms are covered in the current version of BUMEDINST 5210.9.

MEDICAL DEPARTMENT JOURNAL

Medical Department activities afloat are required to keep a journal, referred to as the Medical Department Journal. This journal contains a complete, concise, chronological record of events of importance or historical value concerning the Medical Department (other than medical histories of individuals). It lists personnel entered onto or deleted from the binnacle or sick list; reports of personnel casualties, injuries, and deaths; results of inspections of fresh provisions; training given to nonmedical personnel; stretcher bearers assigned; results of inspections of medical equipment, battle dressing stations, gun bags, and stretchers; receipt of medical supplies; and other general information of significance. The journal is signed daily by the senior medical officer, when assigned, or the senior medical department representative (SMDR). The journal is a permanent record and is retired in accordance with the current version of SECNAVINST 5212.5.

REPORTS TO THE OFFICER OF THE DECK OR DAY (OOD)

In addition to being entered into the Medical Department Journal, any other important occurrences are reported by the senior representative of the medical activity to the OOD (or other proper official) for entry into the duty log or journal of the command. Items such as injuries or death of personnel and damage, destruction, or loss of Medical Department property are reported. The names of patients in serious condition are reported directly to the commanding officer and the OOD, with the information necessary for notification of the patient's next of kin.

SICK CALL TREATMENT LOG

A log referred to as the Sick Call Treatment Log is maintained for each ship or activity. The log contains each patient's reporting date and time, name, rate, social security number, command, division, complaint, diagnosis, treatment, disposition, and departure time from sick call. When full, the log is retired in accordance with SECNAVINST 5212.5.

BINNACLE LIST

The Binnacle List, NAVMED 6320/18, is used to excuse an individual from duty for a period of 24 hours or less. This report is prepared by the senior medical department representative on board and should be submitted to the commanding officer no later than 0930 each day. This form contains a list of individuals recommended to be excused from duty because of illness. The list is approved by the commanding officer, and no names may be added without the CO's permission.

MORNING REPORT OF THE SICK

The Morning Report of the Sick, NAVMED 6320/19, is used to excuse an individual from duty for a period of more than 24 hours. This report contains a list of the sick and injured, including names, diagnoses, and conditions. It is prepared by the senior medical department representative on board and is submitted to the commanding officer by 1000 daily.

When it is necessary to excuse someone from duty after the Morning Report of the Sick is submitted, add the patient's name to the Binnacle List, and submit the appropriate report to the commanding officer. If a patient is still unfit for duty when the next Morning Report of the Sick is submitted, add his name to the NAVMED 6320/19 as of the date on which his name was first entered on the Binnacle List. If a satisfactory diagnosis cannot be established, simply note "Diagnosis undetermined" and indicate the chief complaint. Report suspected cases of malingering to the commanding officer.

TRAINING LOG

All lectures and training periods that are part of the medical training program should be recorded in the Training Log and a notation made in the Medical Department Journal. The entries should include the date, location, type of training (GMT, etc.) or subject matter, and what department personnel received the training (Engineering, Deck, etc.).

IMMUNIZATION LOG

To aid you in annotating health records and filling out monthly medical reports, develop and maintain an immunizations log. As the minimum, the information should include the date; name; rank; social security number; immunization type; duty station; and, for personnel receiving PPDs, a contact phone number. There should also be space for adverse reactions.

WATER TEST LOG

The purpose of the water test log is to record the readings of daily residual chlorine or bromine levels and the weekly bacteriological examinations required on potable water aboard ship and in the field.

APPOINTMENT LOG

The purpose of the appointment log is to track medical consultations and clinical appointments that are scheduled by the Medical Department. When a patient is unable to keep an appointment, a notation indicating both the cancellation and rescheduling of the appointment should be made in the log. Multiple appointment cancellations by the same member should be brought to the attention of the member's chain of command.

DIRECTIVES ISSUANCE SYSTEM

LEARNING OBJECTIVE: *Recall the policies and procedures for maintaining directives, drafting correspondence, and filing.*

As a Hospital Corpsman in an administrative billet, you may be responsible for maintaining your command's files and the CD-ROM library of Navy directives. Refer to SECNAVINST 5215.1 for complete details of your responsibilities.

TYPES AND PURPOSES OF DIRECTIVES

A directive may be an instruction (same as a Marine Corps order), a notice (same as a Marine Corps bulletin), or a change transmittal. Directives prescribe or establish policy, organization, conduct, methods, or procedures; require action; set forth information essential to the effective administration or operation of activities concerned; or contain authority or information that must be promulgated formally.

Instruction

An instruction is a directive containing authority or information having continuing reference value, or requiring continuing action. It remains in effect until superseded or otherwise canceled by the originator or higher authority.

Notice

A notice is a directive of a one-time or brief nature, and it always contains a self-canceling provision. A notice has the same force or effect as an instruction. Notices usually remain in effect for 6 months or less, but never for longer than a year. Any requirement for continuing action contained in a notice (such as submitting a report, using a form, or following a specified procedure) is canceled when the notice is canceled, unless the requirement is incorporated into another document (such as an instruction).

Change Transmittal

A change transmittal is used to transmit changes to manuals, publications, instructions, or, occasionally, notices. Each transmittal describes the nature of the change and gives directions for making it. Changes and corrections are made by inserting new pages, removing obsolete pages, or making pen-and-ink changes in the existing text. When a list of effective pages is included with a change, it is important to check all pages against the checklist. This procedure enables you to determine if your publication is complete and current. In the Marine Corps, comparable changes are made to orders and bulletins.

MAINTAINING DIRECTIVES

Instructions are normally placed in large three-ring binders in numerical sequence according to a standard subject identification code number (SSIC), consecutive number, and issuing authority. At some activities, directives may be maintained in a CD-ROM library. For security purposes, classified directives and documents are generally filed in separate binders and maintained in a safe. Because of their brief duration, notices ordinarily do not need to be filed in the master file (main files of instructions). If it is

necessary to file them temporarily with instructions, tab the notices so that each one may be easily and promptly removed as soon as its cancellation date is reached. Copies may be filed in separate suspense binders when necessary.

Locator Sheets

When directives must be removed from the files, a locator sheet is made up and put in where the directive should be in the binder. This sheet will contain the identity of the issuing authority, the directive's standard subject identification code number, subject title, date removed, and both the location of the directive and the name of the person who has custody of it.

Making Changes

Follow the instructions enclosed in change transmittals to enter changes to directives. Proper notations, such as "CH-1," are entered in the upper right margin of the first page of each directive changed to indicate changes received and incorporated. For publication-type instructions, completed changes are noted on the record of changes sheet in the front of the publication.

List of Effective Instructions

Each year, BUMED conducts a review of all current instructions, then compiles and distributes a consolidated list of effective internal and external instructions via the internet.

CORRESPONDENCE

In addition to maintaining directives and logs and submitting reports, the Hospital Corpsman working in an administrative billet must be able to draft and type correspondence correctly and neatly and be able to file correspondence so that it may be retrieved quickly and efficiently.

Navy official correspondence is usually prepared in the standard naval letter format, referred to as the **standard naval letter**. The standard naval letter is also used when corresponding with certain agencies of the United States Government. Some civilian firms that deal extensively with the Navy also prepare correspondence using the standard naval letter. Instructions for typing standard naval letters are very precise and must be followed to the last detail. All the information to properly prepare naval correspondence can be found in the current version of the *Department of the Navy Correspondence Manual*, SECNAVINST 5216.5. You should consult this manual when you prepare correspondence. You may use approved computer programs for preparing correspondence.

File Number

The size and complexity of the Navy demands a standard method for filing paperwork. This standardization frees personnel from learning new filing systems when moving from one activity to another. The **SSIC system** of coding correspondence through use of a four- or five-digit number representing its subject matter provides an efficient, consistent method of filing and retrieving documents. SSICs are found in *Department of the Navy Standard Subject Identification Codes,* SECNAVINST 5210.11. They serve as file numbers for and are required on all Navy and Marine Corps letters, messages, directives, forms, and reports. SSICs will be discussed in more detail in the upcoming section on filing.

Originator's Code

An originator's code, formed according to local instructions and serving as a basic identification symbol, appears on all outgoing correspondence. It is usually the office symbol of the drafter, but it may be the hull number of the drafter's ship. For example: **LHA 18-80.** This is office/department 80 of ship LHA-18.

Serial Number

Classified correspondence must contain a serial number. Whether unclassified correspondence is also serialized depends on local policy. A command that produces little correspondence probably does not need to serialize. An activity that uses serial numbers starts a new sequence at the beginning of each calendar year and assigns the numbers consecutively. The serial number, when used, is combined with the originator's code. The following format is used: **Ser LHA18-80/0726.** This represents the 726th piece of correspondence produced by office/department 80 of ship LHA-18 during the current calendar year.

There is no punctuation following the serial number and no space before or after the slash. For classified correspondence, the classification letter precedes the serial number (**C** for Confidential, **S** for Secret, **T** for Top Secret). For example: **Ser LHA18-80/C16**. This is the sixteenth piece of

confidential correspondence originating from office/department 80 of LHA-18 since the beginning of the current calendar year.

ELECTRONIC MAIL

Electronic mail (e-mail) lets individuals and activities exchange information by computer. You could use it for informal communications in place of telephone calls or to transmit formal correspondence within DoD.

FACSIMILE TRANSMISSION SERVICE

Facsimile machines (fax) provide a rapid and reliable alternative to the mail service for transmission of documents. Use of fax machines and other electronic media is discussed in the *Navy Correspondence Manual*.

MESSAGES

A message is a written thought or idea, expressed as briefly and precisely as possible, and prepared for transmission by the most suitable means of telecommunication. Details on format, headings, precedence, and addressal of naval messages are contained in the current version of the *Naval Telecommunications Procedures Manual,* NTP 3.

FILING

In the previous section of this chapter, we said that each piece of correspondence requires a file number, derived from the *Department of the Navy Standard Subject Identification Codes,* SECNAVINST 5210.11, and referred to as the **SSIC**. The extent of your knowledge of this standardization system of subject identification will determine the efficiency with which you will be able to retrieve a piece of correspondence from your files.

Numerical Subjects Grouping

SSICs are broken down into 13 major groups:

1000 series—Military Personnel

2000 series—Telecommunications

3000 series—Operations and Readiness

4000 series—Logistics

5000 series—General Administration and Management

6000 series—Medicine and Dentistry

7000 series—Financial Management

8000 series—Ordnance Material

9000 series—Ships Design and Material

10000 series—General Material

11000 series—Facilities and Activities Ashore

12000 series—Civilian Personnel

13000 series—Aeronautical and Astronautical Material

These major groups are subdivided into primary, secondary, and, at times, tertiary (third-level) subdivisions. Primary subjects are designated by the last three digits of the code number, secondary subjects by the last two digits, and tertiary subjects by the last digit. For example: **6224**

6000 Medicine and Dentistry

 6200 Preventive Medicine

  6220 Communicable Diseases

   6224 Tuberculosis

6100 Physical Fitness

6600 Dentistry

Detailed subdivisions can be found in SECNAVINST 5210.11.

Classifying

Classifying, as it is used here, is the process of determining the correct subject group or name-title codes under which correspondence should be filed and any subordinate subjects that should be cross-referenced. Classifying is the most important filing operation because it determines where correspondence is to be filed.

The proper way to subject-classify a document so that it can be readily identified and found when needed is to read it carefully, analyze it, and then select the SSIC that most closely corresponds to the subject.

Cross-Reference Filing

File most official correspondence, reports, or other material under only one standard subject identification code. There are times when more than one code will apply to the contents of the correspondence. In these cases, a system of cross-referencing is desirable to permit you to locate the correspondence quickly. To cross-reference, use a Cross-Reference Sheet, DD Form 334 (filling in the required information about the correspondence), or make a copy of the correspondence and place it in the appropriate cross-referenced file. Instances where you need to use a Cross-Reference Sheet are when

- a document has more than one subject;

- the subject may be interpreted in such a way that it lends itself to filing under more than one specific subject group;

- two or more subject identification codes pertain to the names, places, or items appearing in the document;

- enclosures are separated from the basic correspondence; or

- oversize material is filed in an area that is separate from the file for which intended.

Official Method of Filing

Loose filing of correspondence in standard file folders is the official method because it saves time and material. A label containing identifying data for each folders contents is generally placed on the tab of the folder. Five-drawer, steel, non-insulated, letter-size cabinets are standard equipment in the Navy for filing correspondence and documents. Material that cannot be folded neatly in the intended file should be filed in a suitable cabinet. Note the location of this material on the basic document of a cross-reference sheet. Files containing classified documents or Privacy Act data are to be properly secured in accordance with the current version of OPNAVINST 5510.1. Use of computers to maintain files is also a quick method for retrieval. However, paper and/or backup disk copies of the computer files must also be available.

Terminating Files

General correspondence, as well as most other files, are terminated at the end of each **calendar** year, and new files are begun. Budget and accounting records are also terminated annually, but at the end of each **fiscal** year (30 September). Maintain terminated files in the office for 1 year before they are retired to a storage area where they are maintained until they are eligible for destruction or transfer to a Federal Records Center. The current version of the *Disposal of Navy and Marine Corps Records Manual,* SECNAVINST

5212.5, contains detailed information about terminating files.

DISPOSITION OF RECORDS

The Department of the Navy is producing records with increasing speed and ease. Actions and decisions, both important and unimportant, are being documented at every level of command. Informational papers are being more widely distributed. The records disposal program is designed to identify records for permanent retention or temporary retention and later destruction. One of the goals of the program is to dispose each year of a volume of records at least equal to the volume of records created during that year.

Decisions to save or not save must not be avoided by saving all your files. No matter how firmly you believe that disposing of a file today will mean that someone will need it tomorrow, a decision must be made. If you are in doubt about disposal of certain records, avoid taking it upon yourself either to retain or dispose of them; consult with your superiors to decide what course of action to take. The current version of the *Disposal of Navy and Marine Corps Records Manual,* SECNAVINST 5212.5, discusses the retention period of official files and explains whether they should be destroyed or forwarded to a Federal Records Center for further retention.

ELECTRONIC RECORDS

An electronic record is any information that is recorded in a digital form that only a computer can process. In practice, there is no difference between managing electronic and paper records. The *Navy Correspondence Manual* is an excellent guide to use for handling electronic records.

TICKLER FILES

As we discussed earlier in this chapter, the Medical Department is required to submit a number of reports. These required reports are listed in OPNAVNOTE 5214 (which is published annually) and in NAVMED P-117, chapter 23. To ensure that these reports are submitted in a timely manner, a system has been developed to readily identify what report is due and when it is due. This system is known as the **tickler** system. The manner in which a tickler file is made up may vary with each command. Use a computer to save time since there are many approved programs available to create tickler files. Or, you may use 5" x 8" cards with separators marked with the month (i.e.,

January through December), with the tickler card filed in the month in which the report is due. The tickler file may also be used as a reminder of action required on incoming correspondence, or interim reports on a project with a future completion date. Aboard ship, the tickler file is also required for personnel requiring immunizations, physical examinations, or program evaluation. To ensure that departments submit all reports when due, it is advisable to have a tickler system alerting them in sufficient time before the actual due date. This may be accomplished as follows:

- Put out a monthly listing of reports due.

- Provide each department with a copy of the appropriate tickler card.

To be effective, the tickler file requires daily attention and updating.

MEDICAL DEPARTMENT SUPPORT TO THE FLEET MARINE FORCE (FMF) AND FLEET HOSPITALS

LEARNING OBJECTIVE: *Recognize the medical organization of the Fleet Marine Force and Fleet hospitals.*

To understand the complexity of medical support to FMF and Fleet hospitals, you must first be familiar with its overall organization. We will first discuss the FMF. Medical and dental personnel are not members of the U.S. Marine Corps. They are detailed from the Navy and assigned to the FMF, which is a balanced force of combined air and ground troops trained, organized, and equipped primarily for offensive deployment. The FMF consists of a headquarters, force troops, a force service support group (FSSG), one or more Marine divisions, brigades, and aircraft wings. Each of these units is assigned a specific number of medical support personnel, providing an interrelated network of medical support.

FMF MEDICAL SUPPORT

In general, Medical Department personnel serving with FMF may be divided into two groups:

- Combat personnel, who provide medical and initial first aid to prepare the casualty for further evacuation, and

- Support personnel, who provide surgical and medical aid to those who need early definitive care and cannot be further evacuated.

Medical personnel are an integral part of the combat unit to which they are assigned; they train with their units and live with and accompany them at all times.

All of the units comprising an FMF have Medical Department personnel organic to them. However, the majority of medical support comes from the medical battalion of Force Service Support Group (FSSG). The FSSG is a composite grouping of functional units. These functional units provide combat service support beyond the organic capability of all elements of FMF.

The medical battalion provides combat medical support required for independently deployed battalion landing teams, regimental landing teams, Marine expeditionary units, or Marine expeditionary brigades. The primary mission of the medical battalion is to provide

- casualty collection,

- emergency treatment,

- temporary hospitalization,

- specialized surgery, and

- evacuation.

In addition, medical battalions must plan, supervise, and coordinate timely preventive measures for controlling disease.

The basic organization of a typical medical battalion is shown in figure 14-1. A further breakdown of the organization can be found in chapter 3 of the *Marine Corps Warfighting Publication (MCWP) 4-11.1.*

FMF DENTAL SUPPORT

The mission of FMF dental units is to furnish dental services to a Marine Expeditionary Force. By attaching dental sections and detachments of the task force, battalion personnel maintain dental readiness during exercises, deployments, operations other than war, and combat operations.

In an emergency environment, the dental battalions primary mission is to provide dental health maintenance, with a focus on emergency care. Personnel from these detachments may also provide postoperative, ward, central sterilization, and supply room support, and other medical support as determined to be appropriate by the medical battalion and surgical company commanders.

FLEET HOSPITALS

Initially conceived and developed as facilities to provide medical support during intense combat operations, fleet hospitals are also used in lengthy low-intensity scenarios. Fleet hospitals are transportable, medically and surgically intensive (capable of performing advanced medical and surgical procedures), and deployable in a variety of operational scenarios. Available in sizes ranging from 100 to 500 beds, these health-care assets can be used by a variety of field commanders. Fleet hospitals are designed to be used in long-term operations (60+ days) involving a

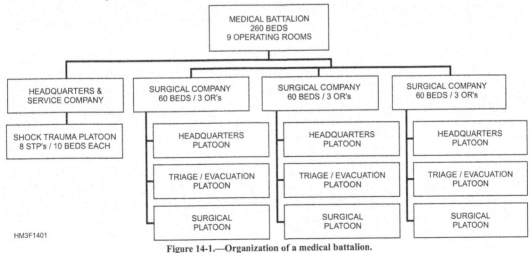

HM3F1401

Figure 14-1.—Organization of a medical battalion.

sizable number of ground forces. Moderately sophisticated care is provided, along with resuscitative medical and surgical care, and selected specialty care. Fleet hospitals are substantially self-supporting and relocatable; however, relocatability varies with the hospital size.

Mission

A fleet hospital's mission depends on its type and the operation in which it will be used. The type is determined by bed size and echelon of care. Fleet hospitals are designed and staffed to provide Echelon III or Echelon IV levels of patient care.

Designation

Fleet hospitals designated as active duty facilities will be manned by active duty personnel, with a command staff assigned from one particular naval hospital using the Medical Augmentation Program (MAP). Naval Reserve fleet hospitals will be staffed by preassigned Naval Reserve personnel. After activation, fleet hospitals are deployed to an operational theater where command and control pass to an operational commander.

Organization

The internal organization of the fleet hospital is similar to a shore-based MTF. It consists of the command staff (commanding officer, executive officer, command master chief, and special assistants) and five directorates (nursing service, medical services, surgical service, ancillary service, and administrative service).

Security and Safety

A deployed fleet hospital must have a security plan that addresses security precautions, threat response, and disaster recovery. The security program covers physical, informational, and classified material aspects normally included in the area of operation (AO) security plan. Physical security for fleet hospitals is both internal and external.

Fleet hospitals will follow the same OPNAV safety program as other operational units. Hospital commanders establish a safety program and an internal organization to address safety issues and appoint a safety officer.

Logistics

Logistics for a fleet hospital include medical supplies, equipment, and services. Logistical requirements can range from acquiring raw material to delivering medical supplies to a field hospital, or returning medical equipment to a theater after a patient evacuation. Tasks of fleet hospital logistics include contracting, host-nation support, equipment management, facilities management, transportation, graves registration, and postal service. All of the fleet hospital supply department operations are conducted in accordance with NAVSUP P-485.

Personnel

Staffing for active duty fleet hospitals comes from several CONUS MTFs, while designated reserve units staff a particular reserve fleet hospital. Each fleet hospital has its own **active manning document** (AMD). Personnel are normally issued TAD orders for less than 180 days. If the operation exceeds 179 days, PCS orders may be issued. Replacements are handled the same way as in any fixed MTF.

Training

BUMED is responsible for monitoring the training of all authorized personnel assigned to fleet hospital mobilization billets. COMNAVSURFRESFOR is responsible for overseeing the training of Naval Reserve personnel assigned to staff Naval Reserve fleet hospitals.

COMMAND MEDICAL READINESS PLAN

LEARNING OBJECTIVE: *Recall the policies and procedures for the drafting of a command medical readiness plan, and recall mobile medical personnel augmentation procedures.*

As you advance in the Hospital Corps, you may be involved in assisting in the development of a command readiness plan. This is the process by which wartime medical requirements are filled by active duty and reserve personnel to bring units to their full or partial wartime allowance.

MEDICAL AUGMENTATION PROGRAM (MAP)

The Medical Augmentation Program is a computer-supported program that provides medical personnel to the operating forces during situations requiring medical personnel augmentation (additional personnel). Inherent in this system is the ability to monitor wartime manning readiness and determine the impact of future personnel requirements. The program also allows for the planning of training for Medical Department personnel. Other aspects that must be considered are the establishment of training requirements, the development of a readiness reporting system, and the phased deployment of personnel.

Augmentation Sources

Through MAP, the requirements of the operational commanders are combined with the active duty resources of the augmentation source commands. The commands that are to be supported by MAP are functional units, typically manned only at a minimum level during peacetime and requiring manpower augmentation in order to fulfill their missions during contingency situations. Current manpower authorization levels are not a factor in defining unit augmentation requirements. The augmentation sourcing units are CONUS-based medical and dental treatment facilities. These medical and dental facilities provide and train the augmentees. The sourcing units' assets are matched with the augmentation requirements.

Program Scope

The scope of the MAP is based on a worst-case scenario involving total augmentation to meet the early support requirements of the operational forces. This means bringing all operational units to their full allowances. Limited augmentation scenarios are also within the scope of this program. Double tasking is not permitted under the MAP. The MMART system is a subset of the MAP and should not be viewed as a separate entity. The MMART surgical/surgical support teams are incorporated into the system as the core of an LHA/LPH/LHD augment. Individuals may have both MMART and LHA/LPH/LHD mission assignments, but these are identical, not dual tasks. Specific unit platforms and training requirements are discussed in detail in the current version of *Medical Augmentation Program (MAP)*, BUMEDINST 6440.5.

MOBILE MEDICAL AUGMENTATION READINESS TEAM (MMART)

The MMART system is a peacetime subset of the MAP. The mission of an MMART is to serve as a force of trained Medical Department personnel capable of rapidly augmenting operational forces for limited, short-term military operations, disaster relief missions, fleet and FMF exercises, and scheduled deployments. During contingencies requiring medical augmentation, the MMART surgical and surgical support teams become the integral augment core for LHA/LPH/LHDs. Other MMART teams dissolve into other augment units.

The MMART is a composite of separate teams manned by medical and dental specialists. The nucleus of the MMART is the surgical team. When combined, a number of distinct specialty teams comprise a single MMART. A full composite MMART consists of one of each of the following component specialty teams:

- Surgical team
- Surgical support team
- Head and neck trauma team
- Neurosurgical team
- Nursing team
- Medical regulating team
- Special psychiatric rapid intervention team (SPRINT)
- Blood bank team
- Preventive medicine team
- Disaster relief/evacuation team

An MMART may be deployed as a full composite team. However, in most situations, an individual specialty team or a combination of specialty teams is all that is required. The personnel and material organization of the MMART may be modified at BUMED direction to meet the specific operation or disaster mission. MMARTs are generally deployed as intact units to an operational commander. These teams may be augmented or reduced as necessary, but they are deployed to a single unit. The exception to this situation is in medical regulating teams, which are fragmented to various ships to set up a medical regulating communications network. For further information about MMART, see the current version of *Mobile Medical Augmentation Readiness Team (MMART) Manual*, BUMEDINST 6440.6.

JOINT MEDICAL OPERATIONAL PLAN

LEARNING OBJECTIVE: *Identify the steps in the development of a joint medical operational plan.*

As a Hospital Corpsman you should be able to assist in the development of a joint medical operational plan. This is a plan that outlines the use of medical assets in support of tactical operations. The tactical mission of the combat forces is the basis for all medical planning. Medical preparation and planning must be initiated early and must be specifically designed to support the tactical operation.

MEDICAL ESTIMATE

A medical estimate is an estimate of personnel and material needed to supply medical services in support of military operations. The steps that are taken in preparing the medical estimate include consideration of the command mission, consideration of the factors affecting the health services (workload, supplies, etc.), and evaluation of proposed courses of action (i.e., listing comparative advantages and disadvantages of each).

Medical Intelligence

The staff surgeon and dental surgeon must be thoroughly informed of all military operations before a proper medical estimate can be made. Some of the items that should be considered are enemy capabilities, friendly capabilities, and environment (terrain, climate, etc.). This information, taken together, becomes **medical intelligence**.

Patient Estimate

Based on the medical intelligence, a preliminary patient estimate can be made of the probable number of patients, types of patients, patient distribution, and the areas of greatest patient density. From these preliminary patient estimates, a calculation is made of the number and types of medical units and the amount and kinds of medical material which will be required. Similar estimates, based on the anticipated health situation, will be required for preventive medicine units.

Evaluation of Course of Action

The staff surgeon must determine the various courses of action that are available and the probable effect of each enemy capability on the success of each course of action, and weigh the advantages and disadvantages of each course of action. The staff surgeon will then decide which course of action promises to be the most successful in accomplishing the mission. A recommendation will be made to the commander for medical requirements, along with where, when, and how medical units should be employed.

PLANNING FACTORS

Basic planning for medical support in joint operations involves four major considerations:

- Plans pertaining exclusively to each medical service

- Plans of each medical service that require coordination with the other elements of the same armed service

- Plans involving joint action among the services

- Plans involving coordination with allied forces

Admission Rates

One of the prerequisites for sound medical planning is an accurate estimate of patients, calculated by applying admission rates to personnel strengths. Admission rates are numerical expressions of the relative frequency with which patients are admitted to hospitals from a specified population over a designated period of time. The particular admission rates used in medical planning represent average rates derived from similar experiences in similar military operations. The three primary categories of patients used in calculating admission rates in an area of military operation are wounded (battle) patients, nonbattle injury patients, and patients who are ill.

Evacuation

Patient evacuation policy is established by the Secretary of Defense, with the advice of the Joint Chiefs of Staff and the recommendation of the theater commander. The policy states, in number of days, the maximum period of noneffectiveness (i.e., hospitalization) that patients may be held within the command for treatment. Any patient who is not expected to return to duty within the number of days expressed in the theater evacuation policy is evacuated. Evacuation plans are greatly influenced by the amount and type of transportation available to medical service.

SUMMARY

In this chapter we discussed medical reports, logs, and records commonly used by the Navy Medical Department. We also covered maintenance and disposal of instructions and notices, preparation of correspondence, and filing procedures. Additionally, the chapter covered the Fleet Marine Force, development of a command medical readiness plan (to include the Mobile Medical Augmentation Readiness Team (MMART) and unit augmentation), and development of a joint medical operational plan.

CHAPTER 15

HEALTHCARE ADMINISTRATION

In the Medical Department, proper records administration is very important. We are charged with administering not only routine personnel records, but also clinical records that may affect the rights and benefits of patients and their dependents years beyond retirement or discharge.

As a Hospital Corpsman, you could be assigned to or responsible for the administrative affairs concerning inpatients or outpatients. This chapter will provide information on the function of healthcare programs you may be involved with or responsible for. We will also discuss the legal implications in medical care, including the various aspects of consent, incident reports, and release or nonrelease of medical information under the Privacy and/or Freedom of Information Acts. Further, guidance concerning your relationship and interaction with law enforcement personnel and the legal community will also be outlined.

PATIENT ELIGIBILITY FOR HOSPITALIZATION AND NONFEDERAL CARE

LEARNING OBJECTIVE: *Recognize the policies and procedures for DEERS, CHAMPUS, and TRICARE.*

The fact that a person seeking treatment is or was connected with the federal government does not automatically entitle him to treatment at a naval medical treatment facility. A number of factors determine eligibility for certain types of medical attention and the source and amount of remuneration for that treatment. The following section deals with eligibility verification by presentation of a valid ID card and utilization of the Defense Enrollment Eligibility System (DEERS). Further guidance can be obtained by familiarizing yourself with the following sources:

- NAVMEDCOMINST 6320.3, *Medical and Dental Care for Eligible Persons at Navy Medical Department Facilities*

- NAVMEDCOMINST 6320.18, *Civilian Health and Medical Program of the Uniformed Services (CHAMPUS) Regulation*

- NAVMED P-5020, *Resources Management Handbook*

DEFENSE ENROLLMENT ELIGIBILITY REPORTING SYSTEM (DEERS)

The Defense Enrollment Eligibility Reporting System (DEERS) was developed to improve distribution and control of military healthcare services. Additionally, DEERS was implemented to assist in the projection and allocation of costs for healthcare programs and to minimize fraudulent healthcare claims. Navy medicine's eligibility for care instruction, NAVMEDCOMINST 6320.3, provides guidance as to who and under what circumstances members can receive medical and dental care at Navy Medical Department facilities; the extent and conditions under which such care may be provided; and the collection process to pay for that care.

Enrollment for all seven uniformed services (i.e., Army, Air Force, Marine Corps, Navy, Coast Guard, Public Health Service, and National Oceanic and Atmospheric Administration) is accomplished through completion and submission of an *Application for Uniformed Services Identification and Privilege Card*, **DD 1172**, for a member's dependent. When a new ID card is obtained for the dependent, the member's DEERS data is updated online. If problems exist within a patient's database, active duty personnel and their dependents must be referred to the sponsor's personnel office. Refer all other beneficiaries (e.g., retired personnel and their dependents) to the nearest personnel office.

Direct Care System Procedures

In addition to providing authorization to standard medical care through inclusion in its membership database, DEERS now includes a dental policy based upon beneficiary information (versus the previous policy based on sponsor information). This change in policy occurred in part because of the increased accuracy of the database as well as the percentage of personnel enrolled.

Although DEERS and the ID card system are related, there are instances when the beneficiary is in possession of a valid ID card and the DEERS system shows the patient as ineligible or not in the database. In these instances, eligibility verification using the ID card shall not override DEERS without some other type of collateral documentation. (See sections on DEERS overrides and exceptions later in this chapter.) It must be stressed that military treatment facilities (MTFs) are to **verify** eligibility. **Establishment** of eligibility is under the cognizance of the respective service personnel offices.

Eligibility

Patients who present for non-emergency treatment without a valid ID card but who are in the DEERS database will **not** be provided medical care without first signing a statement that they are eligible and giving the reason why a valid ID card is not in their possession. If a valid ID card is not provided within 30 calendar days, the patient is referred for billing as a Civilian Humanitarian Non-indigent, in accordance with the *Resources Management Handbook*, NAVMED P-5020. Such billing may be delayed if the commanding officer of the facility is convinced proof is delayed for reasons beyond the control of the patient or sponsor. In all cases where a patient presents without an ID card and does not appear in the DEERS database, **non-emergency** care will be denied.

REASONS FOR INELIGIBILITY.—When a DEERS check is performed and the patient is found ineligible for any of the following reasons, routine non-emergency healthcare will be denied (except as noted later in this section).

- Sponsor not enrolled in DEERS

- Dependent not enrolled in DEERS

- Ineligible due to passed terminal (end) eligibility date

- Sponsor has separated from active duty

- Spouse is divorced from sponsor and is not entitled to benefits as a former spouse

- Dependent child is married

UNDER NO CIRCUMSTANCES WILL THE CLERK PERFORMING THE ELIGIBILITY CHECK DENY THE REQUESTED CARE. Only command-designated supervisory personnel can perform this function.

DEERS ELIGIBILITY OVERRIDES.—The nine "DEERS eligibility overrides" are listed below. Unless otherwise stated, all overrides must be supported by a valid ID card.

1. **DD 1172**—The patient presents an original or copy of the DD 1172 used for DEERS enrollment. There are specific items required for verification, and current service directives must be checked.

2. **All Other Dependents Recently Becoming Eligible for Benefits**—Patients who become eligible for benefits in the previous 120 days may be treated upon presentation of a valid ID card. For children under 10 years of age, a valid ID card of a parent or guardian is acceptable. Upon application for care beyond 120 days, follow the procedure in item 1, above.

3. **New Identification Card**—Patients presenting with a new valid ID card, issued within the previous 120 days, will not be denied care.

4. **Ineligible Due to ID Card Expiration**—When the database shows a patient as ineligible because of ID card expiration, care may be rendered as long as the patient has a new ID card issued within the previous 120 days. After 120 days, follow the procedure in item 1, above.

5. **Sponsors Entering Active Duty Status for a Period of Greater than 30 Days**—A copy of orders ordering a reservist or guardsman to an active duty period of greater than 30 days may be accepted for the first 120 days of the active duty period. After that, follow the procedure in step 1.

6. **Newborns**—Newborns will not be denied care for a period of 1 year following birth. The patient's birth certificate suffices when presented with a parent's valid ID card.

7. **Emergency Care**—This is a medical decision and shall be determined by criteria established within the command.

8. **Sponsor's Duty Station is Outside the 50 United States or has an APO/FPO Address**—Dependents whose sponsors are assigned outside the 50 United States or to a duty station with an APO/FPO address will not be denied care as long as the sponsor is enrolled and eligible in DEERS.

9. **Survivors**—When an eligibility check indicates that a deceased sponsor is not enrolled

in DEERS or the survivor is listed as the sponsor, the survivor will be treated on the first visit and referred to the appropriate personnel office for correction of the DEERS database. For second and subsequent visits, the survivor will be required to follow the procedure in item 1, above.

DEERS ELIGIBILITY EXCEPTIONS.—The following beneficiaries are categorized as "DEERS Eligibility Exceptions." Although authorized care, they may not be authorized to be enrolled in the DEERS system. These beneficiaries will **NOT** be denied care based upon a DEERS check.

- **Secretary of the Navy Designees**—Secretary of the Navy Designees will be treated as indicated on their letter of designation.

- **Foreign Military Personnel**—These personnel and their dependents, assigned through Personnel Exchange Programs or other means, are or may be eligible. Eligible members may also include

  —North Atlantic Treaty Organization (NATO) military personnel and their dependents stationed in or passing through the United States;

  —crew and passengers of visiting military aircraft; and

  —crews of ships of NATO nations that come into port.

Other foreign military personnel may be eligible through Public Law or DoD agreements. As such, they will be treated in accordance with current service directives.

Patients in other organizations, such as Red Cross workers, Secret Service agents, Federal Aviation Administration personnel, and some non-retiree veterans, to name a few, are also in this category. Ensure current eligibility requirements are met for these personnel prior to treatment.

TRICARE

TRICARE is an enhancement of the Civilian Health and Medical Program of the Uniformed Services (CHAMPUS). TRICARE is a medical benefits program established to enhance management of care services in military medical treatment facilities and to cost-share charges for medically necessary civilian services and supplies required in the diagnosis and treatment of illness or injury. TRICARE is also utilized if the required services are not available from the direct care system of the Department of Defense treatment facilities or designated MTFs.

Information pertaining to eligibility, extent of care, providers, cost, and claims is contained in the booklet *Sailing with TRICARE, for Sailors and Their Families*. A copy of this publication, along with the *TRICARE Provider Directory* and other helpful TRICARE information is available at your local TRICARE Service Center. A wealth of guidance is also available via the DoD TRICARE homepage, http://www.tricare.osd.mil.

NAVY MEDICINE'S QUALITY ASSURANCE PROGRAM

LEARNING OBJECTIVE*: Recall the philosophy of Navy medicine's Quality Assurance Program.*

The Quality Assurance Program is used to evaluate the degree of excellence of the results of delivered care and to make improvements so that care in the future will result in a higher degree of quality. Quality assurance activities reflect what patients and providers expect of each other. In past years, various means of reviewing and evaluating patient care have been introduced. In 1979, the JCAH Board of Commissioners imposed the requirement for hospitals to coordinate quality assurance activities and to use an ongoing monitoring system to review and evaluate the quality and need for care. This approach is effective in identifying important patient-related problems and is applicable in every healthcare delivery situation. Many of the principles, standards, and organizational requirements of JCAH have been adopted and are contained in OPNAV 6320.7, *Health Care Quality Insurance Policies for Operating Forces*. BUMEDINST 6010.13, *Quality Assurance Program*, lists the required elements for process improvement (quality assurance) programs of naval hospitals, medical clinics, and dental clinics.

PATIENT RELATIONS AND COMMAND PATIENT CONTACT PROGRAMS

LEARNING OBJECTIVE*: Recall the philosophy of the Patient Relations Program and the Command Patient Contact Program.*

Navy healthcare professionals have long understood the need for good communication and rapport between the patient and the medical department staff. The atmosphere in which patient care is given has a tremendous effect on the patient's perception of the quality of care. The quality of medical care rendered to Navy beneficiaries is superb; however, too frequently the medical care is perceived by the patient to be substandard because personnel in patient contact points are not adequately trained in interpersonal relations. Good patient rapport is an essential element of health care delivery. Many complaints voiced by patients would not occur if personnel manning critical patient contact points presented a courteous, positive, and knowledgeable attitude that reflected a genuine concern for the patient.

To this end, the Patient Relations Program was implemented through BUMEDINST 6300.10, *Health Care Relations Program*. The Patient Relations Program's primary goal is to provide assistance by intervention in and resolution of a patient's complaints or problems. The Patient Contact Program, a subset of the Patient Relations Program, ensures an effective means of resolving such issues before the patient departs the facility. As an adjunct to this goal, both programs strive to enhance the channels of communication between the hospital and the patient population, as well as among the hospital staff.

FAMILY ADVOCACY PROGRAM

LEARNING OBJECTIVE: *Recognize policies and procedures pertaining to the Family Advocacy Program.*

The purpose of the Family Advocacy Program is to identify, treat, and monitor Navy personnel engaging in spouse or child abuse/neglect (whether physical or psychological) and sexual abuse. The program, a responsibility of the Navy Military Personnel Command, is guided by SECNAVINST 1752.3 and, further, by BUMEDINST 6320.70. In each geographical location, a Family Advocacy Representative (FAR), usually a staff member of the Naval Hospital, manages the program. A basewide committee, composed of medical, line, chaplain, and Family Service Center personnel, reviews abuse cases and determines whether each case is established, suspected, or unfounded. Established cases are reported at the central registry at the Bureau of Medicine and Surgery, where service statistics are compiled and the future assignment of established abusers is monitored and controlled.

DRUG AND ALCOHOL ABUSE PREVENTION AND CONTROL PROGRAM

LEARNING OBJECTIVE: *Recognize policies and procedures pertaining to the Drug and Alcohol Abuse Prevention and Control Program.*

The Navy has established a "zero tolerance" standard for drug usage. Although prevention and punishment are still major components of the zero tolerance policy, the major emphasis has shifted to education and training. Routine after-care treatment of addiction is rarely offered to individuals found abusing drugs, and the most likely outcome of drug abuse is appropriate disciplinary action and separation from the service. Levels of alcohol-abuse treatment range from shipboard education programs to inpatient admission. Post-treatment consists of monitoring and support groups, both of which are crucial aspects of the 1-year after-care rehabilitation program.

All individuals with substance abuse problems—whether alcohol- or drug-related—are totally accountable for their actions and the consequences of them in accordance with the Uniform Code of Military Justice (UCMJ) and other relevant federal, state, and local laws. See OPNAVINST 5350.4, *Drug and Alcohol Abuse Prevention and Control*, and SECNAVINST 5300.28, *Military Substance Abuse Prevention and Control*, for additional information and guidance.

Drug and alcohol abuse is costly in terms of lost work hours and unnecessary administrative and judicial processing and is a critical drawdown on morale and esprit de corps. It undermines the very fiber of professional readiness, safety, discipline, judgment, and loyalty. It is not only the abuser who is affected, but the abuser's shipmates as well. "Zero tolerance" recognizes that drug and alcohol abuse is incompatible with the maintenance of high standards of performance, military discipline, and readiness, and is destructive of Navy efforts to instill pride and professionalism in its members.

PREVENTION

Prevention programs are an important aspect of military life. **PREVENT 2000** (Personal Responsibility and Values, Education and Training) is a program designed specifically for the younger Sailor. **ADAMS** (Alcohol and Drug Abuse, Managers and Supervisors) is required for E-5 and above.

Most commands have full-time or collateral-duty **DAPA**s, Drug and Alcohol Program Advisors, who provide the direct liaison between law enforcement, medical, the Family Services Center, and the commanding officer in all matters dealing with intervention, identification, and treatment. The DAPA coordinates on-site training, facilitates Alcohol Anonymous meetings, and provides referrals for outside intervention and inpatient treatment if indicated. Personnel can be identified to the DAPA through aberrant behavioral patterns, suspicious medical findings, and by self-referral to either medical or the chaplain's office.

CONTROL

Medical personnel become professionally involved in substance abuse programs when called upon to withdraw blood or urine from an individual suspected of drug or alcohol abuse. Few areas cause as much concern and confusion to healthcare providers as the question of when those bodily fluids may be lawfully extracted.

At the outset, a few basic facts must be discussed.

1. The healthcare provider should not undertake a fluid extraction procedure when to do so is medically contraindicated.

2. Refusal to perform an extraction in the face of lawful authority could subject the healthcare provider to charges of obstruction of justice or willful disobedience of an order.

3. The healthcare provider is not an arbiter of the law. (In other words, the admissibility of evidence derived from a blood or urine sample is not a matter for Medical Department personnel to decide.)

4. Common sense and cooperation with command and law enforcement officials should be the guideposts in every instance where extraction of bodily fluids is an issue.

The following are the circumstances where withdrawal of blood or urine from active duty military members is authorized:

- **Consensual withdrawal**—If an individual expressly consents to an extraction of bodily fluids and there is a legitimate reason for the extraction, the healthcare provider may perform the procedure.

- **Valid medical purpose**—Specimens may be obtained from an individual for a valid medical examination, provided the individual has expressly or implicitly consented to the examination.

- **Competence for duty examinations**—The Competence for Duty Examination request form (NAVMED 6120/1) contains a block for the submitting authority to request laboratory analysis. See figures 15–1 and 15–2. The following procedures should be used in handling competence for duty requests.

  —The command initiating the request should complete items 1 through 12 of the form. The individual submitting the request must have authority to make the request. Normally, this will be a commanding officer, executive officer, or command duty officer of the initiating command.

  —After proper initiation of the request, the medical officer or other authorized healthcare provider will complete blocks 13 through 49 on the form.

  —If the command has requested laboratory analysis, the patient should first be requested to give written consent to the procedure. If the patient will not give consent but will allow extraction, the sample should be taken. If the patient refuses consent and will physically resist extraction, the requesting command should be notified and no extraction attempted unless a search authorization is issued.

PHYSICAL READINESS PROGRAM

LEARNING OBJECTIVE: *Recognize the policies and procedures pertaining to the Physical Readiness Program.*

COMPETENCE FOR DUTY EXAMINATION
NAVMED 6120/1 (1-70) S/N 0105-LF-208-3050
(Formerly NAVMED 1630)

INSTRUCTIONS FOR THE USE AND PURPOSE OF THIS FORM ARE CONTAINED IN BUMEDINST 6120.20 SERIES.
THIS FORM SHALL NOT BE USED FOR PROCEDURES PERFORMED FOR CLINICAL OR THERAPY PURPOSES.

DEFINITION OF COMPETENCE FOR DUTY

FOR PERSONS IN THE NAVAL SERVICE: The ability to perform fully the naval duties to which the individual normally would be assigned. (Note: A person who has indulged in intoxicating beverages, narcotics or dangerous drugs to such an extent as to impair
sensibly the rational and full exercise of his mental and physical faculties cannot be entrusted with the duties incident to naval
service. The fact that the person is in a patient, leave, or liberty status is immaterial to the determination of his competence
to perform his naval duties.)

FOR ALL OTHERS: The mental and physical ability to perform fully any task or service which the individual may normally be expected to perform.

INSTRUCTIONS
1. Items 1-12 shall be completed in duplicate by the commanding officer or other proper authority requesting examination.
2. Items 13-49 shall be completed by medical officer conducting examination. Under item 13, History, include information provided by examinee as to ingestion and quantity of alcoholic beverage, narcotic, drug substance, or food, and time taken. Note any
evidence of disease or injury (other than the condition prompting this examination) in item 16.
3. When conducting an examination for competence for duty and individual is accused or suspected of an offense, comply with
BuMedInst 6120.20 series.
4. All treatment provided at the time of examination shall be entered on form NAVMED 6150/3, Sick Call Treatment Record.

A. REQUEST FOR EXAMINATION

1. TO:	2. DATE	3. TIME (Hours)

It is requested that a physical examination be given the following individual to determine competence for duty.

4. NAME (Last, first, middle)	5. GRADE OR RATE	6. DUTY STATION

7. REASON FOR REFERRAL

8. SIGNATURE (Requester)	9. GRADE OR RATE	10. TITLE
11. NAME OF REQUESTER (Typewrite or print in ink)		12. DUTY STATION

B. CLINICAL EXAMINATION

13. HISTORY

14. GENERAL APPEARANCE (Include appearance of clothing)	15. MENTAL STATE

16. DISEASES OR INJURIES (Other than the condition prompting this examination, per inst. 2 above)

17. TEMPERATURE	18. PULSE (Rate and character)
19. BLOOD PRESSURE	
20. FACE (Flushed, pallid, cyanotic)	21. TONGUE
	22. BREATH
23. SKIN (Warm, cool, moist, dry, pale)	24. SPEECH (Thick, slurred, ability to repeat words such as Merciful, Pedestrian, Peter Piper)
25. EYES (Size of pupils, reaction to light, conjunctivae, etc.)	

HM3f1501

Figure 15-1.—NAVMED 6120/1, *Competence for Duty Examination request form* (front).

The policies governing this program are outlined in OPNAVINST 6110.1. Currently, physical readiness testing is required for all personnel on a semi-annual basis. Testing, education, and training advice are provided through a network of collateral duty command fitness coordinators. In addition to the requirement for program implementation by each subordinate command, Medical Department responsibilities are

- providing technical assistance to BUPERS,

- conducting lifestyle, fitness, and obesity research,

26. OTHER CONDITIONS	27. SAMPLE OF HANDWRITING
VOMITING	
INCONTINENCE OF URINE	
INCONTINENCE OF FECES	

C. NEUROLOGICAL EXAMINATION

28. REFLEXES	29.	COORDINATION	
HYPERACTIVE	FINGER TO NOSE		ROMBERG TEST
HYPOACTIVE	HEEL TO KNEE		
TREMOR	ABILITY TO APPROACH AND PICK UP OBJECT FROM THE FLOOR		GAIT

D. LABORATORY EXAMINATIONS

30. BLOOD ANALYSIS (Name of test and results expressed as mgm per ml or in other standard units)	31. TIME TAKEN (HOUR)	33. OTHER TESTS (Gastric contents, urine, etc.)	34. TIME TAKEN (HOUR)
	32. DATE		35. DATE

36. SPECIMEN OBTAINED BY (Name of person)   37. RESULTS VERIFIED BY (Name of person)

E. CONCLUSIONS AS TO COMPETENCE FOR DUTY

Check the applicable "YES" or "NO" box to indicate answer.	YES	NO	If the answer to item 38 is NO, also answer items 39 and 40. If the answer to item 39 is YES, describe in block 16 DISEASES or INJURIES. If answer to item 40 is YES describe under block 43.
38. Is examinee competent to perform duty?			
39. Is examinee's condition due to disease or injury?			
40. Is examinee's condition due to the use of drugs or alcohol?			

41. DISPOSITION: ☐ RETURNED TO FULL DUTY   ☐ ADMITTED TO SICKLIST   ☐ RELEASED TO CUSTODY OF (Specify to whom)

WARNING: For copies of Article 31, (a) and (b), Uniform Code of Military Justice, and Paragraph 30b., Manual for Courts-Martial, United States, 1969 (Revised edition), see BUMEDINST 6120.20 series.

42. THE MEMBER ☐ HAS ☐ HAS NOT BEEN WARNED IN ACCORDANCE WITH ARTICLE 31, (a) AND (b), UNIFORM CODE OF MILITARY JUSTICE AND PARAGRAPH 30f, MANUAL FOR COURTS-MARTIAL, UNITED STATES, 1969 (REVISED EDITION).

43. REMARKS (All answers should be as brief as possible. Items requiring more space should be continued in this 'Remarks' block. Specify item continued.)

F. RESPONSE TO REQUESTER

In accordance with the request in Section A, the individual has been examined as set forth above to determine competence for duty.

A signed copy of this report is being inserted in the Health Record of the individual.

44. THE INDIVIDUAL ☐ HAS ☐ HAS NOT RECEIVED A COPY OF THIS REPORT.

45. SIGNATURE (Examiner)	46. GRADE OR RATE	47. DUTY STATION	48.
49. NAME (Typewrite)			TIME _____ DATE _____

NAVMED 6120/1 (1-70) (BACK)   ☆U.S. GOVERNMENT PRINTING OFFICE: 1977—703-173/3216 2-1   6-17264

HM3f1502

Figure 15-2.—NAVMED 6120/1, *Competence for Duty Examination request form* (back).

- reviewing health status and granting waivers for those individuals unable to safely participate in physical fitness testing and training, and

- assisting in the development of exercise prescriptions.

LEGAL IMPLICATIONS IN MEDICAL CARE

LEARNING OBJECTIVE: *Recognize the policies and procedures pertaining to consent for medical treatment, incident reports, and release of medical information.*

There are few aspects of medical administration of treatment that do not have some legal implications. Every time a patient comes into contact with a facility or its staff members, either directly or indirectly, formally or informally, the potential for legal entanglement exists. Although the law has become more and more involved in the operation of hospitals, the exercise of common sense combined with a knowledge of those situations that require special care will protect the hospital and its staff from most difficulties.

This section addresses some of the situations that regularly arise and have legal consequences, including the policy and instructions that apply to those situations. Keep in mind that the law is an inexact science, subject to widely varying circumstances. The information in this chapter cannot substitute for the advice of an attorney. Hospital staff members are encouraged to consult with hospital or area Judge Advocate General (JAG) Corps officers on issues with which they are uncomfortable.

CONSENT REQUIREMENTS FOR MEDICAL TREATMENT

With limited exceptions, every person has the right not to be touched without his having first given permission. This right to be touched only when and in the manner authorized is the foundation of the requirement that consent must be obtained before medical treatment is initiated. Failure to obtain consent may result in the healthcare provider being responsible for an assault and battery upon the patient.

Informed Consent

While the term "consent" in the medical setting refers to a patient's expressed or implied agreement to submit to an examination or treatment, the doctrine of "informed consent" requires that the healthcare provider give the patient all the information necessary for a knowledgeable decision on the proposed procedure. When courts say that a patient's consent must be informed, they are saying that a patient's agreement to a medical procedure must be made with full awareness of the consequences of the agreement. If there is no such awareness, there has been no lawful consent.

The duty to inform and explain rests with the provider. **THIS RESPONSIBILITY CANNOT BE DELEGATED.**

The provider must describe the proposed procedure in lay terms so the patient understands the nature of what is proposed. The risks of the treatment must be explained. If there are any alternative medical options, they should be disclosed and discussed.

For common medical procedures that are considered simple and essentially risk free, a provider is not required to explain consequences that are generally understood to be remote. A determination of what is simple and common should be made from the perspective of appropriate medical standards. Where the harm that could result is serious or the risk or harm is high, the duty to disclose is greater.

Methods should be developed within each hospital department to acquaint patients with the benefits, risks, and alternatives to the proposed treatment. In some departments, prepared pamphlets or information sheets may be desirable. In others, oral communication may be the best method. Some states (e.g., Texas) have laws that are very specific about what is required.

Emergency Situations

Consent before treatment is not necessary when treatment appears to be immediately required to prevent deterioration or aggravation of a patient's condition, especially in life-threatening situations, and it is not possible to obtain a valid consent from the patient or a person authorized to consent for the patient. The existence and scope of the emergency should be adequately documented.

Who May Consent

The determination of who has authority to consent to medical treatment is based on an evaluation of the competency of the patient. If competent, usually the patient alone has the authority to consent. Competency refers to the ability to understand the nature and consequences of one's decisions. In the absence of contrary evidence, it may be assumed that the patient presenting for treatment is competent. If the patient is incompetent, either by reason of statutory incompetence (e.g., a minor) or by reason of a physical or mental impairment, the inquiry must turn to whoever has the legal capacity to consent on behalf of the patient. Parents and guardians will usually have the authority to consent for their minor child or children. In many states, though not all, a husband or wife may give consent for an incompetent spouse. It is the law of the state in which the hospital is located that controls the question of "substitute consent."

Forms of Consent

Consent for medical treatment should be obtained through an open discussion between the provider and patient during which the patient expressly agrees to the procedure. The consent should then be documented by having the patient sign any appropriate forms and by the provider noting any important details of the discussion in the medical record.

In certain limited circumstances, the consent of an individual to simple medical treatment may be implied from the circumstances. Implied consent arises by reasonable inference from the conduct of the patient or the individual authorized to consent for the patient. Reliance on this form of consent is strongly discouraged except in the most routine, risk-free examinations and procedures.

Witness to Consent

Any competent adult may witness the patient's consent. It is preferable that the witness be a staff member of the hospital who is not participating in the procedure. It is not advisable for a relative of the patient to act as a witness.

Duration of Consent

A consent is valid as long as there has been no material change in the circumstances between the date that consent was given and the date of the procedure. It is desirable that a new consent be obtained if there is a significant time lapse or if the patient has been discharged and readmitted due to postponement of the procedure.

INCIDENT REPORTS

When an event occurs that harms an individual, illustrates a potential for harm, or evidences serious dissatisfaction by patients, visitors, or staff, then a risk-management incident has taken place. Examples of such episodes could include the following:

- A patient's family helps him out of bed despite directions to the contrary by staff members. The patient falls and is injured.

- Excessive silver nitrate is put into the eyes of a newborn, impairing vision.

- The mother of the child complains about the care that has been given to her child and informs a staff member that she is going to talk to her lawyer about what has happened.

When a member of the staff becomes aware of an incident, he has a responsibility to make the hospital command aware of the situation. The mechanism for doing this is the **incident report** system. Incident reports are designed to promptly document all circumstances surrounding an event, to alert the commanding officer, quality assurance coordinator, and other involved administrators and clinicians of a potential liability situation, and, in a broader sense, to establish an information base on which to monitor and evaluate the number and types of incidents that take place in the facility.

Because incident reports, by their very nature, contain a great deal of information that would be of interest to persons filing claims or lawsuits against the Navy for alleged substandard medical care, and because the law recognizes the need for hospitals to have a reliable means of discovering and correcting problems, most states have enacted laws that make incident reports confidential. In other words, a person cannot obtain a copy of an incident report to help in their legal action against the hospital.

However, incident reports can lose their "protected" status if they are misused or mishandled. It is important, therefore, to treat these reports like other confidential documents. You must strictly limit the number of copies made and the distribution of the reports. Do not include the report in the patient's treatment record. The report should be limited to the facts and must not contain conclusions. Finally, the report should be addressed and forwarded **directly** to the quality assurance coordinator of the hospital.

Further guidance concerning the Risk Management Program, the program that governs incident reports, can be found in BUMEDINST 6010.21.

RELEASE OF MEDICAL INFORMATION

Two federal statutes, the **Privacy Act** and the **Freedom of Information Act** (FOIA) combine to establish the criteria for collecting, maintaining, and releasing medical treatment records.

Freedom of Information Act

The Freedom of Information Act governs the disclosure of documents compiled and maintained by government agencies. A written request for Department of the Navy records that explicitly or implicitly refers to FOIA must be responded to in accordance with the provisions of the Act. The Department of the Navy will make available to any person all documents, not otherwise exempt, provided the requester reasonably describes the records sought and promises to pay for reasonable search and photocopy costs. Each naval activity is responsible for developing procedures for ensuring the prompt handling, retrieval, and review of requested records. The official having responsibility for the records has 10 working days to respond to the requester.

A naval record will be withheld only when it is exempt from disclosure under FOIA. One basis for exempting a record from disclosure applies to personnel, medical, and similar files, the release of which would constitute a clearly unwarranted invasion of personal privacy. This concern over clearly unwarranted privacy intrusion is reflected in the provisions of the Privacy Act.

Privacy Act

The public's concern over the inner workings and functioning of the government was the reason for the creation of the FOIA. However, it became obvious that a balance had to be made between the public's right to know and other significant rights and interests. One of these competing interests was the protection of an individual's personal right to privacy. In response to this need, the Privacy Act of 1974 was enacted. The stated purpose of the Privacy Act is to establish safeguards concerning the right to privacy by regulating the collection, maintenance, use, and dissemination of personal information by federal agencies.

The Privacy Act requires federal agencies to

- permit an individual to know what records pertaining to him are collected, maintained, used, or disseminated by the agency;

- permit an individual to prevent records pertaining to him and obtained by the agency for a particular purpose from being used or made available for another purpose without the individual's consent;

- permit an individual to gain access to information pertaining to him in federal agency records, have a copy made for all or any portion thereof, and correct or amend such records;

- collect, maintain, use, or disseminate any record of identifiable personal information in a manner that ensures such action is for a necessary and useful purpose, that the information is current and accurate, and that adequate safeguards are provided to prevent misuse of such information;

- permit exemptions from the requirements of the Privacy Act only in those cases where there is specific statutory authority to do so; and

- be subject to civil suits for any damages that occur as a result of willful or intentional violation of any individual's rights under the Privacy Act.

In addition, any officer or employee of an agency who willfully violates certain provisions of the Privacy Act is subject to criminal prosecution and fines.

Under the Privacy Act's provisions concerning disclosure of information, there are several circumstances under which naval treatment records and their contents can be disclosed. Included are disclosures to employees of the Department of the Navy who have a need to know the information. Also included are disclosures to a person under compelling circumstances affecting health or safety, pursuant to a court order, and to another government agency for civil or criminal law enforcement activities. Circumstances under which the release of medical information is appropriate are discussed in chapter 12, *Health Records*, and in the section of this chapter concerning law enforcement personnel.

MEDICAL CONDITIONS AND LAW ENFORCEMENT PERSONNEL

LEARNING OBJECTIVE*: Recognize the policies and procedures pertaining to prisoner patients, victims of alleged sexual assault and rape, substance abuse and control, probable-cause searches, and line-of-duty and misconduct investigations.*

Some medical conditions, by their very occurrence, will result in the involvement of law enforcement personnel. Individuals who are injured while committing a criminal offense; victims of abuse, neglect, or assault; impaired or injured as a result of drug abuse; or injured as a result of a traffic accident will often be the subject of an official investigation. Many times the investigators will want to question the patient or the healthcare providers treating the patient. Often, the medical records of the patient will be requested by the authorities. Occasionally, officials will want to take the patient into custody.

Under the Posse Comitatus Act, a federal statute enacted in 1956 (18 U.S.C. § 1385), it is unlawful for the U.S. military to be used to enforce or assist in the enforcement of federal or state civil laws. There are many exemptions to this act, but the issue for healthcare providers is settled by asking the following question: *"Is the medical procedure being done on this patient for a legitimate medical reason, or is it only being performed to assist civil law enforcement?"* Provided there is a reasonable medical justification for the procedure, the results of the procedure may be shared with civil law enforcement officials under the circumstances discussed below.

Cooperation with law enforcement officials, to the extent possible, is required. Provided there are no medical contraindications, patients who are either suspected of having committed an offense or who are presumed victims of criminal activity will be made available to speak with investigators. As discussed previously, access to medical treatment records is governed by the Privacy Act and FOIA. Generally, records of patients may be made available to U.S. Navy investigators once they have established a need to know the information. This determination will usually be made by the hospital JAG or public affairs officer. Other Department of Defense, federal, state, or local law enforcement officers may have access to treatment records if access is necessary as part of a criminal

investigation and there is no unwarranted violation of the privacy rights of the individual involved. Similarly, local health and social service departments may be provided information from the record. The same guidelines that apply to access to treatment records apply to staff members' discussing with investigating officers the details of the medical treatment provided to a patient.

DELIVERY OF A PATIENT UNDER WARRANT OF ARREST

No patient may be released from treatment before it is medically reasonable to do so. Once it is determined that the individual can be released without significant risk of harm, the following guidelines regarding release to law enforcement authorities apply.

- **Nonactive Duty Patients**—When a nonactive duty patient is released from medical treatment, the facility no longer exercises any degree of control, and normal legal processes will occur. No official action by hospital personnel is required before local authorities take custody of the released patient. There may be occasions, however, when law enforcement officials should be notified of an imminent release of a patient.

- **Active Duty Patients**—The commanding officer is authorized to deliver personnel to federal law enforcement authorities who display proper credentials and represent to the command that a federal warrant for the arrest of the individual concerned has been issued. There are circumstances in which delivery may be refused; however, guidance should be sought from a judge advocate of the Navy or Marine Corps when delivery is to be denied.

Normally, it is the responsibility of the permanent command to take custody and control of an active duty member suspected of committing an offense. If the member is an unauthorized absentee and the command to which he is assigned is not in the same geographic area as the treatment facility, release of the patient should be coordinated with the nearest Transient Personnel Unit or Military Prisoner Escort Unit. Close liaison with the member's permanent command should also be established.

In cases where delivery of an active duty patient is requested by local civil authorities, and the treatment facility is located within the requesting jurisdiction or aboard a ship within the territorial waters of such jurisdiction, commanding officers are authorized to deliver the patient when a proper warrant is presented. Whenever possible, a judge advocate of the Navy or Marine Corps should be consulted before delivery. If the treatment facility is located outside the jurisdiction requesting delivery, only a General Courts-Martial authority (as defined by the Uniform Code of Military Justice, Manual for Courts-Martial, and Navy Regulations) is authorized to arrange for delivery of such the patient. Extradition, return agreements, and other prerequisites to delivery will have to be completed.

When disciplinary proceedings involving military offenses are pending, the treatment facility should obtain legal guidance from a judge advocate before delivering a patient to federal, state, or local authorities. When the commanding officer considers that extraordinary circumstances exist which indicate that delivery should be denied, then the Judge Advocate General of the Navy must be notified of the circumstances by message or phone.

PRISONER PATIENTS

Prisoner patients fall into three categories of eligible beneficiaries:

- Enemy prisoners of war and other detained personnel

- Nonmilitary federal prisoners

- Military prisoners

Enemy Prisoners of War and Other Detained Personnel

Enemy prisoners of war and other detained personnel are entitled to all necessary medical and dental care, subject to the availability of care and facilities.

Nonmilitary Federal Prisoners

Nonmilitary federal prisoners are authorized only emergency medical care. When such care is being provided, the institution to which the prisoner is sentenced must furnish the security personnel to ensure custody of the prisoner and safety of others in the facility. Upon completion of emergency care, arrangements will be made immediately to transfer these individuals to a nonmilitary treatment facility or for return to the institution to which sentenced.

Military Prisoners

Status of Forces policy is to protect, to the maximum extent possible, the rights of U.S. personnel who may be subject to criminal trial by foreign courts and imprisonment in foreign prisons. Active duty members are generally not separated from the service until they have completed their term of imprisonment and returned to the United States. During this confinement, they will normally remain healthcare beneficiaries.

Military prisoners (those sentenced under the Uniform Code of Military Justice) whose punitive discharges have been executed but whose sentences have not expired are authorized medical and dental care. Individuals on appellate leave, awaiting execution of a punitive discharge, are also entitled to care. Military prisoners whose punitive discharges have been executed and who require hospitalization beyond expiration of their sentences are not eligible for care, but they may be hospitalized as civilian humanitarian nonmilitary indigents until disposition can be made to some other facility.

SEXUAL ASSAULT AND RAPE

Sexual assault and rape are criminal offenses, often associated with serious injury. The management of cases involving sexual assault and rape must be a joint medical and legal function. A sexual assault investigation kit, supplied by the Naval Criminal Investigative Service, is used to gather and preserve evidence of a crime. Included in this kit are step-by-step procedures for the examination of the patient, as well as a checklist of specimens to be collected.

In order to safeguard and obtain evidence to be used in possible legal proceedings, liaison between the naval treatment facility, military and civil investigative agencies, and state and local agencies (such as Child and Spouse Protective Services) should be established. It must be kept in mind that medical personnel are not to judge, defend, or prosecute the individuals involved. NAVMEDCOMINST 6310.3, *Management of Alleged or Suspected Sexual Assault and Rape Cases*, provides further guidance for the care, evaluation, and medico-legal documentation of the victim of an alleged rape or sexual assault.

Every effort must be made to treat the patient with respect and courtesy and to provide appropriate privacy. In dealing with alleged victims of sexual assault, careful attention to psychological factors must be given to lessen the impact of the incident. This is especially important when a minor is involved and the reaction of adults may be more harmful than the actual assault itself. Tactful questioning and the use of appropriate terminology are of extreme importance throughout the history taking and examination. OPNAVINST 1752.1, *Sexual Assault Victim Intervention (SAVI) Program,* and SECNAVINST 5800.11, *Victim and Witness Program,* provide guidance for the care and support of victims of sexual assault.

CHILD AND SPOUSE ABUSE AND NEGLECT

The nature of child and spouse abuse and neglect requires a careful patient history and physical examination to identify or rule out past and present injuries caused by abuse or neglect. The policies and guidelines established by the Navy Family Advocacy Program must be followed. This program was discussed earlier in this chapter and is outlined in SECNAVINST 1752.3 and BUMEDINST 6320.70.

SUMMARY

Retaining our high medical standards and the quality healthcare the fleet demands, as well as providing care for military dependents and a constantly expanding retiree database, requires a healthcare administration support structure that is second to none. DEERS management and the determination of patient eligibility are crucial components and only two of the areas discussed in this chapter. Also covered were many of the health-related programs established to benefit and support eligible recipients in the military community. These programs are often meant to eliminate the need for others. Good quality assurance, for example, creates better patient relations, thereby minimizing legal problems; substance abuse and family advocacy programs identify problems before they become unmanageable; and the physical readiness program helps build a healthier Sailor, thus eliminating needless patient visits.

This chapter also provided an overview of the Hospital Corpsman's responsibilities in the area of interaction with legal authorities. Sexual assault, spouse and child abuse, and drug and alcohol incidents require legal and medical teamwork. Many legal battles are lost because of failure to adhere to the proper administrative procedures. As a Hospital Corpsman, you must be aware of these procedures and ensure that they are followed precisely.

CHAPTER 16

DECEDENT AFFAIRS PROGRAM

The Navy's Decedent Affairs Program consists of search, recovery, identification, care, and disposition of remains of deceased personnel for whom the Department of the Navy is responsible. The Decedent Affairs Program is considered a highly visible and extremely sensitive program. Arrangements for the burial of the deceased should be conducted in an expedient but dignified manner, and survivors of the deceased should be given the greatest possible amount of support and assistance.

ASSIGNMENT OF RESPONSIBILITIES

LEARNING OBJECTIVE: *Identify military activities that are responsible for the management of the Navy and Marine Corps Decedent Affairs Program.*

The overall manager of the Navy and Marine Corps Decedent Affairs Program is the Naval Office of Medical/Dental (MEDDEN) Affairs, located at Great Lakes, IL. At the local level, naval hospitals and other naval activities are responsible for inspecting remains, briefing escorts and making travel arrangements, and (for burial at sea) delivering remains to the point of embarkation. Naval hospitals manage deaths that occur at the hospital and in their local catchment (area of responsibility) area. At small independent operational units and on board naval vessels, the responsibility for managing the Decedent Affairs Program falls on the commanding officer or officer-in-charge and the senior Hospital Corpsman. For this reason, Hospital Corpsmen should have a working knowledge of decedent affairs procedures, which are outlined in NAVMEDCOMINST 5360.1, *Decedent Affairs Manual.*

PROGRAMS

LEARNING OBJECTIVE: *Recall the purpose of the Current Death Program, Graves Registration Program, Concurrent Return Program, Return of Remains Program, and the Casualty Assistance Call Program.*

To carry out the various responsibilities of the Decedent Affairs Program, five programs have been established. They are

- the **Current Death Program**,

- the **Graves Registration Program**,

- the **Concurrent Return Program**,

- the **Return of Remains Program**, and

- the **Casualty Assistance Calls Program**.

CURRENT DEATH PROGRAM

The Current Death Program provides professional mortuary services, supplies, and related services incident to the care and disposition of remains of persons eligible for these services. Under this program, remains are shipped to a place designated by the primary next of kin (PNOK), such as a spouse or parents, for permanent disposition. The decedent's personal effects will also be shipped to the legal recipient. The Current Death Program is normally operational on a worldwide basis during peacetime, but may also be used during major conflicts.

GRAVES REGISTRATION PROGRAM

The Graves Registration Program (GR or GRREG) provides for the search, recovery, evacuation (to a temporary cemetery or a mortuary), initial identification, disposition of personal effects found with each deceased, and burial of deceased persons in temporary cemeteries. This program is only operational when authorized by the responsible commander during major military operations. When necessary, the GR program includes the establishment and maintenance of temporary burial sites. Detailed guidance on graves registration procedures are contained in the Navy and Marine Corps publication NAVMED P-5016/NAVMC 2509A, *Handling of Deceased Personnel in Theaters of Operation.*

CONCURRENT RETURN PROGRAM

The Concurrent Return Program combines the Current Death Program and Graves Registration

Program. This program provides for the search, recovery, and evacuation of remains to a processing point; identification and preparation of remains in a mortuary; and shipment, for permanent disposition, to a final destination designated by the PNOK. The Concurrent Return Program normally becomes operational when large numbers of military personnel are committed to a strategic area.

Remains buried in temporary cemeteries (under the GR program or in emergencies) will normally be disinterred and evacuated under the Concurrent Return Program if conditions and capabilities permit.

RETURN OF REMAINS PROGRAM

The Return of Remains Program provides for permanent disposition of remains of persons buried in temporary cemeteries who could not be evacuated under the Concurrent Return Program. The Return of Remains Program is activated only upon the enactment of special legislation. This special legislation may authorize the establishment of one or more permanent American cemeteries in the overseas area and may give PNOK the option of having the remains buried therein or shipped to another place of their choosing. When the Return of Remains Program becomes activated, the Chief, Bureau of Medicine and Surgery (BUMED), is responsible for advising field activities of its activation.

CASUALTY ASSISTANCE CALLS PROGRAM

The Casualty Assistance Calls Program (CACP) is administered by the Commander, Naval Military Personnel Command (COMNAVMILPERSCOM), and the Commandant of the Marine Corps (CMC). Although integrally related, the CACP is not part of the Decedent Affairs Program. The CACP details a Casualty Assistance Calls Officer (CACO), usually a commissioned officer (although senior enlisted personnel may be used), to personally contact the PNOK. The CACO helps the PNOK and SNOK (secondary next of kin—children over 18, brother, etc.) with problems surrounding the death, and provides information on such matters as

- disposition of remains,

- death gratuity and unpaid pay and allowances,

- personal effects of the deceased,

- settlement of the decedent's estate (wills, bank accounts, property, savings bonds, commercial insurance, etc.),

- Servicemen's Group Life Insurance (SGLI), and

- travel of dependents to grave site and to permanent residence.

The Navy and Marine Corps Casualty Assistance Calls Programs are operated differently. The individual service instructions noted below should be consulted for specifics.

- NAVPERS 15560, *Naval Military Personnel Manual* (MILPERSMAN)

- BUPERSINST 1770.3, *The Navy Casualty Assistance Calls Program (CACP) Manual*

- MCO P3040.4, *Marine Corps Casualty Procedures Manual* (MARCORCASPROC-MAN)

ELIGIBILITY FOR DECEDENT AFFAIRS

LEARNING OBJECTIVE: *Identify individuals who are eligible for decedent affairs benefits.*

Navy and Marine Corps members who expire while serving on active duty or active and inactive duty for training are entitled to Decedent Affairs Program benefits. Generally, the following persons under the jurisdiction of the Department of the Navy are entitled to some decedent affair benefits: dependents, retirees, and civilian employees. For details, see NAVMEDCOMINST 5360.1, *Decedent Affairs Manual.*

NOTIFICATION OF DEATH

LEARNING OBJECTIVE: *Identify forms used to report casualties, deaths, and personnel missing or missing in action.*

As soon as possible after it is determined that a casualty has occurred, submit a casualty report in accordance with MILPERSMAN 4210100. When death occurs, complete the "Personnel Casualty Report (Death), Report Symbol NMPC 1770-4

Officer/Enlisted." For missing personnel, complete the "Personnel Casualty Report (Missing/Missing in action), Report Symbol NMPC 1770-4 Officer/Enlisted."

PERSONNEL CASUALTY REPORT

A personnel casualty report must be completed for the following persons who become casualties:

- Active duty Navy

- Retired Navy

- Certain former service members

- Certain military dependents

- Members of other Armed Forces

- Civilians serving with or attached to Navy commands

- Others whose deaths occur on naval reservations or aboard ships

When a member becomes a casualty, his commanding officer should submit a personnel casualty report. However, if a service member becomes a casualty while away from his command, the command or activity that learns of the casualty occurring should submit the personnel casualty report. The member's command should supplement the personnel casualty report that was previously submitted by another command.

METHOD OF REPORTING CASUALTIES

Personnel casualty reports should be sent by priority message.

Action Addressees on Personnel Casualty Reports

The following activities should be action addressees on personnel casualty reports:

1. Commander, Naval Military Personnel Command

2. Chief, Bureau of Medicine and Surgery

3. Casualty Assistance Calls/Funeral Honors Support (CAC/FHS) Program coordinators of the area in which the primary and secondary NOK reside, or the appropriate overseas CAC/FHS program coordinator

4. The Naval Office of Medical/Dental (MEDDEN) Affairs

Information Addressees on Personnel Casualty Reports

The following activities should be listed as information addresses on personnel casualty reports:

1. Secretary of the Navy

2. Navy Finance Center

3. Navy Family Allowance Activity, Cleveland (if the member reported is in a missing status, or if the status is being changed from missing to deceased)

4. The CAC/FHS program coordinator of the area in which the casualty occurred

5. The Chief of Naval Operations (if the casualty is incidental to operations, and on all reports of progress in searches for missing members)

6. The appropriate home port/station, type commander, appropriate operational and administrative commands, and the Enlisted Personnel Management Center (EPMAC)

7. The command or activity designated by the CAC/FHS program coordinator to provide casualty assistance

8. The Fleet Home Town News Center

9. The Naval Safety Center

10. The Judge Advocate General

11. The Appropriate Naval Legal Service Office (if the casualty is the result of other than natural causes)

12. The Armed Forces Institute of Pathology

If the decedent was a Marine Corps member, follow the notification procedures and message formats contained in the MARCORCASPROCMAN, MCO P3040.4.

NOTIFICATION OF NEXT OF KIN

LEARNING OBJECTIVE: *Recall notification of next of kin procedures.*

In cases of death, primary next of kin are personally notified by a uniformed Navy or Marine

Corps representative, as appropriate. Personal notification of the PNOK will normally be made between 0600 and 2200, except under unusual circumstances (e.g., the new media is expected to make a press release; or the member has been hospitalized in serious or very serious condition within CONUS, and the NOK is already aware of the prognosis).

When a death occurs within CONUS, it is the responsibility of the member's commanding officer to make sure that personal notification is made. Outside CONUS, the COMNAVMILPERSCOM will make sure that personal notification is made through the appropriate senior commander overseas.

CONFIRMATION OF THE CASUALTY

Notifications that are not made by telegram should be confirmed by a telegram, unless the PNOK or SNOK has specifically stated that written confirmation is not desired. This follow-up notification should take place within 24 hours of the personal notification.

See MILPERSMAN 4210100 for examples of basic telegram formats for notification and confirmation of death. The formats are presented for guidance only, and rigid adherence is not required.

CONDOLENCE LETTER

Commanding officers are required to write a letter to the appropriate NOK within 48 hours of a casualty. The letter, in addition to expressions of condolence, should contain appropriate details of the casualty; however, no details should be included that are likely to distress the NOK. A copy of the letter is sent to the COMNAVMILPERSCOM and Office of the Judge Advocate General (OJAG)—Investigations Division. Example formats for condolence letters can be found in the *Decedent Affairs Manual*.

AUTOPSY

LEARNING OBJECTIVE: *Determine under what circumstances an autopsy should be performed.*

An autopsy will be performed on the remains of all persons who die on active duty or active duty for training when the commanding officer (CO) deems it necessary. The CO's request may be self-initiated or based upon the recommendation of an investigating officer, other fact-finding body, or a medical officer. An autopsy may be necessary to determine the true cause of death, to get information for completing military records, or to protect the welfare of the military community.

AIRCREW AUTOPSY

The *Manual of the Medical Department* (MANMED), NAVMED P-117, states that when an aircrew member dies while serving as an aircrew member on a military aircraft, the medical officer will recommend to the CO that an autopsy be performed to determine the cause of death. The cause of death in these cases is interpreted to mean any correlation between pathological evidence and the accident cause factor.

REQUESTING PERMISSION FOR AUTOPSY

When an autopsy is desired but not mandatory, the following sentence will be incorporated in the casualty notification message that requests disposition instructions from the PNOK:

"In the interest of medical science and to confirm medical diagnosis, it is requested that your telegram include whether or not permission is granted to accomplish mortem examination."

NONMILITARY AND RETIRED PERSONNEL AUTOPSY

When an autopsy is deemed necessary for retired personnel or nonmilitary persons who die at a naval treatment facility or on a Navy installation, written authorization from the NOK must be obtained before performing the autopsy. The request for permission to perform an autopsy should be incorporated in the casualty notification message, as noted above.

SEARCH, RECOVERY, AND IDENTIFICATION

LEARNING OBJECTIVE: *Recall procedures used to search for, recover, and identify remains.*

The search for, recovery, and identification of remains should be accomplished as soon as possible and should be coordinated with an administrative fact-finding body. Normally, the need for these operations results from acts of violence, such as an aircraft accident, fire, explosion, or natural disaster. The *Manual of the Judge Advocate General* (JAGMAN), JAGINST 5800.7, requires the convening of an administrative fact-finding body when incidents of this nature occur. This responsibility is usually delegated to a naval activity with necessary capabilities at or near the scene of disaster. In establishing identification of remains, search and recovery operations are part of the fact-finding body's functions, with technical assistance furnished by appropriate medical authorities.

SEARCH AND RECOVERY

Every effort should be made to recover all remains. In disasters such as aircraft accidents, fires, explosions, etc., involving the death of naval members and members of other services, notify the Bureau of Medicine and Surgery (BUMED) and MEDDEN Affairs by priority message. This assures immediate interdepartmental cooperation and the early dispatch of necessary supplies, equipment, medical and dental records, and technical personnel. The priority message should include the following information:

- Name, grade or rate, and social security number of all personnel believed dead or missing

- Names of those personnel already identified and method of identification

- Names of those personnel tentatively already positively identified, and whether remains are anatomically intact

- Type and quantity of mortuary supplies, transfer cases, chemicals, and other equipment required

- Whether technical help is desired

Do not release information to the NOK, family, or news media unless specific instructions are received from BUMED and MEDDEN Affairs to do so.

When search, recovery, and identification operations continue for more than 36 hours, chronological progress reports should be dispatched every 24 hours to BUMED and MEDDEN Affairs, with the appropriate information addressees directed by NAVMEDCOMINST 5360.1.

IDENTIFICATION

When the CO is satisfied that identification has been established beyond doubt and documented accordingly, the remains may be considered identified. A minimum of two statements of recognition, substantiated by dental and/or fingerprint comparison or intact remains, will substantiate identification requirements.

MEDDEN Affairs will establish final conclusions and take action required for final disposition of these remains if shipped from outside CONUS to CONUS. Disposition of unidentified remains will be directed by the MEDDEN Affairs or the CMC, as appropriate.

After thorough study of all evidence, final conclusions made by MEDDEN Affairs will result in one of the following determinations:

- Identification of the remains

- Unidentified, but believed to be a specific individual

- Unidentified, unknown

- Group remains, known individuals

- Group remains, unknown individuals

When an autopsy of remains is required or requested, the identification specialist should schedule the autopsy to be performed during the identification process or immediately following. This will preclude any delays in releasing the body for burial and make sure that methods of identification are included in the autopsy report.

Personal effects found on or with remains, after having served all identification purposes, will be disposed of in accordance with current instructions contained in the *Naval Supply Manual*, NAVSUP P-485, or the MARCORCASPROCMAN, MCO P3040.4, as appropriate.

IDENTIFICATION PROBLEMS

All remains, except those that have been positively identified and are anatomically complete, will require additional study and processing by an identification specialist. The MEDDEN Affairs may be requested to provide an identification specialist to visit the activity and make a complete review, to assure that all possible techniques, methods, and procedures have been used to provide a positive identification. The CMC should be an information addressee when members of the Marine Corps may be involved. When members of other services are involved, BUMED and MEDDEN Affairs should be notified by priority message to ensure immediate interdepartmental coordination.

PROCURING MORTUARY SERVICES

LEARNING OBJECTIVE: *Recall mortuary services procurement methods, and recognize primary and secondary burial expenses.*

Mortuary services for the remains of individuals eligible for Decedent Affairs Program benefits outside CONUS are specified in local instructions. Mortuary services within CONUS are provided by naval activities through annual contracts, individual purchase orders, or by private arrangements.

ANNUAL CONTRACTS

Annual contracts are awarded to funeral directors serving the local area of activities anticipating 10 or more deaths per year.

ONE-TIME CONTRACTS

One-time contracts (individual purchase orders) are issued by an activity to a funeral home when an annual contract is not in effect.

PRIVATE ARRANGEMENTS

Private arrangements are made by the PNOK. The PNOK should be advised of services and supplies available through Navy sources and on reimbursement limitations. Reimbursement limitations and reimbursement forms can be obtained by contacting MEDDEN Affairs or the local naval hospital's Decedent Affairs Office.

AUTHORIZED SERVICES

Annual contracts and one-time contracts cover primary funeral expenses but do not include secondary expenses. NOK should be tactfully encouraged to allow the Navy to make all primary-care arrangements, since greater benefits can be furnished throughout procedures. For more information concerning procedures and authorized items, consult NAVMEDCOMINST 5360.1. Primary and secondary funeral expenses are explained in the following sections.

Primary Expenses

Primary expenses are expenses incurred in connection with the recovery, preparation, encasement, and burial of the remains. Primary expenses include

- expenses incurred in the recovery and removal of remains,
- embalmment,
- casket and shipping case,
- cremation,
- interment,
- clothing (e.g., military uniform), and
- delivery of the remains to a common carrier terminal, a local cemetery, or crematorium.

Secondary Expenses

Secondary expenses are expenses incurred in connection with the funeral and burial of remains. Secondary expenses include

- funeral coach,
- transportation of relatives to the cemetery,
- gravesite,
- vault,
- funeral director's services,
- clergyman's services,
- opening and closing the grave,
- floral tribute, and
- obituary notices.

PREPARATION AND PROCESSING REMAINS

LEARNING OBJECTIVE: *Recall procedures for preparing and processing remains.*

It is imperative that preservative treatment be initiated as soon as possible after death. The naval authority with decedent affairs responsibility should maintain close coordination with appropriate military or civilian authorities to ensure the prompt release and delivery of remains to the mortuary facility. Remains must be prepared under approved high standards of the mortuary profession and returned to the final destination in their most normal and lifelike appearance.

INITIAL PREPARATION

Remains may be refrigerated for short periods pending arrival of a transportation vessel or arrival of the government embalmer. To minimize cellular deterioration, remains should be refrigerated above the freezing point at 36° to 40°F (2.2° to 4.4°C).

OVERSEAS FACILITIES

Government mortuary facilities are located in various overseas areas and have the responsibility to furnish mortuary services for all eligible categories of military and civilian personnel. The geographical areas of responsibility are outlined in the CINCPACINST 5360.1, *Geographic Responsibilities for Mortuary Operations.* Also consult NAVMEDCOMINST 5360.1 for locations of overseas mortuaries.

When death occurs in overseas areas not served by facilities listed in NAVMEDCOMINST 5360.1, request assistance from the senior naval command. In some areas, Department of State sources may have the capability to render advice or assistance. The senior naval command may also be able to arrange airlift of remains from the place of death to a point where a government mortuary or a commercial facility is available, or arrange for emergency dispatch of a qualified embalmer from an overseas government mortuary to the place of death.

CERTIFICATE OF DEATH (OVERSEAS)

When remains are transferred from an overseas activity to a CONUS point of entry, three signed copies of DD Form 2064, *Certificate of Death (Overseas),* must accompany the remains. Failure to include the DD Form 2064 may cause delays in providing further transfer within CONUS. Additionally, at least two DD Form 565, *Statement of Recognition,* should be included.

BURIAL CLOTHING

The service dress blue uniform or (if this uniform is not available for deceased personnel) the appropriate winter service dress uniform, with authorized insignia, devices, badges, decorations, underwear, and hose are the only approved items for burial, unless other items are specifically requested by the NOK. Shoes and headgear should also be procured when required or requested. These items may be withdrawn from the deceased's personal effects or purchased from the Navy Exchange, Navy Retail Clothing Store, or Marine Corps Clothing Store. When not available through these sources, procurement through commercial sources is authorized. When suitable items are not available for personnel who die outside the 48 contiguous United States, the U.S. port of entry should be contacted and given estimated uniform sizes, as soon as possible, so burial clothing can be purchased. Funding for uniform items is noted in NAVMEDCOMINST 5360.1.

When requested by the NOK, remains may be attired in a white uniform or civilian clothing consisting of appropriate outer clothing, underwear, hose, and, if specifically requested, shoes. Items of clothing in the individual's possession at the time of death should be used if available and in satisfactory condition.

PLACEMENT OF REMAINS IN CASKET OR TRANSFER CASE

Normally, remains are placed in a specification casket or transfer case in a manner that will create an appearance of rest and composure. Precautions should be taken to ensure maintenance of position during transit.

Each remains returned in a transfer case will be wrapped in a white cotton sheet plus a second wrapping in a polyethylene cover, and sealed with pressure-sensitive tape or heat sealed.

CASKETS

There are two sizes of caskets. Each is an 18-gauge silvertone metal sealer with a cut top. The standard size casket has internal dimensions of 23 x 78 inches (58.4 cm x 1.98 m), while the oversize casket has internal dimensions of 25 x 81 inches (63.5 cm x 2.06 m).

INSPECTION OF REMAINS

After processing or reprocessing and before shipment, all remains should be inspected in accordance with NAVMEDCOMINST 5360.1. The decedent affairs officer (DAO) is responsible for expediting arrangements for transportation. As such, personnel should be available at all times, including Saturdays, Sundays, and holidays, to perform inspections. Before acceptance, the inspector must make sure that all services and supplies meet current specifications.

CREMATION

LEARNING OBJECTIVE: *Recall guidelines for requesting cremation of remains.*

When requested in writing or by telegram, cremation is authorized, subject to compliance with civil regulations. No overt action by naval authorities should be made to encourage the NOK to elect cremation. Cremation will not be permitted if any questions exists concerning an individual's legal right to direct disposition of the remains.

AT-SEA DISPOSITION

LEARNING OBJECTIVE: *Recall burial-at-sea procedures.*

Commanding officers who receive requests for at-sea disposition of remains or cremains (cremated remains) will forward the request to the appropriate fleet commander-in-chief (CINC) and requested port of embarkation. Fleet CINCs are authorized to designate activities to accept remains or cremains on a "not-to-interfere basis." The port of embarkation will coordinate the arrangements. Upon receipt of authorization, the date of committal or dispersion will be determined by the availability of resources. Except under unusual circumstances, civilian personnel will not be authorized to attend services aboard naval ships at sea or aboard naval aircraft. Exceptions that cannot be resolved at the delegated authority level will be referred to the CNO for final determination. Refer to NAVMEDCOMINST 5360.1 for eligibility and specifics.

PUTREFIED REMAINS

When the mortician is unable to arrest the odor of remains, they will not be accepted for burial at sea. The odor generated for such remains will detract from the dignity of the ceremony and will have a detrimental effect on the officers and men of the vessel. Cremated putrefied remains may be accepted.

CEREMONY RECORDS

Since civilians are not normally allowed to attend ceremonies aboard naval ships or aircrafts, photographs and/or video of the ceremony will be taken. Both a letter describing the ceremony and the burial flag will be sent to the NOK, in accordance with NAVMEDCOMINST 5360.1.

CONSIGNMENT AND TRANSPORTATION OF REMAINS

LEARNING OBJECTIVE: *Recall consignment policies and authorized methods of transportation of remains.*

Activities that arrange transportation have the responsibility to provide expeditious transportation and a confirmed schedule as soon as possible by whatever methods meet the requirements. Consideration should be given to any special desires of the NOK, including releasing the remains for transportation that they may wish to provide.

CONSIGNMENT

Remains may only be consigned to a funeral director, the director or superintendent of a national cemetery, or the consignee designated by the MEDDEN Affairs for unclaimed remains. In addition to the above consignees, cremains may be consigned to the PNOK or person designated by the PNOK.

AUTHORIZED METHODS OF TRANSPORTATION WITHIN THE UNITED STATES

Authorized methods of transportation within the United States include government air, commercial air, chartered air taxi, and funeral coach.

Government Air

Government air **is not** authorized within CONUS without approval of the CNO (OP-414). If the circumstances indicate government air, MEDDEN

Affairs should be contacted for guidance and assistance.

Commercial Air

Commercial air may be supplemented by either rail or funeral coach transportation. An escort must travel with the remains. If delays en route or changes in schedule occur, the escort must notify the installation arranging the transportation and the consignee.

Chartered Air Taxi

Chartered air taxi service may be authorized when commercial air is not available to the destination and the use of a funeral vehicle or rail would cause undue delay.

Funeral Coach

The funeral coach method of transportation may be used under any of the following circumstances:

- To transfer remains from the place of preparation to another local funeral home, to a local cemetery, or to a common-carrier terminal

- When common-carrier service is not available

- When a common carrier is available only part of the way to the place designated by the PNOK, then funeral coach service may be used for the remaining portion of the transportation authorized

- When the cost is not in excess of the common-carrier cost

- When the cemetery cannot provide transportation from the terminal to the cemetery, a funeral coach may be used as a continuation of common-carrier service when remains are consigned directly to a national cemetery or a Navy cemetery or plot

- To transfer remains from the common-carrier terminal at destination to the funeral establishment, and to deliver remains to the local cemetery or crematory

- When requested by the NOK, and the family member defrays costs in excess of the method that would have been used by the government

- When the use of a common-carrier service will involve extended layover, and this method will expedite the arrival

TRANSPORTATION OF CREMATED REMAINS

Cremated remains (cremains) of active duty personnel will be hand carried by an escort, and transported using commercial air, rail, a funeral director's vehicle, or other appropriate vehicle. When an escort is not authorized, cremains may be transported by registered mail (preferred method), air, or surface transportation to the PNOK, or to a specified individual designated by the PNOK.

TRANSPORTATION OF REMAINS OF CONTAGIOUS OR COMMUNICABLE DISEASE VICTIMS

When death is the result of a contagious or communicable disease, remains, after embalming, should be placed immediately in a transfer case or casket. The transfer case or casket should be closed immediately and a gummed 2" x 4" label, marked "CONTAGIOUS" should be affixed to the outside of the receptacle at the head end. Information concerning diseases considered contagious may be obtained from local or state health officials. When the remains carry communicable or contagious disease, make sure that the consignment message specifically states that death was due to a contagious or communicable disease.

AUTHORIZED TRANSPORTATION TO OR FROM CONUS

Remains of eligible decedents who die outside the 48 contiguous United States will be transported by the most expeditious U.S. government means; normally, government air (Air Mobility Command (AMC) flights) are used. If such transportation is not available, impractical, or would cause undue delay, commercial air may be authorized by MEDDEN Affairs.

OUTSIDE CONUS DESTINATIONS

When persons eligible for decedent affairs benefits are consigned to a destination outside the 48 contiguous United States, the activity responsible for preparation and transportation will contact the nearest consul of the country concerned to ascertain the requirements for entry, and assure that all requirements are met before arranging transportation of the remains. Failure to do so could lead to serious delays. Three certified copies of the civilian certificate of death should accompany the remains.

ESCORTS

LEARNING OBJECTIVE: *Recall criteria for escort selection, and identify escort duties and responsibilities.*

Escorts are provided to accompany remains to ensure prompt, safe delivery, as a mark of respect to the decedent, and as an indication of the Navy's desire to help the NOK. Only one escort is authorized. More than one may be assigned; however, two escorts may not serve at the same time. Problems concerning arrangements for a Navy escort that cannot be resolved by the responsible command should be referred to MEDDEN Affairs or the area commander outside CONUS. Problems concerning Marine Corps members should be referred to CMC.

INSIDE CONUS ESCORTS

Within CONUS, escorts are detailed to accompany the remains or cremains of each Navy and Marine Corps decedent to their final destination. Furnishing escorts is the responsibility of the activity arranging transportation of the remains or cremains. When selecting an escort for the deceased, the activity arranging transportation is encouraged to consult the last duty station of the deceased.

OUTSIDE CONUS ESCORTS

When remains are consigned to a place outside CONUS where Armed Forces representatives or other government officials are not available to receive, transfer, or otherwise assist in transportation arrangements, military escorts will be provided.

Unless a special escort is requested by the PNOK and approved by MEDDEN Affairs, remains transported by AMC aircraft from a point outside CONUS to a CONUS port of entry will not be accompanied by an escort. The aircraft commander will act as the escort during the time of transport by AMC aircraft. An escort will be detailed by the military activity responsible for transportation arrangements at the CONUS port of entry.

SELECTION OF ESCORTS

Any Navy or Marine Corps member on active duty may serve as an escort. Navy and Marine Corps members who volunteer may be accepted if they meet the criteria for selection. Unless a special escort is requested by the NOK, the escort selected should be of the same branch of service, status, and paygrade of the deceased. The escort should be a friend of the deceased, from the same unit, and preferably of the same religion.

SPECIAL ESCORTS

A special escort is defined as a person requested specifically by the PNOK or by his representative, or a person assigned by an appropriate command because unusual circumstances prevail and such assignment is considered in the best interest of the naval service. All requests for special escorts must be referred to MEDDEN Affairs.

If desired by the PNOK, a civilian or member of another service may be assigned as a special escort. An escort in retired or inactive status should be treated as a civilian. All military special escorts are assigned subject to availability as determined by their CO and, unless closely related to the deceased, generally are not authorized outside CONUS.

DUTIES OF THE ESCORT

A naval escort is a representative of the Navy who will be required to perform services of a very special and personal nature. It is very important that these duties are thoroughly explained to the escort. Providing instructions to the escort is the responsibility of the command arranging for transportation of the remains. The *Manual for Escorts of Deceased Naval Personnel*, NAVPERS 15955, will assist in this function. For additional information, you should consult NAVMEDCOMINST 5360.1.

DISPOSITION OF PERSONAL EFFECTS

LEARNING OBJECTIVE: *Recall disposition of personal effects policies.*

All personal effects of the deceased are to be collected and inventoried, except where the member occupied government or public housing and the spouse requires no assistance. In the event the spouse dies simultaneously with the service member, the CO cooperates with surviving relatives of the deceased and civil authorities by providing protection for the property of the deceased.

The CO appoints an inventory board consisting of two members, of which one member is normally a commissioned officer. The inventory should be recorded on an Inventory of Personal Effects Form, NAVSUP Form 29. An original and four copies will be prepared and signed by the board members. The board will send all five copies with the personal effects to the supply officer for completion, disposition, and signature. The supply officer returns three signed copies. The inventory board sends one copy to the COMNAVMILPERSCOM, files one in the service record of the deceased, and sends one to the officer who appointed the board.

CIVIL CERTIFICATES OF DEATH

LEARNING OBJECTIVE: *Determine when civil certificates are required and where they should be distributed.*

A civil certificate of death must be obtained if a death occurs within one of the 50 United States or the District of Columbia. If a death occurs outside these areas, with the exception of Guam, a *Certificate of Death (Overseas)*, DD 2064, should be prepared. This certificate is in addition to the civil certificate of death; however, the civil certificate of death is not required in all overseas areas. Civil authorities should be consulted to determine local requirements. When a death occurs at a naval activity in any state, territory, or insular possession of the United States, the CO will report the death to civil authorities (usually the coroner or medical examiner). It is a general practice for medical officers to complete a civil certificate of death for all deaths occurring in naval medical treatment facilities.

The medical officer or Medical Department representative of the ship or station where the deceased was attached will obtain the certificate from the civil authorities. If requested by the authorities, the civil certificate of death may be prepared and signed by a naval officer. If problems arise in getting a certificate, request assistance from MEDDEN Affairs. If death occurs abroad and no naval activity is available, the nearest consular officer should be requested to get a certificate. The medical officer or Medical Department representative will prepare and forward a DD 2064 with the civil certificate of death, supporting papers, and the closed health record.

In general (except where the state has retained concurrent jurisdiction with the United States, civil authorities have no jurisdiction over deaths occurring

on naval reservations. However, a transit or burial permit should be obtained from civil authorities to remove the remains from a naval reservation either for shipment or burial. If death of any person for whom the Department of the Navy is responsible occurs outside the limits of a naval reservation, the remains normally will not be moved until permission has been received from civil authorities.

DISTRIBUTION OF DEATH CERTIFICATE FOR DEATHS OCCURRING IN CONUS

When a Navy or Marine Corps death occurs in one of the 50 United States or the District of Columbia, follow local civil requirements. In addition, the following procedures in table 16-1 apply:

DISTRIBUTION OF DEATH CERTIFICATE FOR DEATHS OCCURRING OUTSIDE CONUS

When a Navy or Marine Corps death occurs outside the 50 United States or the District of Columbia, follow the local civil requirements. In

Table 16-1.—Distribution of Death Certificate for Deaths Occurring in CONUS

For CONUS decedents. . .	Send copy of death certificate to. ..
Active Duty	Commanding Officer Naval Medical Information Management Center Bethesda, MD 20814 *(Place one copy in member's closed health record.)*
Inactive Duty	Naval Reserve Personnel Center 4400 Dauphine Street New Orleans, LA 70149
Active/Inactive Marines	Commandant of the Marine Corps (Code MSPA-1) Department of the Navy Washington, DC 20380

addition, a DD 2064 is prepared and copies are distributed as outlined in table 16-2.

DEATH CERTIFICATES FOR SHIPMENT OF REMAINS

When death occurs outside CONUS, three signed copies of DD 2064 will accompany the remains to CONUS. When death occurs within CONUS, three certified copies of the civil certificate of death will accompany the remains from CONUS to outside CONUS, in addition to all other forms required by NAVMEDCOMINST 5360.1.

NOTE: A certificate of death should not be prepared for persons listed as missing.

Table 16-2.—Distribution of Death Certificate for Deaths Occurring in Outside CONUS

For OUTUS decedents. . .	Send copy of death certificate to. . .
Active Duty	Commanding Officer Naval Medical Information Management Center Bethesda, MD 20814 *(The original death certificate is placed in member's closed health record.)*
Inactive Duty	*Navy personnel:* Naval Reserve Personnel Center 4400 Dauphine Street New Orleans, LA 70149 *Marine Corps personnel:* Commandant of the Marine Corps (Code MSPA-1) Department of the Navy Washington, DC 20380
Other deaths	The command indicated if the death occurred aboard a ship, at a naval station, or on a naval aircraft. For full details, see MANMED.

PAYMENTS AND COLLECTIONS

LEARNING OBJECTIVE: *Recall funeral payment and collection procedures.*

Authorized Decedent Affairs Program expenses are chargeable to the special open allotment held by BUMED. In circumstances involving reimbursable transactions, costs may also be initially charged to the open allotment subject to reimbursement. The allotment may be charged by any Navy or Marine Corps activity assigned procurement or payment responsibility. Army and Air Force activities may charge the allotment when arranging for authorized supplies and services at the request of a naval activity.

PRIMARY EXPENSES

If the NOK makes arrangements for disposition of remains, rather than using services of DoD, or completes funeral arrangements before DoD services are offered, the amounts outlined below are allowed toward incurred expenses. The figures quoted are subject to change, so check the latest series of NAVMEDCOMINST 5360.1 for the authorized allowances, or contact the MEDDEN Affairs.

When an Armed Forces contract or mortuary is available (and services were offered to the NOK) but not used, an amount not to exceed what procurement would have cost the Navy is allowed. This includes costs the Navy would have incurred over and above contract expenses. Contact MEDDEN Affairs for current allowance limits.

TRANSPORTATION EXPENSES

If the NOK arranges for transportation of remains, reimbursement may be made in an amount not to exceed what transportation would have cost the government. If the Navy has arranged for transportation and the final destination cannot be reached by common carrier, reasonable costs may be allowed for supplemental transportation by funeral coach or other vehicle.

SECONDARY (INTERMENT) EXPENSES

Secondary expenses will be provided to the NOK whether the remains or cremains are interred in a private cemetery, a national or federal government cemetery, or in a burial at sea. The allowance paid for each method of interment will be in accordance with

NAVMEDCOMINST 5360.1, *Decedent Affairs Manual.*

MEMORIAL SERVICE FOR NONRECOVERABLE REMAINS

When remains of eligible military personnel, whose determination of death has been made, are nonrecoverable, reimbursement to the PNOK (or designee) may be made for memorial service expenditures. A claim for reimbursement may be allowed if presented within the approved time frame after notification of the NOK of the date of death. The PNOK must submit receipted invoices or a certified claim to MEDDEN Affairs.

HEADSTONES AND MARKERS

Personnel serving on active duty at the time of their death are eligible for a headstone or marker provided by the Veterans' Administration (VA). At a national cemetery, the director or superintendent will make the arrangements. In naval plots and cemeteries, the Navy will make the arrangements. In other cemeteries, an application should be submitted to the VA. If a commercial headstone or marker is procured, a limited reimbursement is authorized. A memorial marker may be provided upon request to commemorate the death of a member whose remains were not recovered or were buried at sea.

REIMBURSEMENT PROCEDURES

LEARNING OBJECTIVE: *Recall procedures for reimbursement of funeral costs.*

When the Navy has arranged for primary services and transportation, a claim for payment of the supplemental transportation charges may be submitted to MEDDEN Affairs by the funeral director at the final destination.

DD Form 1375, *Request for Payment of Funeral and/or Interment Expenses*, should be given to the PNOK (or PNOK's designee) to claim reimbursement or payment for primary expenses, transportation, and secondary expenses.

GOVERNMENT SERVICES NOT UTILIZED WITHIN CONUS

Claims relating to primary expenses and transportation costs to a common-carrier terminal for transportation to the final destination will be forwarded to MEDDEN Affairs.

Claims relating to interment (secondary) allowances and supplemental transportation costs will be forwarded to MEDDEN Affairs.

GOVERNMENT SERVICES NOT UTILIZED OUTSIDE CONUS

Area commanders outside CONUS are authorized to make local payment of expenses incurred in areas under their jurisdiction.

Claims in areas outside the jurisdiction of the activities (area commanders) noted in NAVMEDCOMINST 5360.1 should be submitted to BUMED for resolution.

GOVERNMENT SERVICES UTILIZED

When the Navy has arranged for primary services and transportation, submit claims for payment and reimbursement of interment costs or supplemental transportation expenses to MEDDEN Affairs.

REPORTING EXPENSES

LEARNING OBJECTIVE: *Recall reporting procedures for funeral expenses.*

Activities incurring expenses in connection with disposition of remains of Navy and Marine Corps personnel do not report these expenses to BUMED except when indicated on the DD Form 2062, *Record of Preparation and Disposition of Remains (Outside CONUS)*, and DD Form 2063, *Record of Preparation and Disposition of Remains (Within CONUS)*. In arranging for disposition of remains of other services' deceased personnel, activities obtaining services and supplies from commercial sources should forward a letter report, MED 5360-3, *Report of Disposition and Expenditures–Remains of the Dead*, to the service concerned. Costs for which the activity's funds have been cited should be shown on the letter report.

NATIONAL CEMETERIES

LEARNING OBJECTIVE: *Recall services that are available at national cemeteries.*

Except for Arlington National Cemetery (which is under the jurisdiction of the Department of the Army) and a few other exceptions noted in NAVMEDCOM-INST 5360.1, national cemeteries are under the jurisdiction of the Chief Memorial Affairs Director, Department of Memorial Affairs, Veterans' Administration, Washington, DC.

NATIONAL CEMETERY CLASSIFICATIONS

There are three classifications of national cemeteries:

1. **Open (Active)**—Cemeteries with grave spaces available.

2. **Closed (Inactive)**—Cemeteries without grave spaces available.

3. **New (Inactive)**—Cemeteries planned but not yet opened.

ELIGIBILITY FOR INTERMENT

Remains of the following naval and former naval members may be buried in any open national cemetery except at the National Cemetery at Arlington, Virginia:

- Navy or Marine Corps member who was serving on active duty at time of death (other than active duty for training).

- Former Navy or Marine Corps members who were discharged under conditions other than dishonorable.

- Any member of a Navy or Marine Corps Reserve organization whose death occurred under honorable conditions while the individual was

    1. On active duty for training (including authorized travel to and from active duty training),

    2. on inactive duty training (including authorized travel to and from such training), or

    3. hospitalized or undergoing treatment at the expense of the government for injury or disease incurred or contracted during the period covered by 1 and 2, above.

- Members of the Naval Reserve Officers' Training Corps whose death occurred under honorable conditions while they were

    1. attending an authorized training camp or authorized training cruise,

    2. performing authorized travel to and from that camp or cruise, or

    3. hospitalized or undergoing treatment at the expense of the government of the United States for injury or disease incurred or contracted during the period covered by 1 and 2, above.

- Surviving spouse and minor children of individuals covered above.

(For further information on interment eligibility at Arlington, consult NAVMEDCOMINST 5360.1.)

At the discretion of the Chief Memorial Affairs Director, unmarried adult children of eligible individuals may be buried in any open national cemetery (except Arlington) if they were totally disabled either physically or mentally before attaining the age of 21. The Chief Memorial Affairs Director may also authorize the burial of unremarried widows or widowers or eligible deceased members whose remains were either lost at sea or buried at sea not at their own volition, or who were officially determined missing or missing in action and subsequently administratively declared dead for the purpose of terminating missing or missing-in-action status.

HONORS

Military honors for interment in national cemeteries are the responsibility of the member's service. Honors for services at Arlington National Cemetery are coordinated by the superintendent of the cemetery with BUPERS or the CMC, as appropriate.

VAULTS

A metal, asphalt, or concrete vault may be procured at the NOK's expense, if it is preferred. If a vault is privately procured, the superintendent/director must be notified of the outside dimensions to ensure the proper preparation of the grave. The contractor furnishing the vault must also provide necessary equipment and personnel for placing the vault in the grave before the funeral service and for placement of the vault lid after the service.

VIEWING REMAINS

National cemeteries no longer have facilities for viewing remains. If the NOK desires a viewing before interment, the remains must be consigned to a local funeral director.

SCHEDULING

Unless extraordinary circumstances exist with respect to the condition of remains, interment in national cemeteries will not be made on Saturdays, Sundays, or holidays.

NAVAL PLOTS AND CEMETERIES

LEARNING OBJECTIVE: *Recall policy for interment at a naval cemetery.*

With two exceptions, MEDDEN Affairs exercises technical direction of naval plots and cemeteries. Presently, there are only a few active naval cemeteries, so plot availability is extremely limited. For this reason, decedents who are eligible for interment in national cemeteries will not normally be authorized interment in a naval plot or cemetery. However, exceptional or unusual circumstances will be referred to BUMED for determination.

GROUP INTERMENTS

LEARNING OBJECTIVE: *Recall guidelines for group interments.*

When remains of two or more individuals killed in the same incident cannot be individually identified, a priority message detailing the circumstances should be sent to MEDDEN Affairs. MEDDEN Affairs will then determine if there is a need for an identification specialist to be sent. If remains cannot be individually identified, the collective remains will be interred as a group interment. Group interments should be made in a national cemetery, within the 50 United States, as close to the midpoint of the two most widely separated homes of record of known deceased individuals involved, or as otherwise directed by the program managers. MEDDEN Affairs will coordinate with the other services as required. Procedures followed in group interments are:

1. Unidentified remains should be prepared, wrapped and placed into the minimum number of caskets possible without overcrowding. Partially segregated but identifiable remains should be wrapped separately.

2. One or more escorts should be provided, as long as the number of escorts does not exceed the number of deceased persons.

3. The PNOK and two blood relatives of each deceased member in a group interment are authorized round-trip transportation to the place of interment at government expense.

4. The ceremonies should be conducted with full military honors and be in accordance with the religious preferences applicable to all denominations represented within the group. Photographs should be provided to the PNOK, if desired.

5. The headstone or headstones should be inscribed with the names of all known deceased personnel.

SUMMARY

The Decedent Affairs Program consists of the search, recovery, identification, care, and disposition of remains of deceased personnel for whom the Department of the Navy is responsible. Large medical treatment facilities normally manage decedent affairs mattes. However, when a death occurs at small independent operational units, senior Hospital Corpsmen will be responsible for the proper management of this program. For this reason, basic components of the Decedent Affairs Program were covered in this chapter. For further guidance, you should consult the *Decedent Affairs Manual* or contact the Naval office of Medical/Dental Affairs, Mortuary Affairs Section, Great Lakes, Illinois.

HISTORY OF THE HOSPITAL CORPS
UNITED STATES NAVY

ORIGIN AND DEVELOPMENT OF THE CORPS

Few military organizations can look upon their histories with the same degree of pride and awe as the Navy Hospital Corps. Since the establishment of the Navy medical department in Colonial times and the commissioning of the Hospital Corps a century ago, Hospital Corpsmen and their forerunners have proven themselves ready to support Marines and Sailors by giving them aid whenever and wherever necessary. This level of dedication has remained a strong current running through the Corps' history, even as the tools and techniques used by its members have evolved.

REVOLUTIONARY WAR

The first direction given to the organization of Navy medicine consisted of only one article in the *Rules for the Regulation of the Navy of the United Colonies of North America* of 1775. Article 16 stated:

> A convenient place shall be set apart for sick or hurt men, to be removed with their hammocks and bedding when the surgeon shall advise the same to be necessary: and some of the crew shall be appointed to attend to and serve them and to keep the place clean. The cooper shall make buckets with covers and cradles if necessary for their use.

Interestingly, the cooper (or barrel-maker), whose skills could be used to make bedpans, had a more detailed job description than did any kind of trained medical assistant.

A typical medical section was usually limited to two, perhaps three men: the surgeon, the surgeon's mate, and possibly an enlisted man. The surgeon was a physician. The surgeon's mate, usually a doctor as well, held status like that of a modern warrant officer but signed on only for a particular cruise. Although surgeons' mates were historically viewed as part of the Medical Corps, their position and responsibilities appear to be more equivalent to those of today's senior Hospital Corpsmen.

Few things changed in medical techniques and organization between 1775 and 1814, the period covering America's first naval wars. Among the less dramatic responsibilities of caring for the noncombat ill and injured were feeding and personal care of the sick. The simple daily ration of porridge, or "loblolly," was sure to be carried down to those in the medical space by untrained attendants.

SURGEON'S MATES AND LOBLOLLY BOYS

Congress approved an act on March 2, 1799, which copied the words of the Continental Congress' medical department Article 16 of 1775 exactly. As a result, there was still no title or job description for enlisted medical personnel. The nickname "loblolly boy" was in common use for so many years that it became the official title in Navy Regulations of 1814. The loblolly boy's job, described in the Regulations of 1818, included the following:

> The surgeon shall be allowed a faithful attendant to issue, under his direction, all supplies and provisions and hospital stores, and to attend the preparation of nourishment for the sick.... The surgeon's mates shall be particularly careful in directing the loblolly boy to keep the cockpit clean, and every article therein belonging to the Medical Department. . . . The surgeon shall prescribe for casual cases on the gun deck every morning at 9 o'clock, due notice having been previously given by his loblolly boy by ringing of a bell.

SURGEON'S STEWARDS AND LOBLOLLY BOYS

A new senior enlisted medical rate, surgeon's steward, was introduced in the ensuing decades. The term is first seen in 1841 in Navy pay charts, but it appears that the new billet was only allowed on larger ships. By April 1, 1843, the Navy Department issued an order allowing surgeon's stewards to be assigned to brigs and schooners. The relative importance of medical Sailors was hereby increased. Surgeon's stewards ranked second in seniority among the ship's petty officers, next only after the master-at-arms.

SURGEON'S STEWARDS AND NURSES

The year 1861 brought civil war to this country, and—due to the enormous expansion of the Navy because of the war—changes and developments in the medical department ensued. On June 19, 1861, a Navy Department circular order established a new name for the loblolly boy.

> In addition to a surgeon's steward, 1 nurse would be allowed for ships with a complement of less than 200; 2 nurses would be allowed for ships with a complement of more than 200; and sufficient nurses would be allowed on receiving ships in a number proportionate to the necessities of the vessel.

While the shipboard medical department changed the titles of its personnel, new techniques in mass care of the sick and wounded were also developed. A captured sidewheel steamer was repaired and modified to care for patients. Refinements to the ship included bathrooms, kitchens, and laundries—even elevators and the facilities to carry 300 tons of ice. On December 26, 1862, the USS *Red Rover* became the first Navy vessel specifically commissioned as a hospital ship. The medical complement included 30 surgeons and male nurses, as well as four nuns.

APOTHECARIES AND BAYMEN

Postwar reductions in the size of the Navy brought new classifications to enlisted medical personnel. The title "surgeon's steward" was abolished in favor of three grades of apothecaries in 1866. Those selected as apothecaries had to be graduates of a course in pharmacy or possess the same knowledge gained through practical experience. The Apothecary, First Class, ranked with a warrant officer, while the second and third classes were petty-officer equivalents. The three rates were reduced to one petty officer apothecary on March 15, 1869.

"Nurse," as a title for junior enlisted medical personnel, was replaced by the title "bayman" (defined as one who manned the sick bay) in the early 1870s. U.S. Navy Regulations of 1876 used the title officially, and it remained valid for 22 more years.

An apothecary of the 1890s mixed and dispensed all medication aboard a ship. He was responsible for all medical department reports, supply requests, and correspondence, and he helped maintain medical department records. The apothecary administered anesthesia during surgery and was the primary instructor for new baymen.

The apothecaries' responsibilities did not end there, however. (See figure APP-I-1.) During shipboard surgery, the bayman focused an electric light on the incision site while the surgeon did his work on what served as a combination of both writing and operating table. He sterilized surgical instruments by boiling them, then stored them in a solution of 5 percent phenol. Bandages and dressings were sterilized by baking them in a coffee can in the ship's oven. Sick bay itself was prepared for surgery by wiping the entire room down with a chlorine solution. On days when the ship's routine called for scrubbing bags and hammocks, a bayman was responsible for washing those of the sick. When required, he painted the ship's medical spaces.

During the last two decades of the 1800s, many in the naval medical establishment called for reforms in the enlisted components of the medical department. Medicine had by now progressed far more as a science, and civilian hospitals all had teaching schools for their nurses. Foreign navies had trained medical Sailors, and the U.S. Army had established its own Hospital Corps of enlisted men on March 1, 1887. Navy Surgeon General J. R. Tryon argued, in his annual report of 1893, against the practice of assigning landsmen to the medical department with nothing more than on-the-job-training. He advocated the urgent need for an organized hospital corps.

Physicians in the fleet were equally certain of the need for changes. Surgeon C. A. Sigfried of the USS *Massachusetts* made his views known in his report to the Surgeon General in 1897.

> The importance of improving the medical department of our naval service is more and more apparent, in view of the recent advances in the methods and rapidity of killing and wounding. The great want is a body of trained bay men or nurses, and these should be better paid and of better stamp and fiber. Now and then we procure a good man, and proceed with his training as a bay man. He soon finds opportunity for betterment in some one of the various departments of the ship, in the matter of pay and emolument, either in some yeoman's billet or in some place where his meager $18 per month can be suddenly

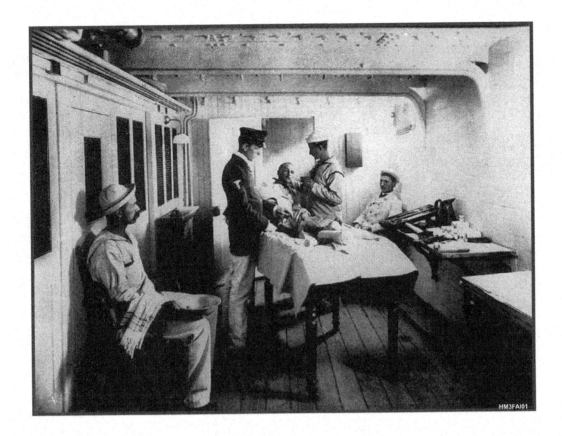

Figure APP-I-1.—An apothecary (petty officer first class) treats a shipmate aboard the USS *Boston* in 1888.

increased to $30, $40, or even $60 per month. The bay man, who should be an intelligent, sober man, and well trained in many things pertaining to nursing, dieting, ambulance, and aids to wounded, and have a moderate amount of education, finds his pay at present among the lowest in the ship's company; even the men caring for storerooms get more per month.

HOSPITAL STEWARDS AND HOSPITAL APPRENTICES

Arguments for a professional, well-trained group of individuals to provide medical care for the Navy finally paid off, although it took the imminent danger of combat in the Spanish-American War to spur Congress into action. Within a bill aimed at building the armed forces was a section to provide for the Navy's long-needed Hospital Corps. It was approved by President William McKinley on June 17, 1898. From that date to the present, either generically or by rating title, medical Sailors have been called "Hospital Corpsmen."

To ensure that the members of the new Hospital Corps were adequately trained in the disciplines pertinent to both medicine and the Navy, a basic school for corpsmen was established at the U.S. Naval Hospital Norfolk (Portsmouth), Virginia. Originally called the School of Instruction, it opened September 2, 1902. Its curriculum included anatomy and physiology, bandaging, nursing, first aid, pharmacy, clerical work, and military drill. The first class of 28 corpsmen was graduated on December 15, 1902. (See figure APP-I-2.)

The school continued for a brief time and was then moved to the Naval Hospital in Washington, D.C., remaining in existence there until 1911. For the next 3 years, there was no basic school for corpsmen, but the concept was revived in 1914. The next two Hospital Corps Training Schools were opened in Newport, Rhode Island, and on Yerba Buena Island, California.

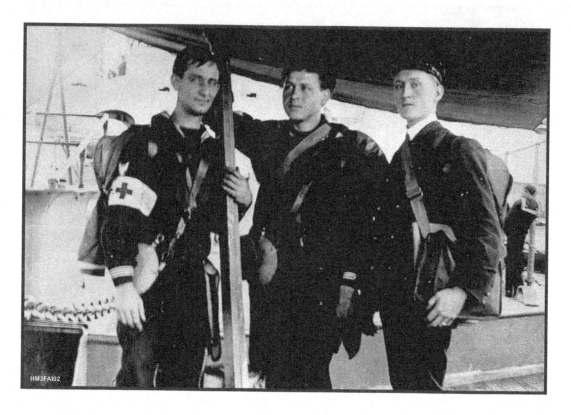

Figure APP-I-2.—A hospital steward (chief petty officer) and two hospital apprentices from a ship's landing party medical section, 1905.

HOSPITAL APPRENTICES AND PHARMACIST'S MATES

The next revision in the structure of the Hospital Corps came by act of Congress on August 29, 1916. Under this plan, the rates were hospital apprentices, second class and first class (both of whom wore a red cross on the sleeve); pharmacist's mates, third, second, and first; and chief pharmacist's mate. The officer contingent of the Hospital Corps included the two warrant officer ranks of pharmacist and chief pharmacist. The reorganization allowed for a massive, fivefold increase in the size of the Hospital Corps.

At the start of 1917, the Hospital Corps counted 1,700 men in its ranks. A concerted effort to recruit and train new personnel enabled the corps to reach its authorized strength of 3 1/2 percent of the Navy and Marine Corps, or 6,000 men. But as these plans came to fruition, the United States entered World War I in April. By the end of 1918, the corps peaked at about 17,000.

PHARMACIST'S MATES IN WORLD WAR I

The massive wartime expansion in Hospital Corps strength necessitated additional schools to train the newcomers. Hospital Corps School, Great Lakes, Illinois, had been established in January 1913. Wartime schools were created in Minneapolis at the University of Minnesota, in New York at Columbia University, and at the Philadelphia College of Pharmacy. A school for Naval Reserve Force Hospital Corpsmen was set up at Boston City Hospital. Other crash-course schools for shipboard personnel were conducted at a number of other civilian hospitals. Hospital Corpsmen who were needed to serve as medical department representatives on small vessels such as destroyers were trained at the Pharmacist's Mate School at Hampton Roads, Virginia, the forerunner of the Independent Duty Hospital Corpsman School.

Hospital Corpsmen were assigned to the multitude of duty types and locations needed to support a Navy involved in a world war. Naval hospitals were opened and staffed. Ships and aircraft squadrons were given medical support. At sea, the dangers of the new war were ever present.

Naval training facilities and shore establishments needed Hospital Corpsmen, as did occupation forces in Haiti and other bases around the world. But World War I provided the Hospital Corps a role that would afford it some of the most dangerous challenges it would ever face: duty with the Marine Corps.

Assignment to Marine Corps units was not completely new. Hospital Corpsmen were serving with Marine occupational forces in Cuba, Haiti, and Santo Domingo at the outbreak of the war, and they had seen other similar service. It was the change of the Marine Corps' role to one of expeditionary forces in a large-scale ground war that changed what Hospital Corpsmen would do. Sick call and preventive medicine were continuous roles that remained unchanged. Facing artillery, mustard gas, and machine gunfire were new experiences.

A heritage of valorous service with the Marines was born, as evidenced by two Hospital Corpsmen receiving the Medal of Honor. Other decorations to Hospital Corpsmen included 55 Navy Crosses, 31 Army Distinguished Service Crosses, 2 Navy Distinguished Service Medals, and 237 Silver Stars. A hundred foreign personal decorations were granted to Navy Hospital Corpsmen, and 202 earned the right to wear the French Fourragère shoulder aiguillette permanently. Their 684 personal awards make the Hospital Corps, by one account, the most decorated American unit of World War I.

PHARMACIST'S MATES IN WORLD WAR II

World War II became the period of Hospital Corps' greatest manpower, diversity of duty, and instance of sacrifice. Between 1941 and 1945, the ranks of this small organization swelled from its prewar levels of near 4,000 to more than 132,000 personnel. This increase came to fulfill new responsibilities with new technologies at new duty stations. In the face of great adversity, the Hospital Corps would cement its reputation for effectiveness and bravery.

The Navy's fleet expanded to thousands of ships, and the Marine Corps grew from a few regiments to six divisions. A two-ocean war produced horrific numbers of casualties, and the Hospital Corps grew to meet the needs of casualty collection, treatment, and convalescence. To educate the influx of new Sailors, Hospital Corps Training School at Portsmouth, Virginia, was augmented by a temporary school at Naval Hospital Brooklyn, New York. The school at Great Lakes was recreated in 1942, and others were started at Farragut, Idaho, and at Bainbridge, Maryland, in 1943. A separate Hospital Corps Training School was established for women (fig. APP-I-3) at Bethesda, Maryland, in January 1944. Specialized schools were opened to train pharmacist's mates for independent duty and for service with the Marines. Additionally, courses were established to instruct personnel on new equipment and techniques in dozens of developing medical fields.

Shore-based duty sent Hospital Corps personnel to hospitals and dispensaries in the United States and abroad. Advance-base hospitals on newly captured Pacific islands formed a crucial link in the chain of evacuation from battle sites. Those facilities in Hawaii or England received casualties from their respective fronts, and wounded service personnel recuperated in Stateside hospitals. Hospital Corpsmen made the treatment of American casualties possible at each of these by providing technical support and direct patient care.

Duty on surface ships afforded Hospital Corpsmen numerous challenges and abundant environments in which to face them. Hospital ships required the services of personnel in much the same way as shore-based hospitals, except that those on ship were afloat and subject to attack. Other classes of vessels, such as landing ships and patrol craft (LSTs and PCERs), became large floating clinics/ambulances which required additional Hospital Corps personnel. Additionally, combatant ships and transports in the Atlantic, Pacific, and Mediterranean theaters took casualties from ships, aircraft, and submarines throughout the war, necessitating the service of well-trained Hospital Corpsmen.

Approximately 300 Hospital Corpsmen sat out all but the early days of the war when they were captured in the Philippines by the invading Japanese. In prisoner-of-war camps and huddled in POW "hell ships," they endured malnutrition, disease, torture, and brutality. One hundred thirty-two Hospital Corpsmen died as prisoners during World War II, a death rate almost 20 percent higher than among other American POWs.

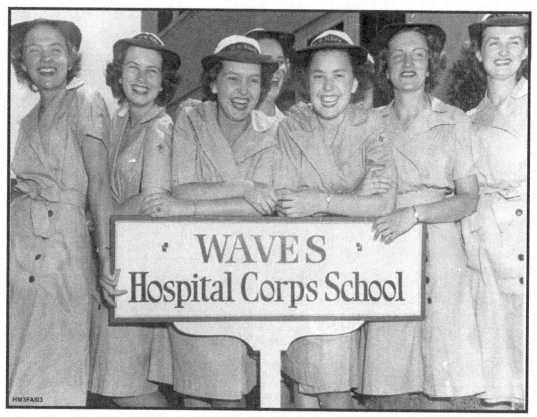
Figure APP-I-3.—Women entered the Hospital Corps in World War II as WAVES.

Hospital Corpsmen served on the beaches not only in the island campaigns of the Pacific, but in Europe as well. Teams of Navy medical personnel formed aid stations with beach battalions at Sicily and Normandy, treating Army and allied wounded under fire. Hospital Corpsmen ensured the survival of these casualties until they could reach hospitals in England.

Of all the Hospital Corpsmen in World War II, Fleet Marine Force personnel endured, perhaps, the most grueling side of war. As they swarmed numerous beaches in the Pacific, they became targets themselves as they braved fire to reach downed comrades. At Guadalcanal, Tarawa, Peleliu, Saipan, Tinian, Kwajalein, Iwo Jima, and Okinawa, Hospital Corpsmen bled and died, often in greater numbers than the Marines for whom they cared. Hospital Corps casualties in the 4th Marine Division at Iwo Jima, for example, were 38 percent.

Members of the Hospital Corps treated some 150,000 combat casualties during the war. This number does not include thousands of others—those plagued by disease and injured in the line of duty—who were aided by their medical shipmates. The cost of this service was high: 1,170 Hospital Corpsmen were killed in action and thousands more were wounded. But their valor was rewarded. Hospital Corpsmen earned 7 Medals of Honor (almost half of those awarded to Sailors in the war), 66 Navy Crosses, 465 Silver Star Medals, and 982 Bronze Star Medals.

A NEW HOSPITAL CORPS

Massive reorganization of the armed forces took place after World War II. A new Department of Defense was established, and the Army-Navy Medical Service Corps Act removed commissioned allied health and medical administration officers from the Hospital Corps. This law also provided for a separate Dental Technician rating, which remained a component of the Hospital Corps until 1972. Women in the Hospital Corps had previously been WAVES, a component of the U.S. Naval Reserve, but the new legislation permitted women to enlist in the Regular Navy.

Effective April 1, 1948, the Navy changed the names and insignia of the Hospital Corps. The new rating titles were hospital recruit, hospital apprentice, hospitalman, hospital corpsmen third, second, and first class, and chief hospital corpsman. The red Geneva cross (fig. APP-I-4), which had marked corpsmen for 50 years, was replaced in the rating badge with the original symbol of the winged caduceus. The rates of senior chief and master chief hospital corpsman were added in 1958.

HOSPITAL CORPSMEN IN KOREA

As part of a United Nations force, Marines were committed to the Korean peninsula when South Korea was invaded by its northern neighbor in the summer of 1950. Within the first year, Hospital Corpsmen had participated in the dramatic landing at Inchon and the frigid retreat from the Chosin Reservoir. Although only one Marine division was involved in the war between 1950 and 1953, the Hospital Corps lost 108 killed in action. Disproportionate to their numbers was their heroism. In Korea, Hospital Corpsmen earned 281 Bronze Star Medals, 113 Silver Star Medals, and 23 Navy Crosses. All five enlisted Navy Medals of Honor were awarded to Navy Hospital Corpsmen serving with the Marines.

HOSPITAL CORPSMEN IN VIETNAM

American military commitment in Southeast Asia grew in the decades following World War II. As early as 1959, a few Hospital Corpsmen provided medical support for U.S. military personnel as part of the American Dispensary at the U.S. Embassy. Four years later, in 1963, Navy Station Hospital, Saigon, was created. Ninety Hospital Corpsmen staffed the facility, and provided care for U.S. and allied (Australian, New Zealand, Filipino, and South Korean) military, as well as South Vietnamese civilians. These medical personnel conducted routine medical care and treated the victims of combat and terrorist actions until the hospital was transferred to the Army in 1966.

Hospital Corpsmen were assigned aboard ships of various kinds, providing offshore medical support to U.S. forces. The largest commitment here was on the hospital ships USS *Repose* and USS *Sanctuary*. Some 200 Hospital Corpsmen, representing the gamut of technical specialties, worked on each ship. Teams of 20 Hospital Corpsmen served on LPH-class

amphibious ships. Others supported the riverine force on APB-class base ships.

U.S. State Department initiatives and the Medical Civic Action Program (MEDCAP) provided medical support for Vietnamese civilians. Beyond routine aid and treatment, the Hospital Corpsmen working through these programs provided guidance in sanitation and preventive medicine throughout South Vietnam.

By far the Hospital Corps' largest contribution in Vietnam was with Marine Corps units. Starting with the 50 who landed with the Marines at Da Nang in 1965, the enlisted medical component would grow to 2,700 Hospital Corpsmen assigned to 1st and 3d Marine Divisions, 1st Marine Air Wing, and other combat support units. Two medical battalions and two hospital companies operated field hospitals, collecting and clearing units, and dispensaries that treated the flow of combat casualties from the field. Closer support was provided at the battalion aid station (BAS) level, where casualties could be stabilized before evacuation to more definitive care. The BAS was often bypassed because of the exceptional medical evacuation capabilities of helicopter medical evacuation (MEDEVAC).

The most dangerous role of the Hospital Corpsman in Vietnam was in the field. Special units (such as Navy SEAL teams and Marine reconnaissance units) took medical Sailors with them, as did the artillery, air, and infantry elements of the Marine Corps. Most of the 53 Hospital Corpsmen assigned to an infantry battalion served with rifle companies, one or two men per platoon of about 40. These Sailors patrolled with their Marines, risked the same dangers, and rendered the aid that saved the lives of thousands.

HOSPITAL CORPSMEN SINCE VIETNAM

Since April 1975, Hospital Corpsmen have continued to serve in the many "hot spots" around the world. Fifteen Hospital Corpsmen were killed in action when the Marine headquarters in Beirut, Lebanon, was attacked and destroyed by a suicide truck bomber on October 23, 1983. Hospital Corpsmen were present at sea and ashore when the United States took military action in Grenada, and then again when they faced both bullets and the needs of a starving populace in Somalia.

The 1990-91 Iraqi invasion of Kuwait gained a strong response from the United States and the world in the form of Desert Shield/Desert Storm. Preparations were made to drive the Iraqi Army out of the tiny country, and corpsmen were readied to respond to the needs of their shipmates. Hospital Corpsmen around the globe reacted, as their ships, stations, and Marines deployed or prepared to receive casualties. In fact, the first Navy casualty of Desert Storm was a Hospital Corpsman. Of the vast number of Naval Reservists called to active duty, the largest single group activated consisted of Hospital Corpsmen. Of an inventory of just more than 12,000 Hospital Corpsmen in the Naval Reserve, some 6,700 were recalled to active duty. The largest group of them, about 4,600, served at medical treatment facilities and casualty receiving centers; approximately 1,100 went to Marine Corps units; about 840 were attached to Fleet Hospitals Six and Fifteen; and some 470 of the reservists were assigned to the hospital ships *Mercy* and the *Comfort*.

HOSPITAL CORPSMEN TODAY

Today's Hospital Corpsmen perform as assistants in the prevention and treatment of disease and injury. They assist with physical examinations, provide patient care, and administer medicinals. They perform general laboratory, pharmacy, and other patient support services. They assist in the administrative, supply, and accounting procedures within medical departments ashore, afloat, and with the Marine Corps. They instruct medical and nonmedical personnel in first aid, self-aid, personal hygiene, and medical records maintenance. They assist in the maintenance of environmental health standards, and they are prepared to assist in the prevention and treatment of CBR casualties and in the transportation of the sick and injured. Senior Hospital Corpsmen perform technical

planning and management functions in support of medical readiness and quality health care delivery.

In addition to their general assignments, Hospital Corpsmen trained as technicians perform specialized functions within the operational forces, clinical specialties, and administrative department, and they may be assigned duties independent of a medical officer. These complex duties require that each Hospital Corpsman have broad-based training and a versatility neither demanded nor expected of other enlisted rating in the Navy.

Wherever you find the Navy, wherever you find the Marine Corps, there you will find Navy Hospital Corpsmen. In times of peace, they toil unceasingly, day and night, providing quality care to numerous beneficiaries. In times of war, they are on the beaches with the Marines, employed in amphibious operations, in transportation of wounded by air, on the battlefield, and on all types of ships, submarines, aircraft carriers, and landing craft. Their innumerable instances of heroism, during which they have consciously exposed themselves to danger to save lives, are not spectacular because the corpsmen were required to act. Rather, their bravery is exceptional because it was not required, but given freely and willingly in service to their country and their fellow humanity, above and beyond the call of duty.

Abridged from "The U.S. Navy Hospital Corps: A Century of Tradition, Valor, and Sacrifice," by HMCS(FMF) Mark T. Hacala, USNR, with permission from the author.

APPENDIX II

COMMONLY USED ABBREVIATIONS

AA . . . . Alcoholics Anonymous

ACTH . . . . adrenocorticotropichormon

ADH . . . . antidiuretic hormone

AIDS . . . . . acquired immunodeficiency syndrome

B-cells. . . . . . lymphocytes produced in the bone marrow

Ba . . . . barium

Bid . . . . 2 times a day

BP . . . . blood pressure

BUMED . . . . . Bureau of Medicine and Surgery

BUN . . blood, urea, nitrogen (test of kidney function)

BW. . . . . biological warfare

C . . . . Celsius (centigrade)

Ca . . . . calcium

CAAC. . . . . . Counseling and Assistance Center

CBC . . . . complete blood count

CBR . . . . . . chemical, biological, and radiological (warfare)

cc . . . . cubic centimeter/1 ml

CCU . . . . coronary care unit

CHF . . . . congestive heart failure

Cl . . . . chlorine

CNS . . . . central nervous system

CO_2 . . . . carbon dioxide

COPD . . . . chronic obstructive pulmonary disease

CSF . . . . cerebrospinal fluid

CVA. . . . . cerebrovascular accident

CW . . . . chemical warfare

D&C . . . . dilation and curettage

DC. . . . . Dental Corps

DCA. . . . . damage control assistant

diff . . . . differential blood count

DME . . . . diving medical examination

DNA. . . . . deoxyribonucleic acid

DOB . . . . date of birth

DOD . . . . Department of Defense

DTs. . . . . delerium tremens (confusion and incoherence brought on by withdrawal from alcohol)

D_x . . . . diagnosis

ea . . . . each

ECG/EKG . . . . electrocardiogram

EM. . . . . electron microscope

ENT . . . . ear, nose, and throat

F . . . . Fahrenheit

FAC . . . . free available chlorine

FBS . . . . fasting blood sugar

FDA. . . . . Food and Drug Administration

Fe . . . . iron

FSC . . . . *Federal Supply Catalog*

FSH. . . . . follicle-stimulating hormone

g/gm . . . . gram

GI . . . . gastrointestinal

gr. . . . . grain

gtt . . . . drops

GTT. . . . . glucose tolerance test

GU . . . . genitourinary

h.s. . . . . at bedtime (*hora somni*)

Hb/Hgb. . . . . hemoglobin

HCG . . . . human chorionic gonadotropin

Hct. . . . . hematocrit

Hg . . . . mercury

HIV . . . . human immunodeficiency virus

hpf . . . . high-power field (microscope)

I. . . . . iodine

I&O . . . . intake and output

ICU . . . . Intensive care unit

IM . . . . intramuscular

IPPB . . . . intermittent positive-pressure breathing (asthma and emphysema therapy)

IUD . . . . intrauterine device

IV . . . . intravenous

IVP . . . . intravenous pyelogram	OBA . . . . oxygen breathing apparatus
JAG . . . . Judge Advocate General	OD . . . . right eye (*oculus dexter*)
K . . . . potassium	OJT . . . . on-the-job training
KUB . . . . kidney, ureter, and bladder	OR. . . . . operating room
(abdominal x-ray)	OS . . . . left eye (*oculus sinister*)
l *or* L . . . . liter	oz . . . . ounce
Lab . . . . laboratory	P . . . . phosphorus
LES . . . . Leave and Earnings Statement	PAYPERSMAN . . . *Pay and Personnel Procedures*
LH . . . . luteinizing hormone	*Manual*
LLQ . . . . left lower quadrant	pc. . . . . after meals (*post cibum*)
LMP . . . . last menstrual period	PDB. . . . . paradichlorobenzene
LP . . . . lumbar puncture	PDR . . . . *Physicians' Desk Reference*
LUQ . . . . left upper quadrant	PH . . . . hydrogen ion concentration
m . . . . meter	(alkalinity and acidity
MANMED . . . . *Manual of the Medical Department*	measurement)
MC. . . . . Medical Corps	PID . . . . pelvic inflammatory disease
MCH . . . . mean corpuscular hemoglobin	po . . . . orally (*per os*)
MCHC . . . . mean corpuscular hemo-	poly. . . . . segmented neutrophil (seg)
globin concentration	post-op . . . . post-operative
MCV. . . . . mean corpuscular volume	ppd. . . . . purified protein derivative
Med Board . . . . Department of Defense	ppm . . . . parts per million
Medical Review Board	pre-op . . . . pre-operative
mg . . . . milligram	prn . . . . as required (*pro re nata*)
MI . . . . myocardial infarction	PSD . . . . Personnel Support Detachment
MILPERSMAN . . . . . . *Naval Military Personnel*	PVC . . . . premature ventricular contraction
Manual	q4h . . . . every 4 hours
ml . . . . milliliter	q6h . . . . every 6 hours
mm . . . . millimeter	qd . . . . every day
MO . . . . medical officer	qh. . . . . every hour
MSC. . . . . Medical Service Corps	qid . . . . 4 times a day
N . . . . nitrogen	qns . . . . quantity not sufficient
Na . . . . sodium	qt. . . . . quart
NAVEDTRA . . . . . Naval Education and Training	Ra . . . . radium
NAVFINCEN . . . . Naval Finance Center	RBC. . . . . red blood cell
NAVMEDCOM . . . . . Naval Medical Command	Rh . . Rh factor (antigen in blood of some individuals)
NC . . . . Nurse Corps	RLQ . . . . right lower quadrant
NDRC . . . . Naval Drug Rehabilitation Center	RUQ . . . . right upper quadrant
NEC . . . . Naval Enlisted Classification	R_x . . . . take (prescription)
ng . . . . nasogastric	sc/sub-q . . . . subcutaneous
NMPC . . . . . Naval Military Personnel Command	SOAP notes . . . . the only accepted method of
npo . . . . nothing by mouth (*nulli per os*)	medical record entries for
NRTC. . . . . nonresident training course	the military. (**S**ubjective;
O_2 . . . . oxygen	**O**bjective; **A**ssessment;
OB . . . . obstetrics	**P**lan)

SOB . . . . shortness of breath

stat . . . . immediately

STD . . . . sexually transmitted disease

T-cells. . . . . lymphocytes produced in the
thymus gland

TAD/TEMADD . . . . . . temporary additional duty

TB . . . . tuberculosis

tbsp . . . . tablespoon

tid . . . . 3 times a day

tpr. . . . . temperature, pulse, and respiration

TSH . . . . thyroid-stimulating hormone

tsp . . . . teaspoon

UIC . . . . unit identification code

URI . . . . upper respiratory infection

USP-NF . . . . United States Pharmacopeia-National
Formulary

VA . . . . Veterans Administration

VD . . . . venereal disease

VDRL. . . . . Venereal Disease Research
Laboratory (an antibody
test for syphilis)

vs . . . . vital signs

WBC . . . . white blood cell

WHO . . . . World Health Organization

YOB . . . . year of birth

APPENDIX III

PREFIXES AND SUFFIXES USED IN MEDICAL TERMINOLOGY

Medical terminology uses components (i.e., prefixes and suffixes) to build words that represent medical conditions and procedures. These words can often seem intimidating until you learn how to break them down into their component parts.

Examples of Combinations of Prefixes and Suffixes

cholecystitis = chole + cyst + itis   (inflammation of the gallbladder)

- chole = gall
- cyst = bladder
- Itis = inflammation

cholelithiasis = chole + lith + iasis   (condition resulting from gallstones)

- chole = gall
- lith = stone
- iasis = condition (resulting from)

odontalgia = odont + algia   (tooth pain; toothache)

- odont = tooth
- algia = pain

rhinoplasty = rhino + plasty   (to form or build up the nose)

- rhino = nose
- plasty = to form or build up

The following are some of the more common prefixes and suffixes used by healthcare providers to describe body conditions and procedures.

PREFIXES

a-; an- . . . . lacking; absence of
ab- . . . . away from

acr/o . . . . extremities
ad- . . . . towards; addition of
adip/o . . . . fat
aer/o . . . . air
amphi- . . . . on both sides
amyl/o . . . . starch
andr/o . . . . male

angi/o . . . . vessel
ankyl/o . . . . crooked; bent; stiff
ante- . . . . before
anter/o; anteri/o . . . . front
anti- . . . . against
aque/o . . . . water
arthr/o . . . . joint
articul/o . . . . joint
atel/o . . . . incomplete
audi/o . . . . hearing
aur/i . . . . ear
auto- . . . . self
axill/o . . . . armpit
bacteri/o . . . . bacteria
bene- . . . . good
bi/o . . . . life
bi- . . . . two
bil/i . . . . gall; bile
brachi/o . . . . arm
brady- . . . . slow
bucc/o . . . . cheek
calc/o . . . . calcium
capit/o . . . . head
carcin/o . . . . cancer
cardi/o . . . . heart
cata- . . . . down
caud/o . . . . tail; lower part of body
caus/o . . . . burn
cauter/o . . . . heat; burn
celi/o . . . . belly; abdomen
cephal/o . . . . head
cerebell/o . . . . cerebellum
cerebr/o . . . . brain; cerebrum
cervic/o . . . . neck; cervix
chem/o . . . . drug; chemical
chol/e . . . . gall
chondr/o . . . . cartilage
chrom/o . . . . color
chron/o . . . . time
cib/o . . . . meals
con- . . . . with; together
contra- . . . . against; opposed to
coron/o . . . . heart

cortic/o . . . . cortex
cost/o . . . . ribs
crani/o . . . . skull
cry/o . . . . cold
crypt/o . . . . hidden
cutane/o . . . . skin
cyan/o . . . . blue
cyst/o . . . . bladder
cyt/o . . . . cell
dacry/o . . . . tear
dactyl/o . . . . fingers; toes
de- . . . . lack of
dent/i . . . . tooth
derm/o; dermat/o . . . . skin
di . . . . complete
dia- . . . . complete; through
diaphor/o . . . . sweat
dist/o . . . . far
dors/o . . . . back (of body)
dys- . . . . difficult; painful
ec-; ecto- . . . . out; outside
em- . . . . in
en- . . . . in; within
encephal/o . . . . brain
endo- . . . . within
enter/o . . . . intestines
epi- . . . . above
erg/o . . . . work
erythr/o . . . . red
eso- . . . . inward
estr/o . . . . female
eti/o . . . . cause
eu- . . . . good
ex- . . . . out
exo- . . . . outside
fibr/o . . . . fibers; fibrous tissue
gastr/o . . . . stomach
gen/o . . . . producing; beginning
germ/o . . . . sprout; seed
gingiv/o . . . . gums
gloss/o . . . . tongue
gluc/o; glyc/o . . . . sugar
gnos/o . . . . knowledge

gravid/o	pregnancy	mon/o	one; single
gynec/o	woman; female	morph/o	shape; form
hem/o; hemat/o	blood	mort/o	death
hemi-	half	my/o	muscle
hepat/o	liver	myel/o	spinal cord; bone marrow
hidr/o	sweat	myos/o	muscle
hist/o; histi/o	tissue	narc/o	stupor; numbness
home/o	same; constant; unchanged	nas/o	nose
hydr/o	water	nat/i	birth
hyper-	above; increase	necr/o	death
hypn/o	sleep	neo-	new
hypo-	under; below	nephr/o	kidney
hyster/o	uterus; womb	neur/o	nerve
immun/o	safe; protection	ocul/o; ophthalm/o	eye
in-	not; in	odont/o	tooth
infra-	below; inferior	olig/o	few; scanty
inter-	between	onc/o	mass; tumor
intra-	within	or/o	mouth
is/o	same; equal	orth/o	straight
kary/o	nucleus	oste/o	bone
kerat/o	horny; hard; cornea	ot/o	ear
kinesi/o	movement	ov/o	egg
labi/o	lips	pachy/o	heavy; thick
lacrim/o	tear; tear duct	pan-	all
lact/o	milk	para-	beside; near; abnormal
lapar/o	abdomen	path/o	disease
laryng/o	larynx; voice box	per-	through
later/o	side	peri-	around
leuk/o	white	phag/o	eat; swallow
lingu/o	tongue	pharyng/o	throat
lip/o	fat	phil/o	like; love; attraction to
lumb/o	lower back; loins	phleb/o	vein
macro-	large	phob/o	fear
mal-	faulty; poor	phot/o	light
mamm/o	breast	physi/o	nature
mast/o	breast	pne/o	breathing; breath
medi/o	middle	pneum/o	lung
melan/o	black	poly-	many; much
meso-	middle	post-	after; behind
meta-	beyond; near; change	pre-	before
metr/o; metri/o	uterus	proct/o	rectum
micr/o	small	prot/o	first
mit/o	thread	proxim/o	near

pseud/o	false	-ase	enzyme
psych/o	mind	-asthenia	lack of strength
py/o	pus	-blast	immature; embryonic
pyr/o	heat; temperature	-capnia	carbon dioxide
re-	back	-cele	tumor; hernia
rect/o	rectum	-cidal	killing
ren/o	kidney	-clast	break
retro-	behind	-coccus (*pl.* -cocci)	berry-shaped
rhin/o	nose	-crine	secrete; separate
rib/o	sugar	-crit	separate
roentgen/o	x-rays	-cyte	cell
sarc/o	flesh (connective tissue)	-cytosis	condition of cells
scop/o	examination (usually visual)	-desis	binding
semi-	half	-ectasia; -ectasis	dilation; stretching
seps/o	infection	-ectomy	removal of
somn/o	sleep	-emesis	vomiting
son/o	sound	-emia	blood
spher/o	round; globe-shaped	-er	one who
sphygm/o	pulse	-esthesia	sensation
spondyl/o	vertebrae (backbones)	-genesis	condition of producing
stomat/o	mouth	-globin; -globulin	protein
sub-	under; below	-gram	record
supra-	above	-graph	instrument for recording
sym-; syn-	together; with	-graphy	process of recording
tachy-	fast	-ia	condition; process
tele/o	far; distant	-iasis	condition (of)
thorac/o	chest	-ic	pertaining to
top/o	position; location; place	-ist	specialist
tox/o; toxic/o	poison	-itis	inflammation
trans-	across	-lith	stone; calculus
ultra-	beyond; excess	-lysis	destruction; break down
vas/o	vessel; duct	-lytic	destruction
ven/o	vein	-malacia	softening
ventr/o	belly side of body	-manometer	used to measure pressure
vir/o	virus; poison	-megaly	enlargement
viscer/o	internal organs	-meter	used to measure
vit/a; vit/o	life	-oid	resembling
xanth/o	yellow	-ole	little; small
xer/o	dry	-ology	study of
		-oma	growth; tumor

SUFFIXES

		-opia	vision
-ac; -al; -ar; -ary	pertaining to	-opsy	view
-algia	pain	-or	one who

-(o)rraphy	repair of
-(o)rrhea	flow; discharge
-osis	condition (of)
-(o)stomy	creation of an opening
-(o)tomy	cutting into
-ous	pertaining to
-para	births (viable offspring)
-pathy	disease
-penia	decreased number
-phagia	eating; swallowing
-pheresis	removal
-philia	attraction for; increase
-phobia	fear; dread
-phonia	voice; sound
-phoria	feeling (mental state)
-phylaxis	protection
-physis	grow; growth
-plasia	formation; growth
-plasty	form; build up
-plegia	paralysis
-pnea	breathing
-porosis	passage
-ptosis	drooping; falling
-rrhea	discharge; flow
-sclerosis	hardening
-scope	instrument used to examine
-scopy	examination (usually visual)
-spasm	contraction of muscles
-stalsis	constriction
-stasis	control; stop
-static	stopping; controlling
-stenosis	tightening; stricture
-sthenia	strength
-therapy	treatment
-thermy	heat
-tic	pertaining to
-tome	instrument to cut
-tomy	process of cutting; incision
-tresia	opening
-tropic; -trophy	growth; nutrition
-ule	little; small
-uric; -uria	urine
-y	condition; process

COMMON PHARMACEUTICALS

	Pharmaceutical Name	Action & Use
Astringents	Aluminum acetate solution (Burrow's solution, Domeboro®)	Aluminum acetate solution is used as a wet dressing for the relief of inflammatory conditions of the skin, such as poison ivy, swellings and bruises, insect bites, athlete's foot, or other environmental skin conditions, and for superficial external otitis.
	Calamine, zinc oxide, glycerine, and bentonite magma in calcium hydroxide (calamine lotion)	Calamine lotion is used to treat various skin afflictions in the same way as aluminum acetate. It is a topical astringent and protectant. It should not be applied to blistered, raw, or oozing areas of the skin.
Emollients	Theobroma oil (cocoa butter)	Cocoa butter is an excellent emollient with a pleasant odor. It is ideal for the treatment of chapped skin and lips, cracked nipples, or minor irritated or abraded skin areas.
	Petrolatum (petroleum jelly)	Petrolatum is a good emollient that also provides a highly occlusive, protective barrier. When petrolatum is used as an ointment base, it may not release some drugs.
	Zinc oxide ointment	Zinc oxide ointment is a white petrolatum containing approximately 20% zinc oxide powder. It is used as an emollient with slightly astringent properties. Because of its opaqueness, zinc oxide ointment is ideal for protecting sensitive skin from the sun.
Expectorants & Antitussives	Guaifenesin and dextromethorphan (Robitussin DM®)	In this drug combination, guaifenesin acts as an expectorant. It may be useful in the symptomatic relief of dry, nonproductive coughs, and in the presence of mucous in the respiratory tract. Dextromethorphan is a synthetic nonnarcotic derivative of codeine that acts as an antitussive. It is used to control nonproductive coughs by soothing minor throat and bronchial irritations.
	Guaifenesin and codeine phosphate (Robitussin AC®)	Guaifenesin and codeine phosphate are combined to relieve the symptoms of a cold. Guaifenesin is an expectorant, and codeine phosphate is a narcotic antitussive. Patients should be advised that this medication contains a narcotic and, if abused, could cause dependency.

HM3fAIva

	Pharmaceutical Name	Action & Use
Nasal Decongestants	Pseudoephedrine hydrochloride (Sudafed®)	Pseudoephedrine hydrochloride (HCl) is indicated for the symptomatic relief of nasal congestion due to the common cold, hay fever, or other upper respiratory allergies.
	Pseudoephedrine hydrochloride and triprolidine hydrochloride (Actifed®)	Pseudoephedrine HCl and triprolidine HCl are a nasal decongestant and antihistamine combination. Pseudoephedrine HCl, a nasal decongestant, reduces congestion and swelling of mucous membranes, and triprolidine HCl, an antihistamine, promotes drying of mucous membranes. This drug combination is indicated for the symptomatic relief of colds, hay fever, etc.
	Phenylpropanolamine and guaifenesin (Entex®LA)	Phenylpropanolamine, a nasal decongestant, and guaifenesin, an expectorant, are combined for the symptomatic relief of nasal congestion due to the common cold, hay fever, or other respiratory allergies.
Antihistamines	Diphenhydramine hydrochloride (Benadryl®)	Diphenhydramine hydrochloride is given for active and prophylactic treatment of motion sickness, as a nighttime sleep aid, and for the symptomatic relief of urticaria, allergic rhinitis, and other allergic conditions.
	Chlorpheniramine maleate (Chlor-Trimeton®)	Chlorpheniramine maleate is used for the symptomatic treatment of urticaria and other allergic conditions.
	Meclizine hydrochloride (Antivert®, Bonine®)	Meclizine HCl is given to prevent and treat nausea, vomiting, and dizziness of motion sickness. Meclizine HCl has a longer duration of action than diphenhydramine hydrochloride.
	Dimenhydrinate (Dramamine®)	Similar to other antihistamines, the greatest usefulness of dimenhydrinate is the prevention and treatment of motion sickness. It may also be used to control nausea and vomiting in connection with radiation sickness.
Histamine H₂ Receptor Antagonists	Cimetidine (Tagamet®)	Cimetidine is used for short-term treatment and maintenance of active duodenal and benign gastric ulcers. Cimetidine may also be used for other medical conditions which cause an excess amount of gastric acid to be produced.
	Ranitidine (Zantac®)	Like cimetidine, ranitidine is used for short-term treatment and maintenance of active duodenal and benign gastric ulcers to promote healing of duodenal ulcers. In addition, ranitidine is used to treat gastroesophageal reflux disease.

HM3fAivb

	Pharmaceutical Name	Action & Use
Antacids	Magnesium hydroxide (Milk of Magnesia USP)	Milk of magnesia is used for the symptomatic relief of upset stomach associated with hyperacidity, treatment and maintenance of duodenal ulcers, and may be used to reduce phosphate absorption in patients with chronic renal failure. Magnesium hydroxide should be taken on an empty stomach with lots of fluids. It should not be used in the presence of abdominal pain, nausea, or vomiting. Prolonged use may result in kidney stones. Magnesium hydroxide also has a laxative effect.
	Aluminum hydroxide gel (Amphojel®)	Aluminum hydroxide gel is used to manage peptic ulcers, gastritis, and gastric hyperacidity. The major advantage of this drug is that no systemic alkalosis is produced. It may, however, cause constipation.
	Alumina and magnesia oral suspension (Maalox®)	Alumina and magnesia oral suspension coats the stomach lining and neutralizes gastric acid. It is less constipating than aluminum hydroxide alone.
	Alumina, magnesia, and simethicone oral suspension (Mylanta®)	Alumina, magnesia, and simethicone oral suspension coats the stomach lining, neutralizes gastric acid, and reduces flatulence.
Antiseptics, Disinfectants, & Germicides	Phenol (carbolic acid)	Historically one of the first antiseptic agents used, phenol is the standard by which all other antiseptic, disinfectant, and germicidal agents are measured in their effectiveness. Because of its highly caustic nature, phenol must be handled with care. The effect of phenol is coincident with the concentration: high concentrations are germicidal and can cause tissue destruction; lower concentrations are antiseptic. Phenol is inactivated by alcohol. Because more effective and less damaging agents have been developed, phenol is no longer used extensively. **NOTE:** Never use phenol to disinfect rubber, cloth, or plastic.
	Povidone-iodine (Betadine®)	Numerous iodine and iodine-complex agents are available for use in disinfection. The most common of these is povidone-iodine (Betadine®). It is used externally to destroy bacteria, fungi, viruses, protozoa, and yeasts. Povidone-iodine is relatively nontoxic, nonirritating, and nonsensitizing to the skin. When used as an antiseptic, the complex breaks down on contact with skin or mucous membranes to release free iodine, which is slowly absorbed. It is most commonly used as a preoperative skin antiseptic. **NOTE:** Check for iodine allergies before using this antiseptic on patients.

HM3fAivc

	Pharmaceutical Name	Action & Use
Antiseptics, Disinfectants, & Germicides (cont.)	Isopropyl alcohol (Isopropanol)	Isopropyl alcohol is used in a 70% solution as a skin antiseptic; it is volatile and also has a drying effect on the skin.
	Hexachlorophene (pHisoHex®)	Hexachlorophene, a synthetic preparation is a bacteriostatic cleansing agent effective against gram-positive organisms. Pus or serum decrease its effectiveness. Hexachlorophene is a neurotoxic agent and must not be used on premature infants, denuded skin, burns, or mucous membranes. It is used as an antiseptic scrub by physicians, dentists, food handlers, and others. Residual amounts can be removed with alcohol.
	Glutaraldehyde (Cidex®)	Glutaraldehyde is effective against vegetative gram-positive, gram-negative, and acid-fast bacteria, bacterial spores, some fungi, and viruses. It is used in an aqueous solution for sterilization of fiber optics, plastics, rubber, and other materials that are not resistant to heat.
	Hydrogen peroxide	Hydrogen peroxide, a germicide, is routinely used to cleans pus-producing wounds and in the treatment of necrotizing ulcerative gingivitis (NUG) (also known as trench mouth). Hydrogen peroxide is an oxidizing agent that is destructive to certain pathogenic organisms, but it is mild enough to be used on living tissue. It is for external use only and is normally available in a 3% solution.
	Silver nitrate	The soluble salts of silver nitrate ionize in water to produce highly concentrated astringent and antiseptic solutions. Silver nitrate in **solid** form is most commonly used to cauterize mucous membranes and to treat aphthous ulcers. The most common side effect of silver nitrate is that the skin turns black where the silver nitrate comes in contact with it. This black area on the skin is not harmful but will resolve slowly. Silver nitrate in **liquid** form is used as eye drops to prevent gonorrheal ophthalmia in newborns. Liquid silver nitrate is also used as a wet dressing. **CAUTION!** When you use silver nitrate as a wet dressing, you should use precautions to keep the dressing from drying out. If the wet dressing dries out, the silver nitrate will precipitate and be absorbed into the skin, which will turn a slate gray. This condition is known as **argyria**. There is no known reversal for this condition.

HM3fAivd

	Pharmaceutical Name	Action & Use
Sulfonamides	Sulfisoxazole (Gantrisin®)	This systemic sulfonamide is bacteriostatic and is indicated to treat urinary tract infections and acute otitis media.
	Trimethoprim and sufamethoxazole (Bactrim®, Septra®)	The combination of trimethoprim and sufamethoxazole is an anti-infective used to treat urinary tract infections and otitis media.
	Sulfacetamide sodium (Sodium Sulamyd®, Bleph-10®)	Sulfacetamide sodium is an ophthalmic bacteriostatic for the treatment of conjunctivitis, corneal ulcer, and other superficial ocular infections. It is available in solutions of various strengths and in an ointment form.
	Silver sulfadiazine (Silvadene Cream®)	Silver sulfadiazine is a topical antimicrobial agent used to treat second- and third-degree burns to prevent wound sepsis. It is water soluble and easily washed off the skin.

	Pharmaceutical Name	Action & Use
Penicillins	Penicillin G, aqueous	Penicillin G, aqueous, is indicated for susceptible infections such as meningococcal meningitis, endocarditis, and gonorrhea. Penicillin G is for parenteral use only.
	Penicillin G benazathine (Botulin®)	Penicillin G benazathine is indicated for conditions such as syphilis and upper respiratory tract infections caused by streptococcal (group A) bacteria.
	Penicillin G procaine, aqueous (Wycillin®)	Penicillin G procaine, aqueous, is indicated for conditions such as uncomplicated pneumonia, middle ear and sinus infections, NUG and pharyngitis, and acute pelvic inflammatory disease (PID). Penicillin G procaine is for parenteral use only, and it has a longer duration of action than most of the other penicillins.
	Penicillin V potassium (Pen-Vee K®, Betapen-VK®, V-Cillin K®)	Penicillin V is used to treat conditions such as upper respiratory tract infection, otitis media, sinusitis, bacterial endocarditis, and mild staphylococcal infection of skin and soft tissue. Penicillin V has the same spectra of activity of penicillin G and is usually the drug of choice for uncomplicated group-A beta-hemolytic streptococcal infections. It is available as oral tablets or powder for reconstitution for oral suspension.
	Dicloxacillin sodium (Dynapen®)	Dicloxacillin sodium is used to treat infections caused by penicillin G-resistant staphylococci. It may be used to initiate therapy in any patient in whom a staphylococcal infection is suspected.
	Ampicillin (Polycillin®)	Ampicillin is used to treat conditions such as shigella, salmonella, escherichia coli, and gonorrhea.
	Amoxicillin (Amoxil®)	The spectrum of amoxicillin is essentially identical to ampicillin, except that amoxicillin is more effective against shigella. Amoxicillin also has the advantage of more complete absorption than ampicillin.

HM3fAive

	Pharmaceutical Name	Action & Use
Cephalosporins	Cefazolin sodium (Ancef®, Kefzol®)	Cefazolin is used to treat a wide range of medical conditions, such as lower respiratory tract infections (pneumonia and lung abscess), septicemia, and bone and joint infections. Cefazolin sodium is also used perioperatively to reduce the chance of certain infections following surgical procedures (such as vaginal hysterectomy, gastrointestinal (GI) surgery, and transurethral prostatectomy).
	Cephalexin (Keflex®)	Cephalexin is indicated for the treatment of infection of the respiratory tract, otitis media, skin and skin structures, and genitourinary system.
	Cefuroxine (Ceftin®, Zinacef®)	Cefuroxine is used to treat pharyngitis, tonsillitis, otitis media, bronchitis, and mixed infections of the skin and skin structure. Mixed infections are infections that include both aerobic and anaerobic pathogenic organisms. This medication is also used preoperatively to prevent the incidence of certain postoperative infections.
Tetracyclines	Tetracycline hydrochloride (Achromycin®, Sumycin®)	Tetracycline hydrochloride (TCN) is used to treat infections caused by rickettsiae (such as Rocky Mountain spotted fever and typhus fever), agents of lymphogranulomas venereum and granuloma inguinale, and the spirochetal agent of relapsing fever. Tetracycline hydrochloride is indicated for severe acne as an adjunctive therapy. Food and some dairy products may interfere with absorption; antacids containing aluminum, calcium, or magnesium impair absorption of the antibiotic as well. This medication should be given 1 hour before or 2 hours after meals.
	Doxycycline hyclate (Vibramycin®)	Doxycycline is active against a wide range of gram-positive and gram-negative microorganisms and has a low affinity for binding with calcium. In addition to the conditions listed under tetracycline, doxycycline is also indicated for the treatment of uncomplicated chlamydial infections and uncomplicated gonococcal infections.
	Minocycline hydrochloride (Minocin®)	Mincycline hydrochloride is indicated for the same conditions as tetracycline hydrochloride and doxycycline hyclate.

	Pharmaceutical Name	Action & Use
Aminoglycosides	Streptomycin sulfate	Streptomycin sulfate is indicated for all forms of *mycobacterium tuberculosis*; it should be used only in conjunction with other antituberculosis drugs, e.g., Rifampin® or isoniazid. Streptomycin sulfate is also used to treat plague, tularemia, chancroid, granuloma inguinale, and some urinary tract infections where the infectious agent has shown to be susceptible to streptomycin and not susceptible to less toxic preparations.
	Gentamicin sulfate (Garamycin®)	Gentamicin sulfate is used to treat serious systemic infections of susceptible gram-negative organisms. While the patient is on gentamicin sulfate, it is necessary to monitor renal and hepatic function to determine if toxic levels have been reached. Gentamicin sulfate is also available as a topical preparation for the treatment of burns and infected wounds, and as an ophthalmic preparation for eye infections.
	Tobramycin sulfate (Nebcin®)	Tobramycin sulfate is used to treat serious infections such as septicemia, meningitis, and peritonitis.
	Neomycin sulfate (Mycifradin Sulfate®)	Neomycin sulfate is used to a topical preparation to treat skin infections, burn wounds, ulcers, and dermatoses. Neomycin sulfate is given orally to reduce intestinal flora prior to surgery involving the bowel or anus.
Macrolides	Erythromycin (E-Mycin®, Ilotycin®, PCE Dispertab®, Eryc®)	Erythromycin is one of the drugs of choice when penicillin is contraindicated. This medication is indicated to treat medical conditions such as gonorrhea; uncomplicated urethral, endocervical, and anal infections; early syphilis; and cases of severe or prolonged diarrhea associated with campylobater enteritis and enterocolitis. Erythromycin is also prescribed, as a prophylactic agent, prior to colorectal surgery. Erythromycin is available in enteric-coated tablets, as an opthalmic ointment, and as a topic preparation for the adjunctive treatment of acne.
	Clindamycin hydrochlorids (Cleocin®)	Clindamycin hydrochloride is used to treat susceptible anaerobic organisms. The use of clindamycin hydrochloride has often been associated with severe colitis and profuse diarrhea; if this condition occurs, the drug should be discontinued. A topical preparation is available for the treatment of acne.
	Vancomycin hydrochloride (Vancocin®)	Vancomycin hydrochloride is indicated in potentially life-threatening infections not treatable with other effective, less toxic antimicrobials, including the penicillins and cephalosporins. Potentially life-threatening infections that vancomycin may be used for include endocarditis, osteomyelitis, pneumonia, and septicemia.

HM3fAivg

	Pharmaceutical Name	Action & Use
Macrolides (cont.)	Spectinomycin (Trobicin®)	Spectinomycin was developed to treat gonorrhea. It is largely bacteriostatic and very effective in treating uncomplicated gonorrhea. Its advantage lies primarily in being a single-dose therapy and for patients who are allergic to penicillin or have penicillin-resistant strains of the causative organism. It is NOT effective in treating syphilis.
Antifungals	Nystatin (Mycostatin®)	Nystatin is primarily used to treat candidal infections. It is fungicidal and fungistatic against a wide variety of yeasts and yeast-like fungi, and is most often used to treat candidiasis. It is sometimes used concurrently with tetracycline to suppress the overgrowth of *Candida* in the bowel.
	Griseofulvin (Gris-PEG®, Fulvicin®)	Griseofulvin is a fungistatic agent given orally to treat fungal infections of the nails, hair, and skin. It is generally reserved for chronic infections that have not responded to topical therapy alone. Because treatment may last for several months, the patient should be instructed to follow the treatment regimen even though symptoms may abate. Inclusion of topical therapy is a must for effective elimination of the infection. Griseofulvin is not indicated to treat superficial fungal infections that can be controlled by topical antifungals. Because of its toxicity, patients should have periodic evaluations of hepatic and renal function. Griseofulvin is contraindicated in patients with hepatic dysfunction.
	Miconazole nitrate (Monistat®, Micatin®)	Miconazole nitrate is a synthetic antifungal that inhibits the growth of common dermatophytes. It is indicated to treat cutaneous fungal infections and vulvovaginal candidiasis.
	Undecylenic acid (Desenex®)	Undeclyenic acid is used primarily to treat and prevent tinea pedis and is often compounded with zinc to act as an astringent. It is available in ointment, dusting powder, solution, and spray.
	Tolnaftate (Tinactin®, Aftate®)	Tolnaftate was the first fungicide synthesized. It is indicated for the topical treatment of tinea pedis, tinea corporis, tinea capitis, and tinea versicolor.
	Clotrimazole (Lotrimin®, Mycelex®)	This is a broad-spectrum antifungal that inhibits the growth of pathogenic dermatophytes, yeasts, and other types of fungus growth, including *Candida albicans*. It is indicated for the treatment of tinea pedis, tinea cruris, tinea corporis, and candidiasis.

HM3fA.ivh

	Pharmaceutical Name	Action & Use
Antiparasitics	Permethrin (Elimite®)	Permethrin is a pediculicide used to treat *Pediculosis capitis* (head lice) and *Phthirus pubis* (crab lice). It is also indicated for scabies. Use with caution, especially in infants, children, and pregnant women, since it penetrates human skin and has the potential for systemic poisoning. This drug is irritating to the eyes and should be discontinued immediately if local irritation occurs.
	Crotomiton (Eurax®)	Crotamiton is a scabicide indicated for the treatment of scabies (*Sarcoptes scabiei*); it also has an antipruritic effect. Keep away from the eyes and mouth; do not apply to inflamed skin.
	Metronidazole (Flagyl®)	Metronidazole is effective in treating amebiasis. It is also used as a trichomonacide.
	Chloroquine phosphate (Aralen®)	Chloroquine phosphate is the drug of choice in treating acute malarial attacks. It is also used in the prevention and suppression of malaria in endemic areas.
	Primaquine phosphate	Primaquine phosphate is the drug of choice for the prevention or relapse of malaria caused by *P. vivax* and *P. ovale*. Primaquine phosphate is contraindicated in G-6-PD-deficient personnel, as it may result in hemolytic anemia.
	Sulfadoxine and pyrimethamine (Fansidar®)	Sulfadoxine and pyrimethamine is used in the curative treatment of strains of malaria that are resistant to chloroquine phosphate. It is also used prophylactically in endemic areas.
	Mebendazole (Vermox®)	Mebendazole is effective in treating infestations of hookworm, roundworm, pinworm, and whipworm.
	Pyrantel pamoate (Antiminth®)	Pyrantel pamoate is regarded as the drug of choice for pinworm and roundworm infestations.
	Thiabendazole (Mintezol®)	Thiabendazole is a vermicide used to destroy pinworms, roundworms, threadworms, hookworms, and whipworms. It is not indicated as a prophylactic agent.

	Pharmaceutical Name	Action & Use
Laxatives	Mineral oil	Mineral oil is an emollient laxative used to lubricate the fecal mass. It is often used in combination with an irritant agent such as phenolphthalein (Ex-Lax®).
	Glycerin suppositories (Sani-Supp®)	Glycerin suppositories are widely used in children. They promote peristalsis through local irritation of the mucous membrane of the colon.
	Bisacodyl (Ducolax®)	Bisacodyl is a relatively nontoxic irritant cathartic that reflexively stimulates the colon on contact. It usually produces softly formed stools in 6 to 12 hours and is normally taken at bedtime. It is often used as a preparatory agent prior to some surgeries and radiological examinations.

HM3fAIvi

	Pharmaceutical Name	Action & Use
Laxatives (cont.)	Magnesium citrate (Citrate of magnesia)	Magnesium citrate is a saline irritant laxative that also inhibits the absorption of water from the intestine. It is preferred by radiology departments for use prior to special x-rays.
	Psyllium hydrophilic mucilloid (Metamucil®)	Psyllium hydrophilic mucilloid is a bulk laxative that works by absorbing water. The effect occurs within 12 to 72 hours. It is provided as a dry powder that is stirred into water or fruit juice. This laxative should be drunk immediately after mixing, while the material is in suspension.
	Ducosate calcium (Surfak®)	Ducosate calcium is a stool softener that promotes water retention in the fecal mass.
	Ducosate sodium (Colace®)	Ducosate sodium has the same action as ducosate calcium.
Antidiarrheals	Kaolin mixture with pectin (Kaopectate®)	Kaolin mixture with pectin is used in the symptomatic treatment of diarrhea. The pectin portion absorbs excess fluid and consolidates the stool. The kaolin portion absorbs irritants and forms a protective coating on the intestinal mucosa.
	Diphenoxylate hydrochloride with atropine sulfate (Lomotil®)	Diphenoxylate hydrochloride with atropine sulfate is used for the symptomatic treatment of diarrhea. This medication reduces peristalsis and intestinal motility by affecting the smooth muscles in the intestine. Because diphenoxylate is chemically related to meperidine hydrochloride (Demerol®), it is classified as a controlled substance. To prevent abuse of the drug, a sub-therapeutic amount of atropine is added.
Diuretics	Hydrochlorothiazide (Esidrix®, Oretic®, HydroDIURIL®)	Hydrochlorothiazide is used for edema associated with congestive heart failure and other edematous conditions. It is also used to manage hypertension as the sole agent or in combination with other antihypertensive agents.
	Chlorthalidone (Hygroton®)	Chlorthalidone is used in the same manner as hydrochlorothiazide.
	Furosemide (Lasix®)	Furosemide, a potent diuretic, is used to treat edema associated with congestive heart failure, cirrhosis of the liver, and renal disease. It is particularly useful when greater diuretic potential is desired, and may be used alone or in combination with other antihypertensive agents to treat hypertension.
	Acetazolamide (Diamox®)	Although classified as a diuretic, the primary indication for this drug is the treatment of glaucoma (to reduce intraocular pressure).

HM3fAivj

	Pharmaceutical Name	Action & Use
Diuretics (cont.)	Triamterene and hydrochlorothiazide (Dyazide®, Maxzide®)	This combination of a potassium-sparing (triamterene) and potassium-depleting diuretic is often more effective than either drug alone. It is used for edema associated with congestive heart failure and other edematous conditions. It is also used in the management of hypertension.
Nonnarcotic Analgesics, Antipyretics, and Anti-inflammatory Agents	Aspirin (ASA, CAMA, Ecotrin®)	Aspirin is still the most economical analgesic, antipyretic, and anti-inflammatory agent available. Some preparations have an antacid-type buffer to assist in the reduction of gastric irritation. It is an analgesic for mild to moderate pain and an effective antipyretic. Aspirin is also indicated for various inflammatory conditions, such as rheumatoid arthritis and bursitis.
	Acetaminophen (Tylenol®)	Acetaminophen, an analgesic and antipyretic, is used to relieve pain and fever accompanying diseases (such as the common cold and influenza). It is also used to relieve pain and discomfort of upper GI disease (ulcer and gastritis), gouty arthritis, a variety of arthritic and rheumatic conditions involving musculoskeletal pain, as well as other painful disorders. Acetaminophen is indicated for patients who are allergic to aspirin.
	Ibuprofen (Motrin®)	Ibuprofen is indicated for the relief of mild to moderate pain, including headaches and menstrual cramps. It is also used as an anti-inflammatory agent to treat arthritis, tendinitis, bursitis, etc. It is not recommended for use in cases of gastrointestinal bleeding or renal impairment, or during the third trimester of pregnancy.
	Indomethacin (Indocin®)	Indomethacin is a potent anti-inflammatory agent with antipyretic and analgesic properties. Because of its potential for adverse reactions, indomethacin should be reserved for cases of chronic rheumatoid arthritis, osteoarthritis, and acute gout.
	Naproxen sodium (Anaprox®)	Naproxen sodium, an analgesic, is indicated for the relief of mild to moderate pain and for the treatment of primary dysmenorrhea, rheumatoid arthritis, osteoarthritis, tendinitis, bursitis, and acute gout. Its effects are similar to those of aspirin and indomethacin, but with fewer and less toxic gastrointestinal side effects; however, it is not indicated for patients with a history of gastrointestinal disease, especially those with a propensity for peptic ulcer disease.
	Tolmetin sodium (Tolectin®)	Tolmetin sodium, an anti-inflammatory agent, is used for treatment and long-term management of acute rheumatoid arthritis and osteoarthritis. It is also used to treat juvenile rheumatoid arthritis.
	Piroxicam (Feldene®)	Piroxicam, an anti-inflammatory agent, is used to relieve the signs and symptoms of acute and chronic osteoarthritis and rheumatoid arthritis.

HM3fAivk

	Pharmaceutical Name	Action & Use
Central Nervous System Stimulants	Methylphenidate hydrochloride (Ritalin®)	Methylphenidate HCl is indicated for use in hyperkinetic children and children with attention deficit disorders. In children, this drug as a central nervous system depressant. Methylphenidate HCl is also indicated for narcolepsy in adults.
	Dextroamphetamine sulfate (Dexadrine®)	Dextroamphetamine is primarily indicated for narcolepsy. However, because of dextroamphetamine's anorexiant effect (it diminishes the appetite), it is occasionally used as an adjunct to diet therapy for obesity caused by overeating.
Central Nervous System Depressants	Phenobarbital (Luminal®)	Phenobarbital is a long-lasting barbiturate frequently used to treat convulsive seizure disorders. This is the drug of choice in petit mal epilepsy, and it is also used as a hypnotic or sedative.
	Pentobarbital (Nembutal®)	Pentobarbital is indicated for short-term treatment of insomnia. It is also used as a preanesthetic medication.
	Secobarbital (Seconal®)	Secobarbital is used in the same manner as pentobarbital and has a rapid hypnotic effect.
	Phenytoin sodium (Dilantin®)	Phenytoin sodium, a nonbarbiturate anticonvulsant, is the drug of choice for the treatment and management of grand mal epilepsy. Because phenytoin sodium possesses no hypnotic properties, it is preferred to phenobarbital in treating seizure disorders. However, phenytoin sodium and phenobarbital are frequently used in combination to more effectively manage certain types of epilepsies.
	Ethyl alcohol (ethanol)	Ethyl alcohol, a controlled substance, is mainly used in compounding various medicinal preparations not normally stocked by pharmacy. In small doses, alcohol stimulates the gastric mucosa, increasing the flow of juices. Continual small doses produce hypnotic effects. Systemically, ethyl alcohol is a sedative.
Opium & Opium Alkaloids	Camphorated opium tincture (Paregoric)	Camphorated opium tincture is used mainly as an intestinal tranquilizer to control diarrhea.
	Morphine sulfate	Morphine sulfate, an opium alkaloid, is indicated for the relief of severe pain. It is used preoperatively to sedate patients and to treat severe pain associated with myocardial infarction. Morphine is contraindicated for patients with head injuries, acute alcoholism, and convulsive disorders.

HM3fAivl

	Pharmaceutical Name	Action & Use
Opium & Opium Alkaloids (cont.)	Codeine sulfate	Codeine sulfate, an opium alkaloid, is like morphine. However, it has only one-sixth of the analgesic power and one-fourth of the respiratory depressant effect of morphine. Codeine is used for moderate to severe pain and as an antitussive.
	Meperidine hydrochloride (Demerol®)	Meperidine hydrochloride is a synthetic analgesic similar to morphine. It is used for moderate to severe pain and as a preoperative medication. Meperidine HCl is not as effective as morphine in its analgesic properties.

	Pharmaceutical Name	Action & Use
Psychotherapeutic Agents	Chlorpromazine hydrochloride (Thorazine®)	Chlorpromazine hydrochloride is indicated for alleviating manifestations of psychosis, tension, and agitation. Dosage is highly individualized depending on the severity of symptoms and degree of response. Chlorpromazine HCl may also be used as an antiemetic.
	Thioridazine (Mellaril®)	Thioridazine is used for antipsychotic purposes and is considered to be a good all-around tranquilizer.
	Prochlorperizine (Compazine®)	Prochlorperizine is most often used in the symptomatic treatment of nausea and vomiting, but it shares all the antipsychotic effects of chlorpromazine.
	Haloperidol (Haldol®)	Haloperidol is indicated in treating schizophrenia with manifestations of acute manic symptoms, social withdrawal, paranoid behavior, and the manic stage of manic-depressive patients.
	Lithium (Eskalith®, Lithonate®)	Lithium is used to treat manic episodes of manic-depressive illness. It is the drug of choice to prevent or diminish the intensity of manic episodes.
	Amitriptyline hydrochloride (Elavil®)	Amitriptyline HCl is an antidepressive mood elevator with mild tranquilizing effects. It is indicated for the long-term treatment of depressive disorders.
	Chlordiazepoxide hydrochloride (Librium®)	Chlordiazepoxide hydrochloride is an antianxiety agent for the treatment of anxiety disorders. It is **not** indicated for the anxiety or tension associated with the stress of everyday activities. Chlordiazepoxide HCl is also indicated in the abatement of acute withdrawal symptoms of alcoholism.
	Hydroxyzine pamoate (Vistaril®, Atarax®)	Hydroxyzine pamoate is a rapid-acting antianxiety and antiemetic with antispasmodic and muscle relaxant effects. It is most often used in pre- and postoperative sedation and in conjunction with meperidine hydrochloride to enhance its effects and reduce nausea.

HM3fAivm

	Pharmaceutical Name	Action & Use
Psychotherapeutic Agents (cont.)	Diazepam (Valium®)	Diazepam is useful in treating mild to moderate depression with anxiety and tension. Because of its muscle relaxant properties, it is also used to treat spastic muscle conditions and convulsive seizure episodes. Diazepam is the drug of choice in status epilepticus.
	Fluoxetine hydrochloride (Prozac®)	Fluoxetine is an oral antidepressant used to treat depression. It may also be useful in treating bulimia nervosa and obsessive-compulsive disorders.
	Temazepam (Restoril®)	Temazepam is a nonbarbiturate sedative and hypnotic indicated for the treatment of insomnia.

	Pharmaceutical Name	Action & Use
Skeletal Muscle Relaxants	Methocarbamol (Robaxin®)	Methocarbamol is used as an adjunct therapy for the relief of discomfort associated with acute, painful musculoskeletal conditions. It may have a beneficial effect in the control of neuromuscular manifestations of tetanus.
	Cyclobenzaprine hydrochloride (Flexeril®)	Cyclobenzaprine hydrochloride is indicated as an adjunct to rest and physical therapy for relief of muscle spasm with acute painful musculoskeletal conditions.
	Chlorzoxazone (Parafon Forte DSC®)	Chlorzoxazone is used in the same manner as cyclobenzaprine HCl.
	Orphenadrine citrate, aspirin, and caffeine (Norgesic®)	This drug combination contains a skeletal muscle relaxant (orphenadrine citrate), an analgesic and anti-inflammatory agent (aspirin), and a CNS stimulant (caffeine). It is used as an adjunct to rest and physical therapy for relief of muscle spasm with acute painful muskuloskeletal conditions.

	Pharmaceutical Name	Action & Use
Cardiovascular Agents	Digoxin (Lanoxin®)	Digoxin is indicated for all degrees of congestive heart failure and for various arrhythmias. It has a direct effect on the myocardium, causing an increase in the force of contractions.
	Quinidine sulfate	Quinidine sulfate is indicated for premature atrial and ventricular contractions and other arrhythmias.

NOTE: Do not confuse this medication with quinine sulfate, an antimalarial. |
| | Amyl nitrite | Amyl nitrite is primarily used for the prevention of erection in adult males following circumcision. Occasionally, this drug is used for cardiac patients. |
| | Nitrogylcerin (Nitrostat®, Nitro-Bid®) | Nitroglycerin is indicated for the treatment and management of acute and chronic angina pectoris. |

HM3fAivn

	Pharmaceutical Name	Action & Use
Cardiovascular Agents (cont.)	Isosorbide dinitrate (Isordil®, Sorbitrate®)	Isosorbide dinitrate is similar to nitroglycerin in its antianginal action.
	Dipyridamole (Persantine®)	Dipyridamole is indicated as an adjunct to warfarin sodium (an anticoagulant) in the prevention of postoperative thromboembolic complications of cardiac valve replacement.
	Procainamide hydrochloride (Pronestyl®, Procan SR®)	Procainamide HCl is indicated for the treatment of premature ventricular contractions, ventricular tachycardia, and atrial fibrillation. It may also be used for cardiac arrhythmias associated with anesthesia and surgery.
	Verapamil (Isoptin®)	Verapamil is indicated for the treatment of angina, essential hypertension (hypertension occurring without an organic cause found), and cardiac arrhythmias.
	Diltiazem (Cardizem®)	Diltiazem is indicated for the treatment of angina pectoris and for the management of essential hypertension.
Vasoconstrictors	Epinephrine (Adrenaline Chloride®, Sus-Phrine®)	When inhaled, epinephrine is used to relieve acute bronchial asthma. When injected, epinephrine relieves respiratory distress in bronchial asthma attacks and relieves bronchospasms in patients with chronic bronchitis, emphysema, and other obstructive pulmonary diseases. It may also be used to treat hypersensitivity reactions to drugs, serums, insect stings, or other allergens. (Symptoms of these reactions may include bronchospasms; urticaria; pruritus; and swelling of the skin, lips, eyelids, tongue, and nasal mucosa; and anaphylactic shock.)
	Tetrahydrozaline hydrochloride (Visine Eye Drops®)	Tetrahydrozaline HCl is an ophthalmic preparation for the symptomatic relief of irritated eyes.
	Phenylephrine hydrochloride (Neo-Synephrine®)	Phenylephrine hydrochloride is used to shrink mucous membranes of the nose and to relieve local congestion.
	Oxymetazoline hydrochloride (Afrin®)	Oxymetazoline HCl is a topical vasoconstrictor used to relieve nasal congestion.
Anticoagulants	Heparin sodium	Heparin sodium is used in prophylaxis and treatment of venous thrombosis (and its expansion) and of pulmonary embolism.
	Warfarin sodium (Coumadin®)	Warfarin sodium is used extensively to treat embolism in the prevention of occlusions.

HM3fAivo

	Pharmaceutical Name	Action & Use
Vitamins	Vitamin A (Retinol)	Vitamin A, a fat-soluble vitamin, is necessary for visual adaptation to darkness. Deficiencies rarely occur in well-nourished individuals, and an excess of vitamin A can be toxic. Conditions which may cause vitamin A deficiency include biliary tract or pancreatic disease, colitis, hepatic cirrhosis, and extreme dietary inadequacy (such as anorexia). Retinoic acid, a degradation product of retinol, is useful to treat acne and pseudofolliculitis barbae.
	Vitamin B_1 (Thiamine hydrochloride)	Vitamin B_1, a water-soluble vitamin, is necessary for carbohydrate metabolism. This vitamin is used to treat patients with appetite loss resulting from dietary disturbances. The deficiency disease is beriberi.
	Vitamin B_2 (Riboflavin)	Vitamin B_2, a water-soluble vitamin, functions in the body as a coenzyme necessary in tissue respiratory processes, e.g., oxidation reduction reactions. Deficiency is associated with cheilosis, glossitis, visual disturbances, or visual fatigue.
	Vitamin B_3 (Niacin)	Vitamin B_3, a water-soluble vitamin, is indicated for the correction of a niacin deficiency and in the prevention and treatment of pellagra.
	Vitamin B_6 (Pyridoxine hydrochloride)	Vitamin B_6, a water-soluble vitamin, is a coenzyme in the metabolism of protein, carbohydrate, and fat. It is most often used during isoniazid (INH) therapy to prevent the development of peripheral neuritis.
	Vitamin B_{12} (Cyanocobalamin)	Vitamin B_{12}, a water-soluble vitamin, is essential to growth, cell reproduction, and blood cell formation. When vitamin B_{12} therapy is used to treat pernicious anemia, the treatment is continued indefinitely, and folic acid is normally included in the therapy protocol.
	Vitamin C (Ascorbic acid)	Vitamin C, a water-soluble vitamin, is necessary for the prevention and cure of scurvy. Vitamin C in high doses is believed to prevent the common cold, and to treat asthma, atherosclerosis, wounds, schizophrenia, and cancer.
	Vitamin D	Vitamin D, a fat-soluble vitamin, is involved in the regulation of calcium and phosphorus metabolism. Vitamin D deficiency leads to rickets in children and osteomalacia in adults.
	Vitamin E (Tocopherol)	Vitamin E, a fat-soluble vitamin, is an antioxidant that prevents the destruction of red blood cells by preventing fatty acids in the red blood cells from taking on too much oxygen. It stimulates the production of an enzyme necessary to cell respiration and protects the cell membrane.
	Vitamin K	The naturally occurring form of vitamin K is fat soluble. However, many of the synthetic forms of vitamin K are water soluble. Vitamin K is involved in the formation of prothrombin and other blood clotting factors. Deficiency results in an increase in blood-clotting time.

HM3fAivp

	Pharmaceutical Name	Action & Use
General & Local Anesthetics	Nitrous oxide	Nitrous oxide, commonly called laughing gas, is used with oxygen in general anesthesia. Nitrous oxide may produce a condition during which the patient may laugh and become quite talkative. It is commonly used in dentistry or as a preinduction agent to other general anesthesias. **CAUTION!** High concentrations of nitrous oxide may cause cyanosis and asphyxia.
	Halothane (Fluothane®)	Halothane can be used for inhalation anesthesia in most operative procedures with patients of all ages. It is nonflammable and nonexplosive. Halothane is contraindicated in obstetrics or in patients with hepatic dysfunction.
	Ketamine hydrochloride (Ketalar®)	Ketamine hydrochloride is a fast-acting general anesthetic agent used as a preinduction agent or for procedures that do not require skeletal muscle relaxation. One significant effect of this agent is that when the patient begins to recover from the drug, they might experience psychological manifestations ranging from pleasant dream-like states to hallucinations to delirium accompanied by confusion and irrational behavior. The effects of these manifestations may be minimized by keeping aural and tactile stimuli to a minimum. Ketamine HCl is contraindicated for patients with hypertensive disease.
	Fentanyl and droperidol (Innovar®)	Fentanyl and droperidol is a combination of a narcotic (fentanyl) and a tranquilizers (droperidol). Because of the self-potentiating combination, it must be used with extreme caution in patients with any respiratory problems.
	Procaine hydrochloride (Novocain®)	Administered only by injection, procaine hydrochloride may be used for many types of anesthesia, including spinal anesthesia. It is available in various solutions for injection.
	Lidocaine hydrochloride (Xylocaine®)	Lidocaine HCl is the standard to which all other anesthetics are compared. Lidocaine HCl may be combined with epinephrine for vasoconstrictive effects. Lidocaine is also used to treat myocardial infarctions to prevent or suppress preventicular contractions. **CAUTION!** Total dosage injected in 24 hours should not exceed 0.05 g per patient when used with epinephrine.

HM3fAivq

	Pharmaceutical Name	Action & Use
General & Local Anesthetics (cont.)	Dibucaine (Nupercainal®)	Dibucaine is used as a topical local anesthetic on mucous membranes and may also be administered parenterally.
	Proparacaine (Ophthetic®, Ophthaine®)	This is a local ophthalmic anesthetic used topically. It is suited for almost every opthalmic procedure. Proparacaine is fairly long lasting.

	Pharmaceutical Name	Action & Use
Oxytocics	Ergonovine maleate (Ergotrate Maleate®)	Ergonovine maleate is used in the prevention and treatment of postpartum and postabortal hemorrhage.
	Oxytocin (Pitocin®)	Oxytocin is indicated for the initiation or improvement of uterine contractions or to control postpartum hemorrhage.

HM3fAivr

APPENDIX V

GLOSSARY

The following terms are explained as used in this manual and as commonly defined.

ABDUCTION—Moving an extremity away from the body.

ABRASION—An area of skin or mucous membrane worn from the body mechanically by some unusual or abnormal process.

ABSCESS—A localized collection of pus.

ACIDOSIS—A condition resulting from acid accumulating in the body.

ADDUCTION—Bringing an extremity toward the body.

ADIPOSE—Of a fatty nature.

ADRENERGIC—Activated by, characteristic of, or secreting epinephrine or similar substance.

ABSORBENT—A drug which "takes up" other substances by absorption.

ADSORPTION—The attachment of one substance to the surface of another.

AEROBIC—Growing only in the presence of oxygen.

AFFECT—*(n.)* Feeling experienced in connection with an emotion.

ALBUMINURIA—Albumin in the urine.

ALIMENTARY—Pertaining to food or digestion.

ALKALOSIS—A pathogenic condition resulting from accumulation of base in, or loss of acid from, the body.

AMBULATORY—Walking or able to walk.

ANABOLISM—The constructive process by which the simple products of digestion are converted by living cells into more complex compounds and living matter for cellular growth and repair.

ANAEROBIC—Growing only in the absence of oxygen.

ANALGESIC—A drug used to relieve pain without producing unconsciousness or impairing mental capacities.

ANATOMY—The science of the structure of the body and the relationship of its parts to each other.

ANEMIA—A decrease in certain elements of the blood, especially red cells and hemoglobin.

ANESTHESIOLOGIST—A physician who specializes in anesthesiology.

ANESTHESIOLOGY—A branch of medicine that studies anesthesia and anesthetics.

ANESTHETIST—A registered nurse trained in administering anesthetics.

ANISOCORIA—Unequal diameter of the pupils.

ANODYNE—A drug that relieves pain.

ANOREXIA—Loss of appetite.

ANTHELMINTIC—A drug that expels, paralyzes, or kills intestinal worms.

ANTIBIOTIC—A synthetic product or a product of living microorganisms that kills or inhibits the growth of undesirable microorganisms.

ANTIDOTE—An agent that counteracts a poison.

ANTIGEN—A substance which, under certain conditions, is capable of inducing the formation of antibodies and reacting specifically with the antibodies in a detectable manner.

ANTIPYRETIC—A drug that lowers elevated body temperature.

ANTISEPTIC—A drug or chemical that inhibits the growth of microorganisms without necessarily destroying them.

APNEA—A temporary cessation of breathing.

ARTICULATION—The place of union or junction between two or more bones of the skeleton.

ASEPTIC—Clean; free of pathogenic organisms.

ASTRINGENT—A drug or preparation that produces shrinkage of body membranes, especially mucous membranes.

ASYMPTOMATIC—Having no symptoms.

AUSCULTATION—The act of listening for sounds within the body, with or without a stethoscope.

AUTOLYSIS—The spontaneous disintegration of tissues or cells by the action of their own serum or enzymes, such as occurs after death and in some pathological conditions.

AVULSED—A forcible separation; also, a part torn from another.

AXILLARY—Pertaining to the area of the armpit.

BACTERICIDE—An agent that destroys bacteria.

BACTERIOSTATIC—An agent that inhibits the growth of bacteria.

BIOLOGICALS—Medicinal preparations made from living organisms and their products, including serums, vaccines, antigens, and antitoxins.

BLANCHING—Turning white.

BLEB—Blister, bubble.

BRADYCARDIA—Abnormally slow heartbeat, evidenced by a pulse rate of 60 or less.

BRADYPNEA—Abnormally slow breathing.

BUBO—An inflamed swelling of a lymphatic gland, especially in the area of the armpit or groin.

BUCCAL—Referring to the cheek.

CARRIER—A person or animal that harbors specific infectious agents in the absence of discernible clinical disease, and serves as a potential source of infection for humans.

CASTS—Urinary sediments formed by coagulation of albuminous material in the kidney tubules.

CATABOLISM—A destructive process in which the complex compounds of the digestive process are reduced to more simple substances.

CATHARTICS—Drugs that promote bowel movement.

CERVICAL—Pertaining to the neck or the neck of any organ or structure.

CHEYNE-STOKES—Breathing characterized by alternating periods of apnea and deep respirations.

COAGULATION—Clotting.

COAPTATION—To fit together, as the edges of a wound or the ends of a fractured bone; category of splint.

COCCYX—Tailbone.

COLATION—The process of straining or filtration.

COMMUNICABLE—Capable of being transmitted from one person to another.

COMMUNICABLE PERIOD—The period of time in which an infectious agent may be passed from an infected animal or man to a receptive host. There may be more than one such period of time during the course of disease.

COMMINUTION—The process of physical reduction of a substance to fine particle size.

CONTACT—A person or animal known to have been associated with an infected person or animal, or a contaminated environment, and to have had the opportunity to acquire the infection.

CONTAMINATION—The presence of an infectious agent or toxin on the surface of a body or inanimate article, such as clothing, dishes, surgical dressings or instruments, as well as in food or water.

CONTRACTURE—A condition of muscle shortening and fibrous tissue development that results in a permanent joint deformity.

CONTUSION—A bruise.

CORROSIVE—A substance that rapidly destroys or decomposes body tissue at point of contact.

CREPITUS—The cracking or grating sound produced by fragments of fractured bones rubbing together.

DEBILITY—The state of abnormal bodily weakness.

DEBRIDEMENT—The removal of all foreign matter and devitalized tissue in or about a wound.

DECANTATION—Separating liquids from solids by letting the solids settle to the bottom and pouring off the liquid.

DECEREBRATE—A person with brain damage that produces certain abnormal neurologic signs.

DECORTICATION—Removing portions of the cortical substance of a structure or organ, such as the brain, kidney, or lung.

DECUBITUS ULCER—Bed or pressure sore.

DESQUAMATE—To shed, peel, or scale off.

DIASTOLE—The dilation or period of dilation of the heart, especially of the ventricles.

DIATHERMY—The generation of heat in tissue by electric current for medical or surgical purposes.

DISINFECTION—The killing of infectious agents outside the body by physical or chemical means applied directly.

concurrent—Done during the treatment of a patient with a communicable disease.

terminal—Done after a patient has been discharged or transferred.

DISINFESTATION—A physical or chemical means of destroying animal or insect pests in a particular area.

DISTILLATION—Converting a liquid to a vapor by applying heat and condensing the vapor back to liquid by cooling.

DIURESIS—Urine excretion in excess of the usual amount.

DIURETICS—Drugs that increase the secretion of urine.

DYSPNEA—Labored or difficult breathing.

ECCHYMOSIS—A small hemorrhagic spot, larger than a petechia, in the skin or mucous membrane, forming a nonelevated, rounded or irregular, blue or purplish patch.

ELECTROLYTE—A substance that dissociates into ions in solution or when fused, thereby becoming capable of conducting electricity.

ELIXIR—An aromatic, sweetened, hydroalcoholic solution containing medicinal substances.

EMBOLUS—A clot or other plug brought by the blood from another vessel and forced into a smaller one, thereby obstructing circulation.

EMETIC—A substance that causes vomiting.

EMOLLIENT—A drug that softens, soothes, or smooths the skin or irritated surfaces.

EMULSION—A liquid preparation containing two unmixable liquids, such as oil and water, one of which is dispersed as globules in the other.

ENCAPSULATED—Enclosed within a capsule.

ENDEMIC—The constant presence of a disease in a given locality.

ENTERIC—Of or within the intestine.

EPIDEMIC—The outbreak of disease in a geographic area in excess of normal expectations.

EPIDEMIOLOGY—The study of epidemics and epidemic diseases.

EPISTAXIS—Nosebleed.

EPIZOOTIC—Attacking many animals in a region at the same time.

ERADICATE—Wipe out; destroy.

ERYTHEMA—Redness.

ERYTHROCYTE—Red blood cell.

EUPNEA—Ordinary, quiet breathing.

EUTAXIA—The liquification of solids mixed in a dry state.

EXSANGUINATION—Extensive loss of blood due to hemorrhage, either internal or external.

EXTENSION—Straightening or unbending, as in straightening the forearm, leg, or fingers.

EXTRAVASATION—A discharge or escape, such as blood from a vessel into the tissue.

EXTRICATION—The process of freeing a victim, such as from a wrecked car or flooded compartment.

FLEXION—Bending, as in bending an arm or leg.

FOMITE—An object, such as a book, wooden object, or an article of clothing, that is not in itself harmful, but is able to harbor pathogenic microorganisms and thus may serve as an agent of transmission of an infection.

FUMIGATION—The destruction of disease-producing animals or insects by gaseous agents.

FUNGICIDE—A drug that kills fungus.

FURUNCLE—An abscess in the true skin caused by the entry of microorganisms through a hair follicle or sweat gland.

FUSION—Melting.

GASTROSTOMY—A surgical opening from the external surface of the body into the stomach, usually for inserting a feeding tube.

GAVAGE—Introducing a substance into the stomach through a tube.

GERMICIDE—An agent that kills germs.

GESTATION—The period of carrying developing offspring in the uterus after conception.

GLYCOSURIA—Glucose in the urine.

GRAM-NEGATIVE—A microorganism that does not retain Gram's crystal violet and is stained by the counterstain.

GRAM-POSITIVE—A microorganism that is stained by Gram's crystal violet.

HEMACYTOMETER—An instrument for estimating the number of blood cells in a measured volume of blood.

HEMATEMESIS—Vomiting bright red blood.

HEMATOCRIT—A determination of the volume percentage of red blood cells in whole blood.

HEMIPLEGIA—Loss of motion and sensation of one side of the body.

HEMOGLOBIN—Iron containing red pigment (heme) combined with a protein substance (globin).

HEMOLYSIN—Substance that breaks down red blood cells, thereby liberating hemoglobin.

HEMOPTYSIS—Coughing up bright red blood.

HEMOSTATICS—Drugs that control external bleeding by forming an artificial clot.

HISTOLOGY—The microscopic study of tissue structure.

HOST—A man or other living animal affording subsistence or lodgment to an infectious agent under natural conditions.

HYDROTHERAPY—The scientific use of water in the treatment of disease.

HYPERGLYCEMIA—Abnormally increased content of sugar in the blood.

HYPERPNEA—Increased rate and depth of breathing.

HYPERTENSION—High blood pressure.

HYPERTHERMIA—Abnormally high body temperature, especially that induced for therapeutic purposes.

HYPOGLYCEMIA—Low blood sugar.

HYPOPNEA—Abnormal shallowness and rapidity of breathing.

HYPOSTASIS—Poor or stagnant circulation in a dependent part of the body or organ, as in venous insufficiency.

HYPOTENSION—Low blood pressure.

HYPOTHERMIA—Abnormally low body temperature.

HYPOVOLEMIA—Abnormally decreased volume of circulating fluid (plasma) in the body.

HYPOXIA—Low oxygen content or tension; deficiency of oxygen in the inspired air.

IMMISCIBLE—Incapable of being mixed.

IMMUNE PERSON—An individual who does not develop clinical illness when exposed to specific infectious agents of a disease, due to the presence of specific antibodies or cellular immunity.

IMMUNITY—A defense mechanism of the body which renders it resistant to certain organisms.

INAPPARENT INFECTION—An infection with no detectable clinical symptoms, even though the causative infectious agent may be identifiable with laboratory examinations. It is also known as an asypmtomatic or subclinical infection.

INCIDENCE RATE—The number of specific disease cases diagnosed and reported in a specific population in a defined period of time. It is usually expressed as cases per 1,000 or 100,000 annually.

INCISION—A cut, or a wound produced by cutting with a sharp instrument.

INCOMPATIBLE—Not suitable for combination or simultaneous administration.

INCONTINENT—Unable to control excretory functions.

INCUBATION PERIOD—The period of time between the initial exposure to an infectious agent and the first clinical symptoms of the disease.

INDURATION—An abnormally hard spot or place.

INFECTION—A condition resulting when pathogens enter body tissues, multiply, and cause injury to cells.

INFECTIOUS AGENT—An organism capable of producing infection or disease.

INFECTIOUS DISEASE—A disease of man and animal resulting from an infection.

INFESTATION—The establishment and multiplication of small animals or arthropods (especially insects and rodents) on the body, clothing, or habitat of individuals or animals.

INGUINAL—Pertaining to the abdomen.

INSTRUCTION—A directive containing authority or information having continued reference value or requiring continuing action.

INTEGUMENTARY (SYSTEM)—The skin and its accessory structures, including hair and nails.

INTRADERMAL—Into the dermis.

INUNCTION—Rubbing in.

ISCHEMIA—The lack of blood supply to specific areas due to constriction or obstruction in the blood vessels.

ISOLATION—Procedures taken to separate infected persons or animals, dispose of their secretions, and disinfect or sterilize the supplies, equipment, utensils, etc., used for their care, in order to prevent the spread of disease to susceptible persons or animals. Different procedures may be required for the specific infectious agent involved.

ISOTONIC—A solution having the same salinity as whole blood.

KERATOLYTIC—Removes horny layers of epidermis.

LACERATED—Torn.

LACERATION—A wound made by tearing and resulting in jagged edges.

LACRIMATION—The secretion of tears.

LACRIMATORS—Tear gases.

LACTATION—The production of milk.

LATENT—Concealed; not manifest; potential.

LAVAGE—The irrigation or washing out of an organ (such as the stomach or bowel).

LESION—Any pathological or traumatic discontinuity of tissue or loss of function of a part.

LEUKOCYTE—White blood cell.

LEUKOCYTOSIS—Abnormally high white blood cell count.

LEUKOPENIA—Abnormally low white blood cell count.

LEVIGATION—Adding a small amount of liquid to a mortar and pestle while triturating.

LIGAMENT—A sheet or band of tough, fibrous tissue connecting two or more bones or cartilages, or supporting an organ, fascia, or muscle.

LINIMENT—Solution or mixture of various substances in oily, alcoholic, or emulsified form, intended for external application.

LUMBAR—Pertaining to the part of the back between the thorax and the pelvis.

LYOPHILIZATION—The creation of a stable preparation of a biological substance (blood plasma, serum, etc.) by rapid freezing and dehydration of the frozen product under high vacuum.

MACERATION—Softening of a solid by soaking.

MAGMAS—Thick, creamy, aqueous suspensions of inorganic substances in a very fine state.

MALAISE—A vague feeling of bodily discomfort.

MASTICATION—Chewing.

MEDICAL ASEPTIC TECHNIQUE—The practice that prevents the spread of pathogens from person to person, place to place, or place to person.

MELENA—Excretion of black tarry stools.

METABOLISM—The sum of all the physical and chemical processes by which living organized substance is produced and maintained. Also, the transformation by which energy is made available to the organism.

METAMORPHOSIS—Change of shape or structure, particularly a transition from one development stage to another, as from larva to adult form.

METROLOGY—The science of weights and measures.

MICROORGANISM—A minute, living organism invisible to the naked eye.

MICTURATION—Voiding; urinating.

MORBIDITY RATE—An incidence rate that includes all persons in a particular population who become ill during a specific period of time.

MORPHOLOGY—The science of forms and structure of organized beings.

MORTALITY RATE—The number of deaths, reported in a particular population, over a specific period of time, divided by the total population, reported as deaths per 1,000 population. If the deaths are from one cause, then it is known as a disease-specific mortality rate.

MOTTLED—Marked with blotches or spots of different colors or shades.

MUCUS—A sticky substance secreted by mucous membranes.

MYDRIATIC—Any drug that dilates the pupil.

MYELIN—A lipid substance that forms a sheath around certain nerve fibers.

MYELINATED—Covered with a myelin sheath.

NECROSIS—The death of tissue, usually in small, localized areas.

NOSOCOMIAL—Originating in a hospital.

NOTICE—A directive of a one-time or limited nature that has a self-canceling provision and the same force or effect as an instruction.

NUTRITION—The total process of providing the body with nutriments, and assimilating and using them.

OINTMENT—A semisolid, fatty, or oily preparation of medicinal substances for external application.

OLFACTORY—Pertaining to the sense of smell.

OLIGEMIA—Deficiency in the volume of blood.

OPHTHALMIC—Pertaining to the eye.

ORGANISM—Any living thing.

OSMOSIS—The diffusion of fluids through a membrane or porous partition.

OSSIFICATION—Changing or developing into bone.

OXIDATION—The union of a substance with oxygen.

PALPABLE—Capable of being touched or felt.

PALPITATION—An abnormal, rapid, regular or irregular beating of the heart, felt by the patient.

PARAPLEGIA—Loss of motion and sensation of the lower half of the body.

PARASITICIDES—Drugs that kill parasites.

PARENTERAL—Administration of drugs by injection.

PARESIS—Slight or partial paralysis.

PAROXYSM—A sudden attack, or intensification of the symptoms of a disease, usually recurring periodically.

PATHOGEN—An organism capable of producing disease or causing infections.

PATHOGENICITY—The capability of an infectious agent to cause disease in a susceptible host.

PERCUSSION—The act of striking a body part with short, sharp blows as an aid in diagnosing the condition by evaluating the sound obtained.

PERIPHERAL—Outward part or surface.

PERSISTENT—Stubborn; persevering.

PETECHIA—(*pl.* petechiae) A round pinpoint, nonraised, purplish red spot caused by hemorrhage in the skin.

pH—Scale measuring the acidity or alkalinity of a solution.

PHAGOCYTOSIS—The ingestion and destruction by phagocytes of cells, microorganisms, and other foreign matter in the blood or tissue.

PHARMACOGNOSY—The study of the action of drugs and their uses.

PHYSIOLOGICAL—Characteristic of or appropriate to an organism's functioning.

PLEXUS—Network.

PRECIPITATION—The quality or state of being separated from solution or suspension by chemical or physical change, usually as an insoluble amorphous or crystalline solid.

PRONE—Lying face down.

PROPHYLACTIC—The prevention of disease; preventive treatment.

PROPORTION—Two equal ratios considered simultaneously.

PROSTRATION—Utter exhaustion.

PRURITIS—Intense itching.

PSYCHOLOGICAL—Belonging to or of the nature of psychology; the mental process.

PURULENT—Pus filled or containing pus.

PUSTULE—A small, inflamed elevation of the skin containing pus.

QUADRAPLEGIA—Loss of motion and sensation below the neck.

RALES—An abnormal sound, either moist or dry, classified by location (e.g., bronchial rales, laryngeal rales).

RATIO—The relationship of one quantity to another of like units.

RESERVOIR—A carrier on which an infectious agent depends primarily for survival.

RESISTANCE—The sum total of body mechanisms that provide barriers to the invasion of infectious agents or their toxic products.

RHINORRHEA—The free discharge of a thin nasal mucus.

RHONCHUS—(*pl.* rhoncii) A rattling throat sound due to partial obstruction; a dry coarse rale in the bronchial tubes.

SACRUM—Triangular bone just below the lumbar vertebrae.

SANITIZATION—The process of cleaning with soap and water or boiling to reduce the number of organisms to a safe level.

SEPSIS—The growth of pathogens in living tissue.

SERUM—(*pl.* serums *or* sera) The watery portion of an animal fluid remaining after coagulation; plasma minus the clotting proteins and clotting cells.

SHOCK—Collapse of the cardiovascular system, characterized by circulatory deficiency and depression of vital functions.

SOLUBILITY—The ability of a solid to dissolve in a given amount of solvent.

SPIRITS—Alcoholic or hydroalcoholic solutions of volatile substances.

SPORE—A microorganism in a resting or dormant state that renders it highly resistant to destruction.

SPRAIN—Injury to the ligaments and soft tissues that support a joint.

STERILE—Free of all living organisms.

STERILIZATION—The process of destroying all organisms on a substance or article by exposure to physical or chemical agents; the process by which all organisms, including spores, are destroyed.

STERNUNTATORS—Vomiting agents.

STERTOROUS—Snoring-type breathing sound.

STRAIN—Forcible overstretching or tearing of a muscle or tendon.

STRIATED—Striped or streaked.

STRIDOR—A harsh, high-pitched respiratory sound such as the inspiratory sound often heard in acute laryngeal obstruction.

SUBCUTANEOUS—Under the skin.

SUBLINGUAL—Under the tongue.

SUPERFICIAL—Of or pertaining to the surface, lying on, not penetrating below.

SUPINE—Lying on the back.

SURGICAL ASEPTIC TECHNIQUE—The practice that renders and keeps objects and areas free from all organisms.

SURGICALLY CLEAN—Clean but not sterile.

SUSCEPTIBLE—Not resistant. A person or animal who may acquire an infection or disease when exposed to a specific agent, because his or her resistance to the agent is lacking or reduced.

SUSPECT—A person who may have acquired a communicable disease; it is indicated by the medical history and clinical presentation.

SUSPENSION—A coarse dispersion of finely divided insoluble material suspended in a liquid medium.

SYNCOPE—Faintness or actual fainting.

SYNERGIST—A medicine that aids or cooperates with another.

SYRUP—Concentrated aqueous solutions of sucrose, containing flavoring or medicinal substances.

TACHYCARDIA—Excessively rapid heart beat, usually over 100.

TAENIAFUGE—A drug that expels tapeworms without necessarily killing them.

TENDON—A fibrous cord by which a muscle is attached to the skeleton.

THORACIC—Pertaining to or affecting the chest.

THROMBUS—A plug or clot in a blood vessel or in one of the cavities of the heart, formed by coagulation of the blood. It remains where it was formed.

TINCTURE—Usually an alcoholic solution of animal or vegetable drugs.

TINNITUS—Ringing in the ears.

TOXEMIA—Poisonous products in the blood.

TOXICOLOGY—The science of poisons.

TOXINS—Poisons.

TRACHEOSTOMY—Surgically creating an opening into the trachea.

TRIAGE—Sorting casualties to determine priority of treatment.

TRITURATION—A process of reducing a solid to a very fine powder by grinding in a mortar and pestle.

URTICARIA—Hives or welts.

UREMIA—A condition resulting from waste products not being removed efficiently by the kidneys so that they remain in the blood.

VASCULAR—Pertaining to blood vessels.

VASOCONSTRICTOR—An agent that constricts the blood vessels.

VASODILATOR—An agent that dilates the blood vessels.

VERMICIDE—A drug that expels worms without necessarily killing them.

VESICANT—A blistering drug or agent.

VESICATION—The process of blistering.

VESICLE—A small blister.

VIRULENCE—The degree of pathogenicity of a microorganism or its ability to invade the tissues of the host.

WATERS—Aqueous solutions of volatile substances.

APPENDIX VI

TRADEMARK COMPANIES

The following is a list of trademarks used in this manual.

ACE®	Becton Dickinson and Company
Achromycin®	Lederle Labs
Actifed®	Warner-Lambert Co.
Adrenalin Chloride®	Parke-Davis
Afrin®	Schering-Plough
Aftate®	Schering-Plough
All-Bran®	Kellogg's®, a registered trademark of Kellogg Company
Amoxil®	SmithKline Beecham
Amphojel®	Wyeth-Ayerst
Anaprox®	Roche Laboratories
Ancef®	SmithKline Beecham
Antiminth®	Pfizer
Antivert®	Pfizer
Aralen®	Sanofi
Atarax®	Pfizer
Bactrim®	Roche Laboratories
Benadryl®	Warner-Lambert Co.
Betadine®	Purdue Frederick
Betapen-VK®	Mead Johnson
Bicillin®	Wyeth-Ayerst
Bleph-10®	Allergan
Bonine®	Pfizer
Bran Buds®	Kellogg's®, a registered trademark of Kellogg Company
Bran Flakes®	Post®, a registered trademark of Kraft Foods Inc.
Cardizem®	Hoechst Marion Roussel

Ceftin®	Glaxo Wellcome
Chlor-Trimeton®	Schering-Plough
CIDEX®	Johnson & Johnson Medical, Inc.
Claforan®	Hoechst Marion Roussel
Cleocin®	Pharmacia & Upjohn
Colace®	Roberts
Compazine®	SmithKline Beecham
Coumadin®	DuPont
Darvon®	Teva Pharmaceuticals USA
Demerol HCl®	Sanofi
Desenex®	Novartis
Desoxyn®	Abbott Pharmaceutical
Dexedrine®	SmithKline Beecham
Diamox®	Lederle Labs
Dilantin®	Parke-Davis
Dispenstir®	Hynson, Westcott, and Dunning, Inc.
Domeboro®	Bayer Corporation
Dramamine®	Pharmacia & Upjohn
Dulcolax®	Novartis Consumer
Dyazide®	SmithKline Beecham
Dynapen®	Bristol-Myers Squibb
Dyrenium®	SmithKline Beecham
E-Mycin®	Knoll Labs
Ecotrin®	SmithKline Beecham
Elavil®	Zeneca
Elimite®	Herbert Pharma
Entex®LA	Proctor & Gamble Pharmaceuticals
Equanil®	Wyeth-Ayerst
Ergotrate® Maleate	Lilly
Eryc®	Warner Chilcott Professional Products
Esidrix®	Ciba-Geigy Pharmaceutical

Eskalith®	SmithKline Beecham
Eurax®	Westwood-Squibb
Ex-Lax®	Novartis Consumer
Fansidar®	Roche Laboratories
Feldene®	Pfizer
Flagyl®	Searle
Flexeril®	Merck
Fluothane®	Wyeth-Ayerst
Fulvicin®	Schering
Gantrisin®	Roche Laboratories
Gentamycin®	Boehringer Ingelheim
Gris-PEG®	Allergan
Haldol®	Ortho-McNeil Pharmaceutical
HydroDIURIL®	Merck
Hygroton®	Rhone-Poulenc Rorer
Ilotycin®	Dista
Indocin®	Merck
Innovar®	Janssen
Isoptin®	Knoll Labs
Isordil®	Wyeth-Ayerst
Kaopectate®	Pharmacia & Upjohn
Keflex®	Dista
Kefzol®	Lilly
Ketalar®	Parke-Davis
Lanoxin®	Glaxo Wellcome
Lasix®	Hoechst Marion Roussel
Librium®	Roche Products
Lithonate®	Solvay
Lomotil®	Searle
Lotrimin®	Schering-Plough
Luminal®	Bayer Corporation

Maalox®	Novartis Consumer
Maxzide®	Bertek
Medicut®	American Diagnostic Corporation
Mefoxin®	Merck
Mellaril®	Novartis Pharmaceuticals
Metamucil®	Proctor & Gamble
Micatin®	McNeil Consumer Products
Minocin®	Lederle Labs
Mintezol®	Merck
Monistat®	Ortho Dermatalogical
Monosticon DRI-DOT®	Organon Teknika Corporation
Motrin®	McNeil Consumer
Multistix®	Ames Company, a division of Miles Laboratories, Inc.
Mycelex®	Bayer
Mycifradin® Sulfate	Pharmacia & Upjohn
Mycostatin®	Westwood-Squibb
Mylanta®	Johnson & Johnson-Merck
Nebcin®	Lilly
Nembutal®	Abbott
Neo-Synephrine®	Sanofi
Nitro-Bid®	Hoechst Marion Roussel
Nitrostat®	Parke-Davis
Norgesic®	3M
Novocain®	Sanofi Winthrop Pharmaceuticals
Nupercainal®	Ciba-Geigy
One Step II Wright-Giemsa Stain Solution®	Criterion Sciences, a division of Cornwell Corporation
Ophthaine®	Bristol-Myers Squibb
Ophthetic®	Allergan
Oretic®	Abbott
Parafon Forte DSC®	Ortho-McNeil Pharmaceutical

PCE Dispertab®	Abbott
Pen-Vee K®	Wyeth-Ayerst
Persantine®	Boehringer Ingelheim
pHisoHex®	Sanofi
Pitocin®	Parke-Davis
Polycillin®	Mead Johnson
Primaquine® Phosphate	Sanofi Winthrop Pharmaceuticals
Procan SR®	Parke-Davis
Pronestyl®	Bristol-Myers Squibb Company
Prozac®	Dista
Pyridium®	Parke-Davis Pharmaceuticals, a division of Warner-Lambert Co.
Restoril®	Novartis
Rifampin®	Hoechst Marion Roussel
Ritalin®	Novartis
Robaxin®	Robins
Robitussin DM® **Robitussin AC®**	Whitehall-Robins Healthcare, a division of American Home Products Corporation
Sani-Supp®	Sandoz
Seconal®	Lilly
Septra®	Glaxo Wellcome
Shredded Wheat®	Post®, a registered trademark of Kraft Food Inc.
Silvadene Cream®	Hoechst Marion Roussel
Sodium Sulamyd®	E. Fougera & Co., a division of Altana Inc.
Sorbitate®	Zeneca
Sudafed®	Warner-Lambert Co.
Sumycin®	Apothecon
Surfak®	Hoechst-Roussel
Sus-Phrine®	Forest
Tagamet®	SmithKline Beecham
Talwin®	Sanofi Winthrop Pharmaceuticals
Thorazine®	SmithKline Beecham

Tinactin®	Schering-Plough
Tolectin®	Ortho-McNeil Pharmaceutical
Trobicin®	Pharmacia & Upjohn
Tylenol®	McNeil Consumer
Unopette® Microcollection System	Becton-Dickinson, a division of Becton, Dickinson and Company
V-Cillin K®	Eli Lilly
Valium®	Roche Products
Vancocin®	Lilly
Vermox®	Janssen
Vibramycin®	Pfizer
Visine Eye Drops®	Pfizer
Vistaril®	Pfizer
Virtual Naval Hospital™	A trademark of The University of Iowa
Wycillin®	Wyeth-Ayerst
Xylocaine®	Astra
Zantac®	Glaxo Wellcome
Zinacef®	Glaxo Wellcome

REFERENCES

NOTE: Although the following references were current when this NRTC was published, their continued currency cannot be assured. Therefore, you need to be sure that you are studying the latest revision.

1995 Accreditation Manual for Hospitals, Joint Commission on Accreditation of Healthcare Organizations, Oakbrook Terrace, IL, 1995.

2000 Emergency Response Guidebook (ERG), RSPA P5800.8, Department of Transportation, Washington, DC, 2000.

Afloat Supply Procedures, NAVSUP P-485, Commander, Naval Supply Systems Command, Mechanicsburg, PA, October 1997.

Ambulance Support, BUMEDINST 6700.42, Chief, Bureau of Medicine and Surgery, Washington, DC, February 1995.

AMPCOR Syphilis RPR, AMPCOR, Bridgeport, NJ. [Product brochure.]

Bacto Gram Stain Set, DIFCO Laboratories, Detroit, MI, 1994. [Product brochure.]

Balows, Albert, ed. in chief, and William J. Hausler, Jr., Kenneth L. Hermann, Henry D. Isenberg, and H. Jean Shadomy, eds., *Manual of Clinical Microbiology*, 5th ed., American Society for Microbiology, Washington, DC, 1991.

Bates, Barbara J., et al, *A Guide to Physical Examination and History Taking*, 6th ed., J.B. Lippincott, Philadelphia, 1995.

Brown, Barbara A., *Hematology: Principles and Procedures*, 6th ed., Lea & Febiger, Philadelphia, PA, 1993.

Browner, Bruce D., Lenworth M. Jacobs, and Andrew N. Pollack, *Emergency Care and Transportation of the Sick and Injured*, 7th ed., Jones & Bartlett Publishers, Sudbury, MA, 1998.

Bureau of Medicine and Surgery (BUMED) Navy Occupational and Health (NAVOSH) Program, BUMEDINST 5100.13A, Chief, Bureau of Medicine and Surgery, Washington, DC, December 1996.

Chandra, Nisha C., and Mary F. Hazinski, eds., *Basic Life Support for Healthcare Providers*, American Heart Association, Dallas, TX, 1994.

Civilian Health and Medical Program of the Uniformed Services (CHAMPUS) Regulation, NAVMEDCOMINST 6320.18, Commander, Naval Medical Command, Washington, DC, October 1988.

Competence for Duty Examinations, Evaluations of Sobriety, and Other Bodily Views and Intrusions Performed by Military Personnel, BUMEDINST 6120.20B, Chief, Bureau of Medicine and Surgery, Washington, DC, 1982.

Damage Controlman 3&2, NAVEDTRA 10572, Naval Education and Training Professional Development and Technology Center, Pensacola, FL, May 1986.

Decedent Affairs Manual, NAVMEDCOMINST 5360.1, Commander, Naval Medical Command, Washington, DC, September 1987.

Dental Infection Control Program, BUMEDINST 6600.10A, Chief, Bureau of Medicine and Surgery, Washington, DC, August 1992.

Dental Technician Training Manual, Vol. 1, NAVEDTRA 12572, Naval Education and Training Professional Development and Technology Center, Pensacola, FL, October 1999.

Dental Technician Training Manual, Vol. 2, NAVEDTRA 12573, Naval Education and Training Professional Development and Technology Center, Pensacola, FL, October 1999.

Department of the Navy (DON) Anthrax Vaccination Implementation Program (AVIP), SECNAVINST 6230.4, Secretary of the Navy, Washington, DC, April 1998.

Department of the Navy Correspondence Manual, SECNAVINST 5216.5D, Secretary of the Navy, Washington, DC, May 1998.

Department of the Navy Disability Evaluation Manual, SECNAVINST 1850.4D, Secretary of the Navy, Washington, DC, December 1998.

Department of the Navy File Maintenance Procedures and Standard Subject Identification Codes (SSIC), SECNAVINST 5210.11D, Secretary of the Navy, Washington, DC, October 1987.

Department of the Navy Freedom of Information Act (FOIA) Program, SECNAVINST 5720.42F, Secretary of the Navy, Washington, DC, January 1999.

Department of the Navy Privacy Act (PA) Program, SECNAVINST 5211.5D, Secretary of the Navy, Washington, DC, July 1992.

Dorland's Illustrated Medical Dictionary, 27th ed., W. B. Saunders Company, Philadelphia, PA, 1988.

Drug and Alcohol Abuse Prevention and Control, OPNAVINST 5350.4C, Chief of Naval Operations, Washington, DC, April 2000.

Drug Facts and Comparisons, 1996 edition, J. B. Lippincott, Philadelphia, PA, 1996.

Ellenhorn, Matthew J., *Ellenhorn's Medical Toxicology : Diagnosis and Treatment of Human Poisoning*, Lippincott, Williams & Wilkins, Philadelphia, PA, 1997.

Emergency War Surgery NATO Handbook, NAVMED P-5059, United States Department of Defense, Washington, DC, 1988.

Family Advocacy Program, BUMEDINST 6320.70, Chief, Bureau of Medicine and Surgery, Washington, DC, June 1999.

Family Advocacy Program, SECNAVINST 1752.3A, Secretary of the Navy, Washington, DC, July 1996.

First Aid for Soldiers, App. A, FM21-11, Headquarters, Department of the Army, Washington, DC, 1988.

Forms and Reports Management Program, BUMEDINST 5210.9, Chief, Bureau of Medicine and Surgery, Washington, DC, August 1991.

Gennaro, Alfonso R., ed., *Remington: The Science and Practice of Pharmacy*, 19th ed., Mack Publishing Company, Easton, PA, 1995.

Goldfrank, Lewis R., Neal E. Flomenbaum, and Neal A. Lewin, *Goldfrank's Toxicologic Emergencies*, McGraw-Hill Professional Publishing, New York, NY, 1998.

Goodman, Louis S., Lee E. Limbird, and Joel G. Hardman, *Goodman & Gilman's The Pharmacological Basis of Therapeutics*, 9th ed., McGraw-Hill, New York, NY, 1996.

Graff, Sister Laurine, *A Handbook of Routine Urinalysis*, J. P. Lippincott, Co., Philadelphia, PA, 1983.

Gray's Anatomy, 37th ed., Churchill Livingston, Inc., New York, NY, 1989.

Guidelines for Controlled Substances Inventory, NAVMEDCOMINST 6710.9, Commander, Naval Medical Command, Washington, DC, May 1986.

Guthrie, Helen A., *Introductory Nutrition*, 7th ed., Times Mirror/Mosby College Publishing, St. Louis, MO, 1989.

Health Care Relations Program, BUMEDINST 6300.10, Chief, Bureau of Medicine and Surgery, Washington, DC, July 1996.

Henry, John B., *Clinical Diagnosis and Management by Laboratory Methods*, 18th ed., W. B. Saunders Company, Philadelphia, PA, 1991.

http://hazmat.dot.gov/gydebook.htm

http://www.tricare.osd.mil

http://www.vnh.org

Immunizations and Chemoprophylaxis, BUMEDINST 6230.15, Chief, Bureau of Medicine and Surgery, Washington, DC, November 1995.

Informed Consent for Medical and Dental Treatment, NAVMEDCOMINST 6320.16, Commander, Naval Medical Command, Washington, DC, August 1988.

Inhalants—The Silent Epidemic, National Inhalant Prevention Coalition, Austin, TX, 1999.

Isselbacher, Kurt J., Eugene Braunwald, Jean D. Wilson, Joseph B. Martin, Anthony S. Fauci, and Dennis L. Kasper, eds., *Harrison's Principles of Internal Medicine*, 13th ed., vols. 1 & 2, McGraw-Hill, Inc., New York, NY, 1994.

Kerschner, Velma L., *Nutrition and Diet Therapy*, 3rd ed., F. A. Davis Company, Philadelphia, PA, 1991.

Kubler-Ross, Elisabeth, M.D., *On Death and Dying: What the Dying Have to Teach Doctors, Nurses, Clergy, and Their Own Families*, Collier Books, New York, NY, 1969.

Leiken, Jerrold B., and Frank P. Paloucek, *Poisoning and Toxicology Compendium*, Lexi Comp, Hudson, OH, 1997.

M-M-R® II (Measles, Mumps, and Rubella Virus Vaccine Live), Merck & Co., Inc., West Point, PA, 1999. [Product insert.]

Management of Alleged or Suspected Sexual Assault and Rape Cases, NAVMEDCOMINST 6310.3, Commander, Naval Medical Command, Washington, DC, April 1989.

Management of Infectious Waste, BUMEDINST 6280.1A, Chief, Bureau of Medicine and Surgery, Washington, DC, June 1994.

Manual for Courts-Martial, Part 3, "Military Rule of Evidence 315, Military Cause/Search and Seizure"; and "Military Rule of Evidence 312, Body Views and Intrusions," United States Army Publishing Company, 1998.

Manual of Clinical Dietetics, 5th ed., The American Dietetic Association, 1996.

Manual of Naval Preventive Medicine, NAVMED P-5010, Chief, Bureau of Medicine and Surgery, Washington, DC, August 1999.

Manual of the Judge Advocate General, chap. 2, "Delivery of Patient Under Warrant of Arrest," and "Line of Duty Misconduct," JAGINST 5800.7A, Department of the Navy Judge Advocate General, Alexandria, VA, October 1990.

Manual of the Medical Department, NAVMED P-117, Chief, Bureau of Medicine and Surgery, Washington, DC, January 2000.

Marine Corps Warfighting Publication (MCWP) 4-11.1, Health Services Support Operations, chapter 3, Commandant, U.S. Marine Corps, Washington, DC, March 1998.

Medical and Dental Care for Eligible Persons at Navy Medical Department Facilities, NAVMEDCOMINST 6320.3B, Commander, Naval Medical Command, Washington, DC, May 1987.

Medical Augmentation Program (MAP), BUMEDINST 6440.5B, Chief, Bureau of Medicine and Surgery, Washington, DC, February 2000.

Medical, Dental, and Educational Suitability Screening and Exceptional Family Member Program (EFMP) Enrollment, BUMEDINST 1300.2, Chief, Bureau of Medicine and Surgery, Washington, DC, 2000.

Medical Support in Joint Operations, NAVMED P-5047, Chief, Bureau of Medicine and Surgery, Washington, DC, 1972.

Meeker, Margaret H., and Jane C. Rothrock, *Alexander's Care of the Patient in Surgery*, 10th ed., Mosby—Year Book, Inc., St. Louis, MO, 1995.

Military Requirements for Petty Officer Third Class, NAVEDTRA 12024, Naval Education and Training Professional Development and Technology Center, Pensacola, FL, 1999.

Military Substance Abuse Prevention and Control, SECNAVINST 5300.28C, Secretary of the Navy, Washington, DC, March 1999.

MILSTRIP/MILSTRAP Desk Guide, NAVSUP P-409, Commander, Naval Supply Systems Command, Mechanicsburg, PA, June 1998.

Mobile Medical Augmentation Readiness Team (MMART) Manual, BUMEDINST 6440.6, Chief, Bureau of Medicine and Surgery, Washington, DC, May 1993.

Mobile Medical Augmentation Readiness Team (MMART) Program, OPNAVINST 6440.1B, Chief of Naval Operations, Washington, DC, August 1991.

Monosticon DRI-DOT, Organon Teknika Corp., Durham, NC, 1986. [Product brochure.]

Morphia Dosage and Casualty Marking, BUMEDINST 6570.2, Chief, Bureau of Medicine and Surgery, Washington, DC, November 1994.

NATO Handbook on the Medical Aspects of NBC Defensive Operations, NAVMED P-5059.

Naval Ships' Technical Manuals, Commander, Naval Sea Systems Command, Arlington, VA.

Naval Supply Systems Command (NAVSUP) Manual, vols. 2 & 5, Commander, Naval Supply Systems Command, Mechanicsburg, PA, 1990.

Naval Warfare Publication: Deployable Health Service Support Platforms (NWP 4-02.4), Part A, Fleet Hospitals, Navy Tactical Support Activity, Washington, DC, August 1996.

Navy and Marine Corps Records Disposition Manual, SECNAVINST 5212.5D, Secretary of the Navy, Washington, DC, April 1998.

Navy Customer Service Manual, NAVEDTRA 12972, Naval Education and Training Professional Development and Technology Center, Pensacola, FL, 1993.

Navy Occupational Safety and Health (NAVOSH) Program Manual, OPNAVINST 5100.23E, Chief of Naval Operations, Washington, DC, January 1999.

Nosocomial Infection Control Program, BUMEDINST 6220.9A, Chief, Bureau of Medicine and Surgery, Washington, DC, September 1998.

O'Keefe, Michael F., ed., *Brady Emergency Care*, 8th ed., Prentice-Hall, Inc., Englewood Cliffs, NJ, 1998.

Occupational Noise Control and Hearing Conservation, NAVMEDCOMINST 6260.5, Commander, Naval Medical Command, Washington, DC, April 1984.

Olson, Kent R., *Poisoning and Drug Overdose*, 3rd ed., McGraw-Hill Professional Publishing, New York, NY, 1999.

One Step II Wright-Giesma Stain Solution, Criterion Sciences, division of Cornwell Corp., Riverdale, NJ, 1997. [Product brochure.]

Patient's Bill of Rights and Responsibilities, enclosure (5) to *Health Care Relations Program*, BUMEDINST 6300.10, Chief, Bureau of Medicine and Surgery, Washington, DC, July 1996.[9 Jul 96]

Physical Readiness Program, OPNAVINST 6110.1F, Chief of Naval Operations, Washington, DC, May 2000.

Physicians' Desk Reference, 53rd ed., Medical Economics Co., Montvale, NJ, 1999.

Poliovirus Vaccine Inactivated—IPOL®, Connaught Laboratories, Inc., Swiftwater, PA, 1997. [Product insert.]

Procedures for Administering and Treating Prisoners and Awardees, NAVMEDCOMINST 6320.11, Commander, Naval Medical Command, Washington, DC, October 1984.

Provision of Standbys During Medical Examinations, BUMEDINST 6320.83, Chief, Bureau of Medicine and Surgery, Washington, DC, November 1991.

Quality Assurance (QA) Program, BUMEDINST 6010.13, Chief, Bureau of Medicine and Surgery, Washington, DC, August 1991.

Recommended Dietary Allowances, 10th ed., Subcommittee on the Tenth Edition of the RDAs, Food and Nutrition Board, Commission on Life Sciences, National Research Council, 1989.

Risk Management Program, BUMEDINST 6010.21, Chief, Bureau of Medicine and Surgery, Washington, DC, October1996.

Sailing with TRICARE, for Sailors and Their Families, TRICARE, April 1999.

Schwartz, George R., ed. in chief, and C. Gene Cayten, Mary Anne Mangelsen, Thom A. Mayer, and Barbara K. Hanke, eds., *Principles and Practice of*

Emergency Medicine, 3rd ed., vols. 1 & 2, Lea & Febiger, Philadelphia, PA, 1992.

Seiverd, Charles E., *Hematology for Medical Technologists*, 5th ed., Lea & Febiger, Philadelphia, PA, 1983.

Sexual Assault Prevention and Response, SECNAVINST 1752.4, Secretary of the Navy, Washington, DC, September 1995.

Sexual Assault Victim Intervention (SAVI) Program, OPNAVINST 1752.1A, Chief of Naval Operations, Washington, DC, December 1993.

Shipboard Medical Procedures Manual, COMNAVSURFLANTINST 6000.1H, Commander, Naval Surface Force, U.S. Atlantic Fleet, Norfolk, VA, February 1997.

Standard First Aid Course, NAVEDTRA 13119, Chief, Bureau of Medicine and Surgery, Washington, DC.

Stoklosa, Mitchell J., and Howard C. Ansel, *Pharmaceutical Calculations*, 10th ed., Lea & Febiger, Media, PA, 1996.

The Merck Manual, 16th ed., Merck & Co., Inc., Rahway, NJ, 1992.

The Navy SEAL Nutrition Guide, Department of Military and Emergency Medicine, Uniformed Services University of Health Sciences, F. Edward Hébert School of Medicine, 1994.

Tilton, Richard C., Albert Balows, David C. Hohnadel, and Robert F. Reiss, eds., *Clinical Laboratory Medicine*, Mosby—Year Book, Inc., St. Louis, MO, 1992.

Timby, Barbara K., *Fundamental Skills and Concepts in Patient Care*, 6th ed., Lippincott-Raven Publishers, Philadelphia, PA, 1996.

Tobacco Use in Naval Medical Department Activities, BUMEDINST 6200.12, Chief, Bureau of Medicine and Surgery, Washington, DC, June 1990.

Treatment of Chemical Agent Casualties and Conventional Military Chemical Injuries, NAVMED P-5041.

Turgeon, Mary Louise, *Immunology and Serology in Laboratory Practice*, 2nd ed., Mosby—Year Book, Inc., St. Louis, MO, 1996.

Typhoid Vi Polysaccharide Vaccine, Connaught Laboratories, Inc., Swiftwater, PA, 1995. [Product insert.]

Unopette Microcollection System, Becton-Dickinson, division of Becton, Dickinson and Co., Rutherford, NJ, 1991. [Product brochure.]

Victim and Witness Assistance Program, SECNAVINST 5800.11A, Secretary of the Navy, Washington, DC, June 1995.

INDEX

Assignment Questions

Information: The text pages that you are to study are provided at the beginning of the assignment questions.

ASSIGNMENT 1

Textbook Assignment: "Anatomy and Physiology," pages 1-1 to 1-48.

1-1. When the body is in the anatomical position, the thumbs point

1. medially
2. laterally
3. anteriorly
4. posteriorly

1-2. A person lying on his/her back is in what position?

1. Prone
2. Erect
3. Supine
4. Lateral recumbent

1-3. The physical and chemical breakdown of the food we eat is called

1. digestion
2. metabolism
3. anabolism
4. catabolism

1-4. The transfer of fluids across the plasma membrane of a cell from an area of lower concentration to an area of higher concentration is a process known as

1. infusion
2. diffusion
3. perfusion
4. osmosis

1-5. Homeostasis is defined as

1. control of bleeding
2. absorption, storage, and use of food products
3. self-regulated control of the body's internal environment
4. the power of voluntary movement

1-6. That portion of a cell containing all the genetic material important in the cell's reproduction is called the

1. plasma membrane
2. nucleus
3. cytoplasm
4. reticulated endothelium

1-7. What type of tissue is known as the lining tissue of the body?

1. Connective
2. Areolar
3. Sebaceous
4. Epithelial

1-8. The secretion of digestive fluids and the absorption of digested foods and liquids is the chief function of which tissue?

1. Columnar
2. Osseus
3. Sercus
4. Squamous

1

1-9. Because this tissue is continuous throughout the body, if an infection were allowed to spread, it could reach every area of the body by moving through which of the following tissues?

1. Areolar
2. Adipose
3. Osseous
4. Fibrous

1-10. Which of the following are the two most prominent mineral elements of bone?

1. Ossein and calcium
2. Phosphorus and calcium
3. Sodium and phosphorus
4. Periosteum and ossein

1-11. The bones of the wrist are classified as which of the following bones?

1. Long
2. Short
3. Flat
4. Irregular

1-12. Bones of the cranium include which of the following?

1. Maxilla
2. Occipital
3. Atlas and axis
4. All of the above

1-13. The appendicular skeleton is composed of the bones of the

1. skull and vertebral column
2. thorax and vertebral column
3. pelvis and thorax
4. upper and lower extremities

1-14. The upper three ribs on each side are known as which of the following types of ribs?

1. True
2. False
3. Floating
4. Sternal

1-15. The head of the humerus is called the

1. scapula
2. acetabulum
3. glenoid falsa
4. epicordyle

1-16. The innominate bone is composed of three parts that are united in adults to form a cuplike structure called the

1. glenoid fossa
2. acetabulum
3. symphysis pubis
4. obturator foramen

1-17. The prominences easily felt on the inner and outer aspects of the ankle are called

1. medial and lateral malleolus
2. medial and lateral condyles
3. greater and lesser tuberosities
4. greater and lesser trochanters

1-18. Bones that develop within a tendon are known as which of the following?

1. Condyloid
2. Sesamoid
3. Vermiform
4. Falsiform

1-19. Moving an extremity away from the body is called

1. flexion
2. extension
3. abduction
4. adduction

1-20. The act of straightening a limb is known as

1. flexion
2. extension
3. abduction
4. adduction

1-21. The primary function of the muscles includes all of the following EXCEPT

1. providing heat during activity
2. maintaining body posture
3. producing red blood cells
4. providing movement

1-22. The ability of muscles to regain their original form when stretched is known as

1. contractiblity
2. elasticity
3. extensibility
4. tonicity

1-23. Actin and myosin are the two protein substances involved in

1. muscle recovery
2. muscle nourishment
3. muscle contraction
4. rigor mortis

1-24. Which of the following properties describes the ability of muscles to respond to a stimulus?

1. Contractility
2. Irritability
3. Extensibility
4. Tonicity

1-25. If a generally sedentary person in less than good physical condition enters a marathon with intent to complete the race, which of the following outcomes can he/she be expected to encounter?

1. If the day is cool, there will be no significant risk
2. Any physical deficiency can be overcome with a carbohydrate-rich diet before the race
3. If stretching exercises are performed before the race, he/she will be ok
4. He/she runs the risk of muscle damage

1-26. Intramuscular injections are frequently given in which of the following muscles?

1. Trapezius
2. Pectoralis majoris
3. Deltoid
4. All of the above

1-27. Intramuscular injections are usually given in which of the following muscles?

1. Quadriceps
2. Sartorius
3. Gastrocnemius
4. Gluteus maximus

1-28. The body's primary thermo-regulatory action is a function of dilating and contracting blood vessels and the

1. stratum germinativum
2. sweat glands
3. sebaceous glands
4. melanin

1-29. The total blood volume in the average adult is in what ranges?

1. 3 to 4 liters
2. 4 to 5 liters
3. 5 to 6 liters
4. 6 to 7 liters

3

1-30. A decreased red blood cell (RBC) count could be the result of a medical condition affecting the

1. compact bone
2. periosteum
3. yellow marrow
4. red marrow

1-31. Blood of the average female adult contains (a) how many million RBCs per (b) what unit?

1. (a) 4.5 (b) mm^3
2. (a) 6.0 (b) cm^3
3. (a) 4.5 (b) l
4. (a) 4.5 (b) low power field

1-32. A white blood cell (WBC) count of 18,000 may indicate what condition?

1. Leukocytosis
2. Normalcy
3. Infection
4. Vetiligo

1-33. In an accident victim suffering from a fibrinogen deficiency, the rescuer may have difficulty performing which of the actions listed below?

1. Controlling hemorrhage
2. Immobilizing a fracture
3. Supporting respiratory function
4. Reducing a dislocation

1-34. In addition to preventing excessive blood loss, the formation of a blood clot serves which, if any, of the following purposes?

1. To convert fibrinogen into blood serum to aid healing
2. To form the foundation for new tissue growth
3. To manufacture leukocytes
4. None of the above

1-35. The valves of the heart include all of the following EXCEPT

1. atrial
2. mitral
3. tricuspid
4. pulmonary

1-36. Oxygenated blood is carried by which of the following vein(s)?

1. Inferior vena cava
2. Superior vena cava
3. Portal
4. Pulmonary

1-37. The contraction phase of the heart is

1. systole
2. tension
3. diastole
4. active

1-38. The pulse pressure is the difference between which of the following measurements?

1. Venous and arterial pressure
2. Resting and active pulse rate
3. Arterial and ventricular pressure
4. Systole and diastole

1-39. The venous system that carries digested materials from the intestinal tract is called the

1. portal
2. pulmonary
3. abdominal
4. pelvic

1-40. Lymph nodes participate in all of the following functions EXCEPT

1. manufacture of white blood cells
2. filtration of bacterial debris
3. production of hormones
4. collection of large protein molecules

1-41. Windpipe is another term for

1. nares
2. larynx
3. trachea
4. pharynx

1-42. The primary muscle of respiration is known as the

1. pleura
2. alveolus
3. diaphragm
4. mediastinum

1-43. Of the following nerves, which, if any, controls the larynx during the process of breathing?

1. Phrenic
2. Intercostal
3. Vagus
4. None of the above

1-44. A nerve cell, or neuron, is composed of all of the following EXCEPT a/an

1. synapse
2. axon
3. cyton
4. dendrite

1-45. The impulse receptors of a nerve are called

1. dendrites
2. Schwann cells
3. ganglia
4. neurons

1-46. The space through which a nerve impulse passes from one neuron to another is called a/an

1. myelin sheath
2. synapse
3. axon
4. ganglion

1-47. Balance, coordination of movement, and harmony of motion are functions of what part of the brain?

1. Cerebral cortex
2. Cerebellum
3. Pons
4. Temporal lobe

1-48. Circulation and respiration are controlled primarily from what area of the brain?

1. Medulla oblongata
2. Pons
3. Cerebellum
4. Cerebrum

1-49. The meninges, membrane layers covering of the brain and spinal cord, are composed of all of the following EXCEPT the

1. dura mater
2. pia mater
3. arachnoid
4. foramen magnum

1-50. In what part of the body is cerebral spinal fluid produced?

1. Ventricles of the brain
2. Spinal cord
3. Meninges
4. Medulla oblongata

1-51. The 12 pairs of cranial and 31 pairs of spinal nerves form what nervous system?

1. Peripheral
2. Central
3. Autonomic
4. Sympathetic

```
A. Facial
B. Trigeminal
C. Hypoglossal
D. Accessory
```

IN ANSWERING QUESTIONS 1-52 THROUGH 1-54, SELECT FROM THE LIST ABOVE THE CRANIAL NERVE THAT PERFORMS THE FUNCTION LISTED IN EACH QUESTION.

1-52. Controls the muscles of the tongue.

1. A
2. B
3. C
4. D

1-53. Transmits sensation of taste.

1. A
2. B
3. C
4. D

1-54. Receives sensory input from the face.

1. A
2. B
3. C
4. D

1-55. The autonomic nervous system is composed of two main divisions: the

1. pons and medulla oblongata
2. voluntary and involuntary systems
3. sympathetic and parasympathetic systems
4. cerebrum and cerebellum

1-56. Conservation and restoration of energy are the result of nerve impulses arising from which, if any, of the following nervous systems?

1. Sympathetic
2. Parasympathetic
3. Voluntary
4. None of the above

```
A. Sympathetic
B. Central
C. Peripheral
D. Parasympathetic
```

IN ANSWERING QUESTIONS 1-57 THROUGH 1-60, SELECT FROM THE LIST ABOVE THE NERVOUS SYSTEM THAT IS MOST RESPONSIBLE FOR THE SYMPTOM OR FUNCTION GIVEN IN THE QUESTION.

1-57. Increased heart rate.

1. A
2. B
3. C
4. D

1-58. Vision.

1. A
2. B
3. C
4. D

1-59. Decreases heart rate to normal.

1. A
2. B
3. C
4. D

1-60.   Reflex arc.

1.   A
2.   B
3.   C
4.   D

1-61.   Hormones secreted by the endocrine system are

1.   secreted directly into the gland, tissue, or organ it influences
2.   directed to the gland, tissue, organ by a duct system
3.   secreted into the circulatory system
4.   typically produced in large quantities

1-62.   The overproduction of which hormone leads to acromegaly?

1.   Somatotropin
2.   Oxytocin
3.   Gonadotropin
4.   Thyroxin

1-63.   Which of the following diseases is characterized by a deficiency of the antidiuretic hormone?

1.   Myxedema
2.   Diabetes insipidus
3.   Hyperthyroidism
4.   Addison's disease

1-64.   An insufficient secretion of thyroxin is characterized by all of the following symptoms EXCEPT

1.   weight gain
2.   fatigue
3.   profuse sweating
4.   slowed heart rate

1-65.   Calcium levels in the blood are controlled by which of the following hormones?

1.   Thyroxin
2.   Vasopressin
3.   Oxytocin
4.   Parathormone

1-66.   Electrolyte balance is a function of the hormone produced by the

1.   posterior lobe of the pituitary gland
2.   anterior lobe of the pituitary gland
3.   cortex of the adrenal gland
4.   medulla of the adrenal gland

1-67.   A metabolic response to epinephrine includes which, if any, of the symptoms listed below?

1.   Decreased heart rate
2.   Increased blood pressure
3.   Respiratory distress
4.   None of the above

1-68.   What hormone is produced by the alpha cells of the islands of Langerhans in the pancreas?

1.   Glucagon
2.   Insulin
3.   Norepinephrine
4.   Androgens

1-69.   The cornea is part of the protective outer layer of the eye called the

1.   sclera
2.   conjunctiva
3.   choroid
4.   crystalline body

1-70. The inner part of the eye derives its nourishment primarily from the vascular structure of what tissue?

1. Conjunctiva
2. Sclera
3. Vitreous humor
4. Choroid

1-71. Dilation of the pupil, a muscular response of the iris, normally occurs as a result of what?

1. Increased intensity of light
2. Decrease intensity of light
3. Irritation to the sclera
4. Irritation to the conjunctiva

1-72. Of the elements listed below, which makes seeing in the dark possible?

1. Rods
2. Cones
3. Iris
4. Choroid

1-73. By what process is three-dimensional vision produced?

1. Accommodation
2. Convergence
3. Refraction
4. Stimulation

1-74. The mechanical transmission of sound from the tympanic membrane to the inner ear is a function of which of the following?

1. Auditory ossicles
2. Eustachian tube
3. Bony labyrinth
4. Organ of Corti

1-75. What structure(s) of the inner ear provide(s) neural stimuli used to maintain equilibrium?

1. Fenestra rotunda
2. Fenestra ovalis
3. Semicircular canals
4. Organ of Corti

ASSIGNMENT 2

Textbook Assignment: "Anatomy and Physiology," chapter 1—continued, pages 48-63; "Fundamentals of Patient Care," chapter 2, pages 2-1 through 2-39.

2-1.   The conversion of mechanical impulses (sound waves) to neural impulses that can be interpreted by the brain is a function of the

1.   endolymph
2.   semicircular canals
3.   organ of Corti
4.   fenestra ovalis

2-2.   The enzymatic action of amylase results in the chemical breakdown of

1.   fats to fatty acids
2.   starches to fats
3.   starches to complex sugars
4.   proteins to complex sugars

2-3.   Absorption of food occurs predominantly in which of the following areas of the intestines?

1.   Duodenum
2.   Jejunum
3.   Ileum
4.   Cecum

2-4.   Of the organs listed below, which function as the accessory organs of digestion for the small intestines?

1.   Pancreas, liver, villae
2.   Spleen, liver, gallbladder
3.   Pancreas, pylorus, spleen
4.   Pancreas, liver, gallbladder

2-5.   The gallbladder performs which of the following purposes?

1.   Stimulates the production of insulin
2.   Stores bile
3.   Metabolizes sugars
4.   Produces antibodies

2-6.   The functional unit of the kidney is called the

1.   nephron
2.   Malpighian body
3.   glomerulus
4.   loop of Henle

2-7.   Which of the following is/are (a) function(s) of the kidneys?

1.   To maintain acid-base balance
2.   To remove certain toxic substances
3.   To remove excess sugar
4.   All the above

2-8.   Blood concentration varies due to which, if any, of the following factors?

1.   Temperature
2.   Water intake
3.   State of health
4.   None of the above

2-9.   What is the approximate total capacity of the adult bladder?

1.   250 ml
2.   300 ml
3.   600 ml
4.   750 ml

2-10. Testosterone production is a function of which of the following glands?

1. Cowper's
2. Prostate
3. Testes
4. Bulbourethral

2-11. Which of the following is/are considered the primary female reproductive organs?

1. Ovaries
2. Fallopian tubes
3. Uterus
4. Endometrium

2-12. Fertilization of an ovum normally takes place in the

1. ovaries
2. fallopian tubes
3. uterus
4. vagina

2-13. The concepts of health include

1. the absence of disease or disability
2. soundness of mind, body, and spirit
3. both 1 and 2 above
4. a feeling of euphoria

2-14. Patient rights and responsibilities are standards addressed by what organization?

1. Commander, Navy Medical Command (formerly Bureau of Medicine and Surgery)
2. American Medical Association (AMA)
3. Joint Commission on Accreditation of Healthcare Organizations (JCAHO)
4. National League of Nursing (NLN)

2-15. The limitations imposed upon a healthcare provider are based on local regulations and which of the following elements?

1. The rating's occupational standards
2. The rate training manual
3. The provider's training and experience
4. All of the above

2-16. In the healthcare field, accountability means that providers

1. are held responsible for their actions
2. must continue their education in the healthcare field
3. are bound by a code of ethics
4. all the above

2-17. A patient requests your advice or opinion concerning the care or proposed care (s)he is undergoing. Which, if any, of the following is the appropriate response?

1. Answer honestly, to the best of your ability
2. Refer the patient to the nurse or physician responsible for his/her care
3. Say you'll ask your supervisor
4. None of the above

2-18. Personal and medical information learned about a patient as the result of your position as a Hospital Corpsman is privileged and must not be divulged to unauthorized individuals.

1. True
2. False

A. Learned and shared
behavior patterns and
standards.

B. How one responds to and
regards others.

C. Inherited characteristics.

D. Belief system.

**TO ANSWER QUESTIONS 2-19 THROUGH
2-21, SELECT FROM THE ABOVE LIST THE
STATEMENT THAT MOST ACCURATELY
DESCRIBES THE TERMS GIVEN IN THE
QUESTION. NOT ALL STATEMENTS WILL
BE USED.**

2-19.   Interpersonal relations.

    1.   A
    2.   B
    3.   C
    4.   D

2-20.   Culture.

    1.   A
    2.   B
    3.   C
    4.   D

2-21.   Race.

    1.   A
    2.   B
    3.   C
    4.   D

2-22.   A patient who is a professed atheist is
placed on the Very Serious List (VSL) with
a poor prognosis for recovery. All of the
following actions by the staff are
considered appropriate and ethical
EXCEPT

    1.   informing the rest of the staff of the
patient's nonreligious beliefs
    2.   informing the rest of the staff of the
patient's condition
    3.   informing pastoral services (chaplain)
of the patient's condition and
nonreligious beliefs
    4.   attempting to convince the patient to
accept a religious belief

2-23.   The communication process takes place
only through the written or spoken word.

    1.   True
    2.   False

2-24.   Communication barriers inhibit the flow of
information and may consist of which of
the following factors?

    1.   Decreased auditory acuity
    2.   Age
    3.   Education
    4.   All the above

2-25.   The most common cause of ineffective
communication and the most difficult
obstacle to identify is which of the
following barriers?

    1.   Psychological
    2.   Physical
    3.   Psychosocial
    4.   Spiritual or religious

2-26. In the communication process, listening is a critical skill and can be improved by developing which, if any, of the following attitudes and behaviors?

1. Anticipating what the patient will say
2. Minimizing distractions
3. Taking notes
4. None of the above

2-27. The purpose of therapeutic communication includes all of the following EXCEPT

1. assessing behavior and modifying if appropriate
2. educating a patient regarding health and health care
3. providing information on how to get to the appropriate clinic for treatment
4. obtaining information to determine a patient's illness

A. Contact point communication

B. Therapeutic communication

TO ANSWER QUESTIONS 2-28 THROUGH 2-31, SELECT FROM THE LIST ABOVE THE TERM THAT MOST APTLY APPLIES TO THE REQUIREMENT PRESENTED.

2-28. Developing a patient's history of a complaint.

1. A
2. B

2-29. Explaining the necessities and methods of personal hygiene to the parent of a young patient.

1. A
2. B

2-30. Providing self-care instructions to a patient released to convalescent leave.

1. A
2. B

2-31. Directing the patient to the pharmacy to fill a prescription.

1. A
2. B

2-32. Which of the following are goals of patient health education?

1. Promoting patient self-care
2. Promoting behavior modification
3. Influencing a patient's attitude toward health and disease
4. All the above

2-33. Patient education is the responsibility of

1. the members of the command education and training department
2. only the physician and nurses for the patient
3. all members of the healthcare team
4. the outpatient staff and clinic supervisor only

Kind(s) of observation(s)

A. Subjective only

B. Objective only

C. Both subjective and objective

TO ANSWER QUESTIONS 2-34 THROUGH 2-38, SELECT FROM THE ABOVE LIST THE TYPE(S) OF OBSERVATION(S) THAT MOST ACCURATELY APPLY(S) TO THE SCENARIO DESCRIBED IN THE QUESTION.

2-34. In the emergency room, you are examining a patient who suddenly vomits and tells you he has been feeling nauseous for the past several hours.

1. A
2. B
3. C

2-35. A patient claims to have swallowed many pills and complains of sleepiness and nausea.

1. A
2. B
3. C

2-36. An EKG performed on a patient is interpreted as normal and the patient's breathing improves with oxygen therapy.

1. A
2. B
3. C

2-37. A patient complains of chest pain and has difficulty breathing.

1. A
2. B
3. C

2-38. When picking up a patient's dinner tray, you notice that only the liquids have been consumed at this meal, although the patient has normally eaten full meals before this.

1. A
2. B
3. C

2-39. A medical patient is prescribed therapeutic bed rest primarily for what reason?

1. To inhibit the development of circulatory problems
2. To prevent depression and apathy
3. To prevent further damage to body systems
4. To inhibit the development of respiratory problems

2-40. A health care provider can reasonably expect that all patients admitted for surgical procedures will exhibit which of the following characteristics?

1. Be very demanding
2. Be apathetic and passive
3. Exhibit violent behavior
4. Be fearful and anxious

2-41. SF 522, Request for Administration of Anesthesia and for Performance of Operations and other Procedures, is normally signed by a parent, legal guardian, or spouse EXCEPT when the patient is

1. able to do so
2. over 16 years of age but under 18
3. over 18 years of age but under 21
4. a member of the Armed Forces

2-42. When a regional anesthetic is administered, the patient can expect what effect?

1. Motor, but not sensory perception will diminish
2. Pain will be reduced or eliminated in the body part injected or swabbed
3. Level of consciousness will decline
4. The entire body will become numb

2-43. In general anesthesia, a stimulation of vital signs is evidence of what level of anesthesia induction?

1. Stage 1
2. Stage 2
3. Stage 3
4. Stage 4

2-44. Dropping a metal basin on the operating room floor may cause a violent response from a general anesthesia patient in what stage of anesthesia?

1. Stage 1
2. Stage 2
3. Stage 3
4. Stage 4

2-45. In the immediate postoperative recovery phase, a patient's skin color may be indicative of all of the following EXCEPT

1. the patient's ability to recover from the anesthetic agent
2. postoperative hemorrhage
3. degradation of respiratory function
4. the development of shock

2-46. When permitted, postoperative patients should be encouraged to ambulate to improve the functions of which of the following physiologic systems?

1. Renal system
2. Digestive system
3. Cardiopulmonary system
4. All of the above

2-47. When caring for a young, otherwise healthy orthopedic patient requiring immobilization, the healthcare provider can anticipate all of the following EXCEPT

1. symptoms of emotional stress
2. frequent complaints of sore or aching pain
3. periods of dizziness associated with disorientation
4. a deterioration of skin tone and function

2-48. Unless otherwise directed by the physician, when one is applying a cast to an arm, the patient's wrists is generally in which of the following positions?

1. Extended about 10 degrees
2. In the neutral position
3. Flexed about 30 degrees
4. In any of the above; specific position is immaterial

2-49. A patient who has been fitted with a cast should be instructed to return to the medical treatment facility as soon as possible under which of the following circumstances?

1. The cast becomes soiled
2. The extremity affected by the cast is numb
3. The itching becomes unbearable
4. The cast gets wet

2-50. In the theory of death and dying, it is suggested that most people exhibit five stages. The stage where the terminal patient becomes concerned about the state of his or her affairs and family members is known as the stage of

1. denial
2. acceptance
3. bargaining
4. depression

2-51. Patient falls may be avoided by taking which of the following preventive measures?

1. Proper use of bed/gurney siderails
2. Keeping floors dry and uncluttered
3. Instructing patients on the proper use of walking aids (crutches, canes, etc.)
4. All of the above

2-52. Electrical and electronic equipment poses significant injury hazards. Of the following, which is the authorized means of reducing this hazard?

1. Repairing frayed cords with electrical tape to prevent shock
2. Informing the staff of defective equipment
3. Having medical repair perform electrical safety checks on all equipment
4. Using only two-prong, nongrounded electrical plugs

2-53. Skin contact burns can be caused by icebags or hypothermia blankets.

1. True
2. False

2-54. During a fire evacuation, which of the following procedures is NOT considered appropriate?

1. Immediately remove patients to safety
2. Close all windows and doors
3. Turn off all oxygen equipment not necessary to sustain life
4. Clear all possible exits

2-55. Because of its nonstatic qualities, the most acceptable material for use in the operating room is

1. wool
2. synthetic fabrics
3. untreated synthetic/cotton blends
4. 100% cotton

2-56. Documentation and analysis of all accidents and injuries is provided for which of the following reasons?

1. To forestall negligence or malpractice suits
2. To identify and punish the responsible person(s)
3. To identify and correct safety deficiencies
4. All of the above

2-57. Environmental hygiene is directed toward producing a healthy environment and includes such practices as maintaining unit cleanliness and

1. providing for adequate ventilation
2. limiting noise levels
3. proper disposal of soiled articles
4. all of the above

2-58. What source is considered the most frequent reservoir of infectious agents pathogenic to man?

1. Soil
2. Animals
3. Man
4. Plants

A. Corpsman's hands
B. Patient
C. Abdominal wound
D. Furuncle

TO ANSWER ITEMS 2-59 THROUGH 2-62, SELECT FROM THE ABOVE LIST THE SITUATIONAL ELEMENT THAT MOST CLOSELY MATCHES THE CHAIN OF INFECTION LINK GIVEN IN THE QUESTION AS IT APPLIES TO THE FOLLOWING SCENARIO.

A corpsman assists a medical officer to perform incision and drainage of a furuncle on a patient's leg. After the I&D procedure, the corpsman changes a postsurgical abdominal dressing on the same patient. A few days later, the surgical wound appears red and swollen and a culture reveals a significant staphylococcal infection.

2-59. Reservoir of the infectious agent.

1. A
2. B
3. C
4. D

2-60. Mode of transmission.

1. A
2. B
3. C
4. D

2-61. Portal of entry.

1. A
2. B
3. C
4. D

2-62. Susceptible host.
1. A
2. B
3. C
4. D

2-63. One essential practice of medical asepsis is washing your hands before and after changing a patient's dressing(s).

1. True
2. False

2-64. Minimizing the spread of an infectious disease can be accomplished by the use of isolation techniques that may include

1. limiting patient contact
2. establishing physical barriers
3. concurrent and terminal disinfection
4. all of the above

2-65. The sterilization method of choice for most articles used in surgery is

1. dry heat
2. steam under pressure
3. ethylene oxide gas
4. soaking in glutaraldehyde

2-66. Which of the following is an important step in using ethylene oxide gas for sterilization?

1. Providing protective masks to the operators
2. Providing an aeration period
3. Including surgical blades and sutures in the pack
4. Ensuring adequate steam pressure in the chamber

2-67. Sterilization of individual strands of suture is acceptable for which of the types listed?

1. All absorbable suture material
2. All nonabsorbable suture material
3. Both 1 and 2 above
4. Stainless steel sutures only

2-68. Which of the following rubber products may be resterilized after use?

1. Disposable surgeon's gloves
2. Latex surgical drains
3. Surgical suction tubing
4. Disposable urinary catheters

2-69. While adding items to a sterile field, you think you may have dragged the corner of a wrapper across part of the field. What should your course of action be?

1. Do nothing. Wrappers are considered clean
2. Tell the scrub technician so he or she can avoid that part of the field
3. Say nothing and continue with what you are doing
4. Dismantle the field and set up a new field

2-70. When setting up a minor surgery case, you notice that the instrument pack is outdated, What should you do?

1. Unwrap and inspect the pack and if usable, resterilize
2. Resterilize the pack without unwrapping
3. Return it to the shelf and let someone else take care of it
4. Use the pack; only the outside is not sterile

2-71. The surgical hand scrub is performed to

1. chemically sterilize the hands and forearms
2. remove all bacteria from the hands and forearms
3. reduce bacterial to a minimum on the hands and forearms
4. remove obvious dirt and grime from the hands and forearms

2-72. Transient and resident bacteria are easily removed from the skin by the friction created during the surgical hand scrub.

1. True
2. False

2-73. What is the preferred method of cleaning an operating room floor between operations?

1. Sponge and disinfectant
2. Broom
3. Mop
4. Wet vacuum

2-74. For effective sterilization of microbiological infectious waste, the temperature of the sterilizing steam must be maintained at _____ for at least _____, at _____ per square inch of gauge pressure.

1. 121° F, 45 minutes, 15 pounds
2. 121° C, 90 minutes, 10 pounds
3. 250° F, 90 minutes, 15 pounds
4. 250° C, 45 minutes, 10 pounds

ASSIGNMENT 3

Textbook Assignment: "First Aid Equipment, Supplies, Rescue and Transportation," chapter 3, pages 3-1 to 3-26; "Emergency Medical Care Procedures," chapter 4, pages 4-1 to 4-37.

3-1.   In first aid situations, the ability to improvise is a highly desirable personal characteristic for a Corpsman.

1.   True
2.   False

3-2.   A typical ambulance emergency bag does NOT contain which of the following items?

1.   Toomey Syringe
2.   Atropine
3.   Airways
4.   Trach Adaptor

A. Spica	E. Barton
B. Figure-eight	F. Triangular
C. Spiral reverse	G. Cravat
D. Four-tailed	

IN ANSWERING QUESTIONS 3-3 THROUGH 3-9, REFER TO THE LIST ABOVE, MATCHING THE TYPE OF BANDAGE WITH THE BODY PART TO WHICH IT IS MOST COMMONLY APPLIED.

3-3. Axilla.

1.   A
2.   B
3.   F
4.   G

3-4.   Ear.

1.   C
2.   D
3.   E
4.   G

3-5.   Head.

1.   F
2.   D
3.   B
4.   A

3-6.   Elbow.

1.   A or B
2.   C or F
3.   E
4.   G

3-7.   Ankle.

1.   D
2.   C
3.   B
4.   A

3-8.   Calf.

1.   A
2.   B
3.   C
4.   D

3-9.   Chin.

1.   C or A
2.   D or E
3.   F or G
4.   G only

3-10. The oxygen breathing apparatus (OBA) is a valuable adjunct in rescue operations for what reason?

1. It can be connected directly to an external air source
2. It provides positive pressure ventilation for the wearer
3. It neutralizes or filters toxic gasses
4. It generates its own oxygen

3-11. When, if ever, should an oxygen source be connected to an air line mask?

1. When entering a carbon dioxide filled compartment or void
2. When entering a compartment or void with fuel oil vapors
3. After the couplings have been cleaned of all oil or grease
4. Never

3-12. The standard gas mask provides effective protection against

1. carbon monoxide and carbon dioxide
2. low oxygen concentrations
3. both 1 and 2 above
4. chemical and biological warfare agents

3-13. When using a lifeline to raise an unconscious person from a compartment, the lifeline should be attached to the victim in what manner?

1. Around the waist and to the belt
2. Around the chest and under the arms
3. Around the hips and the wrists
4. Around the arms and the legs

IN ANSWERING QUESTIONS 3-14 AND 3-15, REFER TO THE FOLLOWING SCENARIO. DETERMINE THE PHASE OF RESCUE OPERATIONS, STAGE OF EXTRICATION, AND/OR RESCUE PROCEDURE INDICATED BY THE QUESTION.

Scenario
There has been a fire and explosion aboard ship and approximately 30 Sailors are trapped below deck. To get to the trapped Sailors, bulkheads are being breached and a large section of the damaged deck is being cut away. Firefighting teams are still fighting a large out of control fire near where you will be working. Passageway ventilation systems are working to remove dense, acrid smoke. Everyone is wearing OBA. Several steam lines have been ruptured and live electrical lines are sparking throughout the area. The DCO has determined that rescue attempts can be conducted.

3-14. Several Sailors have just been reached. Two are unconscious, badly burned, and pinned under an empty wall locker. One is dead.

1. First and third phases/first stage
2. Second phase/third stage
3. Third phase/third stage
4. First and last phases/first stage

3-15. A Sailor is injured and trapped under a fallen metal beam that is wedged tight by a buckled bulkhead. After unsuccessful efforts to move the beam, special cutting and lifting equipment is called for.

1. First phase
2. Second phase
3. Third phase
4. Last phase

3-16. Five burned Sailors walked out of a smoldering compartment. You are administering first aid and transporting them to sickbay.

1. First and second stages
2. Second stage only
3. First and third stages
4. Second and final stages

3-17. A Sailor whose clothes are on fire runs toward you. A small canvas tarp is nearby. Which of the following actions should you take?

1. Throw the victim to the deck and cover the victim head to foot with the tarp
2. Beat out the flames from the head downward to the feet
3. With the victim wrapped in the tarp, roll the victim over very quickly
4. With the victim standing, wrap the victim in the tarp and beat the flames out with your hands

3-18. The ventilators suddenly shut down and sparking has ceased. Rescuers are to enter a darkened compartment. The DCO is supervising the rescue effort. The rescuers should take which of the following precautions?

1. Check for oxygen, gasses, and explosive vapors
2. Wear a lifeline
3. Carry and wear only nonsparking equipment
4. Each of the above

3-19. Which of the stretchers listed below is considered most practical when lifting a casualty from an engine room?

1. Stokes stretcher
2. Army litter
3. Miller Board
4. Improvised blanket and line stretcher

3-20. Which of the following pieces of rescue equipment should be used to carry a person with a suspected back or neck injury?

1. Army litter
2. Spineboard
3. Either 1 or 2, depending on the circumstances
4. Improvised stretcher

3-21. Probably the easiest way to carry an unconscious person is called the

1. fireman's carry
2. tied-hands crawl
3. blanket drag
4. chair carry

3-22. The tied-hands crawl is the most useful when the victim

1. is too heavy to lift
2. must be move long distances
3. is seriously injured
4. must be moved under low structures

3-23. What is the most distinct advantage of the chair carry?

1. The ease of transporting heavy casualties
2. The ease of negotiating stairs
3. Its safety in transporting neck or back injuries
4. Its safety in transporting pelvic injuries

3-24. Which of the following is NOT a factor the Corpsman considers in deciding whether or not to recommend using a helicopter for evacuating patients?

1. The victim's overall condition
2. The tactical situation
3. The affect of pressure changes in flight
4. Cost

3-25. The primary purposes of first aid include all the following EXCEPT to

1. provide definitive medical treatment
2. preserve resistance and vitality
3. save life
4. prevent further injury

3-26. At what point should the preliminary examination of a casualty be done?

1. In the hospital
2. In the ambulance
3. After making the victim comfortable
4. Before moving the casualty

3-27. In a combat scenario, a casualty sustaining numerous superficial shrapnel wounds should be triaged into which of the following groups?

1. Class I
2. Class II
3. Class III
4. Class IV

3-28. In a trauma related incident where a patient has multiple injuries, you should treat which of the following first?

1. Fractures
2. Most obvious injury
3. Most lift-threatening condition
4. Most painful condition

3-29. For warfare in the future where helicopter evacuation may not be viable, personnel in which of the following treatment categories will receive evacuation triage?

1. I and II
2. II and III
3. I and IV
4. III and IV

3-30. What is the basic concept of triage?

1. To sort casualties into treatment categories for transportation
2. To prioritize treatment categories for surgery
3. To save the maximum number of personnel possible
4. To assist medical personnel in saving time and supplies

3-31. What is the purpose of field assessments?

1. To detect and treat life threatening conditions for immediate care
2. To conduct a subjective interview and an objective examination
3. Both a and b, above
4. To identify needed equipment and supplies

3-32. At an emergency scene, you should immediately take which of the following actions?

1. Inform the person in charge that medical personnel have arrived
2. Ensure that someone begins triage, if needed
3. Review patient emergency assessment procedures
4. Make sure the scene is safe for self and patients

3-33. Which of the following actions are a main focus of conducting a primary survey?

1. Making a status decision and formulating priorities
2. Formulating a treatment plan and making a status decision
3. Formulating priorities and making a transport decision
4. Making a status decision and a transport decision

3-34. At the emergency scene, you should delay giving emergency care to life-threatening problems until you have conducted a thorough field assessment of the patient and the environment.

1. True
2. False

3-35. At an emergency scene, which of the following is a purpose for conducting a subjective interview?

1. To gather information from relatives or bystanders
2. To gather information from the patient
3. To reduce patient fear and promote cooperation
4. All of the above

3-36. What pupillary sign is an indication of a central nervous system disorder?

1. Unequal pupils
2. Constricted pupils
3. Unresponsive pupils
4. Dull and unfocused pupils

3-37. On examination of the chest, you detect distinct "crackling" sounds. What condition should you immediately suspect?

1. Flail chest
2. An obstruction
3. A punctured lung
4. An illness involving the respiratory system

3-38. An absent pedal pulse could be caused by all of the following conditions EXCEPT

1. a broken or dislocated bone
2. delayed capillary refill
3. spints or bandages being placed too tightly
4. a pinched or severed major artery

3-39. Evaluation of diagnostic vital signs includes all of the following EXCEPT

1. blood pressure
2. rhythm/regularity of pulse
3. profuse perspiration
4. level of consciousness

3-40. What term identifies the pressure of the pulse wave as it expands the artery?

1. Pulse rhythm
2. Pulse character
3. Tachycardia
4. Pulse force

3-41. What condition or observation may indicate a patient is going into shock?

1. Systolic pressure below 90 mm Hg
2. Hypertension
3. Erratic breathing
4. A sudden rise in blood pressure

3-42. What is the universal distress signal indicating an obstructed airway?

1. Spasmodic coughing
2. Clutching at the throat
3. Hyperventilation
4. Cherry-red coloration of the skin or nail beds

3-43. To open a partially obstructed airway of a victim with a cervical spine injury, which of the following is considered the safest method?

1. Jaw thrust
2. Head tilt
3. Abdominal thrust
4. Chest thrust

3-44. Symptoms of foreign-body airway obstruction include which of the following?

1. Victim stops breathing
2. Victim starts turning blue
3. Victim loses consciousness for no apparent reason
4. All the above

3-45. Artificial ventilation is indicated in which of the following situations?

1. To assist ventilation in partial airway obstruction
2. In carbon monoxide poisoning
3. In lack of respiratory effort
4. In cyanosis

3-46. Dilated pupils in a patient receiving artificial ventilation is an indication of

1. overventilation
2. adequate ventilation
3. insufficient ventilation
4. hypovolemia

3-47. Artificial ventilation of a patient with a badly displaced mandibular fracture is best given

1. by mouth-to-mouth ventilation
2. by mouth-to-nose ventilation
3. with an oxygen mask
4. by the back-pressure arm-lift method

3-48. The major problem you should anticipate when relieving gastric distention is which of the following?

1. Reduced lung volume
2. Internal bleeding
3. Vomiting
4. Cardiac arrest

3-49. When ventilating an adult using the mouth-to-mask method, how do you best obtain an airtight seal?

1. By fitting the apex of the mask over the bridge of the nose
2. By fitting the apex of the mask over the chin
3. By compressing the collar of an adult mask
4. By attaching an oxygen line

3-50. What is the first step in preparing to perform CPR?

1. Check vital signs
2. Determine unconsciousness
3. Locate the sternum
4. Establish a patent airway

3-51. The best place to find the pulse of an unconscious patient is in which of the following arteries?

1. Pulmonary
2. Carotid
3. Apical
4. Radial

3-52. A fracture of the xiphoid tip of the sternum during CPR may cause significant damage to the

1. rib cage
2. lungs
3. spleen
4. liver

3-53. In one-rescuer CPR, the proper compression to ventilation ratio is

1. 15 to 2
2. 2 to 15
3. 1 to 5
4. 5 to 1

3-54. When properly performing CPR on an adult, the depth of compressions is

1. 0.5 to 1.0 inches
2. 1.0 to 1.5 inches
3. 1.5 to 2.0 inches
4. 1.5 to 2.5 inches

3-55. Which of the following is a physiologic result of shock?

1. Increased cardiac output
2. Hypoxia
3. Hyperperfusion of organs
4. Increased urine output

3-56. The signs and symptoms of shock include

1. hot and dry skin, dilated pupils, weak and rapid pulse
2. hot and dry skin, constricted pupils, strong and rapid pulse
3. cool and moist skin, dilated pupils, weak and rapid pulse
4. cool and moist skin, constricted pupils, strong and rapid pulse

3-57. Oligemic shock is another name for

1. cardiogenic shock
2. neurogenic shock
3. septic shock
4. hypovolemic shock

3-58. An oral electrolyte solution can be made from a liter of water and what other components?

1. 1.0 teaspoon of sugar + 0.5 teaspoon of baking powder
2. 0.5 teaspoon sugar + 1.0 teaspoon baking powder
3. 1.0 teaspoon salt + 0.5 teaspoon baking soda
4. 0.5 teaspoon salt + 1.0 teaspoon baking soda

3-59. Treatment for shock may include all of the following EXCEPT

1. opening and maintaining an airway
2. oxygen therapy
3. intravenous fluid therapy
4. keeping the victim cool

3-60. Which of the following is a contraindication for the use of Medical Anti-Shock Trousers (MAST)?

1. Pelvic fracture
2. Pulmonary edema
3. Fractured femur
4. Depressed skull fracture

3-61. When should Medical Anti-Shock Trousers (MAST) be removed from a patient?

1. When blood pressure reaches 100 mm Hg systolic
2. When intravenous fluids are started
3. In a medical treatment facility under a medical officer's supervision only
4. When the patient is in the ambulance and stabilized

3-62. Which of the following is/are a limitation(s) on the use of the bag-valve mask ventilator?

1. Should be used only by experienced individuals
2. Is hard to clean and reassemble
3. Seal at the face is hard to maintain
4. Each of the above

3-63. Which of the following is/are an advantage(s) of using the pocket face mask as opposed to the bag-valve mask?

1. Acts as a barrier device
2. Provides greater air volume
3. Achieves higher oxygen concentrations
4. 1 and 2 only

3-64. Cricothyroidotomy is the process or technique of

1. hyperextending the neck
2. creating an opening to the trachea
3. suctioning the trachea
4. inserting an esophageal obturator airway

3-65. An avulsion injury is defined as a

1. traumatic removal of a limb
2. piercing injury that closes over
3. clean surgical cut
4. traumatic removal of tissue

3-66. In most situations, what is the best and first method to control hemorrhage?

1. Direct pressure
2. Pressure point
3. Elevation
4. Tourniquet

3-67. The following information about pressure points is correct EXCEPT

1. Pressure points are ideal when bleeding must be controlled for extended periods of time
2. Pressure is applied to the pressure point nearest to but proximal to the wound
3. Use of pressure point and elevation can slow hemorrhage until a tourniquet can be applied
4. Use of pressure point and elevation can slow hemorrhage until a direct pressure dressing can be applied

3-68. If one is applying a tourniquet to a traumatic amputation of the hand, where should the tourniquet be applied?

1. Just above the wrist
2. Just below the elbow
3. Just above the elbow
4. Across the biceps at the thickest part

3-69. When a tourniquet is used to control bleeding, which of the following procedures should be followed?

1. Use narrow material so the band bites into the skin
2. Loosen the tourniquet every 15 minutes to allow blood flow
3. Tighten it only enough to stop arterial bleeding
4. Ensure both the wound and tourniquet are covered by the dressings

3-70. Production of bright red blood during coughing is called

1. hematemesis
2. hemoptysis
3. hematochezia
4. epistaxis

3-71. In treating patients with suspected internal injuries, prime consideration should be given to all of the following EXCEPT

1. oral fluids in all cases
2. treating for shock
3. supplemental oxygen therapy
4. transporting to a medical facility as soon as possible

3-72. To grow and multiply, anaerobic bacteria require

1. hemolytic action
2. increased levels of oxygen
3. normal levels of oxygen
4. absence of oxygen

3-73. The body's physiologic response to an irritation or inflammation is characterized by which, if any, of the following symptoms?

1. Redness, warmth, and swelling
2. Redness, coolness, and discomfort
3. Blanching, coolness, and swelling
4. None of the above

3-74. A single pus-filled cavity in the true skin of the nape of the neck would be classified as a

1. carbuncle
2. furuncle
3. lymph node
4. phagocyte

3-75. Which of the following is proper action to take if a metal splinter is embedded in the left eye?

1. Remove the foreign body with sterile forceps
2. Remove the foreign body with a dry cotton swab
3. Patch the left eye and transport to a medical treatment facility
4. Patch both eyes and transport to a medical treatment facility

ASSIGNMENT 4

Textbook Assignment: "Emergency Medical Care Procedures," chapter 4, pages 4-38 to 4-71; "Poisoning, Drug Abuse, and Hazardous Material Exposure," chapter 5, pages 5-1 to 5-26.

4-1. Appropriate treatment for a sucking chest wound includes all of the following EXCEPT

1. giving oral fluids
2. administering oxygen therapy
3. treating for shock
4. placing the victim on the injured side

4-2. Of the following, which is an appropriate treatment for a protruding abdominal wound?

1. Giving oral fluids
2. Replacing the intestines in the abdominal cavity
3. Applying a dry compress
4. Treating for shock

4-3. Which of the following statements is true about the viral disease known as rabies?

1. It is found only in household pets
2. It is usually fatal in man
3. It is treatable with standard antibiotics
4. It is transmittable only through animal bites

4-4. What procedure should be followed with respect to an animal bite?

1. Cauterize to prevent infection
2. Close with nylon sutures
3. Clean with standard antiseptics
4. Clean with soap and water

4-5. Immediate suturing of a wound is contraindicated if the wound has which of the following characteristics?

1. It is a puncture wound
2. There is edema and/or discharge
3. It is a deep or gaping wound
4. Any of the above

4-6. An alternate name for an absorbable suture material is

1. dermalon
2. gut
3. sick
4. nylon

4-7. In administering anesthesia, the preferred method is to inject the agent directly into a vein or artery located within 1/2 inch of a wound.

1. True
2. False

4-8. Which of the following is/are a recommended step(s) in performing a delayed wound closure?

1. Use dressing forceps while suturing
2. Convert jagged edges to smooth before suturing
3. For best cosmetic effect, place sutures further apart
4. 1 and 3 only

4-9. Of the following statements concerning the appropriate length for a splint, which is accurate?

1. A splint should be long enough to reach from the fracture to the joint below the fracture
2. A splint should be long enough to reach from the fracture to the joint above and below the fracture
3. A splint should be long enough to reach past the joints above and below the fracture
4. The length of a splint is immaterial

4-10. After applying a splint to a fractured forearm, you notice the fingers develop a bluish tinge and are cool to touch. What should you do?

1. Elevate the arm
2. Apply warm compresses
3. Loosen the splint
4. Remove the splint

4-11. What is the primary reason for splinting fractures?

1. To prevent further injury
2. To control hemorrhage
3. To reduce swelling
4. To increase blood circulation

4-12. To fit well and provide adequate immobilization, a splint must have which of the attributes listed?

1. Be well padded at body contact areas
2. Be twice as wide as the injured limb
3. Be strong, rigid, and applied tightly
4. Be applied by two people

4-13. The proper first aid treatment for a fracture of the humerus near the shoulder is to

1. apply a splint to the outside and one to the inside of the upper arm, bandage the arm to the body and support the forearm in a sling
2. apply a splint to the outside of the arm, bandage the arm to the body, and support the forearm in a sling
3. place a pad or folded towel in the armpit, bandage the arm to the body, and support the forearm in a sling
4. splint the arm in the position you find it and bandage the arm securely to the body

4-14. When applying a splint to immobilize a fractured patella, where should you place extra padding?

1. Around the knee and under the buttocks
2. Under the knee and above the heel
3. Under the knee and under the thigh
4. Around the knee and under the calf

4-15. What is the most important consideration in treating a mandibular fracture?

1. Immediate immobilization
2. Ensuring a patent airway
3. Realignment of the jaw
4. Control of pain

4-16. Of the following actions, which is of prime importance when dealing with a head injury?

1. Determine if the skull is fractured
2. Assume cervical spine damage
3. Administer pain medication
4. Remove impaled objects

4-17. How should a suspected spinal fracture victim be transported?

1. Ensure immobilization on a rigid backboard
2. Place a pillow or adequate padding under the neck
3. Transport in the shock position
4. Do all of the above

4-18. Deformity at a joint, coupled with pain, discoloration, and immobility of and around the joint, is characteristic of which of the following disorders?

1. Dislocation
2. Simple fracture
3. Compound fracture
4. Displaced fracture

4-19. Of those listed below, which joints are the most frequently dislocated?

1. Sternal ribs, finger, and jaw
2. Knee, hip, and elbow
3. Knee, hip, shoulder, and jaw
4. hip, shoulder, fingers and jaw

4-20. To reduce a dislocated jaw, you should do which of the following?

1. Pull the chin forward and down
2. Have a victim open his or her mouth several times to affect reduction
3. Grasp behind the front teeth and pull forward
4. Press down behind the last molars and lift the chin

4-21. In general, sprains and strains are injuries to

1. joints and muscles
2. nerves and blood vessels
3. bones and blood vessels
4. bones and nerves

4-22. The treatment for strains and sprains includes all of the following EXCEPT

1. radiographic evaluation
2. immediate application of moist heat
3. immobilization and rest
4. elevation

A. 18%
B. 27%
C. 31.5%
D. 36%

IN ANSWERING QUESTIONS 4-23 THROUGH 4-25, USE THE "RULE OF NINES" AND FIGURE 4-48 IN THE TEXT TO DETERMINE THE EXTENT OF INJURY BY BODY SURFACE AREA, AND SELECT THE MOST APPROPRIATE ANSWER FROM THE LIST ABOVE BASED ON THE INFORMATION GIVEN IN THE QUESTION.

4-23. A steam burn to the face, chest, abdomen, and both arms.

1. A
2. B
3. C
4. D

4-24. A sunburn to the back of both legs, both arms, and the back.

1. A
2. B
3. C
4. D

4-25. A thermal burn to the left arm and front of the left leg.

1. A
2. B
3. C
4. D

4-26. First-aid treatment for extensive second degree burns should include which of the following treatments?

1. Anesthetic ointments and transport only
2. Debridement of the wound and dry dressings
3. Intravenous infusion and analgesia
4. Anesthetic ointments and analgesia

4-27. Morphine is an acceptable analgesic in patients with which of the following symptoms?

1. Head injuries
2. Profound respiratory distress
3. Advanced shock
4. Painful skin burns

4-28. The usual treatment for chemical burns is to flush with copious amounts of water. The two exceptions to this rule are in the case of which of the following chemicals?

1. Phosphoric acid and lye
2. White phosphorus and carbolic acid
3. Dry lime and carbolic acid
4. Sulfuric acid and carbolic acid

4-29. A dilute solution of which of the listed substances will neutralize alkali burns to the skin?

1. Alcohol
2. Phenol
3. Vinegar
4. Baking soda

4-30. First aid treatment of white phosphorus burns with partially embedded particles includes

1. wet dressings of copper sulfate
2. superficial debridement while flushing with water
3. neutralization with a dilute vinegar solution
4. neutralization with a dilute solution of baking soda

4-31. Signs and symptoms of heat exhaustion include a weak rapid pulse, nausea, headache, and

1. constricted pupils
2. greatly increased body temperature
3. cool, moist, and clammy skin
4. flushed, red face

4-32. The incidence of heat exposure injuries can be minimized by all of the following EXCEPT

1. education of personnel
2. environmental monitoring
3. daily salt tablets
4. maintenance of exhaust blowers and vents

4-33. What is the most effective method of rewarming a victim of hypothermia?

1. "Buddy warming"
2. Covering the victim with blankets or a sleeping bag
3. Hot water bottles at the neck, armpits, groin, and the chest
4. Immersion in a tub of warm water

4-34. An antiseptic emollient cream should be applied to which, if any, of the following cold injuries?

1. Chilblain
2. Immersion foot
3. All frostbites
4. None of the above. Cold injuries should be kept dry

4-35. For which, if any, of the following reasons should a frostbite injury remain frozen?

1. To minimize the severity of pain
2. Where there is a possibility of refreezing
3. To prevent shock
4. Never. Frostbite should always be rewarmed as quickly as possible

4-36. Which of the following is/are a recommended step(s) in treating deep frostbite?

1. Slowly rewarm frozen areas
2. Break blisters to speed healing
3. Gently rub injured areas to promote blood circulation
4. Comfort victim with hot tea or coffee

4-37. A Corpsman may administer morphine to which of the following patients?

1. With a head injury
2. In shock
3. With burns from inhaled chemicals
4. Hemorrhaging

4-38. Reversal of a syncopal episode can often be accomplished by what action?

1. Sitting with the head between the knees
2. Sitting upright
3. Lying down with the head and shoulders slightly elevated
4. Lying down in the reverse shock position

4-39. Which of the following methods is the quickest and easiest way of determining if an unconscious person is a diabetic?

1. Check for signs of ketoacidosis
2. Determine blood sugar levels
3. Look for signs of insulin use
4. Search for a Medic Alert tag, bracelet, or card

4-40. Of the following actions, which is the immediate treatment for insulin shock?

1. Administer an injection of insulin
2. Place sugar under the victim's tongue
3. Start an intravenous solution of normal saline
4. Administer oxygen

4-41. In addition to monitoring vital signs and making the patient comfortable, treatment for a stroke includes which of the following procedures?

1. Administering analgesics to relieve pain
2. Giving oxygen therapy
3. Giving a rapid infusion of a 5 percent dextrose solution
4. Giving a 0.3cc injection of epinephrine for vasoconstriction

4-42. Initial first aid treatment for an attack of angina pectoris includes reassurance, monitoring of vital signs, and

1. initiating CPR
2. giving sublingual nitroglycerin
3. advise the patient to return to duty when pain abates
4. giving a 0.3cc of epinephrine IM to increase heart rate

4-43. First aid treatment for acute myocardial infarction without cardiac arrest includes all of the following EXCEPT

1. giving oxygen therapy
2. monitoring vital signs
3. starting an intravenous infusion of only normal saline
4. transporting to a medical treatment facility

4-44. Proper first aid treatment for a patient suffering a convulsive seizure episode consists of which of the following procedures?

1. Protecting the victim from injury
2. Immediately starting CPR
3. Muscle massage during periods of rigidity
4. Injecting 75 to 100 mg of Demerol IM to effect relaxation

4-45. The most common psychiatric emergency is probably the suicide gesture or attempt. Basic treatment consists of all of the following EXCEPT

1. presenting a calm and understanding presence
2. leaving the victim alone to reflect on his or her actions
3. assuming all suicide threats are real
4. treating self-inflicted wounds as any other wound

4-46. When, during childbirth, the baby's head presents, why should you apply gentle pressure to the head?

1. To prevent an explosive delivery
2. To avoid compressing the umbilical cord
3. To compress the cord to stimulate the infant's vital function
4. To allow you time to suction the mouth and nose of the infant

4-47. When should the infant's mouth and nose be suctioned?

1. If spontaneous respirations do not occur
2. When the chin clears the vaginal canal
3. After the child has completely emerged
4. After clamping and cutting the umbilical cord

4-48. Emergency first aid treatment for a prolapsed cord during childbirth includes all of the following EXCEPT

1. decompressing the cord as much as possible
2. giving oxygen therapy
3. placing the mother in the shock position
4. clamping and cutting the umbilical cord when it presents

4-49. If a prolapsed cord occurs, which of the following actions should you take?

1. Give the mother oxygen
2. Place the mother in an extreme shock position
3. Get medical assistance
4. Each of the above

4-50. Poisoning is defined as contact with or exposure to a toxic substance.

1. True
2. False

4-51. A patient presents with dilated pupils, fever, dry skin, urinary retention, decreased bowel sounds, and increased heart rate. What toxidrome does this set of symptoms suggest?

1. Narcotic
2. Anticholinergic
3. Withdrawal
4. Non-syndrome syndrome

4-52. Which of the following is the method of choice for a Corpsman to use to induce vomiting?

1. 15-30 cc of syrup of Ipecac
2. 2 teaspoonfuls of dry mustard in water
3. 2 teaspoonfuls of an active charcoal slurry
4. To tickle the back of the victim's throat

4-53. Of the following, which is the most likely area of damage in a victim who has ingested a strong alkali?

1. Stomach
2. Esophagus
3. Liver
4. Colon

4-54. Treatment of a victim who ingested a strong acid includes intravenous infusion therapy and

1. inducing vomiting
2. diluting the stomach contents with water
3. neutralizing the stomach contents with a weak sodium bicarbonate solution
4. gastric lavage

4-55. Which of the following substances, upon ingestion, poses a threat of chemical or aspiration pneumonia?

1. Acid compounds
2. Alkali compounds
3. Petroleum distillates
4. Any of the above

4-56. If you are unable to reach the poison control center or a physician for specific instructions, how should you treat a victim who has ingested turpentine?

1. Induce vomiting and observe
2. Give 1 to 2 ounces of vegetable oil orally
3. Neutralize the poison with vinegar and water
4. Give 1 to 2 tablespoonfuls of milk of magnesia

4-57. Of the following, which, if any, is considered the most common agent in inhalation poisoning?

1. Carbon dioxide
2. Carbon monoxide
3. Freon
4. None of the above

4-58. Treatment for an inhalation poisoning victim includes all of the following EXCEPT

1. removal from the contaminated atmosphere
2. administration of oxygen
3. administration of stimulants
4. treatment for shock

4-59. A patient presents exhibiting signs of anaphylactic reaction to a bee or wasp sting. Of the following, which is NOT considered appropriate treatment?

1. Removal of patient's jewelry
2. Subcutaneous injection of epinephrine
3. Warm packs over the sting site
4. Removal of the stinger by scraping with a dull knife

4-60. The victim of a scorpion sting may safely be given any of the following pharmaceuticals EXCEPT

1. Demerol or morphine
2. Calcium gluconate
3. Valium
4. All the above are acceptable

4-61. Symptoms of a black widow spider bite may include severe pain, dyspnea, and

1. obvious swelling
2. abdominal rigidity
3. a necrotizing lesion
4. fever and chills

4-62. Excision and corticosterod therapy is early treatment for the bite of which of the following?

1. Scorpions
2. Black widow spiders
3. Brown recluse spiders
4. Snakes

4-63. What is the key identifying feature of the coral snake that distinguishes it from other snakes with similar markings?

1. The yellow band is always next to the red band
2. The red band is always next to the black band
3. It has a distinctive bite pattern
4. It has deep pits below the eyes

4-64. On patrol, a member of your unit receives a rattlesnake bite just below the elbow. What first aid treatment should you perform?

1. Place a tourniquet 1 inch proximal to the bite site
2. Place a constricting band 2 inches proximal to the bite site
3. Place a constricting band 2 inches distal to the bite site below the elbow
4. Both 2 and 3 above

4-65. Jellyfish nematocysts can be neutralized with which of the following substances?

1. Formalin
2. Dilute ammonia
3. Vinegar
4. Any of the above

4-66. The most widely abused drug(s) is/are

1. ethanol
2. opiates
3. barbiturates
4. amphetamines

4-67. Signs and symptoms of stimulant intoxication include all of the following EXCEPT

1. hyperactivity
2. increased appetite
3. dilated pupils
4. increased body temperature

4-68. A person may display which of the following symptom(s) after using a hallucinogenic drug?

1. Pin-pointed pupils
2. Decreased heartbeat
3. Flushed face
4. Both 2 and 3 above

4-69. Marijuana falls into which of the following categories of drugs?

1. Barbiturate
2. Physically addicting
3. Hallucinogen
4. Harmless

4-70. Persons who regularly abuse inhalants risk which of the following injuries?

1. Severe brain damage
2. Damaged internal organs
3. Death
4. Each of the above

4-71. In caring for drug-intoxicated persons, the Corpsman should perform what actions as his/her first priority?

1. Check for an adequate airway
2. Keep the victim awake
3. Induce vomiting if the victim is awake
4. Transport to a medical facility

Level	Health Hazard
0	Little or none
1 and 2	Slight
3	Extreme
4	Deadly

IN ANSWERING QUESTIONS 4-72 AND 4-73, REFER TO THE TABLE ABOVE. MATCH THE TOXICITY LEVEL WITH THE PROTECTION LEVEL REQUIRED, AS DESCRIBED IN THE QUESTION.

4-72. Full body protection and sealed equipment.

1. 0
2. 1 and 2
3. 3 and 4
4. 4 only

4-73. Protection level C.

1. 0
2. 1 and 2
3. 3
4. 4

4-74. The Corpsman should give special attention to which of the following requirements while working in the command sub-zone?

1. Work in low geographic areas to avoid toxic fumes
2. Decontaminate victims and equipment outside of the hazard zone
3. Stay upwind and upgrade of the incident site
4. Collect a sample of the hazardous material for later examination

4-75. What patient decontamination procedure is the most frequently used?

1. Absorption
2. Chemical wash
3. Dilution
4. Disposal and isolation

ASSIGNMENT 5

Textbook Assignment: "Pharmacy and Toxicology," chapter 6, pages 6-1 to 6-26; "Common Pharmaceuticals," appendix IV, pages AIV-1 to AIV-18.

5-1.   The actual title of the "blue bible" of pharmacology is

1.   the Physicians' Desk Reference
2.   The United States Pharmacopoeia and National Formulary (USP-NF)
3.   the Pharmacological Basis of Therapeutics
4.   Remington's Pharmaceutical Sciences

5-2.   The most common factor influencing the amount of drug given to a patient is

1.   weight
2.   gender
3.   age
4.   route of administration

5-3.   What would be the proper dose in milliliters of ampicillin for an 8-year old child if the adult dose is 15 ml?

1.   2
2.   6
3.   9
4.   15

5-4.   What is the name of the rule used to determine appropriate dosage of medication based on a child's weight?

1.   Young's Rule
2.   Clark's Rule
3.   Rule of Nines
4.   Minimum Rule

5-5.   Determine the appropriate dose in milligrams of medication for a child weighing 30 pounds if the average dose for an adult dose is 600 mg.

1.   50
2.   100
3.   120
4.   150

5-6.   In computing the amount of drug to be given to an underweight female, what adjustments to the normal dosage would ordinarily be made?

1.   Increase the dosage because of her weight and further increase because of her sex
2.   Increase of dosage because of her weight but decrease because of her sex
3.   Decrease of dosage because of her sex and further decrease because of her weight
4.   Decrease of dosage because of her sex but an increase because of her weight

5-7.   A drug given repeatedly to a patient often has to be increased in dosage to maintain the desired effect. The need for a larger dose is probably caused by

1.   an acquired tolerance from habitual use
2.   an abnormal sensitivity
3.   a cumulative effect from habitual use
4.   an individual idiosyncrasy

5-8. The most common method of administering medications is

1. orally
2. parentally
3. topically
4. intravenously

5-9. Which of the following is an example of a drug injected intradermally?

1. Insulin
2. Procaine hydrocloride
3. Purified protein derivative
4. 2 or 3 above

5-10. Which of the following is NOT a way in which drugs are grouped?

1. By chemical characteristics
2. By their brand names
3. By their source
4. By their action on the body

5-11. Which of the following is a characteristic side effect of antihistamines?

1. Nausea
2. Drowsiness
3. Uricaria
4. Tinnitis

5-12. Agents that inhibit the growth of microorganisms without necessarily killing them are known as

1. germicides
2. fungicides
3. antiseptics
4. astringents

5-13. The drug group most often used to treat dyspepsia is

1. emollients
2. astringents
3. antacids
4. adsorbents

5-14. Patients sensitive to penicillin may also exhibit sensitivity to cephalosporins.

1. True
2. False

5-15. Milk or milk products may interfere with the absorption of which of the following drugs?

1. Cephalexin (Keflex)
2. Tetracycline hydrochloride
3. Streptomycin sulfate
4. Erthromycin

5-16. Macrolides are effective against which of the following organisms?

1. Gram-positive cocci
2. Dermatophytes
3. Parasites
4. Gram-negative

5-17. Supplemental potassium may be required with which of the following categories of drugs?

1. Anti-inflammatories
2. Antidiahrreals
3. Antipyretics
4. Diuretics

5-18. The two most important opium alkaloids are morphine and

1. paraldehyde
2. codeine
3. meperidine
4. cocaine

5-19. Water-soluable vitamins are not excreted in the urine and are stored in the body in moderate amounts.

1. True
2. False

5-20. As used in the Navy, what is the primary purpose of biological agents?

1. Diagnosis
2. Resuscitation
3. Immunization
4. Pest control

5-21. Which of the following organizations is responsible for the licensing of biological agents?

1. Secretary of the Navy
2. Public Health Service
3. American Medical Association
4. Secretary of the Treasury

5-22. With which of the following is the yellow fever vaccine reconstituted?

1. Sterile water, USP
2. Triple distilled water, USP
3. Sterile, 5% dextrose in water, USP
4. Sterile sodium chloride injection, USP

5-23. Which of the following vaccines should not be administered to individuals who are sensitive to egg products?

1. Smallpox
2. Plague
3. Influenza
4. Anthrax

5-24. A poison that is introduced into the body in one location and affects the body in another location is displaying what effect?

1. Local
2. Remote
3. Cumulative
4. Inhibiting

5-25. The correct abbreviations for the metric system of primary units of measure for weight, volume, and linear dimensions are

1. gr, l, cm
2. gr, ml, m
3. g, l, m
4. g, l, cm

5-26. Which of the following is equal to one one-hundredth of a liter?

1. Dekaliter
2. Deciliter
3. Centiliter
4. Milliliter

5-27. The basic unit of weight in the apothecary system is the

1. gram
2. grain
3. dram
4. milliliter

5-28. A prescription requires 2 ounces of a substance stocked in liters. How many milliliters are required to fill the prescription?

1. 0.030
2. 0.060
3. 30.0
4. 60.0

5-29. A compound requires 40 grains of a substance stocked in kilograms. How many grams are required to prepare the compound?

1. 0.62
2. 2.6
3. 4.2
4. 2,400.0

38

5-30. You have 360 grams of a compound. If 54 grams of the compound is silver nitrite, what is the percentage of silver nitrite?

1. 12.5
2. 15.0
3. 17.5
4. 20.0

INFORMATION FOR ITEMS 5-31 AND 5-32 IS AS FOLLOWS: ASSUME THAT THE FOLLOWING IS THE CORRECT FORMULA FOR COMPOUNDING 1,000 ML OF POTASSIUM ARSENATE SOLUTION.

Arsenic trioxide........................... 12.8 g
Potassium bicarbonate.................. 9.8 g
Alcohol..................................... 40.0 ml
Distilled water, q.s. to make 1000..... 0 ml

5-31. You receive a prescription for 285 ml of the preceding formula. How many milliliters of alcohol should you use in compounding the prescription?

1. 9.6
2. 11.4
3. 13.6
4. 15.9

5-32. If you receive a prescription for 1,800 ml of the preceding formula, how many grams of arsenic trioxide will you use?

1. 7.80
2. 19.40
3. 23.04
4. 25.60

5-33. A patient is to receive 1.8 million units of oxycillin IM. Using quantity sufficient sterile water to reconstitute a vial of 2.4 million units to 2 ml, how much of the solution should the patient receive?

1. 1.0 ml
2. 1.25 ml
3. 1.50 ml
4. 1.75 ml

5-34. A patient is to receive a 3/4 gr dose of Phenobarbital. If you dissolve two 1/2 gr tablets of Phenobarbital in 30 ml of water, how much of the solution should the patient receive?

1. 15.0 ml
2. 17.5 ml
3. 20.0 ml
4. 22.5 ml

5-35. How many grams of sodium chloride are required to prepare 1 liter of a 1:5000 solution?

1. 0.2
2. 0.4
3. 2.0
4. 4.0

5-36. Of the following types of pharmaceutical preparations, which incorporates finely powdered medicinal substances into a fatty base?

1. Lotion
2. Suspension
3. Ointment
4. Elixir

5-37. All pharmacies that dispense medications are required to have what Class balance?

1. A
2. B
3. C
4. D

5-38. What drug incompatibility occurs when agents antagonistic to one another are prescribed together?

1. Therapeutic
2. Physical
3. Chemical
4. 1 and 3 above

5-39. Eutexia is an example of what type of drug incompatibility manifestation?

1. Chemical
2. Physical
3. Therapeutic
4. 2 and 3 above

5-40. A properly administered drug dosage that has an unintended and noxious effect on the patient is the definition of which of the following terms?

1. Contraindication
2. Drug interaction
3. Adverse reaction
4. Therapeutic incompatibility

5-41. In the prescription block of DD 1289, what part lists the names and quantities of the ingredients prescribed?

1. Superscription
2. Inscription
3. Subscription
4. Signa

5-42. If, in the course of filling a prescription, you feel that there may be a discrepancy or incompatibility, you should take which of the following actions?

1. Let the patient know that you discovered an error and will be checking with the prescriber before filling the prescription
2. Consult the prescriber to verify the prescription
3. Both 1 and 2
4. Fill the prescription as written

5-43. Which of the following is a schedule III drug?

1. Marijuana
2. An antitussive
3. Amphetamines
4. Nonbarbiturate sedative

5-44. What schedule of drug can never be ordered with refills?

1. II
2. III
3. IV
4. V

5-45. Which of the following is a bronchomucotropic agent?

1. Petrolatum
2. Guaifenesin
3. Benzoate
4. Phenol

5-46. Aluminum acetate, an astringent, is often used to treat which of the following conditions listed below?

1. Athlete's foot
2. External otitis
3. Poison ivy
4. All of the above

5-47. In conjunction with antacids, which of the following is used to treat duodenal ulcers?

1. Dimenhydrinate
2. Diphenhydramine hydrochloride
3. Ranitidine
4. Pseudoephedrine hydrochloride

5-48. Which of the following drugs is administered to control motion sickness?

1. Cimetidine
2. Meclizine hydrochloride
3. Chlorpheniramine maleate
4. Dephenhydramine hydrochloride

5-49. In addition to being an antacid, magnesium hydroxide may be used as a/an

1. emollient
2. laxative
3. demulcent
4. astringent

5-50. Which of the following is an ideal emollient to protect sensitive skin from the sun?

1. Theobroma oil
2. Lanolin
3. Zinc oxide ointment
4. Aluminum acetate

5-51. The standard by which all other antiseptics are measured is

1. betadine
2. phenol
3. isopropyl alcohol
4. hexachlorophene

5-52. An accidential spill of phenol can be neutralized by

1. water
2. silver nitrate
3. hydrogen peroxide
4. alcohol

5-53. The primary pharmacological action of sulfonimides is

1. viricidal
2. parasiticidal
3. bacteriostatic
4. fungistatic

5-54. The most common use for systemic sulfonamides is in the treatment of which of the conditions listed below?

1. Respiratory infections
2. Urinary tract infections
3. Viral infections
4. Furunculosis

5-55. Silver sulfadiazine is used almost exclusively in the treatment of

1. surgical wound sepsis
2. burns
3. prostatitis
4. furunculosis

5-56. Which of the following is for parenteral administration only?

1. Dicloxicillin
2. Ampicillin
3. Penicillin V
4. Penicillin G

5-57. The drug of choice for uncomplicated group A beta-hemolytic streptococcal pharyngitis is

1. Penicillin V potassium
2. Nafcillin
3. Ampicillin
4. Dicloxicillin

5-58. Severe colitis and diarrhea may be adverse side effects of which of the following?

1. Neomycin sulfate
2. Gentamicin sulfate
3. Penicillin G benzathene
4. Clindamycin hydrochloride

5-59. Which of the following is an appropriate substitute for penicillin when penicillin is contraindicated?

1. Doxycycline
2. Cephalexin
3. Erythromycin
4. Streptomycin

5-60. Of the following drugs, which was developed with the sole purpose being the treatment of gonorrhea?

1. Penicillin G benzathene
2. Nitrofurantoin
3. Spectinomycin hydrochloride
4. Doxycycline hyclate

5-61. Undeclyenic acid is used as a/an

1. disinfectant
2. antipyretic
3. analgesic
4. fungicide

5-62. In addition to the treatment of *Phthirus*, which of the following is effective in the treatment of scabies?

1. Nystatin
2. Miconazole nitrate
3. Permethrin
4. Metronidazole

5-63. Trichomonas vaginalis can be treated with

1. crotamiton
2. metronidazole
3. fansidar
4. mebendazole

5-64. Drugs that destroy parasitic worms are known as

1. ambecides
2. vermicides
3. germicides
4. bactericides

5-65. The drug of choice for the treatment and management of grand mal seizures is

1. methylphenidate hydrochloride
2. phenobarbital
3. phenytoin sodium
4. any psychotropic agent

5-66. Prochlorperizine is used mainly to

1. treat symptoms of nausea and vomiting
2. alleviate symptoms of tension, agitation, and psychosis
3. counteract the effects of alcohol withdrawal
4. relieve respiratory distress

5-67. Muscle relaxants include all of the following EXCEPT

1. methocarbamol
2. diazepam
3. cyclobenzaprine hydrochloride
4. temazepam

5-68. Digitoxin increases the force of cardiac contraction by acting on the

1. vagus nerve
2. valves of the heart
3. heart muscle
4. blood vessels

5-69. Of the following, which is an appropriate drug to administer to a patient suffering an asthma attack?

1. Amyl nitrite
2. Epinephrine
3. Phenylephrine hydrochloride
4. Atropine

5-70. The vitamin deficiency associated with night blindness is

1. vitamin A
2. vitamin B_6
3. vitamin B_{12}
4. vitamin K

5-71. A deficiency of which of the following could lead to inflammation, cracking of the lips, or vision problems?

1. Retinol
2. Thiamine
3. Riboflavin
4. Ascorbic acid

5-72. Which of the following is the vitamin involved in absorption and use of calcium and phosphorus?

1. Vitamin A
2. Vitamin B1
3. Vitamin C
4. Vitamin D

5-73. The agent used to treat pernicious anemia is

1. cyanocobalamin
2. ascorbic acid
3. vitamin D
4. vitamin K

5-74. The general anesthesia agent most commonly used in dentistry is

1. halothane
2. nitrous oxide
3. lidocaine hydrochloride
4. procaine hydrochloride

5-75. On what area of the body is proparacaine hydrochloride most widely used as a topical anesthetic?

1. Nose
2. Ears
3. Eyes
4. Throat

ASSIGNMENT 6

Textbook Assignment: "Clinical Laboratory," chapter 7, pages 7-1 to 7-36.

6-1. Which of the following, if any, is considered the most appropriate source for blood specimens obtained for clinical examination?

1. By venipuncture
2. By finger puncture
3. From an artery
4. None of the above

6-2. Using the steps below, determine the correct sequence for obtaining blood by finger puncture.
    a. Clean finger
    b. Lance finger
    c. Milk finger
    d. Collect specimen
    e. Wipe away first drop

1. a, b, c, e, d
2. c, b, e, a, d
3. a, c, b, e, d
4. c, a, b, e, d

6-3. When performing a finger puncture, the first drop should be wiped away to avoid which of the following conditions?

1. Bacterial contamination
2. Clotting at the puncture site
3. Dilution of the specimen with alcohol
4. Dilution of the specimen with tissue fluids

6-4. How would a 5 ml blood specimen be obtained from a patient with an intravenous antibiotic being given through the left arm and blood being received through the right arm?

1. Multiple finger punctures
2. Left arm
3. Right arm
4. Hand or foot

6-5. A tourniquet applied to the arm during venipuncture should provide enough tension to compress the artery, but not the vein.

1. True
2. False

6-6. The correct needle position for venipuncture is (a) what degree angle and (b) with the bevel in what position?

1. (a) 15, (b) up
2. (a) 30, (b) up
3. (a) 15, (b) down
4. (a) 30, (b) down

6-7. A tourniquet is normally applied before and to aid in the process of venipuncture. At what point in the venipuncture procedure should you remove the tourniquet?

1. Just before needle insertion
2. Just after needle insertion, but before vacutainer
3. Once all specimens have been collected
4. After needle removal

6-8. The part of the microscope on which the prepared specimen is placed for examination is called the

1. arm
2. base
3. frame
4. stage

6-9. All of the following are components of the microscope's illumination system EXCEPT

1. internal light source
2. condenser
3. external light source
4. iris diaphragm

6-10. The total magnification available by using the lens color coded red is

1. 1000X
2. 450X
3. 100X
4. 10X

6-11. Light travels from the objective to the ocular lens through what component of the microscope?

1. Body tube
2. Iris diaphragm
3. High-powered lens
4. Revolving nosepiece

6-12. What objective should be used for a detailed study of stained bacterial smears?

1. Low power
2. High dry
3. Oil immersion
4. Either 2 or 3 above

6-13. If necessary, which, if any, of the following substances may be used for cleaning the lenses on a microscope?

1. Alcohol
2. Bleach
3. Xylene
4. None of the above

6-14. A CBC includes which of the following?

1. Total RBC count
2. Hematocrit
3. Differential WBC count
4. All of the above

6-15. The hemacytometer is designed primarily for what purpose?

1. To differentiate between red blood cells and white blood cells
2. To count white blood cells
3. To count red blood cells
4. Both 2 and 3

6-16. The main reason for using the cover glass included with the hemacytometer instead of an ordinary cover glass is because the hemacytometer cover glass

1. is clearer
2. has an even surface
3. is thicker
4. is less likely to break

6-17. A subnormal RBC count may indicate that the patient has which of the following listed conditions?

1. Leukopenia
2. Anemia
3. Dehydration
4. Uremia

6-18. What is the total capacity of the capillary pipette provided in a Unopette® for RBC count?

1. 0.5µl
2. 1.0µl
3. 10.0µl
4. 100.0µl

6-19. Which of the following conditions indicates that the counting chamber is properly loaded?

1. There is a thin, even film of fluid under the coverglass
2. The fluid flows into the grooves at the edges of the chamber
3. Air bubbles are seen in the field
4. The chamber is flooded

6-20. What objective should be used for counting RBCs?

1. Low power
2. High power
3. Oil immersion
4. High dry

6-21. When counting cells, to arrive at a correct count, the cells touching the lines on the_____ and _____are counted in addition to all cells totally within each square.

1. Left, top
2. Left, bottom
3. Right, top
4. Right, bottom

6-22. To arrive at the number of RBCs per mm^3, total the number of cells counted in the five fields and multiply by

1. 0.1
2. 10.0
3. 100.0
4. 10,000.0

6-23. Which of the following factors affect hemoglobin values?

1. Age
2. Sex
3. Altitude
4. All the above

6-24. Both the number of squares and the counting procedure for WBCs is the same as it is for RBCs.

1. True
2. False

6-25. What is the term used for the volume of erythrocytes expressed as a percentage of the volume of whole blood in a sample?

1. Hematocrit
2. Hemoglobin
3. Red blood count
4. Complete blood cell count

6-26. The hematocrit for a normal, healthy female is within what range?

1. 30 to 40 percent
2. 37 to 47 percent
3. 42 to 50 percent
4. 44 to 52 percent

6-27. A shift from leukocytosis toward leukopenia in a patient with a systemic bacterial infection is a good sign.

1. True
2. False

6-28. Select from those listed below the term used to describe an abnormally high WBC count.

1. Leukocytosis
2. Erythrocytosis
3. Leukopenia
4. Pancytopenia

6-29. Which of the following conditions may cause leukopenia?

1. Strep throat
2. Psittacosis
3. Anaphylactic shock
4. Each of the above

6-30. To arrive at the number of white cells per mm^3 of blood, total the number of cells counted in the four fields and multiply by

1. 0.5
2. 5.0
3. 50.0
4. 5000.0

6-31. A differential blood count is the percentage of distribution in the blood of which of the following types of cells?

1. Lymphocytes
2. Monocytes
3. Leukocytes
4. Erythrocytes

6-32. What is the function of leukocytes?

1. To carry oxygen through the blood
2. To control various disease conditions
3. To aid in clotting the blood
4. Each of the above

6-33. What type of leukocyte comprises the largest percentage of cells in the circulating blood?

1. Lymphocyte
2. Neutrophil
3. Erythocyte
4. Thrombocyte

6-34. When viewing a smear for a differential count, you identify the cells with the large, scattered dark blue granules that are darker than their nuclei as

1. lymphocytes
2. monocytes
3. basophils
4. neutrophils

6-35. The largest of the normal WBCs is the

1. monocyte
2. lymphocyte
3. eosinophil
4. basophil

6-36. On a properly prepared slide for a differential count, the smear will

1. extend from one side of the slide to the other
2. be evenly distributed on the entire slide
3. show no wavy or blank spots
4. show smooth even edges

6-37. Properly prepared differential slides require a longer rinse time than stain time.

1. True
2. False

6-38. If a smear used in a differential count is to be saved for reexamination, remove the immersion oil by placing a piece of lens tissue over the slide and moistening the tissue with

1. alcohol
2. water
3. xylene
4. acetone

6-39. A continued shift to the left with a falling total WBC count probably indicates

1. progress toward normal recovery
2. a decrease in immature neutrophils
3. a breakdown of the body's defense mechanism and is a poor prognosis
4. a decrease in parasitic and allergenic conditions

A. Recovery
B. Parasitic infection
C. Breakdown of the body's defense
D. Active tuberculosis

TO ANSWER QUESTIONS 6-40 THROUGH 6-43, SELECT FROM THE ABOVE LIST THE CONDITION THAT MOST APPROPRIATELY CORRESPONDS TO THE LEUKOCYTIC CHARACTERISTIC IN THE QUESTION.

6-40. Increased eosinophils.

1. A
2. B
3. C
4. D

6-41. Increased monocytes.

1. A
2. B
3. C
4. D

6-42. Decreased WBC count with increased juvenile cells.

1. A
2. B
3. C
4. D

6-43. Decreased WBC count with increased mature cells.

1. A
2. B
3. C
4. D

6-44. All of the following are classifications of bacteria EXCEPT

1. Temperature and moisture content
2. Growth requirements and morphologic characteristics
3. Toxins produced and disease-producing ability
4. Gram's stain reaction and colonial morphology

6-45. The difference between anaerobes and aerobes is that anaerobes need oxygen to reproduce.

1. True
2. False

6-46. Autotrophic bacteria require an environment that supplies them with nourishment.

1. True
2. False

6-47. Which of the following structures provides some bacteria with a means of movement?

1. Capsule
2. Spore
3. Spirillum
4. Flagellum

6-48. What type of bacterial toxin completely lyses erythrocytes?

1. Exotoxin
2. Endotoxin
3. Beta hemolysin
4. Alpha hemolysin

A. Impetigo
B. Plague
C. Pneumonia
D. Gas gangrene
E. Strep throat
F. Whooping cough

TO ANSWER ITEMS 6-49 THROUGH 6-53, SELECT FROM THE ABOVE LIST THE CONDITION MOST PROBABLY CAUSED BY THE AGENT LISTED IN THE QUESTION.

6-49.   Bordetella pertussis.

1.   A
2.   C
3.   E
4.   F

6-50.   Streptococcus pneumoniae.
1.   A
2.   B
3.   C
4.   E

6-51.   Yersinia pestis.

1.   B
2.   C
3.   D
4.   E

6-52.   Clostridium perfringens.

1.   A
2.   C
3.   D
4.   F

6-53.   Staphylococcus aureus.

1.   A
2.   D
3.   E
4.   F

6-54.   In the Gram's stain procedure, which of the following chemicals acts as the mordant?

1.   Crystal violet
2.   Safranin
3.   Iodine
4.   Acetone

6-55.   All of the following statements are true about antigens EXCEPT that an antigen

1.   is inherently unstable structurally
2.   must be foreign to the body
3.   possesses a high molecular weight
4.   has a high specificity to stimulate tissues to produce antibodies

6-56.   The Rapid Plasma Reagin test for syphilis is best used with what type of specimen?

1.   Serum
2.   Plasma
3.   Whole blood
4.   Either serum or plasma

6-57. To properly perform the RPR Card Test, the serum sample should be from arterial blood that has been separated from the blood cells as soon after collection as possible.

1. True
2. False

6-58. Which of the following actions is considered appropriate if a patient's RPR is reactive?

1. Give patient penicillin
2. Send patient to lab for further testing
3. Counsel patient against engaging in unsafe sex
4. Report results of RPR to patient's commanding officer

6-59. Which of the following chemical preparations is frequently used to detect fungi?

1. Hydrogen sulfoxide
2. Hydrogen peroxide
3. Potassium hydroxide
4. Potassium sulfate

6-60. The best urine specimen is that taken during which of the following times?

1. First morning
2. Random
3. Fasting
4. 24 hour

6-61. For a 24-hour urine specimen collection, which of the following statements is INCORRECT?

1. Discard the first specimen
2. Add a preservative after the first specimen has been obtained
3. Discard the last specimen
4. Refrigerate the specimen during the collection period

6-62. What purpose does toluene serve when used in conjunction with a urine specimen?

1. It increases the albumin
2. It dissolves unwanted cells
3. It protects the specimen from decomposition
4. It dissolves the albumin

6-63. Which of the following colors would be considered abnormal in a urine specimen?

1. Colorless
2. Amber
3. Straw
4. Red

A. Pyridium®
B. Bile
C. Blood
D. Fats (chyle)

TO ANSWER ITEMS 6-64 THROUGH 6-67, SELECT FROM THE ABOVE LIST THE MOST PROBABLE CAUSATIVE AGENT THAT WOULD PRODUCE THE URINE COLOR STATED IN THE QUESTION.

6-64. Milky.

1. A
2. B
3. C
4. D

6-65. Dark orange.

1. A
2. B
3. C
4. D

6-66. Red-brown.

1. A
2. B
3. C
4. D

6-67. Brown.

1. A
2. B
3. C
4. D

6-68. A report on urine transparency is valid regardless of standing time.

1. True
2. False

6-69. The specific gravity of a liquid or solid is the weight of the substance as compared to an equal volume of

1. ethanol
2. methanol
3. distilled water
4. normal saline

6-70. In the microscopic examination of urine sediment, scan the slide using the low per objective and examine it in detail using which of the following objectives?

1. Low power
2. High dry
3. High power
4. Oil immersion

6-71. The addition of one drop of 5 percent acetic acid to urine sediment will disintegrate

1. white blood cells
2. mucous threads
3. casts
4. red blood cells

6-72. There are seven types of casts or sediments found in urine. Of the four listed below, which may be attributed to lupus?

1. Red cell casts
2. Fatty casts
3. Granular casts
4. Epithelial casts

ASSIGNMENT 7

Textbook Assignment: "Medical Aspects of Chemical, Biological, and Radiological Warfare," chapter 8, pages 8-1 to 8-18; "Diet and Nutrition," chapter 9, pages 9-1 to 9-11; "Emergency Dental Care and Preventive Medicine," chapter 10, pages 10-1 to 10-6.

7-1. Who is responsible for area decontamination of chemical agents aboard ship?

1. Medical officer
2. Supply officer
3. Damage control personnel
4. All hands

7-2. What should be the first priority in the treatment of chemically contaminated casualties?

1. Control of massive hemorrhage
2. Decontamination
3. Treatment of life-threatening shock and wounds
4. Removal of contaminated clothing

7-3. Who, if anyone, is responsible for maintaining adequate supplies for the decontamination and treatment of CBR casualties?

1. Medical officer
2. Damage control officer
3. Supply officer
4. No one

7-4. Nerve agents produce their effect by interfacing with normal transmission of nerve impulses.

1. True
2. False

7-5. The tendency of a chemical agent to remain effective in a contaminated area is known as

1. lethality
2. persistency
3. volatility
4. permeability

7-6. Inhalation of nerve gas characteristically results in which of the symptoms listed below?

1. Local muscular twitching
2. Dry mouth
3. Pinpoint pupils
4. Pulmonary edema

7-7. In a definitive care facility, the indicated treatment of a nerve agent victim includes which of the following therapies?

1. 2 mg atropine and 600 mg 2-PAM chloride every 15 minutes until recovery
2. 2 mg atropine every 15 minutes until the victim has a dry mouth and mild tachycardia
3. 600 mg 2-PAM chloride every 15 minutes until the victim is conscious
4. Respiratory support only

7-8. What part of the body is most sensitive to the effects of mustard gases?

1. Eyes
2. Lungs
3. Liver
4. Skin

7-9. Specific antidotal therapy is available for which, if any, of the following vesicants?

1. Mustard (HD)
2. Nitrogen mustard (HN)
3. Lewisite (L)
4. None of the above

7-10. First aid treatment for blood agents is amyl nitrite ampules followed by which of the compounds listed below?

1. Oral potassium chloride
2. Oral sodium thiosulfate
3. Intravenous potassium chloride
4. Intravenous sodium thiosulfate

7-11. The symbol for phosgene gas is

1. Cl
2. CN
3. CG
4. CK

7-12. Which of the following odors is an early indication of exposure to phosgene gas in casualty-producing amounts?

1. Bitter almonds
2. A freshly mown lawn
3. Geraniums
4. None of the above. Phosgene is undetectable

7-13. The chemical agent that primarily affects the higher regulatory functions of the CNS is represented by which of the following symbols?

1. AC
2. BZ
3. CN
4. CS

7-14. Exposure to fresh air and allowing wind to blow across wide open eyes is generally sufficient treatment for which of the following agents?

1. Psychochemicals
2. Lacrimators
3. Vomiting agents
4. Glycolates

7-15. With exposure to Adamsite, which, if any, of the following actions must be taken to minimize or inhibit the symptoms of exposure?

1. Don a protective mask and continue duties as vigorously as possible
2. Give an intramuscular injection of physostigmine
3. Give an intravenous infusion of sodium thiosulfate
4. Do none of the above

7-16. What is the proper treatment for burning white phosphorus particles embedded in the skin?

1. Surgical removal followed by a copper sulfate wet dressing
2. A copper sulfate rinse then surgical removal
3. A copper sulfate rinse only
4. Allowing them to burn out

7-17. By what means can biological agents can be detected?

1. Physical senses
2. Chemical detectors
3. Laboratory examination
4. All of the above

7-18. When entering an area known to be contaminated with biological agents, which of the following actions should be taken?

1. Put on gloves, if available
2. Button up clothing
3. Put on a protective mask
4. Do all of the above

7-19. What is the appropriate procedure to follow when biological agents are known to have been placed in your drinking water?

1. Double the amount of chlorine in the water
2. Double the time the water is exposed to the chlorine
3. Boil the water before you drink any of it
4. Refrain from drinking the water

7-20. Presenting a serious internal radiation hazard, alpha particles can enter the body through which of the following?

1. The digestive system
2. The respiratory system
3. Open wounds
4. Any of the above

7-21. Of the following, which type of radiation has the greatest penetrating power?

1. Alpha
2. Beta
3. Gamma
4. Neutron

7-22. In the event of a nuclear detonation, what is the best position to assume?

1. Sitting, with the knees drawn up to the chest, facing away from the blast
2. Face down, with your face covered
3. On your side, in a fetal position facing away from the blast
4. Supine, with your face covered

7-23. The treatment of thermal burns from a nuclear detonation differs from more conventional burn wounds in which, if any, of the following ways?

1. Conventional burn wounds are generally less serious
2. Conventional burn wounds are more likely to become infected
3. Burns resulting from a nuclear detonation are more painful
4. There is no difference

7-24. When using antibiotics for victims of radiation injuries, what is the recommended dosage?

1. One-half of the normal dosage
2. The normal dosage
3. Two times the normal dosage
4. Three times the normal dosage

7-25. Approximately what number of calories must be burned or consumed for the average individual to lose or gain one pound?

1. 1,500
2. 2,000
3. 3,500
4. 5,000

7-26. Which of the following nutritive elements are considered the "building blocks" of the body?

1. Fats
2. Carbohydrates
3. Minerals
4. Proteins

7-27. What happens to protein consumed that is in excess of body requirements?

1. Used to supply energy only
2. Changed into fat only
3. Both 1 and 2
4. Excreted from the body through elimination

7-28. What total number of amino acids are obtained solely from the food we eat?

1. 3
2. 7
3. 9
4. 11

7-29. What amount of protein should a non-pregnant person consume on a daily basis?

1. 0.8 g/kg
2. 1.2 g/kg
3. 2.2 lbs
4. There is no specific recommended amount

7-30. Protein deficiency can result in which of the following conditions?

1. Nutritional edema
2. Secondary anemia
3. Restricted growth
4. Each of the above

7-31. The number of calories generated by each gram of protein, fat, and carbohydrate, respectively is

1. 3, 6, 4
2. 4, 9, 4
3. 6, 3, 9
4. 9, 4, 6

7-32. The serum cholesterol level of adults over the age of 30 should be less than

1. 100 mg/dl
2. 150 mg/dl
3. 200 mg/dl
4. 300 mg/dl

7-33. Of the following, which is NOT a source of dietary fat?

1. Rice
2. Whole milk
3. Avocados
4. Egg yolks

7-34. Refined and processed sugars should make up no more than what percent of an individual's total caloric intake?

1. 5
2. 10
3. 15
4. 20

A. Complex carbohydrates
B. Simple carbohydrates
C. Proteins
D. Fats

FOR QUESTIONS 7-35 TO 7-39, USE THE ABOVE LIST TO MATCH THE FOOD IDENTIFIED IN EACH OF THE QUESTIONS TO THE NUTRITIVE ELEMENT PRIMARILY ASSOCIATED WITH IT.

7-35. Fish.

1. A
2. B
3. C
4. D

7-36. Honey.

1. A
2. B
3. C
4. D

7-37. Butter.

1. A
2. B
3. C
4. D

7-38. Eggs.

1. A
2. B
3. C
4. D

7-39. Corn.

1. A
2. B
3. C
4. D

7-40. An otherwise normal, healthy diet is always sufficient to provide an individual with adequate levels of minerals.

1. True
2. False

7-41. Consumption of excessive amounts of certain vitamins can, in some circumstances, be fatal.

1. True
2. False

7-42. Which of the following is sometimes referred to as "the forgotten nutrient"?

1. Selenium
2. Phosphorus
3. Water
4. Fructose

7-43. According to the Dietary Guidelines for Americans, upon which of the following dietary elements should a nutritional diet be based?

1. Fruits and vegetables
2. Complex carbohydrates
3. Fats
4. Dairy

7-44. Fried foods, as long as they are not too crisp, may be included in a soft diet.

1. True
2. False

7-45. When a liquid diet has been ordered by the attending physician or dietician, the feedings should be ____ ounces and administered every ____ hours.

1. 4-6, 3-4
2. 6-8, 2-3
3. 8-10, 6-8
4. 10-12, 2-3

7-46. A high-calorie diet may be effected by modifying the regular diet in which of the following ways?

1. Adding snacks
2. Increasing portions
3. Providing commercial supplements
4. Each of the above

A.	Liquid
B.	High-calorie
C.	High-protein
D.	Low-calorie
E.	Low-protein

FOR QUESTIONS 7-47 TO 7-51, SELECT THE DIET FROM THE LIST ABOVE THAT MOST APPROPRIATELY MATCHES THE MALADY IN THE QUESTION.

7-47. Malnourishment.

1. A
2. B
3. C
4. D

7-48. Hypothyroidism.

1. E
2. D
3. C
4. B

7-49. Inflammatory GI tract.

1. A
2. B
3. C
4. D

7-50.   Low production of antibodies.

1.   E
2.   D
3.   C
4.   B

7-51.   Chronic nephrotic edema.

1.   B
2.   C
3.   D
4.   E

7-52.   Which of the following is appropriate procedure in the administration of a high-residue diet?

1.   Ensure adequate fluid intake
2.   Limit caffeine intake
3.   Provide raw or tender-cooked vegetables
4.   All of the above

A.   High-residue
B.   Low-residue
C.   Low-sodium
D.   Bland
E.   Low-carbohydrate, high-protein

FOR QUESTIONS 7-53 TO 7-57, SELECT THE DIET FROM THE LIST ABOVE THAT MOST APPROPRIATELY MATCHES THE MALADY IN THE QUESTION.

7-53.   Peptic ulcers.

1.   E
2.   D
3.   C
4.   B

7-54.   Hypertension.

1.   A
2.   B
3.   C
4.   D

7-55.   Hemorrhoidectomy.

1.   E
2.   D
3.   C
4.   B

7-56.   Hypoglycemia.

1.   B
2.   C
3.   D
4.   E

7-57.   Spastic colon.

1.   A
2.   B
3.   C
4.   D

7-58.   What is the most common cause of dental caries?

1.   Sugar
2.   Lack of fluoridation
3.   Infrequent dental examinations
4.   Bacterial plaque

7-59.   Severe inflammation of the tooth pulp is known as

1.   acute pulpitis
2.   periapical absess
3.   marginal gingivitis
4.   necrotizing ulcerative gingivitis

7-60.   The most frequent cause of marginal gingivitis is

1.   bacteria
2.   caries
3.   poor oral hygiene
4.   periodontitis

7-61. What is the most frequent cause of periodontal abscesses?

1. A virus
2. An infection
3. Poor oral hygiene
4. Prolonged irritation

7-62. An inflammation of the gingiva around a partially erupted tooth is known as

1. periodontitis
2. periodontal abscess
3. stomatitis
4. pericoronitis

7-63. An inflammation of the oral mucosa is called

1. periocoronitis
2. gingivitis
3. stomatitis
4. periodontitis

7-64. Labial herpes is an infection that results in which of the following conditions?

1. Fever blisters
2. Gingivitis
3. Pericoronitis
4. All the above

7-65. Excruciating, constant pain 3 days after a tooth extraction indicates which of the following conditions?

1. Hemorrhage
2. Osteitis
3. Stomatitis
4. Pericoronitis

7-66. The form used to record dental treatment is the

1. SF 600
2. SF 602
3. EZ 603A
4. NAVMED 6150/20

7-67. In addition to maintaining and promoting good health, personal hygiene is important for which of the following reasons?

1. Inhibits the spread of disease
2. Promotes good morale
3. Decreases the risk of disabling disease
4. All of the above

7-68. Preventive medicine procedures in the Navy are addressed in detail in what publication?

1. SECNAVINST 4061.1
2. NAVMED P-5010
3. NAVMED P-5038
4. Navy Supply Publication 486

7-69. Animals that carry disease and can transmit those diseases to human or animal hosts to cause illness or injury are called

1. pests
2. insects
3. vectors
4. rodents

7-70. Guidance as to appropriate food storage temperatures, storage life of perishable and semi-perishable food items, and safe time limits for keeping food can be found in which of the following publications?

1. SECNAVINST 4061.1
2. NAVMED P-5010
3. NAVMED P-5038
4. Navy Supply Publication 486

7-71. All Navy and Marine Corps food-service facilities must be inspected by a medical department representative and food-service department representative.

1. True
2. False

7-72. Immunizations used within the Armed Forces are required to meet standards set forth by which of the following organizations?

1. Food and Drug Administration
2. Department of Health and Human Services
3. Centers for Disease Control
4. National Institutes of Health

7-73. Instructions for preparing and submitting the Medical Event Report can be found in which of the following publications?

1. SECNAVINST 4061.1
2. NAVMED P-5010
3. NAVMED P-5038
4. Navy Supply Publication 486

7-74. As long as it is clear, tastes good, and is free from odor, water obtained in the field can be considered to be potable.

1. True
2. False

7-75. Marine sanitation devices (MSDs) perform what function(s) aboard ship?

1. Treat sewage before discharge into restricted waters
2. Collect and hold sewage for treatment
3. Treat sewage before discharge into unrestricted waters
4. Both 2 and 3

ASSIGNMENT 8

Textbook Assignment: "Physical Examinations," chapter 11, pages 11-1 to 11-12; "Health Records," chapter 12, pages 12-1 to 12-25; "Supply," chapter 13, pages 13-1 to 13-21.

8-1. Physical examinations of Navy and Marine Corps personnel, whether active or reserve, may be performed by which of the following?

1. Navy medical officers
2. DoD physicians
3. Credentialed civilian contract physicians
4. All the above

8-2. What entity is responsible for setting the physical standards for entry into the U.S. Navy?

1. Bureau of Naval Personnel
2. Department of Defense
3. Bureau of Naval Medicine
4. Chief of Naval Operations

8-3. In which, if any, of the following publications will you find the prescribed intervals for periodic physical examinations?

1. MILPERSMAN
2. NAVMED P-5010
3. NAVMED P-117
4. None of the above

8-4. All of the following are functions of a medical board EXCEPT

1. evaluating and reporting on diagnosis
2. selection of personnel for special duty
3. planning for treatment, rehabilitation, or convalescence
4. estimating the length of further disability

8-5. Family member screening is required even if a servicemember is accepting unaccompanied orders to an overseas duty station.

1. True
2. False

8-6. Medical surveillance examinations are required for certain occupational fields or certain skills or jobs; e.g., people who work with beryllium or mercury. Specific guidelines on what tests are required and the frequency of those tests can be found in

1. BUMEDINST 5100.1
2. COMNAVMEDCOMINST 5100.46
3. OPNAVINST 5100.23
4. SECNAVINST 6200.2

8-7. What report is used when a member is expected to return to full duty status after being placed on limited duty?

1. Limited Duty (LIMDU) Board
2. Formal Medical Board
3. Abbreviated Temporary Limited Duty (TLD) Medical Board
4. Physical Examination Board (PEB)

8-8. Which of the following steps is appropriate when a servicemember is found not fit for duty after an initial TLD period of 6 months, but has a favorable prognosis and is expected to be returned to duty within 4 more months?

1. Administrative separation
2. Extension of 4 months to his TLD
3. Initiation of a second and final 6-month TLD
4. Formal medical board

8-9. What is the maximum length of time an individual may be held on limited duty without convening a formal board?

1. 8 months
2. 16 months
3. 1 year
4. 2 years

8-10. Who is responsible for verifying the content of a medical board?

1. The attending physician
2. The LIMDU Coordinator
3. The Patient Administration Limited Duty Coordinator
4. The convening authority

8-11. A command endorsement is required on a formal medical board.

1. True
2. False

8-12. A Sailor reports for her periodic physical examination and states that no changes have occurred in her medical status since her last physical. What entry, if any, would be appropriate to put in block 25 of her SF 93, Report of Medical History?

1. "N/A"
2. "No changes"
3. "No significant interval history"
4. Nothing; leave block 25 blank

8-13. One method for testing near visual acuity is the

1. Snellen charts
2. Jaeger cards
3. Farnsworth lantern
4. pseudoisochromatic plates

8-14. The preferred method for testing color vision is the

1. Snellen charts
2. Jaeger cards
3. Farnsworth lantern
4. pseudoisochromatic plates

8-15. EKGs are performed routinely as part of a member's physical examination once the member reaches the age of 35.

1. True
2. False

8-16. The health record of a military member may be used for which of the following purposes?

1. Aid in determining claims
2. Determine physical fitness
3. Provide data for medical statistics
4. Do all of the above

8-17. Of the following, which is NOT considered a major category of the primary medical record?

1. DREC
2. HREC
3. IREC
4. OREC

8-18. Secondary medical records, which are held separately from primary medical records, are not normally opened or maintained for active duty personnel. Under which of the following circumstances may a secondary medical record be established for an active member?

1. The member is to undergo surgery
2. The member is to go TAD for medical treatment
3. The member is under investigation for domestic abuse
4. The member is AWOL

8-19. What information should be included on the NAVMED 6150/20 of a member's primary medical record with respect to the existence of a member's secondary medical record?

1. Nature of secondary record
2. Patient's diagnosis
3. Clinic name, address, and phone number
4. Each of the above

8-20. Custody of health records is generally vested in the medical department. On ships without a medical department representative, an individual retains custody of the record until which of the following times, if any?

1. Transfer
2. Transfer with verification every 6 months
3. Transfer with annual verification
4. Never

8-21. Health records are for official use only but are subject to inspection an any time by

1. the commanding officer or his or her superior
2. authorized medical inspectors
3. the fleet medical officer
4. any of the above

8-22. When a member is hospitalized in a foreign nation and the ship departs port, the health record is

1. retained on board
2. turned over to the hospital
3. forwarded to the nearest U.S. consulate or embassy
4. turned over to another U.S. vessel in port

8-23. Although considered privileged, release of information in the health record is required under the Freedom of Information Act.

1. True
2. False

8-24. Under which of the following circumstances may an individual's medical information be released to his authorized representative(s)?

1. When verbally requested by the individual
2. Upon request of the representative when adequate proof of the individual's death can be provided
3. Upon proof that the individual has been declared mentally incompetent
4. Both 2 and 3 above

8-25. A well-known and preeminent research group requests medical information to use as part of the basis of a study it is performing. What action, if any, should be taken prior to release?

1. Commanding officer of MTF should release information immediately
2. Commanding officer of MTF should check with the Judge Advocate General for advice
3. Commanding officer of MTC should forward the request to BUMED for guidance
4. None; an individual's medical information may not be released for research

8-26. The health record jacket of PO3 Walter T. Door, 333-44-5555, would be what color?

1. Blue
2. Almond
3. Orange
4. Pink

8-27. A health record is only opened in which of the following cases?

1. When a member returns to active duty from the retired list
2. When the original record has been lost
3. When first becoming a member of the naval service
4. In all the above cases

8-28. In the record category box on the health record jacket, all active duty military records are identified by what color tape?

1. Blue
2. Black
3. Red
4. White

8-29. The health jackets of flag or general officers should be annotated to reflect their rank.

1. True
2. False

8-30. When a HREC is opened on a service member, the member should be directed to read and sign the Privacy Act Statement inside the back cover of the HREC.

1. True
2. False

8-31. Entries to the Chronological Record of Medical Care, SF 600, when not typewritten, should be made in which color(s) of ink?

1. Blue
2. Black or blue-black
3. Red
4. Ink color is irrelevant

8-32. What is the preferred form on which to record admission to the hospital?

1. SF 509, Medical Record-Progress Report
2. SF 600, Chronological Record of Medical Care
3. NAVMED 6150/4, Abstract of Service and Medical History
4. NAVMED 6150/20, Summary of Care

```
A. SF 600
B. SF 601
C. DD1141
D. NAVMED 6150/2
```

IN ANSWERING QUESTIONS 8-33 THROUGH 8-36, SELECT FROM THE ABOVE LIST THE APPROPRIATE HEALTH RECORD FORM FOR RECORDING THE INFORMATION GIVEN.

8-33. Routine innoculations.

1. A
2. B
3. C
4. D

8-34. Human immune virus testing.

1. A
2. B
3. C
4. D

8-35. Sick call visits for poison ivy.

1. A
2. B
3. C
4. D

8-36. Results of radiation monitoring.

1. A
2. B
3. C
4. D

```
A. NAVMED 6150/4
B. SF 539
C. SF 601
D. DD 771
```

**IN ANSWERING QUESTIONS 8-37
THROUGH 8-39, SELECT FROM THE ABOVE
LIST THE HEALTH RECORD FORM THAT
MOST CLOSELY RELATES TO THE
STATEMENT IN THE QUESTION.**

8-37. Used for ordering corrective lenses.

1. A
2. B
3. C
4. D

8-38. May be used for an active duty patient who is admitted to the hospital for less than 24 hours.

1. A
2. B
3. D
4. E

8-39. A record of prophylactic immunizations and sensitivity tests.

1. A
2. B
3. C
4. D

8-40. Which of the following documents should NEVER be filed in an individual's HREC?

1. FM 8-33
2. PHS-731
3. SF 509
4. NAVMED 6100/1

8-41. In which of the following circumstance should the health record be verified?

1. Upon reporting
2. Upon transfer
3. At the time of a physical examination
4. In all of the above cases

8-42. Under which of the following circumstances would a member's health record NOT be closed?

1. Transfers to a new duty station
2. Transfers to the Fleet Reserve
3. Placed on the retired list
4. Declared missing in action

8-43. On which of the following documents would a notation be made concerning an member's status as a deserter?

1. SF 600
2. NAVMED 6100/1
3. NAVMED 6150/4
4. Both 1 and 3

8-44. A copy of the HREC of a member separated for disability should be given to the member for presentation to the DVA so that the member's claim can be processed expeditiously.

1. True
2. False

8-45. Which of the following types of appropriations is not normally used by the Navy?

1. Multiple-year
2. Annual
3. Continuing
4. Apportioning

8-46. At the end of the second quarter, what is done with the funds that have not been obligated in the previous quarter?

1. The funds are carried over into the next quarter
2. The funds are carried over into the next year
3. The funds are returned to the Treasury
4. The funds are placed in the command's welfare and recreation fund

8-47. The shipboard medical OPTAR may be used to purchase all of the following items EXCEPT

1. x-ray units and film processors
2. medical books and publications
3. gun bags
4. litters and stretchers

8-48. Which of the following characteristics could designate an item as controlled equipage?

1. High cost
2. Liable to pilferage
3. Required for ship's mission
4. Each of the above

8-49. The first four digits of a National Stock Number are known as the

1. Federal Supply Classification code
2. Federal Stock number
3. National Identification number
4. Cognizance symbol

8-50. How many digits are in a National Stock Number?

1. 9
2. 10
3. 12
4. 13

8-51. In which of the following would you find handling or storage codes, a brief description of each item, and a cross-reference of NINs and NSNs?

1. Management Data List (MDL)
2. Identification List (IL)
3. Authorized Medical Allowance List (AMAL)
4. Naval Supply System Command Manual

TO ANSWER ITEMS 8-52 THROUGH 8-54, SELECT FROM THE TABLE BELOW THE LEVEL OF SUPPLY DEFINED IN THE ITEM.

A.	Stockage objective
B.	Identification List (IL)
C.	Operating level
D.	Requisitioning objective

8-52. The quantity of an item required to support operations between the time a requisition is submitted and receipt of material.

1. A
2. B
3. C
4. D

8-53. The minimum amount of an item of material required to support operations.

1. A
2. B
3. C
4. D

8-54. The maximum amount of material in stock and on order to support operations.

1. A
2. B
3. C
4. D

8-55. What is the name of the standard computer supply management system used by shipboard medical departments?

1. Shipboard Automated Medical Supply
2. SNAP Automated Medical System
3. Supply Automated Medical System
4. Shipboard Automated Management System

8-56. Medical journals and books may be ordered on which of the following forms?

1. DD Form 1149, Requisition and Invoice/Shipping Document
2. NAVSUP Form 1250-1, Single-Line Item Requisition Document (manual)
3. DD Form 1348m, DOD Single-Line Item Requisition Document (mechanical)
4. DD Form 1348m, Non-NSN Requisition (manual)

8-57. Who assigns the Urgency of Need Designator (UND) on a requisition?

1. Activity requiring the material
2. Supply depot
3. Stock point
4. Inventory control point

8-58. What is the purpose of a Report of Discrepancy, SF 364?

1. To determine the cause of a discrepancy
2. To effect corrective action on a discrepancy
3. To prevent recurrence of a discrepancy
4. To do all of the above

8-59. Whenever possible and where space permits, aisles in stowage areas should be at least how wide?

1. 18 in
2. 24 in
3. 30 in
4. 36 in

8-60. All of the following locations aboard ship are appropriate stowage areas for hazardous material EXCEPT

1. below the full-load water line
2. adjacent to a magazine
3. near either end of the ship
4. behind watertight doors

8-61. Alcohol should be stowed in a locked container in the paint and flammable liquid storeroom.

1. True
2. False

8-62. What is the primary purpose of an inventory?

1. To locate missing items
2. To determine what items are in a storeroom
3. To ensure balance on hand match stock record cards
4. To balance the OPTAR

8-63. Differences between on-hand quantity, location of stock, or other stock record data should be reconciled in accordance with what publication?

1. NAVSUP 1114
2. NAVSUP P-437
3. NAVSUP P-485
4. NAVSUPINST 4200.85

8-64. Once a stock record card has been totally filled in, a new card should be prepared, following all of the steps listed EXCEPT

1. bring forward demand quantity and frequency demand totals from old card
2. destroy old card, in accordance with local policy
3. bring forward any outstanding requisitions from old card
4. enter the beginning date on the new card

8-65. How often must inventory of controlled substances be conducted?

1. Weekly
2. Monthly
3. Quarterly
4. Semiannually

8-66. In what document would you find the contents of each contingency block outlined?

1. AMAL
2. MAP
3. MMART Manual
4. SPRINT

8-67. At a minimum, how often should all AMALs be reviewed?

1. Monthly
2. Quarterly
3. Semiannually
4. Annually

ASSIGNMENT 9

Textbook Assignment: "Administration," chapter 14, pages 14-1 to 14-14; "Health Care Administration," chapter 15, pages 15-1 to 15-13; and "Decedent Affairs," chapter 16, pages 16-1 to 16-15.

9-1. The Medical Department Journal contains a chronological record of events concerning the Medical Department and should include all of the following EXCEPT

1. reports of personnel casualties, injuries, or deaths
2. personnel entered onto or deleted from the binnacle list
3. medical histories of personnel
4. training lectures to stretcher bearers

9-2. NAVMED 6320/18, Binnacle List, is used to list all personnel falling into what status?

1. Admitted to the hospital
2. Excused from duty for 24 hours or less because of illness
3. Excused from duty for more than 24 hours because of illness
4. Who reported to sick call in the morning

9-3. NAVMED 6320/19 Morning Report of the Sick, must be submitted to the commanding officer daily by what time?

1. 0800
2. 0900
3. 1000
4. 1100

9-4. A member misses his clinical appointment. He has missed two previous appointments. What action, if any, should the Corpsman maintaining the appointment log take?

1. Call the member and reschedule the appointment
2. Notify the member's chain of command that he has missed several appointments
3. Do nothing; when the member is able to reschedule, he will do so

9-5. A notice issued under the Navy Directive Issuance System has the same force and effect as an instruction.

1. True
2. False

9-6. In the process of making changes to directives, which of the following procedures should you follow?

1. Annotate the first page of the directive with "CH-#" (# = change number) to indicate the change has been incorporated into the directive
2. If the directive is removed from the binder or file, replace the directive with a locator sheet
3. If the directive is in the form of a publication, fill out the "Record of Changes" sheet in the front of the book
4. Each of the above

9-7. Routine unclassified correspondence must contain all of the following items in the identification symbol EXCEPT

1. standard subject identification symbol
2. date
3. serial number
4. organization code

9-8. In what publication would you find examples of and instructions for the proper formatting of a naval message?

1. NTP 3
2. SECNAVINST 5210.11
3. Navy Correspondence Manual
4. Navy Message Manual

9-9. A Navy letter carries the subject identification number 5320. What is the major subject of the letter?

1. Military personnel
2. Operations and readiness
3. General administration and management
4. Financial management

9-10. What is the process called that is used to determine the correct subject group under which documents should be filed?

1. grouping
2. coding
3. classifying
4. cross-referencing

9-11. It is prudent to cross-reference a piece of correspondence under which of the following circumstances?

1. The basic correspondence has separate enclosures
2. The document has multiple subjects
3. There is more than one applicable SSIC
4. Each of the above

9-12. Budget and accounting files are terminated and new files begun at what time(s)?

1. Semi-annually, on 31 March and 30 September
2. Annually, at the end of the calendar year
3. Annually, at the end of the fiscal year
4. Every 3 years

9-13. Tickler files are used to determine all of the following EXCEPT

1. when reports are due
2. ship's movement/port schedule
3. when physical examinations are required
4. immunization schedules

9-14. The Marine Corps specially assigns members to the Fleet Marine Force to serve as medical and dental personnel

1. True
2. False

9-15. All of the following are considered part of the primary mission of the medical battalion EXCEPT

1. emergency treatment
2. evacuation
3. immunization
4. temporary hospitalization

9-16. Which of the following could be considered accurate attributes of a fleet hospital?

1. Non-deployable, permanent station for high-intensity situations
2. Transportable, with 100 to 500 beds, providing moderately sophisticated care
3. Designed for short-term (less than 60 days) operations involving large numbers of ground forces
4. Mostly self-supporting and relocatable, with less than 100 beds

9-17. A fleet hospital has what number of directorates?

1. 2
2. 3
3. 4
4. 5

9-18. The operation of fleet hospital supply departments are conducted in accordance with what directive?

1. NAVMED P-5010
2. BUMEDINST 6440.6
3. NAVSUP P-485
4. NAVSUP P-437

9-19. Through use of the Medical Augmentation Program (MAP), it is possible to do all of the following EXCEPT

1. monitor wartime manning readiness
2. augment operational medical personnel, as necessary
3. train medical personnel
4. develop a readiness reporting system

9-20. The Mobile Medical Augmentation Readiness Team is a peacetime version of the Medical Augmentation Program.

1. True
2. False

9-21. Detailed information concerning MMART can be found in what directive or manual?

1. NAVMED P-5010
2. BUMEDINST 6440.6
3. NAVSUP P-485
4. NAVSUP P-437

9-22. Before an accurate determination of the number of personnel and amount of material are needed for a particular military operation, the staff surgeon and dental surgeon must know about enemy and friendly capabilities, as well as environmental factors. What is this information, taken as a whole, called?

1. Medical estimate
2. Planning factors
3. Medical intelligence
4. Command mission

9-23. Who establishes patient evacuation policy?

1. Secretary of the Navy
2. Joint Chiefs of Staff
3. Chief of Naval Medicine
4. Secretary of Defense

9-24. Eligibility for medical care at a military medical treatment facility is established by the _____ and verified by the _____?

1. Personnel office, medical treatment facility
2. Military treatment facility, personnel office
3. Commanding officer, physician on duty
4. Commanding officer, personnel officer

9-25. In a case where DEERS determines that a patient with a valid ID card is ineligible for care, the ID card will always be the determining factor. No other supporting documents are required

1. True
2. False

9-26. Which of the following beneficiaries can receive medical care and can also be enrolled in the DEERS system?

1. Red Cross workers
2. Secretary of the Navy designees
3. Secret Service agents
4. Newborns

9-27. BUMED and OPNAV both have instructions covering healthcare and quality assurance programs?

1. True
2. False

9-28. It is the primary function of which of the following programs to provide a good communication and rapport between the patient and medical department staff?

1. The Patient Contact Program
2. The FOIA
3. The Patient Relations Program
4. The Family Advocacy Program

9-29. What authority has the responsibility of the Family Advocacy Program?

1. BUMED
2. NMPC
3. Family Service Center
4. BUPERS

9-30. A committee consisting of members from what professional areas of the Navy reviews abuse cases?

1. Medical, line, chaplain, security
2. Medical, chaplain, security, Family Service Center
3. Medical, line, chaplain, Family Service Center
4. Medical, line, security, Family Service Center

9-31. The Navy hopes to achieve its drug free "zero tolerance" goal by the use of which of the following methods?

1. Detection
2. Education
3. Deterrence
4. Treatment

9-32. What training prevention program is specifically aimed at the junior Sailor?

1. ADAMS
2. PREVENT 2000
3. Alcoholics Anonymous
4. IMPACT

9-33. What is the primary function of a DAPA?

1. To facilitate shipboard Alcoholics Anonymous meetings
2. To coordinate on-site training for the crew
3. To act as the liaison between civilian authorities and the Commanding Officer
4. To arrange for inpatient treatment

9-34. Which of the following is a true statement concerning competence for duty exams?

1. The Executive Officer can fill out blocks 1 through 13 of NAVMED 6120/1
2. An Independent Duty Corpsman can fill out blocks 12 - 49 of NAVMED 6120/1
3. The patient must give his written consent before a sample of blood can be obtained
4. A search authorization is required only if the patient refuses to cooperate

9-35. Medical has responsibility for which aspects of the Physical Readiness Program?

1. Testing
2. Education and training
3. Legal
4. Obesity research

9-36. The responsibility of informing a patient of the consequences of a non-emergent medical procedure and obtaining informed consent from that patient lies ONLY with the medical provider.

1. True
2. False

9-37. Of the following, who would be the best choice to witness a patient's consent to a medical procedure?

1. A stranger
2. An immediate family member
3. A member of the medical team
4. A relative

9-38. Which is NOT a true statement about an incident report?

1. They are confidential but if misused or mishandled, they can become public
2. The reports must be limited to only facts and a logical conclusion
3. Copies must be limited
4. They must be forwarded only to the quality assurance coordinator

9-39. The Privacy Act governs the disclosure of documents compiled and maintained by government agencies.

1. True
2. False

9-40. Through use of the FOIA an individual can gain access to information pertaining to himself from federal agency records and correct those records, if necessary.

1. True
2. False

FOR QUESTIONS 9-41 THROUGH 9-45, MATCH THE INSTRUCTION WITH ITS CORRESPONDING NUMBER. ALL ANSWERS WILL NOT BE USED.

A. Risk Management Program
B. Physical Readiness Program
C. Patient Relations Program
D. Family Advocacy Program
E. CHAMPUS
F. Quality Assurance Program
G. Sexual Assault Victim Intervention
H. Victim and Witness Program

9-41. OPNAVINST 1752.1.

1. E
2. F
3. G
4. H

9-42. BUMEDINST 6320.70.

1. A
2. B
3. C
4. D

9-43. NAVMEDCOMINST 6320.18.

1. C
2. D
3. E
4. F

9-44. BUMEDINST 6010.21.

1. A
2. B
3. C
4. D

9-45. BUMEDINST 6010.13.

1. C
2. D
3. E
4. F

9-46. Which statement is true concerning the release of an active duty patient under arrest?

1. No official action by hospital personnel is required before local authorities can take custody
2. No patient may be released from treatment before it is medically reasonable to do so
3. The patient must be transported directly to his parent command
4. A federal warrant must be presented before the patient can be released to civilian authority

9-47. The Commanding Officer is authorized to deliver an active duty patient to civilian authorities when a proper warrant is presented under all of the circumstances listed EXCEPT when

1. the ship is within the territorial waters of the requesting jurisdiction
2. the patient refuses to leave and requests a lawyer
3. the patient is outside the jurisdiction if the civilian authority
4. cognizant JAG office has not been contacted

9-48. All of the following are categories of eligible prisoner beneficiaries EXCEPT

1. military prisoners
2. nonmilitary federal prisoners
3. prisoners of war and other detained personnel
4. illegal aliens awaiting deporation or processing

9-49. Which of the following personnel is authorized emergency care ONLY?

1. Enemy prisoners of war
2. Nonmilitary federal prisoners
3. A previously active duty person past his EAOS released from a foreign prison
4. Personnel detained by the US government but not yet charged with a crime or arrested

9-50. Military prisoners are authorized care under all of the following conditions EXCEPT when

1. their discharge has been executed but their sentence has not expired
2. they are on leave, awaiting discharge
3. they require continued hospitalization after their discharge
4. they have been sentenced under the UCMJ only

9-51. Child abuse and spouse neglect is covered in what program?

1. SAVI
2. Family Advocacy
3. Risk Management
4. Child and Spouse Protective Services

9-52. The Decedent Affairs Program consists of the search, recovery, identification, care, and disposition of remains of deceased personnel for whom the Department of the Navy is responsible.

1. True
2. False

9-53. The Casualty Assistance Calls program is administered by the which of the following commands?

1. Commander, Naval Medical Command
2. Commander, Naval Military Personnel Command
3. Office of Medical Affairs
4. Commanding Officer, Naval Hospital

9-54. The Casualty Assistance Calls offier assists the next of kin (NOK) with which of the following item(s)?

1. Disposition of remains
2. Survivor benefits
3. Obtaining the rights and privileges that the NOK is entitle to
4. All of the above

9-55. Which of the following programs can only be activated upon the enactment of special legislation?

1. Return of Remains Program
2. Concurrent Return Program
3. Graves Registration Program
4. Current Decedent Affairs Program

A. Current Decedent Affairs Program
B. Casualty Assistance Calls Program
C. Concurrent Return Program
D. Graves Registration Program

IN ANSWERING QUESTIONS 9-56 THROUGH 9-59, SELECT FROM THE ABOVE LIST THE PROGRAM THAT MOST CLOSELY RELATES TO THE STATEMENT IN THE QUESTION.

9-56. Provides for the search, recovery, evacuation, initial identification, and burial in temporary cemeteries when tactical situation does not permit concurrent return.

1. A
2. B
3. C
4. D

9-57. Provides professional mortuary services, supplies, and related services incident to care and disposition of remains.

1. A
2. B
3. C
4. D

9-58. Is not identified as part of the Decedent Affairs Program.

1. A
2. B
3. C
4. D

9-59. May be activated to support large numbers of military personnel committed to a strategic area.

1. A
2. B
3. C
4. D

9-60. The personnel casualty report of an active duty Navy member shall be submitted by

1. telegram
2. routine precedence message
3. speedletter
4. priority message

9-61. Within CONUS, who is responsible for ensuring the next of kin is notified of a member's death?

1. Office of Medical Affairs
2. The member's commanding officer
3. Naval Military Personnel Command
4. Commander, Naval Medical Command

9-62. The commanding officer will write a condolence letter to the NOK within _____ hours of the death.

1. 24
2. 36
3. 48
4. 72

9-63. When search, recovery, and identification operations continue for more than 36 hours, a progress report will be made to BUMED and MEDDEN Affairs every _____ hours.

1. 8
2. 12
3. 24
4. 36

9-64. After serving all identification purposes, the personal effects of a deceased naval member are disposed of as directed in the

1. NAVSUP Manual
2. Manual of the Medical Department
3. Naval Military Personnel Manual
4. JAGMAN

9-65. Who will be requested to provide an identification specialist to examine unidentified remains?

1. Naval Military Personnel Command
2. Commander, Naval Medical Command
3. Geographic command
4. Naval Office of Medical/Dental Affairs

9-66. What is the minimum number of projected deaths per year required for awarding contracts by naval activities for procuring mortuary services within CONUS?

1. 15
2. 10
3. 8
4. 5

9-67. To minimize cellular deterioration, remains should be refrigerated at _____ C.

1. 0° to 2.2°
2. 2.2° to 4.4°
3. 4.4° to 6.6°
4. 6.6° to 8.8°

9-68. How many copies of DD 2064 must accompany remains being transferred from an overseas activity to a CONUS point of entry?

1. 5
2. 3
3. 2
4. 1

9-69. Once authorization has been obtained for burial at sea, who coordinates the arrangements?

1. Commander, Naval Medical Command
2. Chief of Naval Operations
3. Office of Medical Affairs
4. Appropriate fleet commanders in chief

9-70. If it is desired to transport the uncremated remains by the Air Mobility Command (AMC) within CONUS, prior approval must be obtained from the

1. Commander, Naval Medical Command
2. Chief of Naval Operations
3. Secretary of the Navy
4. Naval Military Personnel Commander

9-71. Problems concerning arrangements for a Navy escort within CONUS should be referred to the

1. Naval Office of Medical/Dental Affairs
2. Decedent Affairs Officer
3. Commandant of the Marine Corps
4. Area commander

9-72. A request by the primary next of kin (PNOK) for a special escort must be referred to

1. Chief of Naval Operations
2. Naval Military Personnel Command
3. Naval Office of Medical/Dental Affairs
4. Commander, Naval Medical Command

9-73. The maximum authorized Government allowance for expenses toward the interment of a deceased active duty member in a private cemetery can be found in which of the following publications?

1. NAVMEDCOMINST 5360.1
2. NAVPERS 15955
3. NAVSUP P-485
4. NAVMED P-5016/NAVMC 2509A

9-74. Who has jurisdiction at the Arlington National Cemetery?

1. State government
2. Department of the Army
3. Department of the Interior
4. Office of Medical Affairs

9-75. When group burials are necessary, round-trip transportation at government expense to the place of burial is provided for

1. the PNOK
2. all members of the immediate family
3. the PNOK and two blood relatives
4. the PNOK and one other close relative

Advancement Handbook
for
Hospital Corpsman

HM3, HM2, HM1, HMC

Advancement Handbook
for
HOSPITAL CORPSMAN

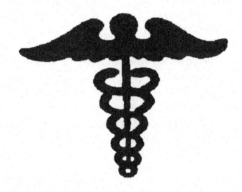

This Advancement Handbook was last reviewed on: July 2002.
There were no changes to the technical content.

PREFACE

The purpose of the Advancement Handbook is to assist Hospital Corpsman in studying for Navywide advancement-in-rating examinations. The bibliographies (BIBs) together with this handbook form a comprehensive examination study package. Since this handbook provides skill and knowledge components for each paygrade of the HM rating, it helps focus study on those areas that will be tested. This feature ensures Sailors will get the most out of their study time.

Each page in Parts 1 through 5 of this Advancement Handbook presents general skill areas, specific skill areas, the knowledge factors associated with each skill area, the pertinent references required to perform each skill, and the types of subject areas you can expect on the examination. Since it would be impractical to test all the tasks that a person in the HM rating is required to perform, you should use this guide as just part of a comprehensive training program.

Part 5 of this guide presents a section of information on the Navy enlisted advancement system (NEAS). The NEAS information covers advancement examination preparation, taking the exam, how exams are scored, how candidates are informed about their standings on exams taken, the final multiple system, when candidates are advanced, and a host of other advancement information useful to all enlisted personnel.

Remember that advancement competition is keen, so your keys to advancement include not only comprehensive advancement examination study but also sustained superior performance.

July 2002 Edition

Published by
Naval Education and Training Professional
Development and Technology Center

CONTENTS

Part 1

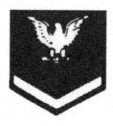

Advancement Handbook for HM3

Advancement Handbook for HM3

General HM *Skill Area*	**Emergency/Field Treatment**
A *skill* you are expected to perform from the General Skill Area above:	**Perform preliminary assessment and treatment of chemical, biological, radiological (CBR)-contaminated patients**
References you should study to gain the knowledge you need to perform this skill:	• NAVEDTRA 14295 • Virtual Navy Hospital Website: http://www.vnh.org/
Exam Expectations. These are subject areas you should know to help you answer exam questions correctly:	You can expect questions on the identification of chemical/biological agents to include: nerve, blister, blood, choking, incapacitants, and harassing agents, and the identification and treatment of chemical injuries to include actions taken before a chemical attack; chemical prophylaxis; chemical decontamination equipment, supplies, and decontamination procedures; identification and treatment of radiological injuries to include actions taken before nuclear explosion, affect on personnel, and treatment of nuclear casualties; radiological decontamination equipment and supplies, decontamination procedures, and minimum requirements for shipboard/field decontamination station design and layout.

Advancement Handbook for HM3

General HM *Skill Area*	**Emergency/Field Treatment**
A *skill* you are expected to perform from the General Skill Area above:	**Treat patients for shock**
Knowledge you should have to perform this skill:	You should be able to: • Recognize and treat the symptoms of shock • Recall the different types of shock and the appropriate treatment • Recall how and when to apply anti-shock garments
References you should study to gain the knowledge you need to perform this skill:	• NAVEDTRA 14295 • *Brady Emergency Care,* current edition • *Emergency Care and Transportation of the Sick and Injured,* current edition • Virtual Navy Hospital Website: http://www.vnh.org/
Exam Expectations. These are subject areas you should know to help you answer exam questions correctly:	You can expect questions on the different types of shock and the associated treatment along with the use of equipment and supplies to treat shock including Pneumatic Counter-Pressure Devices.

Advancement Handbook for HM3

General HM *Skill Area*	**Emergency/Field Treatment**
A *skill* you are expected to perform from the General Skill Area above:	**Perform health care provider basic life support (BLS)**

Knowledge you should have to perform this skill:	You should be able to recognize and treat failures of the respiratory system and heart failure, to include:
	• Airway obstruction
	  - **A**irway/opening airway
	  - **B**reathing/artificial ventilation
	  - **C**irculation/cardiopulmonary resuscitation (CPR)
	• One-rescuer CPR technique
	• Two-rescuer CPR technique

References you should study to gain the knowledge you need to perform this skill:	• NAVEDTRA 14295 • *Brady Emergency Care*, current edition • *Emergency Care and Transportation of the Sick and Injured*, current edition • Virtual Navy Hospital Website: http://www.vnh.org
Exam Expectations. These are subject areas you should know to help you answer exam questions correctly:	You can expect questions on the purpose and method of treating a partial/complete airway obstruction, including the techniques for opening the airway and administering abdominal and chest thrust and the purpose, methods, and procedures for patient assessment, artificial ventilation, and cardiopulmonary resuscitation using both one and two rescuer CPR techniques for an adult, child, and infant.

Advancement Handbook for HM3

General HM *Skill Area*	**Emergency/Field Treatment**
A *skill* you are expected to perform from the General Skill Area above:	**Provide care during emergency child birth**

Knowledge you should have to perform this skill:	You should be able to:
	• Recall procedures required for childbirth
	• Recognize complications of childbirth to include:
	  - Breech delivery
	  - Prolapsed cord
	  - Excessive bleeding
	  - Limb presentation

References you should study to gain the knowledge you need to perform this skill:	• NAVEDTRA 14295 • *Brady Emergency Care*, current edition • *Emergency Care and Transportation of the Sick and Injured*, current edition • Virtual Navy Hospital Website: http://www.vnh.org
Exam Expectations. These are subject areas you should know to help you answer exam questions correctly:	You can expect questions on the procedures for a live birth delivery, the equipment and supplies used and the complications that could occur during childbirth and the treatment for each.

Advancement Handbook for HM3

General HM *Skill Area*	**Emergency/Field Treatment**
A *skill* you are expected to perform from the General Skill Area above:	**Apply tourniquets**
Knowledge you should have to perform this skill:	You should be able to: • Recognize the requirements for a tourniquet • Recall how to apply tourniquets • Recall how to monitor and adjust tourniquets as needed
References you should study to gain the knowledge you need to perform this skill:	• NAVEDTRA 14295 • *Brady Emergency Care*, current edition • *Emergency Care and Transportation of the Sick and Injured*, current edition • Virtual Navy Hospital Website: http://www.vnh.org
Exam Expectations. These are subject areas you should know to help you answer exam questions correctly:	You can expect questions on recognizing the conditions in which a tourniquet is required and the procedures for applying, monitoring, and adjusting tourniquets.

Advancement Handbook for HM3

General HM *Skill Area*	**Emergency/Field Treatment**
A *skill* you are expected to perform from the General Skill Area above:	**Calculate medication dosage requirements**

Knowledge you should have to perform this skill:	You should be able to recall the following dosage information, to include:
	• The need for dosage adjustment using Clark's rule for weight and Young's rule for age and manufacturers' recommendation
	• Measuring equivalents
	• The conversion tables for weights and liquid measures
	• The reducing and enlarging formulas and doses, to include:
	  - Ration and proportion
	  - Fractional method
	• Basic mathematics to include:
	  - Decimals
	  - Fractions
	  - Percentages
	  - Ratio and proportion
	  - Specific gravity

References you should study to gain the knowledge you need to perform this skill:	• NAVEDTRA 14295 • *Brady Emergency Care*, current edition • *Emergency Care and Transportation of the Sick and Injured*, current edition • Virtual Navy Hospital Website: http://www.vnh.org

Exam Expectations. These are subject areas you should know to help you answer exam questions correctly:	You can expect questions on compounding utilizing Clark's and Young's rules along with the manufacturers' dosage recommendation; measuring equivalencies; the conversion tables for weights and liquid measures; the reducing and enlarging formulas and doses using ratio, proportion, and the fractional method; and using basic mathematics including decimals, fractions, and percentages.

Advancement Handbook for HM3

General HM *Skill Area*	**Emergency/Field Treatment**
A *skill* you are expected to perform from the General Skill Area above:	**Inventory and inspect antidote lockers**
Knowledge you should have to perform this skill:	You should be able to recall the following information about antidote lockers, to include: • Its location onboard small ships • Its contents • The procedures for securing the locker
References you should study to gain the knowledge you need to perform this skill:	NAVEDTRA 14295
Exam Expectations. These are subject areas you should know to help you answer exam questions correctly:	You can expect questions on the location, contents, and security of the antidote locker.

Advancement Handbook for HM3

General HM *Skill Area*	**Emergency/Field Treatment**
A *skill* you are expected to perform from the General Skill Area above:	**Perform emergency treatment for soft-tissue injuries**
Knowledge you should have to perform this skill:	You should be able to recall information about emergency treatment of soft-tissue injuries, to include: • Removing superficial foreign bodies from the wound area • The types of wounds and procedures to debride wounds • Administering local anesthetics • The first aid battle dressings required to dress wounds • The need to suture lacerations and the types of sutures material required • Removing sutures and performing follow up care as needed
References you should study to gain the knowledge you need to perform this skill:	• NAVEDTRA 14295 • *Brady Emergency Care,* current edition • *Emergency Care and Transportation of the Sick and Injured,* current edition • Virtual Navy Hospital Website: http://www.vnh.org

Advancement Handbook for HM3

General HM *Skill Area*	**Emergency/Field Treatment**
A *skill* you are expected to perform from the General Skill Area above:	**Perform preliminary assessment and treatment of dental emergencies**
Knowledge you should have to perform this skill:	You should be able to: • Recognize and understand dental terminology • Identify basic dental anatomy. • Recall basic dental histology • Recall the procedures involved in a oral examination • Identify local anesthesia for dental use • Recognize the signs and symptoms of oral diseases and injuries
References you should study to gain the knowledge you need to perform this skill:	• NAVEDTRA 14295 • NAVEDTRA 12570 • *Brady Emergency Care*, current edition • *Emergency Care and Transportation of the Sick and Injured*, current edition • Virtual Navy Hospital Website: http://www.vnh.org
Exam Expectations. These are subject areas you should know to help you answer exam questions correctly:	You can expect questions on dental terminology and basic dental anatomy; procedures involved in an oral examination; the symptoms of oral diseases and injuries; and the local anesthesia for dental use.

Advancement Handbook for HM3

General HM *Skill Area*	**Emergency/Field Treatment**
A *skill* you are expected to perform from the General Skill Area above:	**Perform triage**
Knowledge you should have to perform this skill:	You should be able to recall the following information about performing triage, to include: • The policies and procedures required for performing triage in peacetime and in time of conflict • The policies and procedures to prepare patients for medical evacuations • The requirements to restrain patients • The policies, procedures, equipment, and supplies required to transport patients • The procedures for patient regulating
References you should study to gain the knowledge you need to perform this skill:	• NAVEDTRA 14295 • *Brady Emergency Care,* current edition • *Emergency Care and Transportation of the Sick and Injured,* current edition • Virtual Navy Hospital Website: http://www.vnh.org
Exam Expectations. These are subject areas you should know to help you answer exam questions correctly:	You can expect questions on performing triage in peacetime/conflict based on the patients condition; patient preparation for medical evacuations along with any special situations; the need to restrain patients and the equipment used; the policies, procedures, equipment, and supplies required to transport patients from a field environment using fixed-wing aircraft, and helicopters; transportation of patients ship-to-ship, within a ship or

	submarine, and movement within and between CONUS and OUTUS; and the requirements for patient regulating and tracking.

Advancement Handbook for HM3

General HM *Skill Area*	**Emergency/Field Treatment**
A *skill* you are expected to perform from the General Skill Area above:	**Administer medications in emergency situations**
Knowledge you should have to perform this skill:	You should be able to: • Recall the policies and procedures required for the administration of medications • Recall the procedures for the administration of injections • Recognize anaphylactic reactions • Recall the treatment of anaphylactic reactions
References you should study to gain the knowledge you need to perform this skill:	• NAVEDTRA 14295 • *Brady Emergency Care*, current edition • *Emergency Care and Transportation of the Sick and Injured*, current edition • Virtual Navy Hospital Website: http://www.vnh.org
Exam Expectations. These are subject areas you should know to help you answer exam questions correctly:	You can expect questions on the policies and procedures required for the administration of medications in emergency situations; the procedures, equipment, and supplies used for injections; the recognition of anaphylactic reactions; and the equipment/supplies used for treatment of anaphylactic reactions.

Advancement Handbook for HM3

General HM *Skill Area*	**Emergency/Field Treatment**
A *skill* you are expected to perform from the General Skill Area above:	**Perform basic neurological checks**
Knowledge you should have to perform this skill:	You should be able to recall the procedures for neurological checks to include inspection and palpation.
References you should study to gain the knowledge you need to perform this skill:	• NAVEDTRA 14295 • *Brady Emergency Care*, current edition • *Emergency Care and Transportation of the Sick and Injured*, current edition • Virtual Navy Hospital Website: http://www.vnh.org
Exam Expectations. These are subject areas you should know to help you answer exam questions correctly:	You can expect questions on inspection of mental state; gross deformities, and lacerations; decerebrate posturing; decorticate posturing; and palpation for tenderness and deformities.

Advancement Handbook for HM3

General HM *Skill Area*	**Emergency/Field Treatment**
A *skill* you are expected to perform from the General Skill Area above:	**Perform preliminary assessment and treatment of head and neck injuries**
Knowledge you should have to perform this skill:	You should recall: • The inspection and palpation procedures for the head and neck • The equipment and supplies required for treatment
References you should study to gain the knowledge you need to perform this skill:	• NAVEDTRA 14295 • *Brady Emergency Care*, current edition • *Emergency Care and Transportation of the Sick and Injured,* current edition • Virtual Navy Hospital Website: http://www.vnh.org
Exam Expectations. These are subject areas you should know to help you answer exam questions correctly:	You can expect questions on inspection of the head for hemorrhage, lesions, and contusions; palpation of the head for skull depressions, lumps, and pain; neck inspection procedures looking at the suprasternal notch and trachea; auscultation procedures for sounds; and the equipment and supplies required for treatment.

Advancement Handbook for HM3

General HM *Skill Area*	**Emergency/Field Treatment**
A *skill* you are expected to perform from the General Skill Area above:	**Perform preliminary assessment and treatment of eye injuries**
Knowledge you should have to perform this skill:	You should recall: • The inspection and palpation procedures for eye injuries • The equipment and supplies required for treatment
References you should study to gain the knowledge you need to perform this skill:	• NAVEDTRA 14295 • *Brady Emergency Care,* current edition • *Emergency Care and Transportation of the Sick and Injured,* current edition • Virtual Navy Hospital Website: http://www.vnh.org
Exam Expectations. These are subject areas you should know to help you answer exam questions correctly:	You can expect questions on inspecting the eye for lacerations, foreign matter, pupils size, and pupils reaction; recognizing swelling and lack of sensation through palpation; and recalling the equipment and supplies required for treatment.

Advancement Handbook for HM3

General HM *Skill Area*	**Emergency/Field Treatment**
A *skill* you are expected to perform from the General Skill Area above:	**Perform preliminary assessment and treatment of spinal cord injuries**
Knowledge you should have to perform this skill:	You should recall: • The inspection and palpation procedures for spinal cord injuries • The equipment and supplies required for treatment
References you should study to gain the knowledge you need to perform this skill:	• NAVEDTRA 14295 • *Brady Emergency Care,* current edition • *Emergency Care and Transportation of the Sick and Injured,* current edition • Virtual Navy Hospital Website: http://www.vnh.org
Exam Expectations. These are subject areas you should know to help you answer exam questions correctly:	You can expect questions on spinal range of motion, reflexes, and loss of sensation; muscle tone and paralysis; and on the equipment and supplies required for treatment.

Advancement Handbook for HM3

General HM *Skill Area*	**Emergency/Field Treatment**
A *skill* you are expected to perform from the General Skill Area above:	**Perform preliminary assessment and treatment of orthopedic injuries**
Knowledge you should have to perform this skill:	You should recall • The inspection and palpation procedures for orthopedic injuries • The equipment and supplies required for treatment
References you should study to gain the knowledge you need to perform this skill:	• NAVEDTRA 14295 • *Brady Emergency Care*, current edition • *Emergency Care and Transportation of the Sick and Injured*, current edition • Virtual Navy Hospital Website: http://www.vnh.org
Exam Expectations. These are subject areas you should know to help you answer exam questions correctly:	You can expect questions on fractures, dislocations, sprains, strains, and contusions and the equipment and supplies required for treatment.

Advancement Handbook for HM3

General HM *Skill Area*	**Emergency/Field Treatment**
A *skill* you are expected to perform from the General Skill Area above:	**Perform preliminary assessment and treatment of abdominal injuries**
Knowledge you should have to perform this skill:	You should recall: • The inspection, palpation, and auscultation procedures for abdominal injuries • The equipment and supplies required for treatment
References you should study to gain the knowledge you need to perform this skill:	• NAVEDTRA 14295 • *Brady Emergency Care,* current edition • *Emergency Care and Transportation of the Sick and Injured,* current edition • Virtual Navy Hospital Website: http://www.vnh.org
Exam Expectations. These are subject areas you should know to help you answer exam questions correctly:	You can expect questions on assessment findings and the equipment and supplies required for treatment.

Advancement Handbook for HM3

General HM *Skill Area*	Emergency/Field Treatment
A *skill* you are expected to perform from the General Skill Area above:	**Perform preliminary assessment and treatment of thoracic injuries**
Knowledge you should have to perform this skill:	You should be able to recall: • Inspection, palpation, auscultation, and percussion procedures • The equipment and supplies required for treatment
References you should study to gain the knowledge you need to perform this skill:	• NAVEDTRA 14295 • *Brady Emergency Care,* current edition • *Emergency Care and Transportation of the Sick and Injured,* current edition • Virtual Navy Hospital Website: http://www.vnh.org
Exam Expectations. These are subject areas you should know to help you answer exam questions correctly:	You can expect questions on respiration, chest symmetry, lacerations, punctures, palpation for tenderness, and compression and on recognizing auscultation sounds of heart and lungs and percussion for fluids and lung conditions.

Advancement Handbook for HM3

General HM *Skill Area*	**Emergency/Field Treatment**
A *skill* you are expected to perform from the General Skill Area above:	**Perform preliminary assessment and treatment of genitourinary injuries**
Knowledge you should have to perform this skill:	You should be able to: • Recall the inspection procedures • Recall equipment and supplies required for treatment
References you should study to gain the knowledge you need to perform this skill:	• NAVEDTRA 14295 • *Brady Emergency Care*, current edition • *Emergency Care and Transportation of the Sick and Injured*, current edition • Virtual Navy Hospital Website: http://www.vnh.org
Exam Expectations. These are subject areas you should know to help you answer exam questions correctly:	You can expect questions on observations that you should make during the inspection procedure. Recall the course of action required for treatment. Recall equipment and supplies required for treatment.

Advancement Handbook for HM3

General HM *Skill Area*	**Emergency/Field Treatment**
A *skill* you are expected to perform from the General Skill Area above:	**Perform preliminary assessment and treatment of chemical burns or injuries**
Knowledge you should have to perform this skill:	You should be able to recall: • Types of chemical burns • The inspection procedures • The equipment and supplies required for treatment
References you should study to gain the knowledge you need to perform this skill:	• NAVEDTRA 14295 • *Brady Emergency Care,* current edition • *Emergency Care and Transportation of the Sick and Injured,* current edition • Virtual Navy Hospital Website: http://www.vnh.org
Exam Expectations. These are subject areas you should know to help you answer exam questions correctly:	You can expect questions on the types of chemical burns and locations, the observations made during the inspection procedure; and the equipment and supplies required for treatment.

Advancement Handbook for HM3

General HM *Skill Area*	Emergency/Field Treatment
A *skill* you are expected to perform from the General Skill Area above:	**Conduct preliminary assessment and treatment of thermal burns or injuries**
Knowledge you should have to perform this skill:	You should be able to recall: • The types of burns and degree of burns • The inspection procedures • The equipment and supplies required for treatment
References you should study to gain the knowledge you need to perform this skill:	• NAVEDTRA 14295 • *Brady Emergency Care,* current edition • *Emergency Care and Transportation of the Sick and Injured,* current edition • Virtual Navy Hospital Website: http://www.vnh.org
Exam Expectations. These are subject areas you should know to help you answer exam questions correctly:	You can expect questions on the types of burns, degree of burns; the "Rule of Nines" calculation for given situations; and the equipment and supplies required for treatment.

Advancement Handbook for HM3

General HM *Skill Area*	**Emergency/Field Treatment**
A *skill* you are expected to perform from the General Skill Area above:	**Perform preliminary assessment and treatment of ear, nose, and throat (ENT) injuries**
Knowledge you should have to perform this skill:	You should be able to recall: • Inspection and palpation (mouth/throat only) procedures • The equipment and supplies required for treatment
References you should study to gain the knowledge you need to perform this skill:	• NAVEDTRA 14295 • *Brady Emergency Care,* current edition • *Emergency Care and Transportation of the Sick and Injured,* current edition • Virtual Navy Hospital Website: http://www.vnh.org
Exam Expectations. These are subject areas you should know to help you answer exam questions correctly:	You can expect questions on what observations should be made on inspection of the ear, nose, and throat; palpation procedures for fractures of the mouth/throat, and the equipment and supplies required for treatment.

Advancement Handbook for HM3

General HM *Skill Area*	**Emergency/Field Treatment**
A *skill* you are expected to perform from the General Skill Area above:	**Perform preliminary assessment and treatment of internal hemorrhages**
Knowledge you should have to perform this skill:	You should be able to recall: • Inspection and palpation procedures • The equipment and supplies required for treatment
References you should study to gain the knowledge you need to perform this skill:	• NAVEDTRA 14295 • *Brady Emergency Care*, current edition • *Emergency Care and Transportation of the Sick and Injured*, current edition • Virtual Navy Hospital Website: http://www.vnh.org
Exam Expectations. These are subject areas you should know to help you answer exam questions correctly:	You can expect questions on the inspection and palpation procedures to assess internal hemorrhages and the equipment and supplies required for treatment.

Advancement Handbook for HM3

General HM *Skill Area*	**Emergency/Field Treatment**
A *skill* you are expected to perform from the General Skill Area above:	**Perform preliminary assessment and treatment of environmental injuries**
Knowledge you should have to perform this skill:	You should be able to: • Recognize the types of environmental injuries • Recall the inspection procedures • Recall the equipment and supplies required for treatment
References you should study to gain the knowledge you need to perform this skill:	• NAVEDTRA 14295 • *Brady Emergency Care*, current edition • *Emergency Care and Transportation of the Sick and Injured,* current edition • Virtual Navy Hospital Website: http://www.vnh.org
Exam Expectations. These are subject areas you should know to help you answer exam questions correctly:	You can expect questions on types of environmental injuries and the appearance and treatment of injuries due to heat and cold.

Advancement Handbook for HM3

General HM *Skill Area*	**Emergency/Field Treatment**
A *skill* you are expected to perform from the General Skill Area above:	**Perform preliminary assessment of mental stability**
Knowledge you should have to perform this skill:	You should be able to recall the observation techniques.
References you should study to gain the knowledge you need to perform this skill:	• NAVEDTRA 14295 • *Brady Emergency Care,* current edition • *Emergency Care and Transportation of the Sick and Injured,* current edition • Virtual Navy Hospital Website: http://www.vnh.org
Exam Expectations. These are subject areas you should know to help you answer exam questions correctly:	You can expect questions on the observations that will be made to assess mental stability and the questions and the appropriate responses that should be received during the assessment.

Advancement Handbook for HM3

General HM *Skill Area*	**Emergency/Field Treatment**
A *skill* you are expected to perform from the General Skill Area above:	**Perform preliminary assessment of seizure disorders**
Knowledge you should have to perform this skill:	You should be able to: • Recognize the types of seizure disorders • Recall the treatment for seizure disorders • Recall equipment and supplies required for treatment
References you should study to gain the knowledge you need to perform this skill:	• NAVEDTRA 14295 • *Brady Emergency Care,* current edition • *Emergency Care and Transportation of the Sick and Injured,* current edition • Virtual Navy Hospital Website: http://www.vnh.org
Exam Expectations. These are subject areas you should know to help you answer exam questions correctly:	You can expect questions on the types of seizure disorders, the treatment, and the equipment and supplies required for treatment.

Advancement Handbook for HM3

General HM *Skill Area*	Emergency/Field Treatment
A *skill* you are expected to perform from the General Skill Area above:	**Perform preliminary assessment and treatment of acute drug intoxication's and poisonings**
Knowledge you should have to perform this skill:	You should be able to: • Recognize acute drug intoxication's, poisonings, chemical intoxication's, chemical poisonings, and hazardous material exposures • Recall the treatment procedures • Recall the equipment and supplies required for treatment
References you should study to gain the knowledge you need to perform this skill:	• NAVEDTRA 14295 • *Brady Emergency Care*, current edition • *Emergency Care and Transportation of the Sick and Injured,* current edition • Virtual Navy Hospital Website: http://www.vnh.org
Exam Expectations. These are subject areas you should know to help you answer exam questions correctly:	You can expect questions on the types of drug intoxication's, poisonings, chemical intoxication's, chemical poisonings, and hazardous material exposures; and recall the treatment procedures/protocols and the equipment and supplies required for treatment.

Advancement Handbook for HM3

General HM *Skill Area*	**Emergency/Field Treatment**
A *skill* you are expected to perform from the General Skill Area above:	**Perform preliminary assessment and treatment of cardiovascular conditions**
Knowledge you should have to perform this skill:	You should be able to: • Recognize the types of cardiovascular conditions • Recall the observations that should be made • Recall equipment and supplies required for treatment
References you should study to gain the knowledge you need to perform this skill:	• NAVEDTRA 14295 • *Brady Emergency Care,* current edition • *Emergency Care and Transportation of the Sick and Injured,* current edition • Virtual Navy Hospital Website: http://www.vnh.org
Exam Expectations. These are subject areas you should know to help you answer exam questions correctly:	You can expect questions on, but not limited to, cardiogenic shock, congestive heart failure, "chest pain", angina, and myocardial infarction; the signs and symptoms of each condition; and the equipment and supplies required for treatment.

Advancement Handbook for HM3

General HM *Skill Area*	**Emergency/Field Treatment**
A *skill* you are expected to perform from the General Skill Area above:	**Perform preliminary assessment and treatment of unconscious patients**
Knowledge you should have to perform this skill:	You should be able to recall: • The inspection, palpation, and auscultation procedures • The equipment and supplies required for treatment.
References you should study to gain the knowledge you need to perform this skill:	• NAVEDTRA 14295 • *Brady Emergency Care*, current edition • *Emergency Care and Transportation of the Sick and Injured,* current edition • Virtual Navy Hospital Website: http://www.vnh.org
Exam Expectations. These are subject areas you should know to help you answer exam questions correctly:	You can expect questions on inspection, palpation, and auscultation procedures and the equipment and supplies required for any treatment.

General HM *Skill Area*	Emergency/Field Treatment
A *skill* you are expected to perform from the General Skill Area above:	**Dress wounds**
Knowledge you should have to perform this skill:	You should be able to: • Identify the types of dressings (bandages) used to protect wounds. • Recall how the dressings are applied.
References you should study to gain the knowledge you need to perform this skill:	• NAVEDTRA 14295 • *Brady Emergency Care*, current edition • *Emergency Care and Transportation of the Sick and Injured*, current edition • Virtual Navy Hospital Website: http://www.vnh.org
Exam Expectations. These are subject areas you should know to help you answer exam questions correctly:	You can expect questions on the types of dressings (bandages) used to protect wounds and how the dressings are applied.

Advancement Handbook for HM3

General HM *Skill Area*	**Emergency/Field Treatment**
A *skill* you are expected to perform from the General Skill Area above:	**Perform preliminary assessment and treatment of dermatological conditions**
Knowledge you should have to perform this skill:	You should be able to recall: • Inspection procedures • The equipment and supplies required for treatment
References you should study to gain the knowledge you need to perform this skill:	• NAVEDTRA 14295 • *Brady Emergency Care,* current edition • *Emergency Care and Transportation of the Sick and Injured,* current edition • Virtual Navy Hospital Website: http://www.vnh.org
Exam Expectations. These are subject areas you should know to help you answer exam questions correctly:	You should expect questions on the types of **dermatological** conditions, the inspection procedures, and the equipment and supplies required for treatment.

Advancement Handbook for HM3

General HM *Skill Area*	**Patient Care**
A *skill* you are expected to perform from the General Skill Area above:	**Measure fluid intake/output**
Knowledge you should have to perform this skill:	You should be able to recall: • The procedures for measuring and recording fluid intake and output • The purpose for measuring fluid intake and output
References you should study to gain the knowledge you need to perform this skill:	• NAVEDTRA 14295 • *Lippincott Fundamental Skills and Concepts in Patient Care,* current edition • Virtual Navy Hospital Website: http://www.vnh.org
Exam Expectations. These are subject areas you should know to help you answer exam questions correctly:	You can expect questions on the procedures for measuring and recording fluid intake and output and the purpose for measuring fluid intake and output.

Advancement Handbook for HM3

General HM *Skill Area*	**Patient Care**
A *skill* you are expected to perform from the General Skill Area above:	**Perform preliminary assessment and assist in treatment of orthopedic conditions**
Knowledge you should have to perform this skill:	You should be able to recall: • The different types of orthopedic conditions and the treatment for each • The different types of orthopedic appliances. • How to apply orthopedic appliances • How to perform circulation checks for patients with orthopedic appliances • How to remove orthopedic appliances
References you should study to gain the knowledge you need to perform this skill:	• NAVEDTRA 14295 • *Lippincott Fundamental Skills and Concepts in Patient Care,* current edition • Virtual Navy Hospital Website: http://www.vnh.org
Exam Expectations. These are subject areas you should know to help you answer exam questions correctly:	You can expect questions on the different types of orthopedic conditions and treatments; the types of orthopedic appliances and how to apply them; how to perform circulation checks for patients with orthopedic appliances; and removing orthopedic appliances.

Advancement Handbook for HM3

General HM *Skill Area*	**Patient Care**
A *skill* you are expected to perform from the General Skill Area above:	**Conduct range of motion exercises**
Knowledge you should have to perform this skill:	You should be able to: • Recall the range of motion positions • Recognize range motion limitations • Recall procedures for recording range of motion
References you should study to gain the knowledge you need to perform this skill:	• NAVEDTRA 14295 • *Lippincott Fundamental Skills and Concepts in Patient Care, current* edition • Virtual Navy Hospital Website: http://www.vnh.org
Exam Expectations. These are subject areas you should know to help you answer exam questions correctly:	You can expect question on the range of motion positions, limitations, and procedures for recording range of motion.

Advancement Handbook for HM3

General HM *Skill Area*	**Patient Care**
A *skill* you are expected to perform from the General Skill Area above:	**Assist in opening and draining incisions, infected areas and irrigation of infected areas**
Knowledge you should have to perform this skill:	You should be able to recall the polices and procedures for: • Assisting in opening and draining incisions • Assisting in opening and draining infected areas • Irrigation of infected areas
References you should study to gain the knowledge you need to perform this skill:	• NAVEDTRA 14295 • *Lippincott Fundamental Skills and Concepts in Patient Care, current* edition • Virtual Navy Hospital Website: http://www.vnh.org
Exam Expectations. These are subject areas you should know to help you answer exam questions correctly:	You can expect questions on the policies and procedures for opening and draining incisions, infected areas, and irrigation of infected areas.

Advancement Handbook for HM3

General HM *Skill Area*	**Patient care**
A *skill* you are expected to perform from the General Skill Area above:	**Administer medications**
Knowledge you should have to perform this skill:	You should be able to: • Recall the policies and procedures for administering medications • Recognize Physician and Nurse written orders for medication • Recognize side effects of treatments or medications • Recall the policies and procedures to report side effects of treatments or medications
References you should study to gain the knowledge you need to perform this skill:	• NAVEDTRA 14295 • *Lippincott Fundamental Skills and Concepts in Patient Care, current* edition • Virtual Navy Hospital Website: http://www.vnh.org
Exam Expectations. These are subject areas you should know to help you answer exam questions correctly:	You can expect questions on the policies and procedures for administering medications; recognition of Physician and Nurse written orders for medication; recognizing the side effects of treatments or medications; and recalling the policies and procedures to report side effects.

Advancement Handbook for HM3

General HM *Skill Area*	**Patient Care**
A *skill* you are expected to perform from the General Skill Area above:	**Treat febrile conditions**
Knowledge you should have to perform this skill:	You should be able to: • Recognize a febrile patient • Recall the treatment for a febrile patient
References you should study to gain the knowledge you need to perform this skill:	• NAVEDTRA 14295 • *Lippincott Fundamental Skills and Concepts in Patient Care, current* edition • Virtual Navy Hospital Website: http://www.vnh.org
Exam Expectations. These are subject areas you should know to help you answer exam questions correctly:	You can expect questions on the signs, symptoms, and treatment of a febrile patient.

Advancement Handbook for HM3

General HM *Skill Area*	**Patient Care**
A *skill* you are expected to perform from the General Skill Area above:	**Perform preliminary assessment of laboratory results**
Knowledge you should have to perform this skill:	You should be able to: • Recall normal lab values for basic laboratory test • Recall the policies and procedures for recording laboratory results
References you should study to gain the knowledge you need to perform this skill:	• NAVEDTRA 14295 • *Lippincott Fundamental Skills and Concepts in Patient Care, current* edition • Virtual Navy Hospital Website: http://www.vnh.org
Exam Expectations. These are subject areas you should know to help you answer exam questions correctly:	You can expect questions on normal lab values and the policies and procedures for recording laboratory results.

Advancement Handbook for HM3

General HM *Skill Area*	**Patient Care**
A *skill* you are expected to perform from the General Skill Area above:	**Prepare and sterilize instruments and other materials**
Knowledge you should have to perform this skill:	You should be able to: • Recall preparation and sterilization procedures • Identify equipment and supplies required for sterilization
References you should study to gain the knowledge you need to perform this skill:	• NAVEDTRA 14295 • *Lippincott Fundamental Skills and Concepts in Patient Care, current* edition • Virtual Navy Hospital Website: http://www.vnh.org
Exam Expectations. These are subject areas you should know to help you answer exam questions correctly:	You can expect questions on preparation and sterilization procedures and the equipment and supplies required for sterilization.

Advancement Handbook for HM3

General HM *Skill Area*	**Patient Care**
A *skill* you are expected to perform from the General Skill Area above:	**Don and remove sterile surgical gowns and gloves**
Knowledge you should have to perform this skill:	You should be able to recall the policies and procedures for putting on and taking off sterile surgical gowns and gloves
References you should study to gain the knowledge you need to perform this skill:	• NAVEDTRA 14295 • *Lippincott Fundamental Skills and Concepts in Patient Care,* current edition • Virtual Navy Hospital Website: http://www.vnh.org
Exam Expectations. These are subject areas you should know to help you answer exam questions correctly:	You can expect questions on the policies and procedures for putting on and taking off sterile surgical gowns and gloves.

Advancement Handbook for HM3

General HM *Skill Area*	**Patient Care**
A *skill* you are expected to perform from the General Skill Area above:	**Perform postprocedure cleaning of treatment rooms and equipment**
Knowledge you should have to perform this skill:	You should be able to recall the policies and procedures for performing post medical/surgical procedure cleaning of treatment rooms and equipment
References you should study to gain the knowledge you need to perform this skill:	• NAVEDTRA 14295 • *Lippincott Fundamental Skills and Concepts in Patient Care,* current edition • Virtual Navy Hospital Website: http://www.vnh.org
Exam Expectations. These are subject areas you should know to help you answer exam questions correctly:	You can expect questions on the policies and procedures for performing post medical/surgical procedure cleaning of treatment rooms and equipment.

Advancement Handbook for HM3

General HM *Skill Area*	**Patient Care**
A *skill* you are expected to perform from the General Skill Area above:	**Set up oxygen equipment and provide oxygen therapy**
Knowledge you should have to perform this skill:	You should be able to: • Recall the different types of oxygen equipment • Recall the policies and procedures required to set up oxygen equipment • Recall the procedures to provide oxygen therapy
References you should study to gain the knowledge you need to perform this skill:	• NAVEDTRA 14295 • *Lippincott Fundamental Skills and Concepts in Patient Care,* current edition • Virtual Navy Hospital Website: http://www.vnh.org
Exam Expectations. These are subject areas you should know to help you answer exam questions correctly:	You can expect questions on the different types of oxygen equipment; the policies and procedures required to set up oxygen equipment; and the procedures to provide oxygen therapy.

Advancement Handbook for HM3

General HM *Skill Area*	**Patient Care**
A *skill* you are expected to perform from the General Skill Area above:	**Set up and operate suction equipment**
Knowledge you should have to perform this skill:	You should be able to: • Recognize the different types of suction equipment • Recall the policies and procedures to set up and operate suction equipment
References you should study to gain the knowledge you need to perform this skill:	• NAVEDTRA 14295 • *Lippincott Fundamental Skills and Concepts in Patient Care,* current edition • Virtual Navy Hospital Website: http://www.vnh.org
Exam Expectations. These are subject areas you should know to help you answer exam questions correctly:	You can expect questions on the different types of suction equipment and the policies and procedures to set up and operate suction equipment.

Advancement Handbook for HM3

General HM *Skill Area*	**Patient Care**
A *skill* you are expected to perform from the General Skill Area above:	**Set up humidifiers or vaporizers**
Knowledge you should have to perform this skill:	You should be able to: • Recognize the different types of humidifiers and vaporizers • Recall the policies and procedures to set up humidifiers and vaporizers
References you should study to gain the knowledge you need to perform this skill:	• NAVEDTRA 14295 • *Lippincott Fundamental Skills and Concepts in Patient Care,* current edition • Virtual Navy Hospital Website: http://www.vnh.org
Exam Expectations. These are subject areas you should know to help you answer exam questions correctly:	You can expect questions on the different types of humidifiers and vaporizers and the policies and procedures to set up humidifiers and vaporizers.

Advancement Handbook for HM3

General HM *Skill Area*	**Patient Care**
A *skill* you are expected to perform from the General Skill Area above:	**Perform urinary catheterization**
Knowledge you should have to perform this skill:	You should be able to recall: • Basic male and female anatomy. • The policies and procedures to perform urinary catheterization • The equipment and supplies required
References you should study to gain the knowledge you need to perform this skill:	• NAVEDTRA 14295 • *Lippincott Fundamental Skills and Concepts in Patient Care,* current edition • Virtual Navy Hospital Website: http://www.vnh.org
Exam Expectations. These are subject areas you should know to help you answer exam questions correctly:	You can expect question on basic male and female anatomy; the policies/procedures to perform urinary catheterization; and the equipment and supplies required.

Advancement Handbook for HM3

General HM *Skill Area*	**Patient Care**
A *skill* you are expected to perform from the General Skill Area above:	**Administer enemas**
Knowledge you should have to perform this skill:	You should be able to recall: • Basic anatomy • The policies and procedures to administer enemas • The equipment and supplies required
References you should study to gain the knowledge you need to perform this skill:	• NAVEDTRA 14295 • *Lippincott Fundamental Skills and Concepts in Patient Care,* current edition • Virtual Navy Hospital Website: http://www.vnh.org
Exam Expectations. These are subject areas you should know to help you answer exam questions correctly:	You can expect question on basic anatomy; the policies and procedures to administer enemas; and the equipment and supplies required.

Advancement Handbook for HM3

General HM *Skill Area*	**Patient Care**
A *skill* you are expected to perform from the General Skill Area above:	**Perform intravenous (IV) therapy**
Knowledge you should have to perform this skill:	You should be able to recall: • Basic anatomy • The policies and procedures to perform intravenous (IV) therapy • The equipment and supplies required
References you should study to gain the knowledge you need to perform this skill:	• NAVEDTRA 14295 • *Lippincott Fundamental Skills and Concepts in Patient Care,* current edition • Virtual Navy Hospital Website: http://www.vnh.org
Exam Expectations. These are subject areas you should know to help you answer exam questions correctly:	You can expect questions on basic anatomy; the policies/procedures to perform intravenous (IV) therapy; and the equipment and supplies required.

Advancement Handbook for HM3

General HM *Skill Area*	**Patient Care**
A *skill* you are expected to perform from the General Skill Area above:	**Monitor dressings for hemorrhaging**
Knowledge you should have to perform this skill:	You should be able to recall the procedures to monitor dressings for hemorrhages
References you should study to gain the knowledge you need to perform this skill:	<ul><li>NAVEDTRA 14295</li><li>*Lippincott Fundamental Skills and Concepts in Patient Care,* current edition</li><li>Virtual Navy Hospital Website: http://www.vnh.org</li></ul>
Exam Expectations. These are subject areas you should know to help you answer exam questions correctly:	You can expect questions on what to observe when monitoring dressings for hemorrhages.

Advancement Handbook for HM3

General HM *Skill Area*	**Patient Care**
A *skill* you are expected to perform from the General Skill Area above:	**Take and monitor vital signs**
Knowledge you should have to perform this skill:	You should be able to recall: • Basic anatomy • The policies and procedures to obtain and monitor vital signs to include: - **Temperature** - **Pulse** - **Respiration** • The equipment and supplies required
References you should study to gain the knowledge you need to perform this skill:	• NAVEDTRA 14295 • *Lippincott Fundamental Skills and Concepts in Patient Care,* current edition • Virtual Navy Hospital Website: http://www.vnh.org
Exam Expectations. These are subject areas you should know to help you answer exam questions correctly:	You can expect questions on basic anatomy; the policies/procedures to obtain and monitor vital signs; and the equipment/supplies required.

General HM *Skill Area*	**Patient Care**
A *skill* you are expected to perform from the General Skill Area above:	**Perform patient isolation techniques**
Knowledge you should have to perform this skill:	You should be able to: • Recall the policies and procedures to perform patient isolation techniques • Recall the equipment and supplies required
References you should study to gain the knowledge you need to perform this skill:	• NAVEDTRA 14295 • *Lippincott Fundamental Skills and Concepts in Patient Care,* current edition • Virtual Navy Hospital Website: http://www.vnh.org
Exam Expectations. These are subject areas you should know to help you answer exam questions correctly:	You can expect questions on the policies and procedures to perform patient isolation techniques and the equipment and supplies required.

Advancement Handbook for HM3

General HM *Skill Area*	**Patient Care**
A *skill* you are expected to perform from the General Skill Area above:	**Counsel patients on treatment and self-care**
Knowledge you should have to perform this skill:	You should be able to recall the policies and procedures required to counsel patients on treatment and self-care
References you should study to gain the knowledge you need to perform this skill:	<ul><li>NAVEDTRA 14295</li><li>*Lippincott Fundamental Skills and Concepts in Patient Care,* current edition</li><li>Virtual Navy Hospital Website: http://www.vnh.org</li></ul>
Exam Expectations. These are subject areas you should know to help you answer exam questions correctly:	You can expect questions on the policies and procedures required to counsel patients on treatment and self-care.

Advancement Handbook for HM3

General HM *Skill Area*	**Patient Care**
A *skill* you are expected to perform from the General Skill Area above:	**Annotate inpatient records/charts and annotate medical records/charts using subjective, objective, diagnosis assessment, and treatment plan (S.O.A.P.) format**
Knowledge you should have to perform this skill:	You should be able to: Recall the policies and procedure for annotations in inpatient records/charts. Recall the procedure for annotation and annotate medical records and charts using subjective, objective, diagnosis assessment, and treatment plan (S.O.A.P.) format
References you should study to gain the knowledge you need to perform this skill:	• NAVEDTRA 14295 • *Lippincott Fundamental Skills and Concepts in Patient Care,* current edition • Virtual Navy Hospital Website: http://www.vnh.org
Exam Expectations. These are subject areas you should know to help you answer exam questions correctly:	You can expect questions on inpatient records and charts. Recall the procedure for S.O.A.P. note format.

Advancement Handbook for HM3

General HM *Skill Area*	**Patient Care**
A *skill* you are expected to perform from the General Skill Area above:	**Liaise between doctor, staff, and patient to facilitate problem resolution**
Knowledge you should have to perform this skill:	You should be able to recall basic communications skills
References you should study to gain the knowledge you need to perform this skill:	<ul><li>NAVEDTRA 14295</li><li>*Lippincott Fundamental Skills and Concepts in Patient Care,* current edition</li><li>Virtual Navy Hospital Website: http://www.vnh.org</li></ul>
Exam Expectations. These are subject areas you should know to help you answer exam questions correctly:	You can expect questions dealing with doctor, staff, and patient problem solving situations.

Advancement Handbook for HM3

General HM *Skill Area*	**Patient Care**
A *skill* you are expected to perform from the General Skill Area above:	**Prepare patient for examinations**
Knowledge you should have to perform this skill:	You should be able to: • Recall the policies and procedures for examination preparation • Recognize the different types of examinations and the requirements for each
References you should study to gain the knowledge you need to perform this skill:	• NAVEDTRA 14295 • *Lippincott Fundamental Skills and Concepts in Patient Care*, current edition • Virtual Navy Hospital Website: http://www.vnh.org
Exam Expectations. These are subject areas you should know to help you answer exam questions correctly:	You can expect questions on the policies and procedures for examination preparation, the different types of examinations, and the requirements for each.

Advancement Handbook for HM3

General HM *Skill Area*	**Patient Care**
A *skill* you are expected to perform from the General Skill Area above:	**Perform electrocardiograms (EKG)**
Knowledge you should have to perform this skill:	You should be able to: • Recall the policies and procedures for performing EKGs • Recall the equipment and supplies required
References you should study to gain the knowledge you need to perform this skill:	• NAVEDTRA 14295 • *Lippincott Fundamental Skills and Concepts in Patient Care*, current edition • Virtual Navy Hospital Website: http://www.vnh.org
Exam Expectations. These are subject areas you should know to help you answer exam questions correctly:	You can expect questions on the policies and procedures for performing EKGs and the equipment and supplies required.

Advancement Handbook for HM3

General HM *Skill Area*	**Patient Care**
A *skill* you are expected to perform from the General Skill Area above:	**Perform audiograms**
Knowledge you should have to perform this skill:	You should be able to: • Recall the policies and procedures for performing audiograms • Recall the equipment and supplies required
References you should study to gain the knowledge you need to perform this skill:	• NAVEDTRA 14295 • *Lippincott Fundamental Skills and Concepts in Patient Care,* current edition • Virtual Navy Hospital Website: http://www.vnh.org
Exam Expectations. These are subject areas you should know to help you answer exam questions correctly:	You can expect questions on the policies and procedures for performing audiograms, and the equipment and supplies required.

Advancement Handbook for HM3

General HM *Skill Area*	**Patient Care**
A *skill* you are expected to perform from the General Skill Area above:	**Obtain cultures**
Knowledge you should have to perform this skill:	You should recall: • The policies and procedures for obtaining cultures • The equipment and supplies required
References you should study to gain the knowledge you need to perform this skill:	• NAVEDTRA 14295 • *Lippincott Fundamental Skills and Concepts in Patient Care,* current edition • Virtual Navy Hospital Website: http://www.vnh.org
Exam Expectations. These are subject areas you should know to help you answer exam questions correctly:	You can expect questions on the policies and procedures for obtaining cultures, physical locations on the body to obtain cultures, and the equipment and supplies required.

Advancement Handbook for HM3

General HM *Skill Area*	**Patient Care**
A *skill* you are expected to perform from the General Skill Area above:	**Assess and treat bites and stings (human, animal, or insect)**
Knowledge you should have to perform this skill:	You should recall: • The policies and procedures for assessing and treating bites/stings, along with any special reporting requirements • The equipment and supplies required
References you should study to gain the knowledge you need to perform this skill:	• NAVEDTRA 14295 • *Lippincott Fundamental Skills and Concepts in Patient Care,* current edition • Virtual Navy Hospital Website: http://www.vnh.org
Exam Expectations. These are subject areas you should know to help you answer exam questions correctly:	You can expect questions on the policies and procedures for assessing and treating bites/stings, along with any special reporting requirements and the equipment and supplies required.

Advancement Handbook for HM3

General HM *Skill Area*	**Patient Care**
A *skill* you are expected to perform from the General Skill Area above:	**Order eyeglasses or optical inserts**
Knowledge you should have to perform this skill:	You should recall: • The current policy and procedure for ordering eyeglasses or optical inserts • The required forms
References you should study to gain the knowledge you need to perform this skill:	NAVEDTRA 14295
Exam Expectations. These are subject areas you should know to help you answer exam questions correctly:	You can expect question on the current policy and procedure for ordering eyeglasses or optical inserts and the required forms.

Advancement Handbook for HM3

General HM *Skill Area*	**Patient Care**
A *skill* you are expected to perform from the General Skill Area above:	**Screen patients (sick calls, physical exams, etc.)**
Knowledge you should have to perform this skill:	You should recall: • The procedures to obtain height and weight of a patient • The procedure for obtaining vital signs • The procedure to perform color perception tests • The procedure to measure visual acuity • The equipment and supplies required
References you should study to gain the knowledge you need to perform this skill:	• NAVEDTRA 14295 • *Lippincott Fundamental Skills and Concepts in Patient Care,* current edition • Virtual Navy Hospital Website: http://www.vnh.org
Exam Expectations. These are subject areas you should know to help you answer exam questions correctly:	You can expect questions on the procedures to obtain height and weight of a patient, vital signs, perform color perception tests, and measure visual acuity and the equipment and supplies required.

Advancement Handbook for HM3

General HM *Skill Area*	**Patient Care**
A *skill* you are expected to perform from the General Skill Area above:	**Assess wounds for signs of infection and healing**
Knowledge you should have to perform this skill:	You should be able to recognize the signs of infection and healing at a wound site
References you should study to gain the knowledge you need to perform this skill:	• NAVEDTRA 14295 • *Lippincott Fundamental Skills and Concepts in Patient Care,* current edition • Virtual Navy Hospital Website: http://www.vnh.org
Exam Expectations. These are subject areas you should know to help you answer exam questions correctly:	You can expect questions on the signs of infection and healing at a wound site.

Advancement Handbook for HM3

General HM *Skill Area*	**Patient Care**
A *skill* you are expected to perform from the General Skill Area above:	**Perform preliminary assessment and assist in treatment of eye conditions**
Knowledge you should have to perform this skill:	You should recall: • The inspection and palpation procedures for eye conditions • The equipment and supplies required for treatment
References you should study to gain the knowledge you need to perform this skill:	• NAVEDTRA 14295 • *Lippincott Fundamental Skills and Concepts in Patient Care,* current edition • Virtual Navy Hospital Website: http://www.vnh.org
Exam Expectations. These are subject areas you should know to help you answer exam questions correctly:	You can expect questions on inspecting the eye for lacerations, foreign matter, pupils size, pupils reaction; recognizing abnormal conditions through palpation; swelling, lack of sensation; and the equipment and supplies required for treatment in an inpatient setting.

Advancement Handbook for HM3

General HM *Skill Area*	**Patient Care**
A *skill* you are expected to perform from the General Skill Area above:	**Perform preliminary assessment and assist in treatment of abdominal and thoracic conditions**
Knowledge you should have to perform this skill:	You should recall: • The inspection, palpation, and auscultation procedures for abdominal and thoracic conditions • The equipment and supplies required for treatment
References you should study to gain the knowledge you need to perform this skill:	• NAVEDTRA 14295 • *Lippincott Fundamental Skills and Concepts in Patient Care,* current edition • Virtual Navy Hospital Website: http://www.vnh.org
Exam Expectations. These are subject areas you should know to help you answer exam questions correctly:	You can expect questions on respiration, chest symmetry, lacerations, and punctures; palpation for tenderness; compression; auscultation sounds of heart and lungs, percussion for fluids and lung conditions; and the equipment and supplies required for treatment in an inpatient setting.

Advancement Handbook for HM3

General HM *Skill Area*	**Patient Care**
A *skill* you are expected to perform from the General Skill Area above:	**Perform preliminary assessment and assist in treatment of respiratory conditions**
Knowledge you should have to perform this skill:	You should recall: • The inspection, palpation, and auscultation procedures for respiratory conditions • The equipment and supplies required for treatment
References you should study to gain the knowledge you need to perform this skill:	• NAVEDTRA 14295 • *Lippincott Fundamental Skills and Concepts in Patient Care,* current edition • Virtual Navy Hospital Website: http://www.vnh.org
Exam Expectations. These are subject areas you should know to help you answer exam questions correctly:	You can expect questions on respiration, chest symmetry, recall palpation for tenderness, and compression; auscultation sounds of lungs, and percussion for fluids and lung conditions; and the equipment and supplies required for treatment in an inpatient setting.

Advancement Handbook for HM3

General HM *Skill Area*	**Patient Care**
A *skill* you are expected to perform from the General Skill Area above:	**Perform preliminary assessment and assist in treatment of gastrointestinal (GI) conditions**
Knowledge you should have to perform this skill:	You should recall: • The inspection procedures • The equipment and supplies required for treatment
References you should study to gain the knowledge you need to perform this skill:	• NAVEDTRA 14295 • NAVMED P-5010 • *Lippincott Fundamental Skills and Concepts in Patient Care,* current edition • Virtual Navy Hospital Website: http://www.vnh.org
Exam Expectations. These are subject areas you should know to help you answer exam questions correctly:	You can expect questions on observations that you should make during the inspection procedure including investigation of food borne illness; the course of action required for treatment; and the equipment and supplies required for treatment.

Advancement Handbook for HM3

General HM *Skill Area*	**Patient Care**
A *skill* you are expected to perform from the General Skill Area above:	**Perform preliminary assessment and assist in treatment of genitourinary conditions**
Knowledge you should have to perform this skill:	You should recall: • The inspection procedures • The equipment and supplies required for treatment
References you should study to gain the knowledge you need to perform this skill:	• NAVEDTRA 14295 • *Lippincott Fundamental Skills and Concepts in Patient Care,* current edition • Virtual Navy Hospital Website: http://www.vnh.org
Exam Expectations. These are subject areas you should know to help you answer exam questions correctly:	You can expect questions on observations that you should make during the inspection procedure; the course of action required for treatment and the equipment and supplies required for treatment.

General HM *Skill Area*	**Patient Care**
A *skill* you are expected to perform from the General Skill Area above:	**Perform preliminary assessment and assist in treatment of dermatological conditions**
Knowledge you should have to perform this skill:	You should recall: • The inspection procedures • The equipment and supplies required for treatment
References you should study to gain the knowledge you need to perform this skill:	• NAVEDTRA 14295 • *Lippincott Fundamental Skills and Concepts in Patient Care, current* edition • Virtual Navy Hospital Website: http://www.vnh.org
Exam Expectations. These are subject areas you should know to help you answer exam questions correctly:	You should expect questions on the types of dermatological conditions; the inspection procedures; and the equipment and supplies required for treatment.

Advancement Handbook for HM3

General HM *Skill Area*	**Patient Care**
A *skill* you are expected to perform from the General Skill Area above:	**Perform preliminary assessment and assist in treatment of ENT conditions**
Knowledge you should have to perform this skill:	You should recall: • The inspection and palpation (mouth/throat only) procedures • The equipment and supplies required for treatment
References you should study to gain the knowledge you need to perform this skill:	• NAVEDTRA 14295 • *Lippincott Fundamental Skills and Concepts in Patient Care,* current edition • Virtual Navy Hospital Website: http://www.vnh.org
Exam Expectations. These are subject areas you should know to help you answer exam questions correctly:	You can expect questions on what observations should be made on inspection of the ear, nose, and throat; the palpation procedures for fractures of the mouth/throat; and the equipment and supplies required for treatment in an inpatient setting.

Advancement Handbook for HM3

General HM *Skill Area*	**Patient Care**
A *skill* you are expected to perform from the General Skill Area above:	**Perform preliminary assessment and assist in treatment of diabetic conditions**
Knowledge you should have to perform this skill:	You should be able to: • Recall the types of diabetes • Recognize diabetic coma and insulin shock • Recall the equipment and supplies required for treatment
References you should study to gain the knowledge you need to perform this skill:	• NAVEDTRA 14295 • *Lippincott Fundamental Skills and Concepts in Patient Care,* current edition • Virtual Navy Hospital Website: http://www.vnh.org
Exam Expectations. These are subject areas you should know to help you answer exam questions correctly:	You can expect questions on the types of diabetes, diabetic coma, and insulin shock and the equipment and supplies required for treatment.

Advancement Handbook for HM3

General HM *Skill Area*	**Patient Care**
A *skill* you are expected to perform from the General Skill Area above:	**Perform minor incisions (toe nail resections, lancing, etc.)**
Knowledge you should have to perform this skill:	You should recall: • Basic anatomy • The policies and procedures to perform minor incisions and any invasive procedure • The equipment and supplies required
References you should study to gain the knowledge you need to perform this skill:	• NAVEDTRA 14295 • *Lippincott Fundamental Skills and Concepts in Patient Care,* current edition • Virtual Navy Hospital Website: http://www.vnh.org
Exam Expectations. These are subject areas you should know to help you answer exam questions correctly:	You can expect questions on basic anatomy; the policies and procedures for any invasive procedure; and the equipment and supplies required.

Advancement Handbook for HM3

General HM *Skill Area*	**Patient Care**
A *skill* you are expected to perform from the General Skill Area above:	**Administer immunizations**
Knowledge you should have to perform this skill:	You should be able to: • Recall the most current policies and procedures required for the administration of immunizations • Recall the procedures for the administration of injections • Recognize anaphylactic reactions • Recall the treatment of anaphylactic reactions
References you should study to gain the knowledge you need to perform this skill:	• NAVEDTRA 14295 • *Lippincott Fundamental Skills and Concepts in Patient Care,* current edition • Virtual Navy Hospital Website: http://www.vnh.org
Exam Expectations. These are subject areas you should know to help you answer exam questions correctly:	You can expect questions on the policies and procedures required for the administration of immunizations in inpatient setting situations; the procedures, equipment, and supplies used for injections; and anaphylactic reactions and the equipment/supplies used for treatment of the reactions.

Advancement Handbook for HM3

General HM *Skill Area*	**Patient Care**
A *skill* you are expected to perform from the General Skill Area above:	**Administer and assess intradermal skin tests and record the results**
Knowledge you should have to perform this skill:	You should be able to: • Recall current policies and procedures required for the administration of an intradermal skin test • Recall the procedures for the administration of injections • Recognize positive and negative reactions • Record the results of the skin test • Recall the equipment and supplies required
References you should study to gain the knowledge you need to perform this skill:	• BUMEDINST 6224.8 • NAVEDTRA 14295 • *Lippincott Fundamental Skills and Concepts in Patient Care,* current edition • Virtual Navy Hospital Website: http://www.vnh.org
Exam Expectations. These are subject areas you should know to help you answer exam questions correctly:	You can expect questions on the most current policies and procedures required for the administration of an intradermal skin test; the procedures for the administration of injections; positive and negative reactions; and the equipment and supplies required.

Advancement Handbook for HM3

General HM *Skill Area*	**Patient Care**
A *skill* you are expected to perform from the General Skill Area above:	**Organize inpatient records/charts**
Knowledge you should have to perform this skill:	You should be able to: • Recall the procedures for establishing an inpatient record/chart • Recall policies and procedures for obtaining medical history of patients • Record medical history of patients • Recall the policies and procedures for the disposition of the record/chart
References you should study to gain the knowledge you need to perform this skill:	• NAVEDTRA 14295 • NAVMED P-117 • *SECNAVINST 5210.11* • *Lippincott Fundamental Skills and Concepts in Patient Care,* current edition • Virtual Navy Hospital Website: http://www.vnh.org
Exam Expectations. These are subject areas you should know to help you answer exam questions correctly:	You can expect questions on the procedures for establishing an inpatient record/chart; obtaining medical history of patients; recording medical history; and the disposition of records and charts.

Advancement Handbook for HM3

General HM *Skill Area*	**Patient Care**
A *skill* you are expected to perform from the General Skill Area above:	**Set up and maintain a sterile field**
Knowledge you should have to perform this skill:	You should recall: • The policies and procedures required for setting up and maintaining a sterile field • The policies and procedures for putting on and taking off sterile surgical gowns and gloves • The equipment and supplies required
References you should study to gain the knowledge you need to perform this skill:	• NAVEDTRA 14295 • *Lippincott Fundamental Skills and Concepts in Patient Care,* current edition • Virtual Navy Hospital Website: http://www.vnh.org
Exam Expectations. These are subject areas you should know to help you answer exam questions correctly:	You can expect questions on the policies and procedures required to set up/maintain sterile field; for putting on and taking off sterile surgical gowns and gloves; and the equipment and supplies required.

Advancement Handbook for HM3

General HM *Skill Area*	**Patient Care**
A *skill* you are expected to perform from the General Skill Area above:	**Perform preliminary assessment and assist in treatment of cardiovascular conditions**
Knowledge you should have to perform this skill:	You should be able to: • Recognize the types of cardiovascular conditions • Recall the observations that should be made • Recall equipment and supplies required for treatment
References you should study to gain the knowledge you need to perform this skill:	• NAVEDTRA 14295 • *Lippincott Fundamental Skills and Concepts in Patient Care,* current edition • Virtual Navy Hospital Website: http://www.vnh.org
Exam Expectations. These are subject areas you should know to help you answer exam questions correctly:	You can expect questions on, but not limited to, cardiogenic shock; congestive heart failure; "chest pain"; angina; myocardial infarction; the signs and symptoms of each; and the equipment and supplies required for treatment in an inpatient setting.

Advancement Handbook for HM3

General HM *Skill Area*	**Patient Care**
A *skill* you are expected to perform from the General Skill Area above:	**Perform preliminary assessment and assist in treatment of thermal burns or injuries**
Knowledge you should have to perform this skill:	You should recall: • The types of burns and degree of burns • The equipment and supplies required for treatment
References you should study to gain the knowledge you need to perform this skill:	• NAVEDTRA 14295 • NAVMEDCOMINST 6260.12 • *Lippincott Fundamental Skills and Concepts in Patient Care,* current edition • Virtual Navy Hospital Website: http://www.vnh.org
Exam Expectations. These are subject areas you should know to help you answer exam questions correctly:	You can expect questions on the types and degree of burns; the "Rule of Nines" calculation for given situations; and the equipment and supplies required for treatment in an inpatient setting.

Advancement Handbook for HM3

General HM *Skill Area*	**Patient Care**
A *skill* you are expected to perform from the General Skill Area above:	**Perform preliminary assessment and assist in treatment of chemical burns or injuries**
Knowledge you should have to perform this skill:	You should recall: • The types of chemical burns • The inspection procedures • The equipment and supplies required for treatment
References you should study to gain the knowledge you need to perform this skill:	• NAVEDTRA 14295 • *Lippincott Fundamental Skills and Concepts in Patient Care,* current edition • Virtual Navy Hospital Website: http://www.vnh.org
Exam Expectations. These are subject areas you should know to help you answer exam questions correctly:	You can expect questions on the types and locations of chemical burns and the equipment and supplies required for treatment.

Advancement Handbook for HM3

General HM *Skill Area*	**Patient Care**
A *skill* you are expected to perform from the General Skill Area above:	**Perform preliminary assessment and assist in treatment of head and neck conditions**
Knowledge you should have to perform this skill:	You should recall: • The inspection and palpation procedures for the head and neck • The equipment and supplies required for treatment
References you should study to gain the knowledge you need to perform this skill:	• NAVEDTRA 14295 • *Lippincott Fundamental Skills and Concepts in Patient Care,* current edition • Virtual Navy Hospital Website: http://www.vnh.org
Exam Expectations. These are subject areas you should know to help you answer exam questions correctly:	You can expect questions on inspection of the head; palpation of the head; neck inspection; auscultation procedures; and the equipment and supplies required for treatment in an inpatient setting

Advancement Handbook for HM3

General HM *Skill Area*	**Patient Care**
A *skill* you are expected to perform from the General Skill Area above:	**Perform preliminary assessment and assist in treatment of unconscious patients**
Knowledge you should have to perform this skill:	You should recall: • The inspection, palpation, and auscultation procedures • The equipment and supplies required for treatment
References you should study to gain the knowledge you need to perform this skill:	• NAVEDTRA 14295 • *Lippincott Fundamental Skills and Concepts in Patient Care,* current edition • Virtual Navy Hospital Website: http://www.vnh.org
Exam Expectations. These are subject areas you should know to help you answer exam questions correctly:	You can expect questions on inspection, palpation, and auscultation procedures and the equipment and supplies required for any treatment in an inpatient setting.

Advancement Handbook for HM3

General HM *Skill Area*	**Patient Care**
A *skill* you are expected to perform from the General Skill Area above:	**Perform preliminary assessment and assist in treatment of internal hemorrhages**
Knowledge you should have to perform this skill:	You should recall: • The inspection and palpation procedures • The equipment and supplies required for treatment
References you should study to gain the knowledge you need to perform this skill:	• NAVEDTRA 14295 • *Lippincott Fundamental Skills and Concepts in Patient Care,* current edition • Virtual Navy Hospital Website: http://www.vnh.org
Exam Expectations. These are subject areas you should know to help you answer exam questions correctly:	You can expect questions on the inspection and palpation procedures to assess internal hemorrhages and the equipment and supplies required for treatment in an inpatient setting.

Advancement Handbook for HM3

General HM *Skill Area*	**Patient Care**
A *skill* you are expected to perform from the General Skill Area above:	**Perform preliminary assessment and assist in treatment of spinal cord injuries**
Knowledge you should have to perform this skill:	You should recall: • The inspection and palpation procedures for spinal cord injuries • The special equipment and supplies required for treatment
References you should study to gain the knowledge you need to perform this skill:	• NAVEDTRA 14295 • *Lippincott Fundamental Skills and Concepts in Patient Care,* current edition • Virtual Navy Hospital Website: http://www.vnh.org
Exam Expectations. These are subject areas you should know to help you answer exam questions correctly:	You can expect questions on spinal range of motion; reflexes; loss of sensation; muscle tone; paralysis; and the special equipment and supplies required for treatment in an inpatient setting.

Advancement Handbook for HM3

General HM *Skill Area*	**Patient Care**
A *skill* you are expected to perform from the General Skill Area above:	**Perform preliminary assessment and assist in treatment of acute drug and chemical intoxication's or poisonings**
Knowledge you should have to perform this skill:	You should be able to: • Recognize acute drug intoxication's, poisonings, chemical intoxication's, chemical poisonings, and hazardous material exposures • Recall the treatment procedures • Recall equipment, supplies, and medications required for treatment
References you should study to gain the knowledge you need to perform this skill:	• NAVEDTRA 14295 • *Lippincott Fundamental Skills and Concepts in Patient Care,* current edition • Virtual Navy Hospital Website: http://www.vnh.org
Exam Expectations. These are subject areas you should know to help you answer exam questions correctly:	You can expect questions on the types of drug intoxication's, poisonings, chemical intoxication's, chemical poisonings, and hazardous material exposures and the treatment procedures/protocols, equipment, supplies, and medications required for treatment in an inpatient setting.

Advancement Handbook for HM3

General HM *Skill Area*	**Ancillary services**
A *skill* you are expected to perform from the General Skill Area above:	**Perform basic laboratory diagnostic tests (UA, KOH, etc.)**
Knowledge you should have to perform this skill:	You should be able to: • Recall the different types of laboratory test • Identify the types of specimens required • Recall the policies and procedures for obtaining the types of specimens • Recall the procedure to verify labels of laboratory specimens • Recall the procedures for performing laboratory tests • Identify the equipment and supplies required
References you should study to gain the knowledge you need to perform this skill:	• BUMEDINST 6222.10 • NAVEDTRA 14295
Exam Expectations. These are subject areas you should know to help you answer exam questions correctly:	You can expect questions on, but not limited to, the different types of laboratory tests (UA, CBC, KOH, and STDs); types of specimens required; the policies and procedures for obtaining the types of specimens; the procedure to verify labels of laboratory specimens; the procedures for performing laboratory tests; and the equipment and supplies required.

Advancement Handbook for HM3

General HM *Skill Area*	**Ancillary Services**
A *skill* you are expected to perform from the General Skill Area above:	**Dispense medications**
Knowledge you should have to perform this skill:	You should be able to: • Recall how to reconstitute medications for administration • Convert between generic and trade name equivalency of drugs • Recognize the need for dosage adjustment utilizing Clark's rule for weight and Young's rule for age, and manufacturers' recommendation • Recall measuring equivalents • Recall the conversion tables for weights and liquid measures • Recall the reducing and enlarging formulas and doses, to include: - Fractional method - Ratio and proportion • Recall basic mathematics, to include: - Decimals - Fractions - Percentages - Ratio and proportion - Specific gravity • Identify drug interactions, contraindications, and adverse drug effects • Recall the policies and procedures for filing prescriptions

References you should study to gain the knowledge you need to perform this skill:	- NAVEDTRA 14295 - *Brady Emergency Care*, current edition - *Emergency Care and Transportation of the Sick and Injured,* current edition - Virtual Navy Hospital Website: http://www.vnh.org
Exam Expectations. These are subject areas you should know to help you answer exam questions correctly:	You can expect questions on, but not limited to, reconstituting medications for administration; converting between generic and trade name equivalency of drugs; compounding utilizing Clark's and Young's rules along with the manufacturers' dosage recommendation; measuring equivalencies; the conversion tables for weights and liquid measures; the reducing and enlarging formulas and doses utilizing ratio, proportion, and the fractional method; using basic mathematics including decimals, fractions, and percentages; identifying drug interactions, contraindications, and adverse drug effects; and the policies and procedures for filing prescriptions.

Advancement Handbook for HM3

General HM *Skill Area*	**Preventive/Occupational Medicine**
A *skill* you are expected to perform from the General Skill Area above:	**Sort, collect, package, and dispose of biomedical waste**
Knowledge you should have to perform this skill:	You should recall: • The policies and procedures required for the handling and disposition of biomedical waste ashore and afloat • The equipment and supplies required
References you should study to gain the knowledge you need to perform this skill:	• BUMEDINST 6230.15 • BUMEDINST 6280.1 • NAVEDTRA 14295 • NAVMED P-5010 • NAVMED P-5038 • *NAVMEDCOMINST 6230.1* • *Lippincott Fundamental Skills and Concepts in Patient Care,* current edition • Virtual Navy Hospital Website: http://www.vnh.org
Exam Expectations. These are subject areas you should know to help you answer exam questions correctly:	You can expect questions on the policies and procedures required for handling/disposing of biomedical waste ashore/afloat and the equipment and supplies required.

Advancement Handbook for HM3

General HM *Skill Area*	**Preventive/Occupational Medicine**
A *skill* you are expected to perform from the General Skill Area above:	**Assess and treat external parasite infestations (lice, crabs, scabies, etc.)**
Knowledge you should have to perform this skill:	You should be able to: • Recognize the types of external parasite infestations • Recall the policies and procedures for treating external parasites • Recall the equipment and supplies required
References you should study to gain the knowledge you need to perform this skill:	• NAVEDTRA 14295 • NAVMED P-5010 • *Lippincott Fundamental Skills and Concepts in Patient Care,* current edition • Virtual Navy Hospital Website: http://www.vnh.org
Exam Expectations. These are subject areas you should know to help you answer exam questions correctly:	You can expect questions on the types of external parasites; policies and procedures for treating external parasites; and the equipment and supplies required.

Advancement Handbook for HM3

General HM *Skill Area*	**Preventive/Occupational Medicine**
A *skill* you are expected to perform from the General Skill Area above:	**Conduct preliminary interviews of personnel exposed to communicable diseases (other than STD)**
Knowledge you should have to perform this skill:	You should recall: • The policies and procedures for conducting interviews • The reporting requirements for communicable diseases
References you should study to gain the knowledge you need to perform this skill:	• BUMEDINST 6220.9A • BUMEDINST 6220.12 • BUMEDINST 6230.1 • NAVEDTRA 14295 • NAVMED P-5010 • *Lippincott Fundamental Skills and Concepts in Patient Care,* current edition • Virtual Navy Hospital Website: http://www.vnh.org
Exam Expectations. These are subject areas you should know to help you answer exam questions correctly:	You can expect questions on the policies and procedures for conducting interviews and the reporting requirements for communicable diseases.

Advancement Handbook for HM3

General HM *Skill Area*	**Preventive/Occupational Medicine**
A *skill* you are expected to perform from the General Skill Area above:	**Conduct preliminary STD interviews**
Knowledge you should have to perform this skill:	You should recall: • The policies and procedures for conducting interviews • The reporting requirements for Sexually Transmitted **D**iseases (STD)
References you should study to gain the knowledge you need to perform this skill:	• NAVEDTRA 14295 • NAVMED P-5010 • Virtual Navy Hospital Website: http://www.vnh.org
Exam Expectations. These are subject areas you should know to help you answer exam questions correctly:	You can expect question on the policies, procedures, and reporting requirements for conducting Sexually **T**ransmitted **D**isease interviews.

Advancement Handbook for HM3

General HM *Skill Area*	Preventive /Occupational Medicine
A *skill* you are expected to perform from the General Skill Area above:	**Perform heat stress index tests**
Knowledge you should have to perform this skill:	You should recall: • The policies and procedures to perform heat stress index test • The current flagging system • The PHEL charts • The use of the WBGT meter • Related heat casualty reports and forms
References you should study to gain the knowledge you need to perform this skill:	• NAVEDTRA 14295 • NAVMED P-5010 • Virtual Navy Hospital Website: http://www.vnh.org
Exam Expectations. These are subject areas you should know to help you answer exam questions correctly:	You can expect questions on the policies and procedures to perform heat stress index tests; the flagging system; PHEL charts; use of the WBGT meter; and related heat casualty reports and forms.

Advancement Handbook for HM3

General HM *Skill Area*	**Preventive/Occupational Medicine**
A *skill* you are expected to perform from the General Skill Area above:	**Fit and issue noise protection devices**
Knowledge you should have to perform this skill:	You should recall: • The policies and procedures for fitting and issuing noise protection devices • The equipment and supplies required
References you should study to gain the knowledge you need to perform this skill:	• NAVEDTRA 14295 • NAVMED P-5010 • OPNAVINST 5100.23E • Virtual Navy Hospital Website: http://www.vnh.org
Exam Expectations. These are subject areas you should know to help you answer exam questions correctly:	You can expect questions on the policies and procedures for fitting and issuing noise protection devices and the equipment/supplies required.

Advancement Handbook for HM3

General HM *Skill Area*	**Preventive/Occupational Medicine**
A *skill* you are expected to perform from the General Skill Area above:	**Test water samples**
Knowledge you should have to perform this skill:	You should recall: • The policies and procedures to test water ashore and afloat • The procedures to determine a source of water contamination • The related reports and forms • The equipment and supplies required
References you should study to gain the knowledge you need to perform this skill:	• BUMEDINST 6240.10 • BUMEDINST 6270.8 • NAVEDTRA 14295 • NAVMED P-5010 • Virtual Navy Hospital Website: http://www.vnh.org
Exam Expectations. These are subject areas you should know to help you answer exam questions correctly:	You can expect questions on the policies and procedures to test water ashore and afloat; the procedures to determine a source of water contamination; related reports and forms; and the equipment/supplies required.

Advancement Handbook for HM3

General HM *Skill Area*	**Preventive/Occupational Medicine**
A *skill* you are expected to perform from the General Skill Area above:	**Inspect messing/food service facilities and perform pest control inspections**
Knowledge you should have to perform this skill:	You should recall: • The policies and procedures to inspect messing and food service facilities Ashore and afloat • The policies and procedures required performing pest control inspections ashore and afloat • The related reports and forms • The equipment and supplies required
References you should study to gain the knowledge you need to perform this skill:	• BUMEDINST 6250.12 • BUMEDINST 6250.14 • NAVEDTRA 14295 • NAVMED P-5010 • OPNAVINST 6250.4 • SECNAVINST 4061.1 • SECNAVINST 6210.2A • Virtual Navy Hospital Website: http://www.vnh.org
Exam Expectations. These are subject areas you should know to help you answer exam questions correctly:	You can expect questions on policies and procedures to inspect messing/food service facilities; performing pest control inspections; completing reports/forms, and the equipment and supplies required.

Advancement Handbook for HM3

General HM *Skill Area*	Training/Administration/Logistics
A *skill* you are expected to perform from the General Skill Area above:	**Inventory medical department equipment and supplies**
Knowledge you should have to perform this skill:	You should recall: • The policies and procedures for stocking medical supplies and equipment according to authorized medical allowance list (AMAL) • The procedures for inspecting medical equipment, instruments, and supplies for serviceability • The procedures to store medical supplies ashore and afloat • The procedures to inventory Battle Dressing Stations (BDS)
References you should study to gain the knowledge you need to perform this skill:	• BUMEDINST 6440.5 • BUMEDINST 6440.6 • BUMEDINST 6700.13G • BUMEDINST 6710.63 • NAVMED P-117 • NAVEDTRA 14295 • 632Virtual Navy Hospital Website: http://www.vnh.org
Exam Expectations. These are subject areas you should know to help you answer exam questions correctly:	You can expect questions on the policies and procedures for stocking medical supplies and equipment according to AMAL; inspecting medical equipment, instruments, and supplies for serviceability; the procedures to store medical supplies ashore and afloat and inventorying BDS.

Advancement Handbook for HM3

General HM *Skill Area*	Training/Administration/Logistics
A *skill* you are expected to perform from the General Skill Area above:	**Conduct first aid and health training for non-medical personnel**
Knowledge you should have to perform this skill:	You should be able to recall policies and procedures for first aid/health-related training conducted for medical and non-medical personnel
References you should study to gain the knowledge you need to perform this skill:	<ul><li>BUMEDINST 1500.15</li><li>BUMEDINST 1500.22</li><li>BUMEDINST 1510.18</li><li>BUMEDINST 6224.8</li><li>BUMEDINST 6440.6</li><li>BUMEDINST 6700.42</li><li>SECNAVINST 1500.10</li><li>SECNAVINST 4061.1</li><li>NAVMED P-117</li><li>NAVMED P-5010</li><li>NAVEDTRA 14295</li></ul>
Exam Expectations. These are subject areas you should know to help you answer exam questions correctly:	You can expect questions on health related training that is conducted for medical and non-medical personnel

Advancement Handbook for HM3

General HM *Skill Area*	**Training/Administration/Logistics**
A *skill* you are expected to perform from the General Skill Area above:	**Prepare and review laboratory requests**
Knowledge you should have to perform this skill:	You should be able to recall the policies and procedures for preparing and review laboratory request
References you should study to gain the knowledge you need to perform this skill:	NAVEDTRA 14295
Exam Expectations. These are subject areas you should know to help you answer exam questions correctly:	You can expect questions on the policies and procedures for preparing and reviewing laboratory request.

Advancement Handbook for HM3

General HM *Skill Area*	Training/Administration/Logistics
A *skill* you are expected to perform from the General Skill Area above:	**Open, make entries, verify, and close medical and dental records**
Knowledge you should have to perform this skill:	You should be able to: • Recall the policies and procedures for opening, making entries, verifying, filing, and closing health and dental records • Recall the current instructions pertaining to health and dental records • Recognize the required forms comprising health and dental records • Recall the disposition of health and dental records upon transfer, commissioning, discharge, and death
References you should study to gain the knowledge you need to perform this skill:	• BUMEDNOTE 6150 • NAVMED P-117 • NAVEDTRA 14295 • SECNAVINST 5211.5 • SECNAVINST 5212.5
Exam Expectations. These are subject areas you should know to help you answer exam questions correctly:	You can expect questions on the policies and procedures for opening, making entries, verifying, and disposition of records; the current instructions pertaining to records; the forms comprising health and dental records; policies and procedures for custody; chargeout control; terminal digit filing of records; and the disposition of records upon transfer, commissioning, discharge, and death

Advancement Handbook for HM3

General HM *Skill Area*	Training/Administration/Logistics
A *skill* you are expected to perform from the General Skill Area above:	**Enter and retrieve patient data from automated medical information systems (CHCS, DEERS, etc.)**
Knowledge you should have to perform this skill:	You should recall: • The policies and procedures required entering and retrieving patient data from automated medical information systems • The current instructions pertaining to medical data • The security measures for medical data
References you should study to gain the knowledge you need to perform this skill:	• NAVMED P-117 • NAVEDTRA 14295 • SECNAVINST 5212.5 • SECNAVINST 5216.5 • SECNAVINST 5510.30 • Virtual Navy Hospital Website: http://www.vnh.org
Exam Expectations. These are subject areas you should know to help you answer exam questions correctly:	You can expect questions on the policies and procedures required for entering and retrieving patient data from automated medical information systems; the current instructions; different types of data entries; and security requirements.

Advancement Handbook for HM3

General HM *Skill Area*	Training/Administration/Logistics
A *skill* you are expected to perform from the General Skill Area above:	**Prepare, serialize, and mail a standard naval letter**
Knowledge you should have to perform this skill:	You should be able to identify standard letter format elements to include: • Margins • Identification symbols • From, To, Via, Subject, Reference, and Enclosure lines • Text and paragraph structuring • Signature block • Copy to block • Page numbering • Envelope preparation
References you should study to gain the knowledge you need to perform this skill:	SECNAVINST 5216.5
Exam Expectations. These are subject areas you should know to help you answer exam questions correctly:	You can expect questions on the individual elements of a standard naval letter; placement of the identification symbols; subject line; how to list various references; the number of required spaces; size of margins; the signature block for an official signing "by direction"; numbering pages; how to vary the format; the use with a window envelope; and correspondence policies contained in the Correspondence Manual.

Advancement Handbook for HM3

General HM *Skill Area*	Training/Administration/Logistics
A *skill* you are expected to perform from the General Skill Area above:	**Prepare general/special medical reports and forms (binnacle list, medical event reports, etc.)**
Knowledge you should have to perform this skill:	You should recall: • The policies and procedures for preparing general and special medical reports • The different types of reports and forms • Current instructions and reporting requirements
References you should study to gain the knowledge you need to perform this skill:	• DMRSMAN EPMAC 1080 • BUMEDINST 6010.13 • BUMEDINST 6010.20 • BUMEDINST 6120.20 • BUMEDINST 6220.12 • BUMEDINST 6224.8 • BUMEDINST 6300.10 • BUMEDINST 6310.3 • BUMEDINST 6320.3B • BUMEDINST 6440.6 • BUPERSINST 1770.3 • NAVMED P-117 • NAVMED P-5010 • NAVMED P-5055 • NAVMEDCOMINST 1300.1 • NAVMEDCOMINST 5360.1 • OPNAVINST 17522 • NAVMEDCOMINST 6320.3 • NAVMEDCOMINST 6320.72 • NAVMEDCOMINST 6470.10 • NAVMEDCOMINST 6820.1 • OPNAVINST 1000.16

	• OPNAVINST 1754.2 • OPNAVINST 5100.23 • OPNAVINST 6250.4 • SECNAVINST 5210.11 • SECNAVINST 5212.5 • SECNAVINST 5215.1 • SECNAVINST 5216.5
Exam Expectations. These are subject areas you should know to help you answer exam questions correctly:	You can expect questions on policies and procedures for preparing reports and forms; the different types of reports and forms, including but not limited to: medical accident/incident, manpower/personnel reporting, birth and death certificates, decedent affairs reports, issuance of nonavailability reports, overseas screening reports, TB control program reports, patient regulating, medical augmentation, supply, logistics, casualty assistance, etc.; and current instructions and reporting timelines.

Part 2

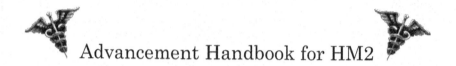

Advancement Handbook for HM2

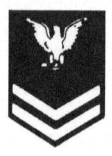

You are responsible for information contained in:
Part 1-HM3

Advancement Handbook for HM2

General HM *Skill Area*	**Emergency/Field Treatment**
A *skill* you are expected to perform from the General Skill Area above:	**Coordinate medical evacuations**
Knowledge you should have to perform this skill:	You should be able to: • Recall the policies and procedures required performing triage in peacetime and in time of conflict • Recall the policies and procedures to prepare patients for medical evacuations • Recognize the requirements to restrain patients • Recall the policies, procedures , equipment, and supplies required to transport patients • Recall procedures for patient regulating
References you should study to gain the knowledge you need to perform this skill:	• NAVEDTRA 14295 • *Brady Emergency Care,* current edition • *Emergency Care and Transportation of the Sick and Injured,* current edition • Virtual Navy Hospital Website: http://www.vnh.org
Exam Expectations. These are subject areas you should know to help you answer exam questions correctly:	You can expect questions on performing triage; patient preparation for MEDEVAC; recognizing the need to restrain patients; the policies, procedures, equipment, and supplies required for transporting patients; and the requirements for patient regulating and tracking.

Advancement Handbook for HM2

General HM *Skill Area*	**Preventive/Occupational Medicine**
A *skill* you are expected to perform from the General Skill Area above:	**Conduct preliminary investigation of food-borne illnesses**
Knowledge you should have to perform this skill:	You should recall: • The policies and procedures to inspect messing/food service facilities and conduct habitability inspections, ashore and afloat • The policies and procedures required performing pest control inspections and water testing ashore and afloat • The related reports and forms, equipment, and supplies required
References you should study to gain the knowledge you need to perform this skill:	• BUMEDINST 6250.12 • BUMEDINST 6250.14 • NAVEDTRA 14295 • NAVMED P-5010 • OPNAVINST 6250.4 • SECNAVINST 4061.1 • Virtual Navy Hospital Website: http://www.vnh.org
Exam Expectations. These are subject areas you should know to help you answer exam questions correctly:	You can expect questions on policies and procedures to inspect messing/food service facilities; conduct habitability and pest control inspections; required reports/forms; and the equipment and supplies required.

Advancement Handbook for HM2

General HM *Skill Area*	**Training/Administration/Logistics**
A *skill* you are expected to perform from the General Skill Area above:	**Conduct instruction and training on health care related items including health benefits counseling**
Knowledge you should have to perform this skill:	You should be able to recall policies and procedures for first aid/health-related training and benefits conducted for medical and non-medical personnel
References you should study to gain the knowledge you need to perform this skill:	<ul><li>BUMEDINST 1500.15</li><li>BUMEDINST 1500.22</li><li>BUMEDINST 1510.18</li><li>BUMEDINST 1510.19</li><li>BUMEDINST 1553.1</li><li>BUMEDINST 5220.3</li><li>BUMEDINST 6224.8</li><li>BUMEDINST 6440.6</li><li>NAVEDTRA 14295</li><li>NAVMED P-117</li><li>NAVMED P-5010</li><li>NAVMEDCOMINST 1520.40</li><li>NAVMEDCOMINST 3040.1</li><li>NAVMEDCOMINST 6700.42</li><li>SECNAVINST 1500.10</li><li>SECNAVINST 4061.1</li></ul>
Exam Expectations. These are subject areas you should know to help you answer exam questions correctly:	You can expect questions on health related training and benefits that are conducted for medical and non-medical personnel.

Advancement Handbook for HM2

General HM *Skill Area*	**Training/Administration/Logistics**
A *skill* you are expected to perform from the General Skill Area above:	**Prepare/Review general/special medical reports and forms (binnacle list, medical event reports, etc.)**
Knowledge you should have to perform this skill:	You should recall: • The policies and procedures for preparing general and special medical reports • The different types of reports, forms, and claims • Current instructions and reporting requirements
References you should study to gain the knowledge you need to perform this skill:	• DMRSMAN EPMAC 1080 • BUMEDINST 6010.13 • BUMEDINST 6010.20 • BUMEDINST 6120.20 • BUMEDINST 6220.12 • BUMEDINST 6224.8 • BUMEDINST 6440.6 • BUPERSINST 1770.3 • NAVMED P-117 • NAVMED P-5010 • NAVMED P-5055 • NAVMEDCOMINST 1300.1 • NAVMEDCOMINST 5360.1 • NAVMEDCOMINST 6320.18 • OPNAVINST 1752.2 (Series) • NAVMEDCOMINST 6320.3 • NAVMEDCOMINST 6320.72 • NAVMEDCOMINST 6470.10 • OPNAVINST 1000.16 • OPNAVINST 1754.2 • OPNAVINST 5100.23

	<ul><li>OPNAVINST 6250.4</li><li>SECNAVINST 5210.11</li><li>SECNAVINST 5212.5</li><li>SECNAVINST 5216.5</li></ul>
Exam Expectations. These are subject areas you should know to help you answer exam questions correctly:	You can expect questions on policies and procedures for preparing reports/forms; the different types of reports/forms, including, but not limited to: medical accident/incident, manpower/personnel reporting, birth and death certificates, decedent affairs reports, third-party claims, issuance of nonavailability reports, heat casualty reports, overseas screening reports, TB control program report, patient regulating, medical augmentation, supply, logistics, casualty assistance, etc.; and current instructions and reporting timelines.

Part 3

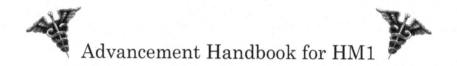

Advancement Handbook for HM1

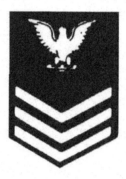

You are responsible for the information contained in:
Part 1-HM3
Part 2-HM2

Advancement Handbook for HM1

General HM *Skill Area*	**Emergency/Field Treatment**
A *skill* you are expected to perform from the General Skill Area above:	**Direct battalion aid station (BAS) operations**
Knowledge you should have to perform this skill:	You should recall: • The policies and procedure for a BAS • The health support and personnel requirements • The equipment and supplies required • The BAS inspection procedures
References you should study to gain the knowledge you need to perform this skill:	• BUMEDINST 6280.1 • BUMEDINST 6440.6 • BUMEDINST 6710.62 • BUMEDINST 6710.63 • NAVMED P-117
Exam Expectations. These are subject areas you should know to help you answer exam questions correctly:	You can expect questions on policies and procedure for a BAS; health support; personnel requirements; equipment; supplies; and BAS inspection procedures.

Advancement Handbook for HM1

General HM *Skill Area*	Ancillary Services
A *skill* you are expected to perform from the General Skill Area above:	**Inventory controlled drugs and substances**
Knowledge you should have to perform this skill:	You should be able to recall the policies and procedures for the inventory of controlled drugs and controlled substances
References you should study to gain the knowledge you need to perform this skill:	NAVMED P-117
Exam Expectations. These are subject areas you should know to help you answer exam questions correctly:	You can expect questions on policies and procedures, board membership, reports/forms, and periodicity for the inventory.

Advancement Handbook for HM1

General HM *Skill Area*	Training/Administration/Logistics
A *skill* you are expected to perform from the General Skill Area above:	**Review general/special medical reports and forms (decedent affairs reports, medical event reports, etc.)**
Knowledge you should have to perform this skill:	You should recall: • The policies and procedures for preparing general and special medical reports • The different types of reports and forms • Current instructions and reporting requirements
References you should study to gain the knowledge you need to perform this skill:	• DMRSMAN EPMAC 1080 • BUMEDINST 6010.13 • BUMEDINST 6010.20 • BUMEDINST 6120.20 • BUMEDINST 6220.12 • BUMEDINST 6224.8 • BUMEDINST 6440.6 • BUPERSINST 1770.3 • NAVMED P-117 • NAVMED P-5010 • NAVMED P-5055 • NAVMEDCOMINST 1300.1 • NAVMEDCOMINST 5360.1 • NAVMEDCOMINST 6320.18 • OPNAVINST 1752.2 (Series) • NAVMEDCOMINST 6320.3 • NAVMEDCOMINST 6320.72 • NAVMEDCOMINST 6470.10 • OPNAVINST 1000.16 • OPNAVINST 1754.2 • OPNAVINST 5100.23 • OPNAVINST 6250.4

	• SECNAVINST 5210.11 • SECNAVINST 5212.5 • SECNAVINST 5216.5
Exam Expectations. These are subject areas you should know to help you answer exam questions correctly:	You can expect questions on policies and procedures for preparing reports/forms; the different types of reports/forms, including, but not limited to: medical accident/incident, manpower/personnel reporting, birth and death certificates, decedent affairs reports, issuance of nonavailability reports, overseas screening reports, TB control program report, patient regulating, medical augmentation, supply, logistics, casualty assistance, etc.; and current instructions and reporting timelines.

Advancement Handbook for HM1

General HM *Skill Area*	**Training/Administration/Logistics**
A *skill* you are expected to perform from the General Skill Area above:	**Assist in drafting command medical readiness plans.**
Knowledge you should have to perform this skill:	You should recall: • The policies and procedures for monitoring command medical readiness, enlisted distribution, and medical personnel augmentation • Total force manpower policies and procedures
References you should study to gain the knowledge you need to perform this skill:	• BUMEDINST 6440.5 • BUMEDINST 6440.6 • EDVERMAN 1080 • OPNAVINST 1000.16
Exam Expectations. These are subject areas you should know to help you answer exam questions correctly:	You can expect questions on policies and procedures for monitoring command medical readiness, enlisted distribution, medical personnel augmentation, and manpower.

Part 4

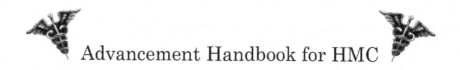

Advancement Handbook for HMC

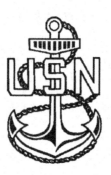

You are responsible for information contained in:
Part 1-HM3
Part 2-HM2
Part 3-HM1

Advancement Handbook for HMC

General HM *Skill Area*	**Training/Administration/Logistics**
A *skill* you are expected to perform from the General Skill Area above:	**Monitor command medical readiness plans**
Knowledge you should have to perform this skill:	You should recall: • The policies and procedures for monitoring command medical readiness • The policies and procedures for enlisted distribution • The policies and procedures for medical personnel augmentation • Total force manpower policies and procedures
References you should study to gain the knowledge you need to perform this skill:	• BUMEDINST 6440.5 • BUMEDINST 6440.6 • EDVERMAN 1080 • OPNAVINST 1000.16
Exam Expectations. These are subject areas you should know to help you answer exam questions correctly:	You can expect questions on policies and procedures for monitoring command medical readiness, enlisted distribution, medical personnel augmentation, and manpower.

Advancement Handbook for HMC

General HM *Skill Area*	Training/Administration/Logistics
A *skill* you are expected to perform from the General Skill Area above:	**Assist in drafting, monitoring, and coordination of joint medical operational plans**
Knowledge you should have to perform this skill:	You should be able to recall the policies and procedures required to draft, monitor, and coordinate joint medical operational plans
References you should study to gain the knowledge you need to perform this skill:	• BUMEDINST 6230.15 • BUMEDINST 6270.8 • BUMEDINST 6440.6 • NAVMED P-117 • NAVMED P-5010 • NAVMED P-5038 • NAVMED P-5055 • NAVMEDCOMINST 5360.1 • SECNAVINST 5510.30
Exam Expectations. These are subject areas you should know to help you answer exam questions correctly:	You can expect question on policies and procedures for joint medical operational plans; the numerical organization of different units; medical requirements; evacuation; patient regulating; potential HAZMAT situations; MMART; health service support; and logistical and supply requirements including chemoprophalaxis.

Advancement Handbook for HMC

General HM *Skill Area*	Training/Administration/Logistics
A *skill* you are expected to perform from the General Skill Area above:	**Inventory controlled medicinals**
Knowledge you should have to perform this skill:	You should be able to recall the policies and procedures for the inventory of controlled medicinal
References you should study to gain the knowledge you need to perform this skill:	NAVMED P-117
Exam Expectations. These are subject areas you should know to help you answer exam questions correctly:	You can expect questions on policies and procedures, board membership, reports/forms, and periodicity for the inventory.

Advancement Handbook for HMC

General HM *Skill Area*	Training/Administration/Logistics
A *skill* you are expected to perform from the General Skill Area above:	**Coordinate the medical organizational performance improvement program**
Knowledge you should have to perform this skill:	You should be able to recall the policies and procedures for advising command on performance improvement
References you should study to gain the knowledge you need to perform this skill:	• BUMEDINST 6010.13 • OPNAVINST 6320.7
Exam Expectations. These are subject areas you should know to help you answer exam questions correctly:	You can expect questions on the policies and procedures for performance improvement and the quality assurance program.

Appendix 1

References Used in This HM Advancement Handbook

Rating	Short Title	Long Title	Chapters/ Paragraphs	Stocking Point
HM3				
	BUMEDINST 1500.15	Resuscitation Training	All	Note 2
	BUMEDINST 1500.22	Review and Evaluation of Operational Readiness Training Programs for Medical and Dental Personnel	All	Notes 2, 4
	BUMEDINST 6220.9A	Nosocomial Infection Control Program	All	Note 2
	BUMEDINST 6010.20	Issuance of Nonavailability Statements	All	Notes 2, 4
	BUMEDINST 6222.10	Sexually Transmitted Disease (STD) Clinical Management Guidelines	All	Notes 2, 4
	BUMEDINST 6224.8	Tuberculosis Control Program	All	Notes 2, 4
	BUMEDINST 6230.15	Immunizations and Chemoprophylaxis	All	Notes 2, 4
	BUMEDINST 6240.10	Standards for Potable Water	All	Notes 2, 4
	BUMEDINST 6250.12	Pesticide Applicator Training and Certification for Medical Personnel	All	Notes 2, 4
	BUMEDINST 6250.14	Procurement of Deratting/Deratting Exemption Certificates	All	Notes 2, 4
	NAVMEDCOMINST 6260.12	Prevention of Cold Injuries	All	Note 2
	BUMEDINST 6270.8	Procedures for Obtaining Health Hazard Assessments Pertaining to Operational Use of Hazardous Materials	All	Notes 2, 4
	BUMEDINST 6300.10	Customer Relations Program	All	Notes 2, 4
	BUMEDINST 6310.3	Management Of Alleged or Suspected Sexual Assault and Rape Cases	All	Notes 2, 4
	BUMEDINST 6320.3B	Medical and Dental Care for Eligible Persons at Navy Medical Department Facilities	All	Notes 2, 4
	BUMEDINST 6440.5	Medical Augmentation Program	All	Notes 2, 4
	BUMEDINST 6440.6	Mobile Medical Augmentation Readiness Team (MMART) Manual	All	Notes 2, 4
	BUMEDINST 6700.42	Ambulance Support	All	Notes 2, 4

	BUPERINST 1770.3	Navy Casualty Assistance Calls Program	All	Note 1
	NAVEDTRA 14295	Hospital Corpsman	All	Note 4
	NAVEDTRA 14274	Dental Technician, Vol 1	All	Note 4
	NAVMEDCOMINST 1300.1	Suitability Processing for Overseas Assignment of Navy and Marine Corps Members and Their Accompanying Dependents	All	Note 2
	NAVMEDCOMINST 5360.1	Decedent Affairs Manual	All	Note 2
	OPNAVINST 1752.2 (Series)	Family Advocacy Program	All	Notes 1
	NAVMEDCOMINST 6820.1	Professional Medical Reference Materials and Publications		Notes 2, 4
	NAVMED P-117	Manual of the Medical Department	All	Note 4
	NAVMED P-5010	Manual of Naval Preventive Medicine	All	Notes 4
	NAVMED P-5038	Control of Communicable Disease in Man	All	Note 4
	NAVMED P-5055	Radiation Health Protection Manual	All	Note 4
	OPNAVINST 5100.23E	Naval Occupational Safety and Health (NAVOSH) Program Manual	All	Note 1
	SECNAVINST 1500.10	Basic Life Support (BLS) Training	All	Note 1
	SECNAVINST 4061.1	Food Sanitation Training	All	Note 1
	SECNAVINST 5210.11D	Department of the Navy File Maintenance Procedures and Standard Subject Identification Codes (SSIC)	All	Note 1
	SECNAVINST 5211.5	Department of the Navy Privacy Act (PA) Program	All	Note 1
	EMERGENCY CARE	Brady Emergency Care, current edition	All	Commercial Publication
	EMERGENCY CARE AND TRANSPORTATION	Emergency Care and Transportation of the Sick and Injured, current edition	All	Commercial Publication
	PATIENT CARE	Lipponcott Fundamental Skills and Concepts in Patient Care, current edition	All	Commercial Publication
	http://www.vnh.org/	Virtual Naval Hospital Web Site	All	Internet Access Required
HM2 You Are Responsible For References Contained In HM3				
	BUMEDINST 6010.13	Quality Assurance Program	All	Notes 2. 4
	BUMEDINST 6120.20	Competence For Duty Examinations	All	Notes 2,4
	BUPERSINST 1750.3	Command Defense Enrollment Eligibility	All	Notes 2, 4

		Report System (DEERS)		
	NAVMEDCOMINST 6320.18	Civilian Health and Medical Program of the Uniformed Services (CHAMPUS) Regulation	All	Notes 2, 4
	NAVMEDCOMINST 6320.72	Non-Naval Medical and Dental Care	All	Notes 2, 4
	NAVMEDCOMINST 6470.10	Initial Management of Irradiated or Radioactively Contaminated Personnel	All	Notes 2, 4
	OPNAVINST 1000.16	Manual of Navy Total Force Manpower Policies and Procedures	All	Note 1
	OPNAVINST 1754.2	Exceptional Family Member Program	All	Note 1
HM1 **You Are Responsible For References Contained in HM2 &HM3**				
HMC **You Are Responsible For References Contained in HM1, HM2, and HM3**				
	OPNAVINST 6320.7	Healthcare Quality Assurance for Operating Forces	All	Note 1

LEGEND:

Note 1—INTERNET: http://neds.nebt.daps.mil/

Note 2—INTERNET: http://navymedicine.med.navy.mil/instructions/

Note 3— INTERNET: http://www.advancement.cnet.navy.mil/

Note 4— CD-ROM: Send name, rank, and mailing address to:
     Virtual Naval Hospital
     Electric Differential Multimedia Lab
     200 Hawkins Drive, 5716 GH
     Iowa City, IA 52242

CPSIA information can be obtained
at www.ICGtesting.com
Printed in the USA
BVOW04s2016020417

480088BV00010BA/278/P

9 780982 147696